Failure to Thrive and Pediatric Undernutrition

Failure to Thrive and Pediatric Undernutrition

A Transdisciplinary Approach

edited by

Daniel B. Kessler, M.D.
Children's Health Center
St. Joseph's Hospital and Medical Center
Phoenix, Arizona

and

Peter Dawson, M.D., M.P.H.
University of Colorado School of Medicine
Denver, Colorado

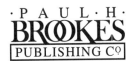

·P A U L·H·
BROOKES
PUBLISHING Cº

Baltimore · London · Toronto · Sydney

Paul H. Brookes Publishing Co.
Post Office Box 10624
Baltimore, Maryland 21285-0624

www.pbrookes.com

Typeset by Barton Matheson Willse & Worthington, Baltimore, Maryland.
Manufactured in the United States of America by
The Maple Press Company, York, Pennsylvania.

Most of the case studies that are described in this book are completely fictional. Any similarity to actual individuals or circumstances is coincidental, and no implications should be inferred. Selected case studies are composites that are based on the authors' experiences; these case studies do not represent the lives or experiences of specific individuals, and no implications should be inferred. Case studies that are based on real people or circumstances are presented herein only with the individuals' written consent.

Any information about medical treatments is in no way meant to substitute for a physician's advice or expert opinion; readers should consult a medical practitioner if they are interested in more information.

Purchasers of *Failure to Thrive and Pediatric Undernutrition: A Transdisciplinary Approach* are granted permission to photocopy the forms on pages 346–348, 382, 554, 555, 558–567, 570, and 580–583 for clinical purposes. Although photocopying for clinical purposes is unlimited, none of these pages may be reproduced to generate revenue for any program or individual. Photocopies must be made from an original book.

Photographs by Peter Dawson.

Library of Congress Cataloging-in-Publication Data

Failure to thrive and pediatric undernutrition : a transdisciplinary approach / edited by
   Daniel B. Kessler and Peter Dawson.
      p.   cm.
   Includes bibliographical references and index.
   ISBN 1-55766-348-3
   1. Failure to thrive syndrome.   2. Malnutrition in children.
   I. Kessler, Daniel B.   II. Dawson, Peter, 1938–   .
   [DNLM: 1. Child Nutrition Disorders.   2. Failure to Thrive.   3. Developmental Disabilities.
   WS 115F1607   1998]
   RJ135.F33   1999
   618.92'39—dc21
   DNLM/DLC
   for Library of Congress   98-35858
                                                                                                        CIP

British Library Cataloguing in Publication data are available from the British Library.

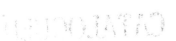

Contents

About the Editors

Daniel B. Kessler, M.D., Director, Developmental and Behavioral Pediatrics, Children's Health Center, St. Joseph's Hospital and Medical Center, 124 West Thomas Road, Phoenix, Arizona 85013; Clinical Associate Professor of Pediatrics, University of Arizona College of Medicine, Tucson; DannyDR@aol.com

Dr. Kessler directs clinical and teaching services in developmental and behavioral pediatrics at the Children's Health Center of St. Joseph's Hospital and Medical Center. Dr. Kessler trained in child abuse and neglect with Eli H. Newberger, M.D., and in child development with T. Berry Brazelton, M.D., both at Children's Hospital, Boston, after completing his pediatric residency training at the New York University Medical Center. Dr. Kessler participated in the first hospital-based, multidisciplinary FTT Team at Children's Hospital, Boston (1980–1983). After his fellowship in Boston, he directed the Carl C. Icahn Center for the Prevention of Child Abuse at The New York Hospital-Cornell Medical Center and directed the FTT Protocol at the Pediatric Clinical Research Center. Dr. Kessler is on the Executive Committee of the Section of Developmental and Behavioral Pediatrics of the American Academy of Pediatrics. He has written and lectured extensively about problems of pediatric undernutrition, problems of behavior and learning, and child abuse. He has consulted to the Social Security Administration, the New York City Human Resources Administration, Southwest Human Development, the Arizona Child Abuse Prevention Fund, the Arizona Department of Health Services, the Children's Justice Task Force, and Share Our Strength.

Peter Dawson, M.D., M.P.H., Pediatrician, Colorado Mental Health Institute at Fort Logan, 3520 West Oxford Avenue, Denver, Colorado 80231, and People's Clinic, Boulder; Clinical Associate Professor, Preventive Medicine and Pediatrics, and Senior Instructor in Psychiatry, University of Colorado School of Medicine, Denver; Peter.Dawson@uchsc.edu

Dr. Dawson practices pediatrics at the People's Clinic in Boulder, Colorado, and at the Colorado Mental Health Institute at Fort Logan in Denver. He developed his knowledge of child development and families by teaching at the JFK Child Development Center of the University of Colorado School of Medicine, working for 17 years in multidisciplinary child development clinics, studying parent support by paraprofessional home visitors, and serving on the board of directors of the Family Resource Coalition of America. He learned about public health by working with public health nurses, serving in several positions in the Maternal and Child Health Section of the American Public Health Association, and founding the Boulder County Consortium on Access to Health Care. He teaches pediatrics and public health at the University of Colorado School of Medicine. He has published 15 articles in professional journals and has received awards from the Department of Maternal and Child Health of the University of North Carolina, American Public Health Association, Boulder Valley Education Association, Boulder *Daily Camera,* and Voices for Children.

Drs. Dawson and Kessler met while they both were Fellows with ZERO TO THREE: National Center for Infants, Toddlers and Families and have collaborated extensively since that time in the area of pediatric undernutrition.

Contributors

Marion Taylor Baer, Ph.D., R.D.
Adjunct Associate Professor
Department of Community Health Services
University of California–Los Angeles
School of Public Health
Associate Professor of Clinical Pediatrics
University of Southern California
School of Medicine
Los Angeles, California

Cynthia Taft Bayerl, M.S.
Director
Perinatal and Pediatric Nutrition Program
Massachusetts Department of Public Health
Bureau of Family and Community Health
Boston, Massachusetts

Julie Berenson-Howard, Ph.D.
Psychologist
Baltimore, Maryland

Rahel Berhane, M.D.
Austin Diagnostic Clinic
Austin, Texas

Carol D. Berkowitz, M.D.
Professor of Clinical Pediatrics
University of California–Los Angeles
School of Medicine
Harbor–UCLA Medical Center
Torrance, California

Marian Birch, D.M.H.
Psychologist
Port Angeles, Washington

William G. Bithoney, M.D.
Senior Vice President
Brookdale University Hospital and Medical Center
Chairman
Ambulatory Care Services
Professor of Pediatrics
State University of New York
Health Science Center at Brooklyn
Brooklyn, New York

Maureen M. Black, Ph.D.
Professor
Department of Pediatrics
University of Maryland School of Medicine
Baltimore, Maryland

T. Berry Brazelton, M.D.
Professor Emeritus
Harvard Medical School
Children's Hospital
Boston, Massachusetts

J. Larry Brown, Ph.D.
Alexander McFarlane Professor and Director
Center on Hunger, Poverty and Nutrition Policy
Tufts University
Medford, Massachusetts

A. Wesley Burks, M.D.
Chief
Pediatric Allergy and Immunology
Professor of Pediatrics
University of Arkansas for Medical Sciences
Arkansas Children's Hospital
Little Rock, Arkansas

Patrick H. Casey, M.D.
Harvey and Bernice Jones Professor of
    Developmental Pediatrics
Department of Pediatrics
University of Arkansas for Medical Sciences
Little Rock, Arkansas

Irene Chatoor, M.D.
Professor of Psychiatry
George Washington University School of Medicine
Vice Chair and Director
Infant Psychiatry
Department of Psychiatry
Children's National Medical Center
Washington, D.C.

Nick Claxton, C.Q.S.W.
Clinical Social Worker
Shriners Hospitals for Children
Philadelphia Unit
Philadelphia, Pennsylvania

Robert Cole, Ph.D.
Clinical Associate Professor of Psychiatry
University of Rochester
Rochester, New York

Elizabeth R. Crais, Ph.D.
Associate Professor
Division of Speech and Hearing Sciences
University of North Carolina
Chapel Hill, North Carolina

Nancy Creskoff, B.S.
Registered Occupational Therapist
The Children's Hospital
Denver, Colorado

Kathy F. Cunningham, M.Ed., R.D.
State Nutritionist for Children with Special Health
    Care Needs
Massachusetts Department of Public Health
Boston, Massachusetts

Pamela L. Cureton, R.D., L.D.
Dietitian
Growth and Nutrition Clinic
Baltimore, Maryland

Diana Becker Cutts, M.D.
Medical Director
Children's Growth and Nutrition Project
Hennepin County Medical Center
Minneapolis, Minnesota

William H. Dietz, M.D., Ph.D.
Director
Division of Nutrition and Physical Activity
National Center for Chronic Disease Prevention
    and Health Promotion
Centers for Disease Control and Prevention
Atlanta, Georgia

Dennis Drotar, Ph.D.
Professor and Chief
Behavioral Pediatrics and Psychology
Rainbow Babies and Children's Hospital
Cleveland, Ohio

Deborah A. Frank, M.D.
Associate Professor of Pediatrics
Boston University School of Medicine
Boston, Massachusetts

Sheila Gahagan, M.D.
Clinical Associate Professor of Pediatrics and
    Communicable Diseases
University of Michigan
Assistant Research Scientist
Center for Human Growth and Development
University of Michigan
Ann Arbor, Michigan

Joni Geppert, M.P.H., R.D., L.N.
Pediatric Research Coordinator
Minneapolis Medical Research Foundation
Minneapolis, Minnesota

Edward Goldson, M.D.
Professor
Department of Pediatrics
University of Colorado Health Sciences Center
The Children's Hospital
Denver, Colorado

Kathleen S. Gorman, Ph.D.
Assistant Professor of Psychology
Psychology Department
University of Vermont
Burlington, Vermont

Joshua Greenberg, J.D.
Assistant Professor
Boston University School of Medicine
Boston, Massachusetts

Angela Haas, M.A.
Speech-Language Pathologist
The Children's Hospital
Denver, Colorado

Catherine A. Hess, M.S.W.
Executive Director
Association of Maternal and Child Health
    Programs
Washington, D.C.

John M. James, M.D.
Colorado Allergy and Asthma Centers
Fort Collins, Colorado

Harriet Kitzman, Ph.D.
Loretta C. Ford Professor of Nursing
University of Rochester
Rochester, New York

Nancy F. Krebs, M.D., M.S.
Assistant Professor
Department of Pediatrics
Section of Nutrition
University of Colorado School of Medicine and
    The Children's Hospital
Denver, Colorado

Fima Lifshitz, M.D.
Chief of Staff
Miami Children's Hospital
Miami, Florida
Professor of Pediatrics
State University of New York
Health Science Center at Brooklyn
Brooklyn, New York

Ida S. Mabry, R.N., M.S.
Failure to Thrive Coordinator and Case Manager
La Rabida Children's Hospital
Chicago, Illinois

Andrea Maggioni, M.D., Ph.D.
Director, Inpatient Services
Miami Children's Hospital
Miami, Florida
Assistant Professor of Pediatrics
State University of New York
Health Science Center at Brooklyn
Brooklyn, New York

Jayne D.B. Marsh, M.S.N., M.P.P.M.
Research Associate, Project Director
Edmund S. Muskie School of Public Affairs
Child and Family Institute
Portland, Maine

Mary McLaughlin, M.P.H., R.D.
Nutritionist
Frances Stern Nutrition Center
New England Medical Center
Boston, Massachusetts

P.J. McWilliam, Ph.D.
Research Investigator
Frank Porter Graham Child Development Center
University of North Carolina at Chapel Hill
Chapel Hill, North Carolina

Elizabeth Metallinos-Katsaras, Ph.D., R.D.
Director of Pregnancy and Pediatric Nutrition
Nutrition Projects Manager
Massachusetts Department of Public Health
Boston, Massachusetts

James Oleske, M.D., M.P.H.
Department of Pediatrics
Children's Hospital of New Jersey
University of Medicine and Dentistry of
    New Jersey
Newark, New Jersey

Elizabeth A. Rider, M.S.W., M.D.
Clinical Instructor in Pediatrics
Instructor in Medical Education
Harvard Medical School
Boston, Massachusetts

Jane Robinson, M.S.
Case Western Reserve University
Cleveland, Ohio

Patience Sampson, L.I.C.S.W.
Clinical Social Worker
Growth and Nutrition Clinic
Boston Medical Center
Boston, Massachusetts

Ellyn Satter, M.S., R.D., M.S.S.W., B.C.D.
Family Therapist and Eating Specialist
Family Therapy Center of Madison
Madison, Wisconsin

Joel I. Shalowitz, M.D., M.M.
Professor and Director
Health Services Management
Kellogg Graduate School of Management
Northwestern University Medical School
Evanston, Illinois

Madeleine U. Shalowitz, M.D.
Post-Doctoral Fellow
Institute for Health Services Research and Policy
    Studies
Northwestern University
Evanston, Illinois
Formerly Director, Failure to Thrive Program
Assistant Professor, Clinical Pediatrics
University of Chicago
Pritzker School of Medicine
Chicago, Illinois

Bettylou Sherry, Ph.D.
Epidemiologist
Division of Nutrition and Physical Activity
National Center for Chronic Disease Prevention
    and Health Promotion
Centers for Disease Control and Prevention
Atlanta, Georgia

Andrew P. Sirotnak, M.D.
Assistant Professor of Pediatrics
Director
Kempe Child Protection Team
University of Colorado School of Medicine
The Children's Hospital
Denver, Colorado

Lynne Sturm, Ph.D.
Clinical Psychologist
Riley Child Development Center
Riley Hospital for Children
Indianapolis, Indiana

Laura Taylor, D.O.
Developmental and Behavioral Pediatrician
University of Oklahoma College of Medicine
Tulsa, Oklahoma

Mary J. Ward, Ph.D.
Associate Research Professor
Cornell University Medical College
New York, New York

Karen Welford, B.S.N., M.P.A.
Director of Early Intervention Field Services
Massachusetts Department of Public Health
Boston, Massachusetts

Harland S. Winter, M.D.
Associate Professor of Pediatrics
Harvard Medical School
Boston, Massachusetts

Donna Wittmer, Ph.D.
Associate Professor
University of Colorado School of Education
Denver, Colorado

Frieda Wong, B.A.
Doctoral Candidate
University of Massachusetts
Amherst, Massachusetts

Marlene Wüst, M.D.
Attending Pediatrician
New York Hospital
Cornell Medical Center
New York, New York

H. Lorrie Yoos, Ph.D., C.P.N.P.
Associate Professor of Clinical Nursing
Pediatric Nurse Practitioner
University of Rochester School of Nursing and
    Medical Center
Rochester, New York

Foreword

The publication of this book marks a major milestone in the recognition and treatment of pediatric undernutrition (failure to thrive). In this rapidly evolving area, this book clearly represents the most substantive compilation of knowledge to date. The text is broadly construed and filled with critical thinking and consistently demonstrates an appreciation of the subtleties and interactions that result in children's failure to grow and to gain weight.

Unlike most books, this book represents a truly transdisciplinary effort. One of the major problems facing the evolution of knowledge in the area of pediatric undernutrition has been that most researchers approach it from only their own perspectives. For instance, physicians may conduct clinical research aimed at elucidating diseases that contribute to childhood malnutrition, whereas psychologists or social workers may elaborate in detail the social factors. In this book, however, all of the appropriate specialists' perspectives are included. The problem is viewed from the developmental-behavioral perspective, as well as from the medical research perspective.

It has seemed to many physicians and other health care professionals that failure to thrive is a multifaceted disorder. The contribution of the child was a necessary adjunct to our previous thinking, for blaming the victim (the anxious parent) did not provide an effective therapeutic approach. By the time the child was showing growth problems, any caring parent was frantic and anxious. Hence, a multifaceted approach was necessary to evaluate the difficulty in the parent–child interaction affecting feeding. Health professionals have unique opportunities to listen to parents and support the growth of young families. New knowledge of child development, such as that provided in this book, can help professionals better understand children and families and solidify the parent–professional relationship.

Of great interest is the authors' approach to classification. In the past, the tendency to classify cases of failure to thrive simply as either organic or nonorganic has resulted in much confusion in the scientific literature. This has confounded data analysis and many of the most basic studies undertaken in this area. A much more effective approach is the simultaneous assessment of risk factors in multiple domains. Furthermore, the failure to incorporate other disciplines into both clinical practice and research protocols may have resulted routinely in misclassification of the etiology of pediatric undernutrition. For example, typically, a pediatrician may not be able to adequately diagnose problems associated with oral-motor deficits or swallowing difficulties and may therefore choose to classify a child as experiencing "nonorganic failure to thrive" when indeed the child has a swallowing difficulty as the etiology of this undernutrition. Furthermore, social services providers classifying children as having nonorganic failure to thrive may miss the fact that problems that are subtle, such as anemia or lead poisoning, may substantially contribute to the child's undernutrition.

Our concern should begin with the intrauterine experience of the fetus. Many of the children whom we have seen are fragile at birth. They may have been nutritionally deprived or exposed to known or unknown toxins. But their threshold for taking in, incorporating, and responding to information (stimuli) as neonates and infants might identify them as potentially fragile and at risk. Unusual crying as a sign of hypersensitivity (even gastrointestinal hypersensitivity) and easy disorganization are symptoms of fragility in the first few months. These infants often contribute to their own "failure" in the parent–infant system. Their general disorganization is identifiable by a newborn behavioral examination, such as the Neonatal Behavioral Assessment Scale. The seeds for later problems in growth and development might have been there from the beginning. Hence, a multidimensional approach is critical as one assembles the information necessary for diagnosis and therapy. This book approaches the disorder of pediatric undernutrition with that perspective for the first time.

In approaching the older child, one needs to recognize that the child's individual behavioral style or temperamental contribution to the parent–child interaction is a critical one. Intake for feeding and assimilation must be based on the child's autonomous cooperation. It is necessary to recognize that feeding, if it is to succeed, must respect separation-individuation; this book promotes that approach.

Physicians and nurses commonly use the Touchpoints protocols to sensitize themselves to the importance of evaluating feeding and other developmental issues and of their relationships with parents. Reading this book, they will extend that approach. They will find the sections on parent–infant relationships and psychological issues necessary to their comprehensive evaluations of families. This book presents a clear discussion of various types of feeding disorders, such as disorders of homeostasis and oppositional feeding disorders. Feeding is a line of development in which the child's autonomy must necessarily be uppermost. The authors are also clear about the need for concrete services for children who are experiencing undernutrition and the need for community services. Programs such as the Special Supplemental Nutrition Program for Women, Infants and Children (WIC) and food stamps are explained in detail. Finally, the book turns to a discussion of advocacy for underserved families who require improved access to food and nutrition services.

In the early 1980s at Boston Children's Hospital, a group of clinicians led by Dr. Jennifer Rathbun, a child psychiatrist, formed the first multidisciplinary team for the treatment of so-called failure to thrive. Many of the contributors to this book were involved in those early efforts, and many more have contributed to the organization of other teams at numerous hospitals and medical schools across the United States. These programs have used a multidisciplinary approach incorporating physicians, nurses, child developmentalists, psychologists, child psychiatrists, social workers, nutritionists, physical and occupational therapists, and speech-language pathologists, working with community agencies, in the care of malnourished children. The publication of this book shows that this transdisciplinary approach can and should become the national norm.

It is with great pride and enthusiasm that we recommend this text as the best volume to assist clinicians and parents in improving the health status of children who are experiencing pediatric undernutrition.

William G. Bithoney, M.D., F.A.A.P.
Senior Vice President
Brookdale University Hospital and Medical
*   Center*
Chairman
Ambulatory Care Services
Professor of Pediatrics
State University of New York
Health Sciences Center at Brooklyn

T. Berry Brazelton, M.D., F.A.A.P.
Professor Emeritus
Harvard Medical School
Children's Hospital
Boston

Preface

Failure to thrive (FTT), or pediatric undernutrition, means inadequate nutrition that impairs growth during the first 2–3 years of life. It is a significant public health concern in both developed and developing countries. It is important because it may, along with other factors, have long-term effects not only on children's growth but also on their cognitive and social development. Workers from many fields are needed to address it. Although several good review articles have been written, we see a need for a comprehensive book on this topic.

OUR ASSUMPTIONS AND EMPHASES

We believe that FTT, or pediatric undernutrition, may be produced by a variety of factors and so must be addressed at the clinical level by a variety of professionals: dietitians, medical and nursing clinicians, rehabilitation specialists, and mental health professionals. We all must embrace the complexity that multiple issues may present, and clinicians must learn parts of or gain appreciation for one another's skills, working together in a transdisciplinary approach. To this end, we asked chapter authors to provide material that would interest readers in their own fields and to make it accessible to readers in other fields. In many instances, working with a family around nutrition may lead one to discover other needs that may even be more important and should be addressed. We believe that it is important to work closely and collaboratively with families, as early intervention programs do. Because information contained in this book may also be of interest to nonmedical (or nonprofessional) people, medical terms are either explained in the text or printed in bold and defined in the glossary at the end of the book.

We also believe that child nutrition should be treated not only at the level of individual children and families but also at the level of community-wide programs. Inadequacies of public policies toward children and families in the United States contribute to undernutrition and must be confronted. Accordingly, we have included chapters to address issues of managed care, community programs, and social policy.

TERMINOLOGY

The title of the book contains both "failure to thrive" and "pediatric undernutrition." The need for two terms reflects some of the confusion in the field. Both are generally defined in terms of inadequate growth. The term *failure to thrive*, used widely in clinical work, implies either a disease process or a mixture of social causes, often incompletely understood and implying blame of the parents. The term *pediatric undernutrition* (PUN) refers more specifically to growth impairment and, we believe, is less pejorative. Although the term *failure to thrive* is more familiar to the professionals who are likely to see this book, the editors have long felt that a more useful and less pejorative term would be preferable. We have used both terms in the title so that professionals will not only identify the historical significance of the work but also recognize our intention to move past easily identified labels to acknowledge complex realities. *Pediatric undernutrition* is closer to what we really mean.

SECTIONS OF THE BOOK

Section I provides the reader with introductory information—a base to understand what follows. Chapter 1 gives our view of the condition and provides further discussion of definition and terminology in historical context. Chapters 2 and 3 tell why the condition is important. Chapter 4 provides important information about working with families. Chapter 5 provides the information necessary to critically examine the basis for our current imperfect understanding of pediatric undernutrition.

Sections II and III provide information that is important to assessing the underlying causes of the condition. Section II starts with a basic discussion of nutrition and moves into the new areas of feeding behavior and the relationship aspects of feeding. Section III discusses the more traditional medical aspects of undernutrition. Chapters 9 and 10 will help the clinician approach and sort out which cases of poor growth and undernutrition are due to medical factors. Chapters 11–18 then address specific medical factors (based on organ systems) that may impair growth. The section ends with four chapters that address issues of terminology (coding) and the organization of medical services.

Section IV addresses issues of child development: oral-motor function and sensation, communication difficulties, and early intervention programs. In Section V, we seek to aid the clinician in better understanding the important cultural, family, and mental health issues that often contribute to undernutrition and may also affect the success of efforts at intervention. Although much research has been conducted in some of these areas, there is little information available to guide treatment approaches.

Sections VI and VII move the discussion to the levels of community services and social policy. The appendixes include clinical tools: special growth charts, questionnaires, and methods of assessing feeding and family interactions.

We hope that this book will help many people do their work better, will move the field forward, and will help improve the lives of undernourished children and their families.

Acknowledgments

This book is the work of many people. We thank the contributors. We admire their expertise, we have enjoyed getting to know them, and we appreciate their dedication and hard work.

We thank Share Our Strength and ZERO TO THREE: National Center for Infants, Toddlers and Families for their encouragement and support for the duration of this project from its earliest inception to its completion.

Dr. Kessler acknowledges the early financial support of the Carl C. Icahn Foundation, as well as support from a Social and Behavioral Sciences Research Grant from the March of Dimes Birth Defects Foundation (No. 12-183) and the Clinical Research Centers (Grant No. RR-00047). He also thanks many individuals for their critical support and encouragement, including Felicia Axelrod, Emilia Sedlis, Sol Zimmerman, Eli H. Newberger, Carolyn Moore Newberger, T. Berry Brazelton, Christine Brazelton, Jennifer Rathbun, William G. Bithoney, Mary Jo Ward, H. Jonathan Polan, John J. Ferry, Maria I. New, Joseph M. Gertner and the staff of the Pediatric Clinical Research Center, Irwin R. Redlener and the staff and fellows of the Division of Behavioral Pediatrics and Child Development, and Ambulatory Pediatrics at The New York Hospital-Cornell Medical Center, Carl C. Icahn, Gail Golden, Michael S. Kappy, John Olsson, Kay Rauth-Farley, Charles Daschbach, and Gifford Loda.

Dr. Dawson thanks Share Our Strength for funding a growth and nutrition project at People's Clinic, his colleagues there, and the families with whom he worked, some of whom appear in photographs in the book. He also thanks Barbara Beasley, Beth Landry-Murphy, Melinda Morris, Alexander Pérez, Clara Pérez-Mendez, Eileen Saunders, Betsy Sprague, and Lucy Warner.

For their help in various ways, we thank Janet Dean, Emily Fenichel, Karen Peterson, William M. Moore, Robert J. Kuczmarski, plus many others whom we may have forgotten to name.

We thank the staff of Brookes Publishing Company for their hard work. Theresa Donnelly first contacted us with the idea for this volume and guided us in planning the book, Heather Shrestha carried it through, and Christa Horan kindly accommodated our thoroughness in editing. We also thank Dave Cantrell of the Division of Biomedical Communications at the University of Arizona Health Sciences Center for his artwork.

Happy families are all alike;
every unhappy family is
unhappy in its own way.

Leo Tolstoy, *Anna Karenina*, 1875

There is no finer investment
for any community than
putting milk into babies.

Sir Winston Churchill, 1943

Section I

Introduction

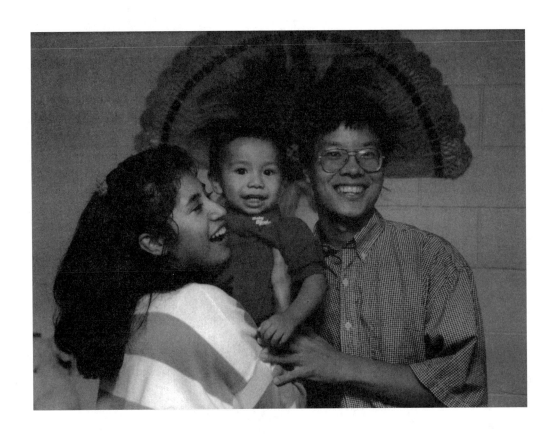

Chapter 1

Failure to Thrive and Pediatric Undernutrition
Historical and Theoretical Context

Daniel B. Kessler

Failure to thrive is a clinical label that is frequently used to describe infants and young children, generally 3 years of age and younger, who fail to grow as expected based on established growth standards for age and gender. After the age of 3 years, other clinical conditions that are associated with growth delay, including psychosocial dwarfism, hyperphagic short stature (Skuse, Albanese, Stanhope, Gilmour, & Voss, 1996), constitutional delay of growth, and familial short stature, are more likely to be diagnosed (see Chapter 15). Although the term *failure to thrive* (or, more common, *FTT*) is used as though it were a specific diagnosis, the disorder may be described more accurately as a clinical syndrome. As with other clinical syndromes, growth "failure" in early childhood, or pediatric undernutrition, is more likely to originate from multiple factors rather than from a single factor.

Why should there be concern when a child exhibits problems of growth and undernutrition? Undernutrition triggers an array of health problems in children, many of which can become chronic in nature and most of which have far-reaching medical as well as social and developmental consequences (see Chapters 2 and 3). Pediatric undernutrition may be associated with decreased immunologic resistance, diminished physical activity, and long-term impairments in cognitive development, academic performance, and socio-

The author acknowledges Peter Dawson, William Bithoney, Karen Peterson, Patrick Casey, Lynne Sturm, and Deborah Frank, whose patience and persistence in expressing their separate perspectives have contributed greatly to this chapter. The author also thanks Gil Foley for his assistance in locating references regarding transdisciplinary work and in reviewing those sections of the chapter.

affective competence. Perhaps even more important, how children are fed and cared for is a reflection of society's values.

DEFINITION

The definition of a condition is critical to the diagnostic process. How a condition is defined has important implications for assessment and treatment. Despite nearly a century of clinical description, there is no universally accepted definition for or understanding of this complex clinical syndrome; thus, there continue to be inconsistencies in the way in which the term is applied and a general lack of clarity that both clouds and distorts its diagnostic value. Historically, the definition of *failure to thrive* has been based on either diagnostic categories or anthropometric criteria. Diagnostic characterization of the syndrome continues to evolve (see Chapter 19), and a consensus involving anthropometric criteria for undernutrition has emerged (see Chapters 2 and 10). Controversy continues regarding the diagnostic application of the term *failure to thrive* as a clinical syndrome in general and of *growth faltering* in specific (K. Peterson, personal communication, May 1997).

Non-uniform diagnostic terminology and criteria also seriously hinder attempts to study the cause and course of this common clinical condition. Criteria for defining growth deficiency or undernutrition in infancy have varied along several important dimensions, including physical growth (e.g., attained weight or length or both, rate of weight gain, importance of weight gain in hospital), duration of growth faltering, physical risk (e.g., acute or chronic illness, prematurity or small-for-gestational-age status), and psychological status (e.g., behavior difficulties, developmental delay or psychosocial disruption). There is disagreement particularly over whether disorders of behavior and development are important aspects of the syndrome of growth deficiency in infancy, or what has been called *failure to thrive*. In the past, the occurrence of social or developmental delay was an important component of the diagnosis, but its relationship to the problem of growth is inconsistent and dependent largely on the etiology of the latter. The editors of this book do not believe that the existence of these secondary phenomena, as important as they are, is necessary to the diagnosis of this condition.

Clinical Categories

Failure to thrive historically has been dichotomized along an organic versus nonorganic axis. *Organic failure to thrive* (OFTT) is believed to result from a major organ system illness or dysfunction. There hardly is a major systemic illness or chronic condition that will not cause growth disturbance in a young child. The term *nonorganic failure to thrive* (NFTT) is used when no organic reason for the FTT can be found and has become a diagnosis of exclusion. A third category of causation, *mixed FTT,* has been added to the alphabet soup with the hope that clinicians will recognize that many cases of organic etiology are compounded by psychosocial difficulty (Homer & Ludwig, 1981). There is, however, a growing consensus, which the editors of this book endorse, that suggests that this approach is both time consuming and overly simplistic (Skuse, 1985, 1993). Traditional categorization or use of the mixed terminology fails to provide guides to intervention; thus, this approach has proved to be clinically inadequate for patient management.

Concept of *Failure to Thrive*

In their commentary *The Concept of Failure to Thrive,* Smith and Berenberg (1970) warned of the dangers of confusing a description of poor growth with a diagnosis. That warning has gone unheeded. Despite a growing knowledge base and recognition on the part of many clinicians that use of the term *failure to thrive* adds little to the understanding of this condition and does much to obscure the condition's complexity, the term appears entrenched, for now, in the medical lexicon. Many (Bithoney, Dubowitz, & Egan, 1992; Goldbloom, 1987; Stickler, 1984) have suggested its abandonment. Parents also are acutely aware of the implication of the term, which may lead to confusion and a sense of failure on their part and thus may impede successful therapeutic intervention. A more useful diagnostic terminology needs to be identified.

Differences in definition explain some of the confusion in the burgeoning pediatric and psychiatric literature that deals with FTT and account for some of the heterogeneity with respect to research findings (see Chapter 5). Because the editors of this book have found useful insights into this condition from studying a variety of clinical populations, this book is more inclusive and broad in its discussion. Included are cases that involve food refusal and feeding difficulties even when those problems have not yet resulted in growth difficulties. Understanding these conditions more generally will help with both prevention and treatment efforts. In this book, the term *failure to thrive* is used in its historical sense and is applied interchangeably with the terms *pediatric undernutrition* and *growth deficiency* (and, sometimes, *growth failure*). This book provides the reader with up-to-date viewpoints on this common and complex syndrome. A review of historical and theoretical perspectives in this chapter provides background for a more practical clinical approach to pediatric undernutrition.

TRANSDISCIPLINARY APPROACH

There is confusion regarding use of the terms *multidisciplinary, interdisciplinary,* and, more recent, *transdisciplinary* (Foley, 1985). In the multidisciplinary model, professionals from a variety of disciplines come together to work as a team; and although each team member is viewed as important, members function as independent specialists rather than as interactive team members. Peterson compared the interaction among team members to parallel play in young children: "side by side, but separate" (1987, p. 484). The child or the family may be assessed individually by several disciplines but generally at the discretion of the team leader, usually a physician in medical settings or a psychologist or a team coordinator in educational or early intervention settings (Foley, 1990).

In interdisciplinary teams, a more formal structure for interaction and communication between individual team members is provided. Although the team members may come together as a whole to discuss their individual assessments and develop a joint service plan, each team member still is responsible solely for his or her unidisciplinary assessment and for developing those aspects of the treatment plan that are related to his or her professional discipline.

The transdisciplinary approach as a "service delivery model" has its origin in the provision of services to infants and toddlers who have developmental disabilities (Foley, 1990). As originally described by Hutchison (1974), the transdisciplinary approach involves a "deliberate pooling and exchange of information, knowledge and skill, crossing and re-crossing traditional disciplinary boundaries by various team members" (United Cerebral Palsy Associations, 1976, p. 1). This model has as one of its goals increasing the opportunity for family members to make meaningful decisions and participate in early intervention. The model also involves team members' sharing roles: Each specialist helps other members to acquire skills that are related to the specialist's area of expertise. This requires both role release (accepting that others can do what the specialist was trained specifically to do) and role expansion (allowing that one's job can include more than what one was trained specifically to do). Transdisciplinary service delivery encourages a whole-child and whole-family approach, allows for the efficient use of the primary team members (i.e., the child and the family do not always need to see many different specialists), and fosters skill development among team members (the early childhood interventionists, in this model). The transdisciplinary model is a natural outgrowth of and complement to the transactional theory of development (Foley, 1990; Sameroff & Chandler, 1978).

This book has been described as providing a *transdisciplinary perspective. Transdisciplinary* is meant not as an alternative to the interdisciplinary or multidisciplinary nature of many teams, with each discipline providing an important component of the assessment (although the emphasis presented here may provide the impetus for just such a realignment), but rather in an educational context to describe how information is being provided in this book. Ultimately, it is expected that it will be used in a therapeutic context as well. Each professional who uses this book will not only enhance his or her own skills but also learn something about and gain an appreciation for the work and contribution of colleagues in other disciplines. A full multidisciplinary team may not always be available (e.g., in rural settings; in Special Supplemental Nutrition Program for Women, Infants and Children [WIC] offices; in child care centers). By using this book as a resource and by interacting with a team over a period of time, professionals will learn to apply new insights from the skills and training paradigms of colleagues and use them to the benefit of families and other professionals with whom they come in contact. In this context, *transdisciplinary* invokes a kind of professional cross-training.

Excellent clinicians always have used a transdisciplinary paradigm, working alongside and learning from their colleagues in nursing, social work, psychiatry, psychology, nutrition, education, and physical, occupational, and speech-language therapy to name just a few. The physician works in a transdisciplinary manner when he or she inquires sensitively about mealtime routines and the lack or the availability of adequate refrigeration and meal preparation facilities for the family. The dietitian or the nutritionist works in a transdisciplinary manner when he or she asks about interpersonal stresses and behavior problems that make it harder for parents to feed their children. Clinicians learn from each other in their discussions of the complex clinical and family situations that compose a large proportion of their work.

PREVALENCE OF PEDIATRIC UNDERNUTRITION

The etiology of pediatric undernutrition is diverse, and the actual prevalence of the condition is difficult to determine accurately. Although much information clearly is out of date (see Chapter 2 for current data on prevalence), it has been estimated that pediatric undernutrition has a prevalence of between 5% and 10% in both rural and urban settings (Altemeier, O'Connor, Sherrod, & Vietze, 1985; Mitchell, Gorrell, & Greenberg, 1980) and accounts for between 1% and 5% of hospitalizations of young children (Berwick, 1980), although this may have declined since the 1980s as a result of the existence of specialized outpatient clinics (see Chapter 9). The number of undiagnosed children who have this syndrome may be higher still. In many developing countries, nutritional deprivation among young children, generally referred to as protein-energy malnutrition (PEM), is endemic.

PEDIATRIC UNDERNUTRITION: THE END RESULT OF MULTIPLE FACTORS

Pediatric undernutrition should be viewed in its larger ecological context in which the condition is the result of any number of factors or interaction of factors. These factors may be viewed in the context of ever-increasing concentric circles around first the infant, then the infant–caregiver interaction, then the larger family environment, and finally the wider social context in which this family or all families are embedded.

Infant Mental Health

Is the syndrome of pediatric undernutrition an emotional disorder or a disorder of growth? Problems of growth may be viewed as the most concrete and, hence, the most accessible measure of impaired infant functioning in a variety of areas, particularly in socioemotional development (Lieberman & Birch, 1985); however, as acknowledgment of the mental health needs of young children and their families has grown (Zeanah, 1993), so, too, has the understanding that the difficulties of infants must be examined in context. So widely accepted is this notion that it has found its way into social policy with the explicit emphasis on families in the Education of the Handicapped Act Amendments of 1986 (PL 99-457) (reauthorized in 1997 [PL 105-17]). Thus growth "failure" may be viewed as at least two failures. On the micro level, it may reflect an adaptational failure to attain a mutually satisfactory regulation of the relationship between infant and caregiver (Lieberman & Birch, 1985; see Chapter 29). On the macro level, it may represent both the failure to understand adequately the complex causative factors that are related to undernutrition and a failure of policy to allow clinicians to safeguard more adequately the health and nutritional status of children from low-income backgrounds (Frank & Drotar, 1994).

Hunger and Poverty

Is the combination of undernutrition and growth deficiency, then, a disease of the poor? In most studies in the United States, undernourished children are drawn disproportionately from low-income families. Although backgrounds of economic well-being clearly fail to protect children from growth or feeding disorders (pediatric undernutrition occurs at all levels of society), poverty continues to be the greatest single risk factor for growth deficiency (Frank & Drotar, 1994; see Chapter 37).

HISTORICAL ORIGINS OF PEDIATRIC UNDERNUTRITION

The term *failure to thrive* has a long, though mixed, usage. The term has been linked to specific disorders of organic origin (Lightwood, 1952), but it also has been used to imply that no organic explanation has been found (Glaser, Heagarty, Bullard, & Pivchik, 1968). In their commentary and historical review of the concept of *failure to thrive,* Smith and Berenberg (1970) identified the verb *thrive* in the first edition of Holt's (1899) *The Diseases of Infancy and Childhood.* In his description of "Malnutrition in Infants (Marasmus)," Holt described this chronic disorder of children:

> The history in severe cases is strikingly uniform. The following is the story most frequently told. "At birth the infant was plump and well-nourished and continued to thrive for a month or six weeks while the mother was nursing him; at the end of that period *circumstances* [emphasis added] made weaning necessary. From that time on the child *ceased to thrive* [emphasis added]. He began to lose weight and strength, at first slowly then rapidly, in spite of the fact that every known infant food was tried." As a last resort the child, wasted to a skeleton, is brought to the hospital. (as cited in Smith & Berenberg, 1970, p. 661)

Although this description remained unchanged in the eight editions that followed, which spanned a period of 34 years, a "considerable restatement" of the condition was identified by Smith and Berenberg (1970) in the tenth edition (Holt & McIntosh, 1933). In the updated discussion of this disorder, now simply referred to as *Marasmus,* the paragraph that was just quoted is unchanged; however, the expanded discussion of "Etiology" now ends with

> Finally it must be admitted that it is not always possible to find why certain infants *fail to thrive* [emphasis added]. Such instances are regarded as due to some congenital weakness of constitution, a concept which is still far from satisfactory. A considerable number of premature infants fall into this group. (as cited in Smith & Berenberg, 1970, p. 661)

The condition of chronic malnutrition, believed by Holt (1899) to have occurred with "striking regularity" as a consequence of early weaning and later (Holt & McIntosh, 1933) to have meant something more, did not immediately come to be known as *failure to thrive.* In the 50 years that followed publication of the tenth edition, other general terms were used to describe such infants, including *chronic nutritional disturbance* (Blackfan, as cited in Smith & Berenberg, 1970). In those early descriptions, it was more common to see the term attached to growth deficiency that was thought to reflect emotional rather than physical causes. Glaser and her colleagues described 50 children in whom "an organic diagnosis could not be established" and listed nine other references "emphasizing the role of environmental causes" (1968, p. 690).

Causes of Failure to Thrive

The characterization of the syndrome of FTT as being of either organic or nonorganic origin or the use of a third mixed category of causation still fails to answer the question, "What is causing the growth failure?" Several theories have been posited, including emotional deprivation, underfeeding, and abuse.

Emotional Deprivation

The view with the longest historical tradition equates NFTT with emotional deprivation (Bakwin, 1949), although it also has been described variously as cachexia of hospitalism (Chapin, 1915a), isolation (Lowrey, 1940), affect hunger (Goldfarb, 1945), anaclitic depression (Spitz, 1946), maternal deprivation (Bowlby, 1952), environmental retardation (Coleman & Provence, 1957), sensory deprivation (Casler, 1961), psychologic malnutrition (Talbot, 1963), idiopathic hypopituitarism (Powell, Brasel, & Blizzard, 1967), environmental failure to thrive (Barbero & Shaheen, 1967), deprivation dwarfism (Silver & Finkelstein, 1967), psychosocial dwarfism (Reinhart & Drash, 1969), reversible somatotropin deficiency (Wolff & Money, 1973), psychosocial deprivation (Patton & Gardner, 1975), and reactive attachment disorder of infancy (American Psychiatric Association, 1980). Terms such as *psychosocial deprivation* were merely euphemisms for maternal neglect (Lieberman & Birch, 1985). The presumption of causation was that the absence of the mothering figure, either literally (e.g., institutionalized infants) or figuratively (e.g., anaclitic depression in the home [the mother was emotionally unavailable to the infant]), led to neuroendocrine disturbance despite adequate food intake (Talbot, Sobel, Burke, Lindemann, & Kaufman, 1947). As is evidenced later in this chapter, this assumption proved to be incorrect.

The notion that a physical problem such as growth deficiency can have as its basis a problem in the child's environment has itself an interesting history. In the beginning of the 20th century, the problem of "institutional deprivation" appears to have been recognized first by a pediatrician, Henry Dwight Chapin (1915b) of New York City. Chapin recognized the limitations of institutional care for children who had acute illnesses and were placed in a hospital and children who were abandoned and placed in foundling homes. He established that with more adequate home environments the death rates among these infants, which historically approached 100% for infants younger than 1 year (Cupoli, Hallock, & Barness, 1980), could be reduced dramatically (Chapin, 1908). Chapin's observations were prophetic (Goldbloom, 1982) for later understanding of the complex interactions of nutritional and environmental factors and the critical need for a nonjudgmental approach toward managing these children and families.

Some 30 years later, clinicians were influenced profoundly by the classic studies of Spitz (1945, 1946) and his descriptions of children in institutions as suffering the results of maternal deprivation. Although not without significant criticism (Pinneau, 1955), Spitz's work was instrumental in solidifying for many the connection between the clinical syndromes that he called *hospitalism* and *anaclitic depression* (and, ultimately, *failure to thrive* as well) and the separation of mother and child.

In his work with institutionalized infants, Chapin (1908, 1915a) was also concerned about the link between malnutrition and infection (see Chapter 13). Thirty years later, this link also was observed by another New York City pediatrician, Harry Bakwin (1949), in the emotional deprivation experienced by hospitalized infants who were isolated for infection control. Although the emotional deprivation was initially attributed to the adverse effects of "malnutrition or marasmus," attention turned to the possible role of infections when the application of advances in nutrition failed to solve the problem. This, in turn, led to elaborate methods of asepsis and isolation with the handling of infants reduced to an absolute minimum. Bakwin suspected that "hospitalism" was in "some vague way related to the infant's psyche" (1949, p. 515) and that the ill effects often were ameliorated by the presence of the mother herself or by someone in a mothering role (as in his own institution, that of interns assigned to provide "tender loving care" often to the benefit of both infant and intern). Rather than increase the incidence of infections in hospital, such practices often were associated with a decrease in cross-infections and dramatic falls in mortality rates even prior to the availability of modern chemotherapeutic and antibiotic agents.

In the years that followed, the constellation of associated findings (including suppression of affect and developmental and intellectual retardation) that were described by Spitz, Bakwin, and others in children who were in institutions were increasingly recognized in some children who were cared for in their own homes (Coleman & Provence, 1957); however, the insight that the growth deficiency experienced by institutionalized infants could also occur in home environments appears to have been made first by Talbot and his colleagues (Talbot et al., 1947). Although they were describing a group of children who were between 2½ and 15 years of age and were referring primarily to short stature ("dwarfism"), they postulated the link between poor growth (without indication of organic cause) and deprivation. The description of such children and the later implication of possible endocrine disturbances as they may relate to growth disturbance in early childhood continue to be areas of controversy, as does the relationship between growth disturbance in infancy and later childhood.

In their comprehensive evaluation of these children, Talbot et al. (1947) described a majority as having long histories of feeding difficulty often beginning in infancy. Early onset of feeding disturbance and difficulties in the social environment of the children were common in those "dwarfs" who were undernourished as well as small. Their conclusion was that the children's undernutrition, based as it was on decreased caloric intake, was secondary to "anorexia due to emotional disturbances or mental deficiency or because of a combination of such disturbances and poverty and ignorance on the part of the parents" (Talbot et al., 1947, p. 789). Although it remained for Powell and his associates (Powell et al., 1967) 20 years later to provide specific evidence for the link, their observations also led them to postulate that hypopituitarism was the cause of the poor growth (although for Talbot, this reflected a homeostatic or adaptive reaction to the malnutrition rather than a direct cause of the growth disturbance).

Underfeeding

The second most important historical trend, which has received increasing support, relates growth deficiency directly to inadequate caloric intake. In this regard, the work of Whitten and his colleagues (Whitten, Pettit, & Fischoff, 1969) has been most influential despite obvious limitations (e.g., small sample size, lack of defined study design; see Chapter 5). Once again, however, the inadequate caloric intake was linked intrinsically to failures in the mothering role.

Whitten and his colleagues challenged the prevailing hypothesis of the day, which linked growth failure to "psychological factors, possibly mediated through either diminished intestinal absorption, inefficient utilization of calories, or abnormal endocrine function" (1969, p. 1675). They did this, in an ironic twist on history, by simulating emotionally depriving home environments in a hospital. By comparing weight gain under conditions of high and low environmental stimulation in a controlled hospital setting, they established that adequate calories rather than quality of environmental stimulation was the key factor in weight gain.

The researchers sought to support their findings further by demonstrating accelerated weight gain in a second group of infants prior to hospitalization by providing their mothers with a measured diet and having the mothers feed the children under the observation of the research staff. Whitten and his colleagues (1969) showed that, whether at home or in a sterile hospital environment, when provided adequate calories, children with growth deficiency demonstrated significant weight gain. These same children would continue to demonstrate this accelerated growth rate even when returned home to presumably emotionally or maternally deprived environments if and only if adequate caloric intake could be ensured by the research staff.

Although not without its critics (e.g., Leonard & Solnit, 1970; Thompson & Blizzard, 1970), this study was the first to acknowledge the importance of providing and ensuring adequate caloric intake for growth in children who demonstrate growth deficiency. It should be noted, however, that Whitten and his colleagues (1969) were able to do little to alter the environment to which the children were returned (which led to inadequate caloric intake initially) and so were unable to implement meaningful and long-lasting change in growth outcomes.

Another illustration of the importance of the caregiving environment comes from the work of Ashworth (1969) and her colleagues in Jamaica. In their work with children who had severe PEM, astonishingly rapid rates of catch-up growth were observed when these children were provided with extra calories and protein to sustain growth (see Chapters 6 and 10). These children demonstrated recovery rates that were 15 times those of normal children of the same age and 5 times those of normal children of similar height and weight. This growth rate slowed as did their intake only as they approached normal weight for height. If they had been fed amounts that were appropriate to their size instead of these increased amounts, then catch-up growth would not have been sustained.

Abuse

While clinicians and researchers were debating the relative contributions of underfeeding and maternal deprivation in the etiology of growth problems in young children, Kempe and his colleagues in Denver, Colorado (Kempe, Silverman, Steele, Droegemueller, & Silver, 1961), were providing evidence for the physical abuse of children by their parents. This was followed by the recognition of the wider spectrum of maltreatment (Helfer & Kempe, 1968) including emotional abuse and neglect and, more recently, sexual abuse. In addition, with the 1960s and 1970s came laws that required that medical personnel and others report incidents of suspected child abuse to the appropriate state and local authorities including child protective services and local law enforcement agencies. The definition of *abuse* in these laws often included acts of omission, including the withholding of food (Krieger, 1974; Shapiro, Fraiberg, & Adelson, 1976), as well as commission. Extreme instances of food deprivation (Adelson, 1963) appear to be more the exception than the rule in children who are evaluated in most large clinical settings. To place emphasis and resources on these rather atypical situations would be to "miss the forest for the trees."

Relationship Between Failure to Thrive and Protein-Energy Malnutrition

Although they have been described in separate literatures, both FTT and PEM reported in developing countries constitute the single syndrome of childhood malnutrition. Although the prominence and degree of interaction may vary depending on the setting, the broad categories of risk appear similar for the two conditions (Peterson & Chen, 1990; Rathbun & Peterson, 1987). Long-term sequelae for either disorder are likely to reflect individual differences in onset, duration, and severity as well as in family, environmental, and cultural variables. Despite these similarities, the search for etiological factors has diverged widely with these two conditions. The source of this divergence may prove instructive. The developed countries of the West have taken a largely "blame the parent" perspective, which is reflected strongly in the "maternal deprivation" tradition; however, the assumptions behind this perspective have been based on studies of small, generally highly biased hospitalized samples (see Chapter 5). Wolke (1996) and his colleagues have questioned the basis for many of the early assumptions regarding these children and their families. In his population-based study (in London), only 17% of the children who were underweight were referred for pediatric evaluation, and those had a high rate of organic illness and family dysfunction. Rather than being hospital based, studies of malnutrition in developing countries frequently used large community-based samples and, as a result, drew far different conclusions regarding etiology. The conceptualization of growth "failure" in the developed world has much to benefit from the complex multifactorial model that has long been used in describing malnutrition in the developing world.

INTERACTIONAL DISORDER OR INTERACTION OF DISORDERS?

The more traditional approach to FTT has given way to a broadened conceptualization of risk status. In this model, positive indicators of risk may coexist in any of a number of interacting systems, including but not limited to the child, the parents, and the larger social environment (Bithoney & Rathbun, 1983; Casey, 1988) in which the child and the family coexist. Increased attention has also been given to the presumed interactional nature of this growth disturbance (Casey, 1983; Kessler, Ward, Auerbach, & Altmann, 1988) as well as to the important nutritional factors that may serve as a final common pathway for the inadequate growth, which is a basic determining feature of this syndrome. Although not all children with problems of growth in infancy have feeding disturbances and although the direction of causality may be uncertain, there is a growing recognition that feeding difficulties of one form or another are central to the development of the syndrome for many children and their parents (Chatoor, Dickson, Schaefer, & Egan, 1985).

Interactional Disorder

Glaser and Lieberman (1984) described an interactional model in which infants are not merely passive recipients of their caregivers' ministrations but active contributors to their growth and development. Infant attributes are viewed not only as important in their own right but also as having a powerful effect in shaping the interaction between infant and parent. Other factors also may influence the parental contribution to the interaction. In Belsky's (1984) process model, parental competence is influenced by three sets of factors. The first is parental resources, especially early developmental experiences and personality. The second is child characteristics, such as temperament, physical health, and illness. The third is the family and social context of parent–child relationships, including the parents' relationship, the family's social networks, and employment and community resources. Several novel maternal difficulties have been described as contributing to disorders of infant growth (Daly & Fritsch, 1995; McGilchrist, Wolkind, & Lishman, 1994). Cultural factors (see Chapter 26) undoubtedly play important roles in the way in which parents and children interact around feeding. A parent's own history of having been parented and the sense of relationship (or attachment) that he or she experienced and may be reproducing with his or her own child may have important implications as well (see Chapter 30).

Interaction of Disorders

At the most basic level, growth deficiency that is based on undernutrition must be related to disturbance or inadequacy of one of the several factors that are described in Table 1, although there are many variations on the themes that are suggested. There are many reasons that an infant is not given or does not take adequate nutrition, and the goal of assessment is to clarify these with an eye toward intervention.

Any of these factors may be the trigger for a "vicious cycle" that perpetuates the growth disturbance (i.e., pediatric undernutrition as an "interaction of disorders"). In addition, each risk factor may itself be modified by the presence of any other risk factor. Clearly, interactional influences exist at multiple levels. As described previously, growth may be influenced both by prematurity and by parental stature (see Chapter 10). Deficiencies of several micronutrients such as zinc or iron (see Chapter 6) also can hinder growth. Iron can have its effect directly by depleting the oxygen supply to growing cells or indirectly by increasing infant irritability and affecting the quality of infant–caregiver interac-

Table 1.   The role of nutritional adequacy

Nutritional adequacy may be impeded by	Possible contributing factors
Inadequate food being offered	Quiet baby or depressed mother, unusual dietary beliefs, lack of knowledge, poverty, substance abuse
Inadequate intake	Anorexia or food refusal, obstructing tonsils or adenoids, oral-motor malformation or dysfunction, dental caries
Inadequate retention	Vomiting, reflux, or diarrhea
Inadequate absorption	Cystic fibrosis or short gut (foul-smelling stools, abdominal distention)
Decreased growth efficiency	Hypothyroidism, congenital heart disease, chronic lung disease, chronic infections, HIV, obstructing tonsils or adenoids
Increased caloric needs	Hyperthyroidism, thermal stress, chronic illness, malignancy, renal failure

tion (Oski & Honig, 1978). Iron deficiency may also predispose the child to lead poisoning (Bithoney, 1986) by increasing intestinal absorption of lead and other heavy metals. Increasing lead levels lead to constipation, abdominal pain, and anorexia (Frank & Drotar, 1994), which lead to further impairment in dietary intake and disorders of growth (see Chapter 11). Diets that are deficient in iron and zinc may result in anorexia, further limiting dietary intake (see Chapter 3).

Undernourished children often find themselves trapped in an infection–malnutrition cycle (see Chapter 13). Malnutrition that is significant enough to result in growth disturbance often impairs immune function and results in frequent otitis, gastrointestinal, and respiratory infections. With each new illness, the child's appetite and intake decrease just as nutritional requirements increase (from fever, diarrhea, or vomiting). Cumulative nutritional deficits leave the child increasingly vulnerable to even more severe and possibly prolonged infections and even more compromised growth (Frank & Drotar, 1994).

A transactional model of development (Sameroff & Chandler, 1978) may be useful for understanding the role and interplay of causative factors in pediatric undernutrition. In this model, undernutrition and its sequelae result from a spectrum of biological and social risk factors that not only interact but also modify one another over time. For most children, undernutrition is the endpoint of a chronic process involving both biological (or medical or nutritional [i.e., organic]) and psychological (or social or environmental [i.e., nonorganic]) influences. Just as serious psychosocial problems may be associated with children's being diagnosed as experiencing organic growth disturbances, all children with nonorganic growth problems have a significant organic disorder: malnutrition.

IMPORTANCE OF PARENTS

Consistent with the influence of the transdisciplinary model is an increasing recognition of the important role of parents (Kessler, 1987; see also Chapter 4) but not just from an etiological ("blame the victim") perspective. It is increasingly clear that parents' involvement is critical to both the diagnostic and the therapeutic process (Frank & Drotar, 1994). Parents are the experts regarding their own children, and all parents who are given equal access to information and resources want only what is best for their children. Obtaining accurate and complete information about a child and his or her world and early consideration of environmental and psychosocial factors in the etiology of growth disturbance requires the establishment of rapport between program staff and family (see Chapter 4) as well as the time and skill for detailed and serial interviews with parents that permit the development of a trusting alliance. Rapport definitely will not be established if the staff takes a stance that blames the parents. Parents should be invited as full members if not, in fact, as the leaders of assessment teams.

FAILURE TO THRIVE OR *PEDIATRIC UNDERNUTRITION:* WHAT'S IN A NAME?

Labels influence perspective. How a condition is defined and characterized has important implications for assessment and treatment. Although the complex interplay of factors that contribute to problems of growth and undernutrition has been discussed, a suitable diagnostic taxonomy has not. It is not for a lack of trying, however (see Chapter 19). Clinicians and other professionals have been surprisingly resistant when asked to consider a replacement for this problematic yet persistent clinical label of FTT. For some, it is habit and familiarity. This term allows them to communicate with colleagues and parents and express a level of concern and, possibly, alarm. For others, it conveys their belief that the term represents a regular pattern of undernutrition that is associated with psychosocial adversity. This is not convincing. Rarely does the term provide either diagnostic clarity or a guide to rational or reasoned intervention.

The challenge that both investigators and clinicians face is to become "increasingly more specific in identifying and describing each of the multiple contributing factors" (Lieberman & Birch, 1985, p. 260) to problems of growth in children. To do so would allow a clarification and a better understanding of the great variety of etiological pathways that affect the children and the families whom clinicians serve. It would allow provision of scant treatment resources with a greater degree of specificity. In an era in which *managed care* and *cost containment* (see Chapters 20 and 21) are the new buzzwords in both health care and human services, increasingly more sophisticated information is needed on what works for children. It is already known that in many centers the availability of interdisciplinary outpatient clinics for the diagnosis and management of growth disorders in young children has greatly reduced the need for hospitalization. Bithoney and his colleagues (1991) have provided evidence that children who are treated in family-focused, multidisciplinary growth and nutrition clinics experience better growth than children who are managed in primary care clinics.

THE NEED TO "EMBRACE COMPLEXITY"

Because the assessment of pediatric undernutrition is best performed using a risk analysis approach, the careful clinician must consider organic and nonorganic factors simultaneously. The process of risk analysis, however, typically generates multiple diagnoses. This is quite different from the dominant medical tradition, which is influenced heavily by a unidimensional and linear model. This tradition is most easily recognized in the "germ theory" of disease causation. The premise of the germ theory, popular since the time of Pasteur, is simple and very seductive: one germ, one disease, one cure. All that has to be done is identify the germ, isolate it, and eradicate it. The risk analysis approach and the simultaneous consideration of multiple diagnoses also run counter to the scientific tradition of parsimony (which states that the simplest explanation that is consistent with a data set should be chosen over more complex explanations); however, it is more in tune with current scientific efforts to understand complex biological systems.

Sally Provence, a widely known pediatrician who had worked at the Yale Child Study Center and was a founding board member of ZERO TO THREE: National Center for Clinical Infant Programs (now ZERO TO THREE: National Center for Infants, Toddlers and Families), advised physicians who were concerned with young children and their families to "embrace complexity" rather than avoid it. The resulting ambiguity, however, can heighten anxiety for even the most experienced clinician. Pressure to come up with an answer, often by the parents themselves, may lead to premature diagnostic closure and counterproductive labeling. A history of family stress or a hostile parent may result in the label of NFTT and limit the investigation of potentially significant organic influences on growth. Similarly, the reluctance of a clinician to accept the importance of environmental etiologies or even of their interaction with organic factors over time may lead to uncritical acceptance of borderline physical or laboratory evidence as proof of an organic etiology and preclude further investigation of important social and environmental concerns. The use of teams of concerned and involved professionals (whether they are transdisciplinary, interdisciplinary, or multidisciplinary) and ongoing comprehensive assessment that is open constantly to the development of new information, as well as the information provided in this volume, provide an adaptive approach to this diagnostic ambiguity.

Clinicians also need to embrace the notion that children and families do not live in a vacuum. Just as the search for the reasons behind a child's growth problems needs to expand beyond the level of the individual, so do the interventions. Although clinicians must start at the individual level to serve children and their families more effectively, they must take a community-wide perspective in their solutions. This volume provides the concerned professional with the tools to do so.

REFERENCES

Adelson, L. (1963). Homicide by starvation: The nutritional variant of the "battered child." *Journal of the American Medical Association, 186,* 104–106.

Altemeier, W.A., O'Connor, S.M., Sherrod, K.B., & Vietze, P.M. (1985). Prospective study of antecedents for non-organic failure to thrive. *Journal of Pediatrics, 106,* 360–365.

American Psychiatric Association. (1980). *Diagnostic and statistical manual of mental disorders* (3rd ed.). Washington, DC: Author.

Ashworth, A. (1969). Growth rates in children recovering from protein-calorie malnutrition. *British Journal of Nutrition, 23,* 835–845.

Bakwin, H. (1949). Emotional deprivation in infancy. *Journal of Pediatrics, 35,* 512–521.

Barbero, G.H., & Shaheen, E. (1967). Environmental failure to thrive: A clinical view. *Journal of Pediatrics, 71,* 639–644.

Belsky, J. (1984). The determinants of parenting: A process model. *Child Development, 55,* 83–96.

Berwick, D.M. (1980). Nonorganic failure to thrive. *Pediatrics in Review, 1,* 265–270.

Bithoney, W.G. (1986). Elevated lead levels in children with nonorganic failure to thrive. *Pediatrics, 78,* 891–895.

Bithoney, W.G., Dubowitz, H., & Egan, H. (1992). Failure to thrive/growth deficiency. *Pediatrics in Review, 13,* 453–460.

Bithoney, W.G., McJunkin, J., Michalek, J., Snyder, J., Egan, H., & Epstein, D. (1991). The effect of a multidisciplinary team approach on weight gain in nonorganic failure-to-thrive children. *Journal of Developmental and Behavioral Pediatrics, 12,* 254–258.

Bithoney, W.G., & Rathbun, J. (1983). Failure to thrive. In M.D. Levine, W.B. Carey, & A.C. Crocker (Eds.), *Developmental-behavioral pediatrics* (pp. 557–571). Philadelphia: W.B. Saunders.

Bowlby, J. (1952). Maternal care and mental health. *WHO Monograph Series, 2.*

Casey, P.H. (1983). Failure to thrive: A reconceptualization. *Journal of Developmental and Behavioral Pediatrics, 4,* 63–66.

Casey, P.H. (1988). Failure to thrive: Transitional perspective. *Journal of Developmental and Behavioral Pediatrics, 8,* 37–38.

Casler, L. (1961). Maternal deprivation: A critical review of the literature. *Monographs of the Society for Research in Child Development, 26,* 1–64.

Chapin, H.D. (1908). A plan of dealing with atrophic infants and children. *Archives of Pediatrics, 25,* 491–496.

Chapin, H.D. (1915a). Are institutions for infants necessary? *Journal of the American Medical Association, 6,* 1–3.

Chapin, H.D. (1915b). A plea for accurate statistics in infants' institutions. *Archives of Pediatrics, 32,* 724–726.

Chatoor, I., Dickson, L., Schaefer, S., & Egan, J. (1985). A developmental classification of feeding disorders associated with failure to thrive: Diagnosis and treatment. In D. Drotar (Ed.), *New directions in failure to thrive: Implications for research and practice* (pp. 235–258). New York: Plenum.

Coleman, R., & Provence, S. (1957). Environmental retardation (hospitalism) in infants living in families. *Pediatrics, 19,* 285–292.

Cupoli, J.M., Hallock, J.A., & Barness, L.A. (1980). Failure to thrive. *Current Problems in Pediatrics, 10,* 1–43.

Daly, J.M., & Fritsch, S.L. (1995). Case study: Maternal residual attention deficit disorder associated with failure to thrive in a two-month old infant. *Journal of the American Academy of Child Psychiatry, 34,* 55–57.

Drotar, D. (1988). Failure to thrive. In D.K. Routh (Ed.), *Handbook of pediatric psychology* (pp. 71–107). New York: Guilford Press.

Education of the Handicapped Act Amendments of 1986, PL 99-457, 20 U.S.C. §§ 1400 *et seq.*

Foley, G. (1985). *Principles of the transdisciplinary approach.* Unpublished manuscript.

Foley, G. (1990). Portrait of the arena evaluation: Assessment in the transdisciplinary approach. In B. Gibbs & D. Teti (Eds.), *Interdisciplinary assessment of infants: A guide for early intervention professionals* (pp. 271–286). Baltimore: Paul H. Brookes Publishing Co.

Frank, D.A., & Drotar, D. (1994). Failure to thrive. In R.M. Reece (Ed.), *Child abuse: Medical diagnosis and management* (pp. 298–324). Philadelphia: Lea & Febiger.

Glaser, H.H., Heagarty, M.C., Bullard, D.M., & Pivchik, E.C. (1968). Physical and psychological development of children with early failure to thrive. *Journal of Pediatrics, 73,* 690–698.

Glaser, M., & Lieberman, A.F. (1984). Failure to thrive: An interactional perspective. In L. Zegans, L. Temoshok, & C. Van Dyke (Eds.), *Emotions in health and illness* (pp. 199–207). San Diego: Grune & Stratton.

Goldbloom, R.B. (1982). Failure to thrive. *Pediatric Clinics of North America, 29,* 151–156.

Goldbloom, R.B. (1987). Growth failure in infancy. *Pediatrics in Review, 9,* 57–61.

Goldfarb, W. (1945). Psychological privation in infancy and subsequent adjustment. *American Journal of Orthopsychiatry, 15,* 247–255.

Helfer, R.E., & Kempe, C.H. (1968). *The battered child.* Chicago: University of Chicago Press.

Holt, L.E. (1899). *The diseases of infancy and childhood.* New York: D. Appleton and Co.

Holt, L.E., Jr., & McIntosh, R. (1933). *Holt's diseases of infancy and childhood* (10th ed.). New York: D. Appleton-Century Company.

Homer, C., & Ludwig, S. (1981). Categorization of etiology of failure to thrive. *American Journal of Diseases of Children, 135,* 848–851.

Hutchison, D. (1974). A model for transdisciplinary staff development: A monograph (Technical Report No. 8). In *The first three years: Programming for atypical infants and their families.* New York: United Cerebral Palsy Associations.

Individuals with Disabilities Education Act Amendments of 1997, PL 105-17, 20 U.S.C. §§ 1400 *et seq.*

Kempe, C.H., Silverman, F.N., Steele, B., Droegemueller, W., & Silver, H.K. (1961). The battered-child syndrome. *Journal of the American Medical Association, 181,* 17–24.

Kessler, D.B. (1987, March). *Failure to thrive: Whose failure? Infant, parent or professional?* Paper presented at the National Center for Clinical Infant Programs Regional Conference, Long Island, NY.

Kessler, D.B., Ward, M.J., Auerbach, W., & Altmann, S.C. (1988, May). *Failure-to-thrive: An interactional disorder or an interaction of disorders?* Paper presented at the Society for Behavioral Pediatrics, Washington, DC.

Krieger, I. (1974). Food restriction as a form of child abuse in ten cases of psychosocial deprivation dwarfism. *Clinical Pediatrics, 13,* 126–133.

Leonard, M.F., & Solnit, A.J. (1970). Growth failure from maternal deprivation and undereating. *Journal of the American Medical Association, 212,* 882.

Lieberman, A.F., & Birch, M. (1985). The etiology of failure to thrive: An interactional developmental approach. In D. Drotar (Ed.), *New directions in failure to thrive: Implications for research and practice* (pp. 259–277). New York: Plenum.

Lightwood, R. (1952). Idiopathic hypercalcemia with failure to thrive. *Archives of Diseases of Childhood, 27,* 302–303.

Lowrey, L. (1940). Personality distortion and early institutional care. *American Journal of Orthopsychiatry, 10,* 576–585.

McGilchrist, I., Wolkind, S., & Lishman, A. (1994). "Dyschronia" in a patient with Tourette's syndrome presenting as maternal neglect. *British Journal of Psychiatry, 164,* 261–263.

Mitchell, W.G., Gorrell, R.W., & Greenberg, R.A. (1980). Failure to thrive: A study in a primary care setting: Epidemiology and follow-up. *Pediatrics, 65,* 971–976.

Oski, F.A., & Honig, A.S. (1978). The effects of therapy on the developmental scores of iron-deficient infants. *Journal of Pediatrics, 92,* 21–25.

Patton, R.G., & Gardner, L.I. (1975). Deprivation dwarfism (psychosocial deprivation): Disordered family environment as cause of so-called idiopathic hypopituitarism. In L.I. Gardner (Ed.), *Endocrine and genetic causes of diseases of childhood and adolescence* (2nd ed., pp. 85–98). Philadelphia: W.B. Saunders.

Peterson, K.E., & Chen, L.C. (1990). Defining undernutrition for public health purposes in the United States. *Journal of Nutrition, 120,* 933–942.

Peterson, N. (1987). *Early intervention for handicapped and at-risk children: An introduction to early childhood special education.* Denver: Love Publishing Co.

Pinneau, S.R. (1955). The infantile disorders of hospitalism and anaclitic depression. *Psychological Bulletin, 52,* 429–453.

Powell, G.F., Brasel, J.A., & Blizzard, R.M. (1967). Emotional deprivation and growth retardation simulating idiopathic hypopituitarism: I. Clinical evaluation of the syndrome. *New England Journal of Medicine, 267,* 1271–1278.

Rathbun, J.M., & Peterson, K.E. (1987). Nutrition in failure to thrive. In R.J. Grand, J.L. Sutphen, & W.H. Dietz (Eds.), *Pediatric nutrition: Theory and practice* (pp. 627–643). Boston: Butterworth-Heinemann.

Reinhart, J.B., & Drash, A.I. (1969). Psychosocial dwarfism: Environmentally induced recovery. *Psychosomatic Medicine, 31,* 165–172.

Sameroff, A.J., & Chandler, M.J. (1978). Reproductive risk and the continuum of caretaking casualty. In F.D. Horowitz (Ed.), *Review of child development research* (pp. 187–244). Chicago: University of Chicago Press.

Shapiro, V., Fraiberg, S., & Adelson, E. (1976). Infant–parent psychotherapy on behalf of the child in a critical nutritional state. *The Psychoanalytic Study of the Child, 31,* 461–491.

Silver, H.K., & Finkelstein, M. (1967). Deprivation dwarfism. *Journal of Pediatrics, 70,* 317–324.

Skuse, D. (1985). Non-organic failure to thrive: A reappraisal. *Archives of Disease in Childhood, 60,* 173–177.

Skuse, D. (1993). Epidemiological and definitional issues in failure to thrive. *Child and Adolescent Psychiatric Clinics of North America, 2,* 37–59.

Skuse, D., Albanese, A., Stanhope, R., Gilmour, J., & Voss, L. (1996). A new stress-related syndrome of growth failure and hyperphagia in children, associated with reversibility of growth-hormone insufficiency. *The Lancet, 348,* 353–358.

Smith, C.A., & Berenberg, W. (1970). The concept of failure to thrive. *Pediatrics, 46,* 661–663.

Spitz, R.A. (1945). Hospitalism: An inquiry into the genesis of psychiatric conditions in early childhood. *The Psychoanalytic Study of the Child, 1,* 53–74.

Spitz, R.A. (1946). Anaclitic depression: An inquiry into the genesis of psychiatric conditions in early childhood. *The Psychoanalytic Study of the Child, 2,* 313–342.

Stickler, G.B. (1984). "Failure to thrive" or failure to define. *Pediatrics, 74,* 559.

Talbot, N.B. (1963). Has psychologic malnutrition taken the place of scurvy in contemporary pediatric practice? *Pediatrics, 31,* 909–918.

Talbot, N.B., Sobel, E.H., Burke, B.S., Lindemann, E., & Kaufman, S.B. (1947). Dwarfism in healthy children: Its possible relation to emotional, nutritional and endocrine disturbances. *New England Journal of Medicine, 236,* 783–793.

Thompson, R.G., & Blizzard, R.M. (1970). Growth failure, deprivation and undereating. *Journal of the American Medical Association, 211,* 1379.

United Cerebral Palsy Associations. (1976). *Staff development handbook: A resource for the transdisciplinary process.* New York: Author.

Whitten, C.F., Pettit, M.G., & Fischoff, J. (1969). Evidence that growth failure from maternal deprivation is secondary to undereating. *Journal of the American Medical Association, 299,* 1675–1682.

Wolff, G., & Money, J. (1973). Relationship between sleep and growth in patients with reversible somatotropin deficiency (psychosocial dwarfism). *Psychological Medicine, 3,* 18–27.

Wolke, D. (1996, July–December). Failure-to-thrive: The myth of maternal deprivation. *The Signal: Newsletter of the World Association for Infant Mental Health, 4,* 1–6.

Zeanah, C.H., Jr. (1993). *Handbook of infant mental health.* New York: Guilford Press.

Chapter 2

Epidemiology of Inadequate Growth

Bettylou Sherry

This chapter addresses the epidemiology of inadequate growth among infants and children. For clarity, the term *inadequate growth* is used in preference to *undernutrition* because the chapter focuses on physical growth indices rather than on direct measures of specific nutrient deficiencies. In addition, use of the general term *inadequate growth* allows for a broader perspective that includes both a public health and a clinical context because adequacy of growth is assessed in surveys and surveillance programs. In contrast, the term *failure to thrive* (FTT) usually is reserved for clinical situations.

Inadequate growth during infancy or childhood is characterized by a complex etiology and is thought to result from medical (e.g., congenital heart disease) or environmental (e.g., abnormal parental health beliefs) causes or a combination of these (Frank, Silva, & Needlman, 1993). Both the complex etiology and the research methodology have limited the understanding of inadequate growth. For example, no standard growth reference or cutoff criteria have been used to define *inadequate growth,* especially with reference to FTT; these inconsistencies in the definition of *inadequate growth* hamper the comparison of available studies (Wilcox, Nieburg, & Miller, 1989). In addition, growth indices provide little information to suggest whether inadequate growth has been caused by primary malnutrition that results from the lack of food or secondary malnutrition due to the disease process (World Health Organization Expert Committee on Physical Status, 1995). Other factors, such as poverty or parental behaviors, also can be viewed as risk factors for inad-

The author thanks Laurence Grummer-Strawn, Ph.D., and James Mendlein, Ph.D., for their thoughtful reviews of this chapter.

This chapter was written by a government employee within the scope of her duties and, as such, shall remain in the public domain.

equate growth, but assessing their relative importance from an epidemiological point of view is a daunting task. Unfortunately, there is little information in the literature describing how various risk factors act alone or in concert to cause inadequate growth.

This chapter suggests a way of defining inadequate growth and reviews the epidemiology of this important problem. Recommendations are made for future research to improve the understanding of the epidemiology and public health impact of inadequate growth.

DEFINING INADEQUATE GROWTH

This section describes the growth references, anthropometric indices, and criteria that are most commonly used to evaluate inadequate growth.

Growth References

A *growth reference* is a chart that enables one to compare children's growth with that of a well-nourished population. It should be based on a sample that is representative of the population and that is large enough to provide stable estimates of the various percentiles in each age group and gender group. The 1977 growth charts that were developed by the National Center for Health Statistics/Centers for Disease Control (NCHS/CDC) (NCHS, 1977) have been the most generally accepted of the growth references because they have met these criteria. Because of their widespread use, these references have facilitated comparisons between studies in many countries and, in the process, have increased understanding of inadequate growth. In addition, the World Health Organization (WHO) advocated their use (Waterlow et al., 1977).

The 1977 NCHS/CDC growth charts (Hamill et al., 1979) are being revised to address a number of concerns that have arisen since the charts were developed (Roche, 1994). These concerns focus primarily on the infant charts. Specifically, in the 1977 NCHS growth charts, data from the Fels Research Institute were used for birth to 3 years because at the time that these charts were constructed, national survey data were insufficient. In the revised growth charts, the Fels data will be replaced with national survey data. This and a number of other changes will provide an improved instrument to evaluate size and growth in infants, children, and adolescents, using more comprehensive national survey data and improved statistical procedures. The primary purpose of the revisions to the charts is to provide a better instrument for health care professionals who evaluate the growth status of children in the United States. For international applications, the WHO has stated its intent to develop specialized growth charts based on exclusively or predominantly breast-fed infants (de Onis, Garza, & Habicht, 1997); however, such a project will require several years to collect and analyze the data. Although the revised growth charts were not available when this book went to press, the NCHS has announced that the completed charts will be available on the World Wide Web (http://www.cdc.gov/nchswww).

Other growth references (e.g., from less-developed countries, for a specific disease) have not been accepted generally for use because they are based on populations that generally are not well-nourished, the sample sizes are too small to provide statistically stable estimates, or they are based on a single ethnic group. As for differences in growth by racial or ethnic status, there appear to be small yet significant variations in both the size and the patterns of growth (WHO Expert Committee on Physical Status, 1995).

Anthropometric Indices

The three anthropometric indices that are most commonly used to screen for inadequate growth are height-for-age, weight-for-height, and weight-for-age. Height-for-age reflects skeletal growth and, therefore, is a long-term indicator of growth status. Weight-for-height describes body proportionality and is sensitive to current caloric adequacy but also can reflect long-term status. In developing countries, data on height often are unavailable, and weight-for-age is the index that is most commonly used. Unfortunately, it is the least useful of the three indices; skeletal growth and proportionality are the phenomena of interest, but weight-for-age is not a clear indicator of either phenomenon. (See Chapter 10 for a more detailed discussion of these indicators.)

Other anthropometric indices that are not reviewed in this chapter include head circumference, which is used in the clinical setting to assess brain growth; mid–upper-arm circumference (MUAC), which is used internationally to screen for nutritional status in emergency situations; and body mass index and skinfold measurements, which are used in clinical practice or research settings to evaluate adequacy of fat deposits.

Scaling Systems for Anthropometric Indices

Three scaling systems—percentiles, z-scores, and percent of the median—are used to classify anthropometric indices. A natural phenomenon of growth is that height-for-age and weight-for-height have relatively normal, or "bell-shaped," distributions. The growth distributions have been normalized so that there is a one-to-one correspondence between the percentile and the z-score scales (Dibley, Goldsby, Staehling, & Trowbridge, 1987); however, as is explained later, the percent of the median does not correspond directly to these scales.

The percentile system is based on an ordinal rank order scale. Because it has a nonlinear distribution, absolute differences in height, for example, are not uniform between percentile intervals of equivalent distance, for example, between the 5th and 10th and the 25th and 30th. Thus, calculation of the mean percentile of a population is not appropriate (WHO Working Group, 1986). Percentiles are commonly used in the clinical setting because they indicate simply and clearly where a child fits in the context of the reference population. For example, if a child has a weight-for-height at the third percentile, then 97% of the population at that age who are the same gender and height weigh more than that child.

The z-score scale, which is linear, is computed by the following equation:

$$z\text{-score} = \frac{(\text{Observed Value}) - (\text{Reference Mean Value})}{\text{Standard Deviation of the Reference}}$$

Z-scores facilitate the monitoring of change; for example, unlike the case with the other two scaling systems, an increase of 1.0 centimeter (cm) in a height-for-age z-score depicts the same increase in height regardless of where the change occurs on the scale. Because it is linear, the z-score scale can be subjected to statistics of central tendency and dispersion such as the mean and standard deviation when assessing population data (WHO Expert Committee on Physical Status, 1995). The z-score scale has many advantages and is preferred because it facilitates the monitoring of change and lends itself to summary statistics that can be used for studies of populations (Dibley et al., 1987; Gorstein et al., 1994; Waterlow et al., 1977; WHO Expert Committee on Physical Status, 1995; WHO Working Group, 1986).

The third system that is used is percent of the median for a specific age and gender. The disadvantage of the percent of the median is that the median and the distribution of the reference population vary by age and gender in ways that differ for each of the indices, so there is no equivalent interpretation across indices (Waterlow et al., 1977; WHO Expert

Committee on Physical Status, 1995). For example, a 6-year-old girl who is 104 cm tall and weighs 15 kilograms (kg) is at 91% of the median for both height-for-age and weight-for-height; but in height-for-age this is equal to the 1.5 percentile, whereas in weight-for-height this is equal to the 16th percentile, making interpretation more difficult between indices. Percent of the median does not take into consideration the distribution of the indices around the median (Gorstein et al., 1994), whereas both the percentile and the z-score scales do account for this. Percent of the median is commonly used in the clinical setting, and clinicians either need to consider these scaling differences when evaluating a child's growth status or are advised to base their evaluation of growth on percentiles or on z-score scales in which interpretation is consistent across indices.

Inadequate growth also can be assessed by examining growth faltering, which refers to a downward trend of the growth indices across percentile lines; however, no standard criteria for magnitude of the growth inadequacy or the time period within which it occurs have been established. The two methods that are most commonly used are comparing a child's weight or length gain for a given period of time with one of the two incremental growth references, either the one that is based on serial data for children from the Fels Study (Roche & Himes, 1980) or the reference that is based on the Iowa and the Fels Study (Guo et al., 1991; see Appendix F) to monitor weight or length gain or by documenting a downward trend of growth indices across major percentile lines (e.g., the 50th, 25th, 10th, and 5th) within a specific time period. Although the z-score is not used commonly to assess growth faltering, it is a more appropriate scale than percentiles because a change of 1.0 z-score, for example, would be standard across the spectrum of the scale.

Another problem with defining *growth faltering* is that the severity of the problem varies by where a child plots on the growth distribution. For example, a weight loss of 0.4 kg between the 6- and 7-month measurements for a male infant who was at the 87th percentile in weight-for-height would place him at the 75th percentile; in contrast, this same weight loss over the same time period for a male infant who was at the 10th percentile at 6 months would place him at the 4th percentile in weight-for-height. The latter example is of much greater clinical concern. (See Chapter 10 for further discussion.)

Criteria and Cutoffs for Anthropometric Indices

For all three anthropometric indices, when the NCHS/CDC/WHO growth reference distribution is used, *inadequate growth* is commonly defined as a value below the fifth percentile when the percentile scaling system is used and below -2 when the z-score is employed (equals a percentile of 2.3). The 5th percentile, which is equivalent to a z-score of -1.65, is recommended for children in the United States (Hamill et al., 1979). For research purposes and studies, especially in less-developed countries, the standard of a z-score that is less than -2 has been recommended (WHO Expert Committee on Physical Status, 1995). As the long-term physical, psychosocial, and developmental impacts of growth deficits become better known, this cutoff may need to be adjusted. Two computer software programs that are in the public domain, Anthro[1] (Sullivan & Gorstein, 1990) and Epi Info[2] (Dean et al., 1997), are available to evaluate growth using z-scores, percentiles, and percent of the median.

---

[1] Available from Centers for Disease Control and Prevention, National Center for Chronic Disease Prevention and Health Promotion, Division of Nutrition and Physical Activity, Maternal and Child Nutrition Branch, 4770 Buford Highway, NE, Atlanta, GA 30341.

[2] Available from Centers for Disease Control and Prevention, Division of Surveillance and Epidemiology, Epidemiology Program Office, Atlanta, GA 30333; www.cdc.gov/epo/epi.

DESCRIPTIVE STUDIES OF INADEQUATE GROWTH

Descriptive studies provide valuable information regarding characteristics that are common to children who exhibit inadequate growth. These characteristics then can be included in etiological studies to evaluate whether they are risk factors for inadequate growth. This section describes large-scale studies of the prevalence of inadequate growth and food insecurity. Children who do not have food security could be at risk for primary malnutrition. In addition, case reports and case series describe common characteristics of children with poor growth.

National Prevalence Studies of Inadequate Growth

Several surveys have provided information on the prevalence of inadequate growth and the characteristics of children who have this problem. Data from the first three National Health and Nutrition Examination Surveys (NHANES I, II, and III) (Mcdowell, Engel, Massey, & Maurer, 1981; NCHS, 1973, 1994) reveal that prevalence rates of both low height-for-age and low weight-for-height are relatively close to the expected 5% among 2- to 5-year-olds and that there have been no major changes in prevalence over the three survey periods (see Table 1) (Federation of American Societies for Experimental Biology, Life Sciences Research Office, 1995b).

The Pediatric Nutrition Surveillance System (PedNSS) (Centers for Disease Control and Prevention, 1992), managed by the CDC, uses the same cutoff points as the NHANES and has found similar prevalence of inadequate growth for 2- to 5-year-old low-income children participating in publicly funded nutrition and public health programs. In 1980, the prevalence of low height-for-age in children was 8.9%; in 1996, it had decreased to 5.8%. In 1980, the prevalence of low weight-for-height was 2.8%; in 1996, it was 2.6% (CDC, 1997). A much larger decline in the prevalence of low height-for-age was observed among Asian children: Those from 1 to 23 months of age showed a dramatic progressive decline in the prevalence rate of low height-for-age from a peak of 24.8% in 1982 to a low of 13.5% in 1989 (Yip, Scanlon, & Trowbridge, 1992).

In 1996, the PedNSS data, which are based predominantly on children who are less than 5 years of age, documented that infants from birth to age 2 months had the highest prevalence by age group on both indicators—12.0% for low height-for-age and 4.1% for low weight-for-height (CDC, 1997); African Americans had higher rates for each of the indicators than any other racial or ethnic group.

Studies of Food Security

The lack of food (food insecurity) should be related to poor growth at least when hunger and malnutrition are present; however, according to Allen (1990), food insecurity is not

Table 1.   Prevalence (%) of low height-for-age and low weight-for-height for 2- to 5-year-olds examined in the National Health and Nutrition Examination Surveys (NHANES) I, II, and III

Growth indices	NHANES I (1971–1974)	NHANES II (1976–1980)	NHANES III (1988–1991)
Low ht/age[a]	4.4%	7.0%	5.2%
Low wt/ht[a]	2.0%	2.2%	2.7%

From Federation of American Societies for Experimental Biology, Life Sciences Research Office. (1995). *Third report on nutrition monitoring in the United States* (Vols. 1 and 2). Washington, DC: U.S. Government Printing Office.

[a]Less than the 5th percentile on the NCHS/CDC growth reference.

associated strongly with poor growth in the United States. More research is needed to understand the relationship between the spectrum of food insecurity and hunger and the differential patterns of growth in the United States. At this point, however, it is of interest to include estimates of the prevalence of food insecurity and hunger. The 1995 Food Research and Action Center report estimated that 4 million low-income children in the United States were hungry and that another 9.6 million were at risk for hunger. *Hunger* was identified by a positive response to five of eight questions regarding food insufficiency; *at risk for hunger* was identified by a positive response to between one and four of these eight questions. Analysis of the NHANES III data showed that 3.3% of the overall U.S. population sometimes did not have enough to eat, but rates for certain groups were much higher. For example, the rate of food insufficiency—an inadequate amount of food as a result of the lack of money or resources—for households with incomes less than 131% of the federal poverty threshold (in 1990, the threshold was $13,359 for a family of four) was 10.7%; for households below the poverty threshold, it was 13.2% (Federation of American Societies for Experimental Biology, Life Sciences Research Office, 1995a). The National Center for Children in Poverty (1996) reported that 25.1% of U.S. children were living in poverty in 1994, up from 18% in 1975.

The two previous surveys used definitions of *hunger* and *food insufficiency* that have evolved over time into a clearer concept of food security and insecurity. *Food security* is defined as the access by all people at all times to enough food for an active, healthy life; *food insecurity* is the lack of access at all times to nutritionally adequate food from normal channels; and *hunger* is the uneasy or painful sensation caused by the lack of food that may be caused by food insecurity (Anderson, 1990). On the basis of this clear definition, a food security module and scaling system was developed and added to the U.S. Bureau of the Census Current Population Survey in 1995. Results indicated that 11.9% of households experienced food insecurity with or without hunger in the 12-month period prior to April 1995 (Hamilton et al., 1997).

Case Reports and Case Series

There are numerous case reports and case series that relate to the problem of inadequate growth; much of the American literature concerns infants or other children who are less than 5 years of age. Case reports and series are useful for identifying characteristics of infants and children who are exhibiting inadequate growth in FTT. These characteristics then can be evaluated as potential risk factors in etiological studies that include a control group for comparison. The common characteristics that are mentioned in these reports have been various medical factors (including low birth weight), feeding difficulties and dietary inadequacies, and social and psychological factors.

Medical Characteristics

The most common medical characteristic that is associated with inadequate growth is low birth weight. Using the 5th percentile cutoff for the NCHS/CDC growth reference, Gayle and colleagues found that 20%–40% of low height-for-age in a large sample of low-income children who were younger than 2 years was attributable to low birth weight (Gayle, Dibley, Marks, & Trowbridge, 1987), albeit correcting for gestational age probably would have reduced the percentages. One study (Yip & Mei, 1996) found that children with low birth weights do not fully catch up to full-term infants on the height-for-age index until the age of 5 years. Because infants with low birth weight are smaller in size than infants with normal birth weight, they are identified when they are screened for growth adequacy as exhibiting inadequate growth; however, this does not mean that their growth is inadequate but rather, for many of these cases, they simply are smaller and have more growing to do to attain the size of an infant with normal birth weight. When infants with low birth weight exhibit inadequate growth, it likely is because of medical complications.

Among the chronic diseases or disorders that are cited in case reports or case series on children who have FTT and/or inadequate growth are cancer (Morris, Lough, & Weinberger, 1990), heart disease (Lax, Butto, Leonard, Ring, & Dunnigan, 1989; Poskitt, 1993), obstructive sleep apnea (Marcus et al., 1994), Duchenne's muscular dystrophy (Rapisarda, Muntoni, Gobbi, & Dubowitz, 1995), and cystic fibrosis (Bines & Israel, 1991). Chronic middle-ear effusion (Granot, Matoth, & Feinmesser, 1990) and persistent infectious disease such as acquired immunodeficiency syndrome (AIDS) (Elias-Jones, Larcher, & Price, 1987) and congenitally acquired syphilis (Janner, 1990) have also been reported in this literature, as have enzyme deficiencies (e.g., methyl crotonyl-coenzyme A carboxylase deficiency) (Tuchman, Berry, Thuy, & Nyhan, 1993) and endocrine abnormalities such as transient hypothyroidism (Jain, Isaac, Gottschalk, & Myers, 1994). Syndromes that are associated with FTT include fragile X syndrome (Goldson & Hagerman, 1993), Brachmann-de Lange syndrome (Bull, Fitzgerald, Heifetz, & Brei, 1993), and congenital renal salt-losing syndrome (Chua, Hewitt, & Hobday, 1986).

Feeding Difficulties and Inadequate Diet

Difficulties in breast-feeding that may be risk factors for inadequate growth include obstructive positioning during feeding (Morton, 1992), excessive consumption of foremilk associated with changing breasts before the infant can empty the breast (Woolridge & Fisher, 1988), and nursing caries (Acs, Lodolini, Kaminsky, & Cisneros, 1992). Dietary inadequacies may arise from exclusive breast-feeding for 12 months (Weston et al., 1987) and excess fruit juice consumption (Smith & Lifshitz, 1994).

Insufficient milk syndrome in breast-fed neonates may be a risk factor for inadequate growth. This syndrome may be a result of problems with milk production or extraction (Hill, 1992; Livingstone, 1990); other factors that may result in this syndrome include maternal postpartum hemorrhage (Willis & Livingstone, 1995) and restriction of dietary protein or energy sources (Motil, Sheng, & Montandon, 1994).

Social and Psychological Factors

Review of several reports suggests that social and psychological factors may be important for explaining inadequate growth in some instances. In a study of social factors, researchers retrospectively reviewed the charts of 16 U.S. children who were younger than 18 months with primary protein-energy malnutrition without predisposing disease or other physiological abnormalities and found that being the most recent child in a large sibship and having a teenage mother were common characteristics (Listernick, Christoffel, Pace, & Chiaramonte, 1985). These findings need to be corroborated in an etiological study that includes an appropriate comparison group and an adequate sample to assess *a priori* designated differences between those with this sort of malnutrition and those without.

Child abuse may be associated with inadequate growth. A report of a series of 260 abused children revealed that 26% experienced growth impairment (defined as less than or equal to a -2 z-score in height-for-age or weight-for-age or an improvement during follow-up with appropriate care of at least an increase of 0.5 z-score status in height-for-age or weight-for-age) (Taitz & King, 1988). Psychosocial dwarfism, which is an impairment of growth hormone production as a result of stress (Swanson, 1994), and abnormal interpersonal behavior (Powell & Low, 1983) also have been cited in case reports as explanations for FTT.

The inappropriate health beliefs of parents or their undue fear of obesity might be risk factors for inadequate growth. A report on a case series of seven children who were less than 2 years of age and who experienced FTT found that their caloric intake had been limited by parents who were having them follow diets that are advocated for adults who are at increased risk for cardiovascular disease (Pugliese, Weyman-Daum, Moses, & Lifshitz, 1987). After the children were given an age-appropriate diet, their growth became normal for their age and gender.

Although various reports have supported the notion that behavior, particularly that of parents, may affect a child's growth, research is needed to determine more precisely the causative elements. Interpretation of relevant studies has been made more difficult by a lack of comparison groups, small sample sizes, and problems in selecting appropriate measures for assessment (Boddy & Skuse, 1994; Drotar, 1990; Kotelchuck & Newberger, 1983). In addition, reports frequently do not reveal whether the behavior of interest (e.g., abuse) preceded the growth impairment—and, thus, might have caused it—or followed it, in which case it might have been a consequence. (See Chapter 10 for further discussion.)

One important study reported by Peterson and Chen (1990) sought to examine patterns of medical characteristics and the presence of social or psychosocial problems by the diagnostic category of FTT. They examined the characteristics of a case series of 1,275 children, which they stratified by organic FTT (OFTT), nonorganic FTT (NFTT), mixed (organic and nonorganic) FTT, and normal growth. They found that low birth weight and prematurity were more common in the medical histories of the groups that were labeled as having OFTT and mixed FTT. The proportion of children who were living in households with incomes less than 100% of the poverty threshold was approximately 50% or more in the NFTT, mixed, and normal groups in contrast to only 29% in the OFTT group. Two-parent households existed for 76% of the OFTT category, whereas the other strata had 52%–59% of both parents in the home. In each of the strata, fewer than 10% of the mothers were younger than 20 years. The authors concluded that there were different social patterns associated with the different categories of FTT. Clearly, the OFTT group was different from the others; however, as mentioned previously, to confirm the role of these characteristics as risk factors for inadequate growth, they need to be evaluated in etiological studies.

ETIOLOGICAL STUDIES

Although descriptive studies have provided numerous clues as to which risk factors might be important in inadequate growth, analyses that incorporate comparisons with a control group are needed to make more definitive judgments about causation. This section reviews both univariate and multivariate analyses; these latter analyses are particularly useful because they assess the relative importance of different risk factors and interactions between them in the same statistical model. Studies that are reported in this section were selected because they focused on inadequate growth in children who were diagnosed with FTT, represented either current or classic work, had more rigorous designs with more clearly defined risk factors and outcomes, and/or had a larger sample than other studies.

Univariate Analyses

In a classic work, Pollitt and Eichler (1976) found that children with FTT came from families that, compared with a control group, had lower per capita income and maternal education; as infants, they were more likely to have feeding difficulties or erratic meal patterns (see Table 2). Three other studies also are summarized in Table 2; in one, a retrospective

Table 2. Summary of studies using univariate analysis of variables to assess risk factors for FTT

Study	Definition of FTT	Design and sample size	Variables	Major findings
Pollitt and Eichler (1976)	≤3rd percentile for height-for-age and weight (specific indices weight-for-height or weight-for-age not specified) (Harvard Standards)	Case-control • Hospital outpatient pediatric clinic • Cases, 19 FTT (12–60 months), consecutively enrolled • Controls, 19 normal growth matched on age ±3 months, gender, race • Inclusion criteria: singleton, birth weight ≥2,500 gr, gestational age ≥36 weeks, no physical abnormality/birth complication, maternal height ≥154.5 cm	• Gross yearly income • Per capita income • Mother's education • Household density • Total family size • Number of siblings • Feeding difficulties • Meal patterns	FTT group had: • Lower per capita income ($1,557 vs $2,848, $t = 2.77$, $p = 0.01$) • Lower mean maternal education (11 vs 12 years, $t = 1.88$, $p = 0.05$) • Greater number with feeding difficulties (10 vs 2, $\chi^2 = 5.97$, $p < 0.02$) • Greater number who skipped or ate skimpy meals (16 vs 6, $\chi^2 = 8.74$, $p < 0.01$)
Mitchell et al. (1980)	• Weight-for-age <80% of median (Harvard Standards): a) <24 months if previous weight-for-age >80%, b) at first recording if child not premature, or • FTT noted on medical record before 24 months	Retrospective cohort • Rural primary care center clinics: 312 2- to 5-year-olds (FTT = 30)	• Prevalence • Race • Birth order • Neonatal problems • Well-child clinic visits • Immunizations • Maternal marital status and employment • Household composition	• Prevalence of FTT = 9.6% • FTT group had 1. significantly more neonatal problems (30% vs 15%, $p < 0.05$) 2. incomplete immunizations (47% vs 28%, $p < 0.01$) 3. family problems noted more often in the medical record (37% vs 11%, $p < 0.01$)

(continued)

Table 2. (continued)

Study	Definition of FTT	Design and sample size	Variables	Major findings
Herman-Staab (1992)	*All* of the following: • Weight-for-age ≤5th percentile at >6 months • Weight-for-height ≤25th percentile • Deceleration in weight-for-age between 3 and 7 months with one measurement >5th percentile (NCHS/CDC reference)	• Retrospective cohort: WIC • FTT cohort, *n* = 23 • Comparison cohort, randomly selected non-FTT, *n* = 69 • Eligibility criteria: 1983–1986 birth, on WIC from birth to 12 or 24 months, gestational age ≥36 weeks, maternal height ≥60 inches, birth weight >6.5 lbs (female) or 6.8 lbs (male), head circumference >5th percentile for age or <5th percentile if head circumference percentile approximates height-for-age percentile, no chronic disease/ congenital anomalies, normal hemoglobin	• Maternal: age, education, gravida, parity, perinatal complications, chronic illness, breast-feeding • Infant: birth weight, birth length, birth order, ethnic origin, gender • Environmental: Medicaid status, area of residence, short interconceptual periods, type of delivery, trimester prenatal care began	FTT had a higher percentage of • Children who were never breast-fed (41% vs 7%, Fisher's Exact, $p < 0.05$) • Males (78% vs 49%, $\chi^2 = 4.78$, $p < 0.03$)
Gayle et al. (1987)	Height-for-age <5th percentile (NCHS/CDC reference)	• Cross-sectional study • CDC PedNSS for 1983 • Children <2 years, *n* = 374,554	Low birth weight (<2,500 g)	• Population attributable risk of low height-for-age due to low birth weight is 20%–40% during first 2 years of life depending on age of assessment. • Mean proportion of low height-for-age attributable to low birth weight between birth and 2 years of age is 28.9% in whites, 27.6% in blacks, and 21.3% in Hispanics.

t = students' *t*-test (*t*-test assesses differences between means); *p* = probability.

analysis of a cohort of children attending a rural primary care clinic, researchers found that children with FTT had more neonatal problems, incomplete immunizations, and notations of family problems in the medical record than did controls (Mitchell, Gorrell, & Greenberg, 1980). In a retrospective analysis of records of the Special Supplemental Nutrition Program for Women, Infants and Children (WIC), those with FTT were more likely to be male and to have been breast-fed (Herman-Staab, 1992). The author recommended further research to substantiate and explain these findings. Finally, as noted previously in the discussion of medical characteristics, 20%–40% of the cases of low height-for-age in a group of low-income children were attributed to low birth weight, depending on the age and racial/ethnic group (Gayle et al., 1987). The extremely large sample size in this study enhances its utility; conversely, failure to stratify or control for prematurity and gestational age status is a concern. As noted, lower percentages probably would have been found if data had been corrected for gestational age. It also may have been found that the children with low birth weight may not have been exhibiting inadequate growth but simply may have been small in size.

Multivariate Analyses

In Table 3, summaries are presented of three studies that used multivariate analyses to assess the relative importance of risk factors for inadequate growth. In a case-control study that continued the Pollitt and Eichler study (Kotelchuck & Newberger, 1983), researchers documented that case families (those in which the child had FTT) had more health problems, less social support especially in regard to a less-friendly neighborhood, and a greater difference between the education levels of the parents than control families. In a well-designed retrospective study of a cohort of 438 mothers (Stier, Leventhal, Berg, Johnson, & Mezger, 1993), the researchers found that the children of younger mothers (18 years or younger at the time of the child's birth) were not significantly more likely to experience inadequate growth than were the children of mothers who were older than 18. In another clinic-based study, which involved eight university hospitals, researchers confined their analysis to infants with low birth weight ($N = 914$) who were delivered at 37 or fewer weeks of gestational age, a group that may face higher risk of inadequate growth if they have medical complications (Kelleher et al., 1993). Methodological strengths of this study included defining FTT clearly; limiting subject attrition; and collecting data on biological, psychological, and environmental risk factors. Another strength of this study was limiting study subjects to premature infants with low birth weight, thus limiting the confounding effect of combining infants who had normal and who had low birth weight. Almost one fifth ($n = 180$) of the infants were classified as having FTT; six factors were found to be significant: a small-for-gestational-age infant, maternal education greater than college graduate, abnormal or suspect neurological exam, maternal height less than 62.5 inches, birth weight less than 1,500 g, and father in the home. Advanced maternal education and the presence of the father in the home as risk factors for FTT are unique to this study.

DISCUSSION AND SUMMARY

Knowledge of the epidemiology and the etiology of inadequate growth in the United States is very incomplete; however, on the basis of descriptive epidemiology, prevalence can be documented, the issue of the age group that is at highest risk can be addressed, and trends in prevalence can be shown. In terms of low height-for-age for children 2–5 years old, the prevalence was 5.2% in the NHANES III and 5.8% in the 1996 PedNSS. The prevalence of low weight-for-height in the NHANES III was 2.7%, similar to the 1.9% prevalence

Table 3. Summaries of studies using multivariate analysis to assess risk factors for FTT

Study	Definition of FTT	Design and sample size	Variables	Major findings
Kotelchuck and Newberger (1983)	≤3rd percentile for height-for-age and weight-for-age (Harvard Standards)	• Case-control • Hospital inpatients • Cases, 42 FTT (12–48 months) • Controls, 42 normal growth, matched on age ±3 months, gender, race • Inclusion criteria: singleton, birth weight ≥2,500 gr, gestational age ≥36 weeks, no physical abnormality/birth complication, maternal height ≥154.5 cm	• Demographics • Family structure • Social class characteristics • Number and cause of mother–child separation • Child-centered problems • Family and neighborhood support • Maternal stress (e.g., broken home, illness) • Health index/problems	By discriminant function analysis, FTT group had • A higher health index (more health problems) ($t = -5.94$, $p = 0.001$) • Less-friendly neighborhood ($t = -3.75$, $p = 0.001$) • Greater discrepancy between parents' education ($t = -2.24$, $p = 0.03$) • R^2 for 3-variable model is 43.6%
Stier et al. (1993)	• Weight-for-age percentiles decrease across two major percentile curves (95th, 90th, 75th, 50th, 25th, 10th, 5th) • Weight-for-age <5th percentile and if weight-for-age or weight-for-height <90% median (NCHS/CDC reference)	• Retrospective cohort • Hospital • Study group mothers ≤18 years at child's birth ($n = 219$) • Control mothers >18 years at child's birth ($n = 219$) • Inclusion criteria: singleton birth at hospital October 1979–December 1981, at least two visits to this primary care center before 6 months and one after 10 months of age	• Maternal age • Poor growth • Maltreatment • Change in primary caregiver	• Young maternal age was not associated significantly with an outcome of poor growth (Risk Ratio [RR] = 1.67, 95% CI = 0.75–3.73)

| Kelleher et al. (1993) | All following criteria:
• Coded as FTT in developmental assessment
• Weight-for-age <5th percentile at more than two points in time when corrected for gestational age (NCHS/CDC reference)
• Rate of weight gain in preceding months less than average for gender and corrected for gestational age (incremental growth curves [Roche & Himes, 1980]) | • Nine-month prospective cohort
• Eight large university hospitals in the United States participating in the Infant Health and Development Program
• Cohort of 914 low birth weight (FTT = 180)
• Inclusion criteria: birth weight ≤2,500 g, ≤37 weeks gestational age, singleton or twin birth, lived >48 hours, hospitalized ≤60 days after 40 weeks' gestational age attained, oxygen support ≤90 days
• Exclusions: severe neurologic abnormality or sensory impairment, chromosome-multiple anomaly syndrome, maternal drug or alcohol abuse, maternal inability to communicate in English | • Child: gender, low birth weight for gestational age, weight, height, head circumference, body mass index, neonatal health index, development, behavior
• Parents: maternal age, ethnicity, education, marital status, height, use of prenatal care
• Environment: presence of other siblings, father in the home, family stress score, household density, social support, and family income | By logistic regression analysis, the following factors were significant for FTT:
• Small for gestational age (RR = 2.62, 95% CI = 1.72–3.98)
• Abnormal/suspect neurologic exam (RR = 1.82, 95% CI = 1.21–2.75)
• <1,500 g birth weight (RR = 1.60, 95% CI = 1.01–2.55)
• Maternal education ≥college (RR = 2.12, 95% CI = 1.09–4.13)
• Maternal height <62.5 inches (RR = 1.78, 95% CI = 1.16–2.73)
• Father in home (RR = 1.60, 95% CI = 1.07–2.40) |

R = coefficient of determination; CI = confidence interval; RR = risk ratio.

found in the 1996 PedNSS. These low prevalences of low height-for-age and low weight-for-height are close to the expected prevalence of 5% based on the NCHS/CDC growth reference. A decline in prevalence since 1987, at least as documented in the PedNSS, suggests that the prevalence of inadequate growth is declining over time.

There does not appear to be a single age group that is at greatest risk for inadequate growth. In the CDC's PedNSS, the only group that had a remarkably higher prevalence of low height-for-age and low weight-for-height is the birth to 2-months-old age group; and their high prevalence is, at least in part, due to their higher prevalence of low birth weight status. Because infants with low birth weight are small in size, they will be assessed as having a low height-for-age, in particular, and possibly low weight-for-height on the basis of the NCHS/CDC growth screening criteria. Their being categorized as exhibiting inadequate growth, however, is due to their small size in most cases rather than inadequate growth; thus, evidence suggests that this age group is not at higher risk for inadequate growth. If infants with low birth weight exhibit inadequate growth, then it likely is the result of medical complications.

The prevalence of food insufficiency or insecurity that was documented in the NHANES III is 3.3%. In contrast, the prevalence for those living below poverty was higher (13.2%). This is not surprising because a lack of access to food is more likely to occur among those living in poverty; however, more research is needed to understand how the food security scale relates to inadequate growth. It also should be noted that children in poverty are at relatively greater risk for low birth weight (National Center for Children in Poverty, 1996) and poor access to an adequate diet and are more likely to experience delays in physical, cognitive, language, and emotional development (Klerman & Parker, 1990; Kotch & Shackelford, 1989; Society for Research in Child Development, 1994).

With regard to risk factors for inadequate growth, on the basis of etiological studies, potential risk factors can be classified by those for which there is convincing evidence, some evidence, and suggestive evidence. Review of the literature suggests various medical problems (e.g., chronic diseases, persistent infectious diseases, enzyme deficiencies, endocrine abnormalities, certain syndromes) as potential risk factors. Medical problems can negatively affect adequacy of dietary intake and/or intestinal absorption of food eaten, both of which can result in inadequate growth; however, more information is needed on the relative risk of various diseases in regard to their impact on inadequate growth. Only then can studies to investigate specific linkages between various diseases and the prevalence of inadequate growth be carried out.

Feeding difficulties, inappropriate meal patterns, and parents' beliefs about diet all seem reasonable to advance as possible causes of inadequate growth. Perhaps the strongest argument could be made for feeding difficulties as several case reports about abnormal growth have noted the presence of feeding problems, and a small case-control study found feeding problems to be a risk factor. The argument for this risk factor is strengthened by the plausibility of the argument that feeding difficulties cause an unsatisfactory diet that is followed by inadequate growth. Child abuse also may be related to inadequate growth. Taitz and King's (1988) finding that 26% of abused children in a large case series experienced growth impairment should inspire further study of this risk factor.

To make progress in understanding inadequate growth, well-designed studies need to be conducted with adequate sample sizes to provide appropriate statistical power to evaluate the hypothesis of interest. Variables that have been identified in descriptive epidemiological studies or etiological studies all need to be assessed. Because the prevalence of inadequate growth is low, case-control studies are the most efficient way of evaluating the significance of potential risk factors. Once a body of evidence regarding risk factors for inadequate growth becomes available, these results need to be corroborated with a large, community-based, prospective study of inadequate growth in infants and children. This study should examine all of the potential risk factors so that their relative importance can be assessed in the same model. In addition, a prospective study is needed to document the temporal sequence of the potential risk factors in relation to the development of inadequate growth.

Finally, more research is needed to identify the mechanisms by which various medical, social, and behavior problems cause inadequate growth. Only when the risk factors for inadequate growth are understood will this public health problem be preventable. The goal of public health practitioners needs to be to promote the growth and development of children to reach their maximum capacity.

REFERENCES

Acs, G., Lodolini, G., Kaminsky, S., & Cisneros, G.J. (1992). Effect of nursing caries on body weight in a pediatric population. *Pediatric Dentistry, 14,* 302–305.

Allen, L.H. (1990). Functional indicators and outcomes of undernutrition. *Journal of Nutrition, 120,* 924–932.

Anderson, S.A. (Ed.). (1990). Core indicators of nutritional state for difficult-to-sample populations. *Journal of Nutrition, 120*(Suppl. 11), 1559–1599.

Bines, J.E., & Israel, E.J. (1991). Hypoproteinemia, anemia, and failure to thrive in an infant. *Gastroenterology, 101,* 848–856.

Boddy, J.M., & Skuse, D.H. (1994). Annotation: The process of parenting in failure to thrive. *Journal of Child Psychology and Psychiatry and Allied Disciplines, 35,* 401–424.

Bull, M.J., Fitzgerald, J.F., Heifetz, S.A., & Brei, T.J. (1993). Gastrointestinal abnormalities: A significant cause of feeding difficulties and failure to thrive in Brachmann-de Lange syndrome. *American Journal of Medical Genetics, 47,* 1029–1034.

Centers for Disease Control and Prevention. (1992). Pediatric Nutrition Surveillance System—United States, 1980–1991: CDC surveillance summaries. *Morbidity and Mortality Weekly Report, 41*(SS-7), 1–24.

Centers for Disease Control and Prevention. (1997). [Pediatric Nutrition Surveillance System]. Unpublished raw data.

Chua, H.L., Hewitt, I.K., & Hobday, J.D. (1986). Congenital renal salt-losing syndrome and failure to thrive in infancy. *Australian Paediatric Journal, 22,* 145–146.

de Onis, M., Garza, C., & Habicht, J.P. (1997). Time for a new growth reference. *Pediatrics* [Online], *100*(5). Available: http://www.pediatrics.org/cgi/content/full/5/e8

Dean, A.G., Dean, J.A., Coulombier, D., Burton, A.H., Brendel, K.A., Smith, D.C., Dicker, R.C., Sullivan, K.M., & Fagan, R.F. (1997). Epi Info (Version 6.04b): A word-processing, database, and statistics program for public health on IBM-compatible microcomputers [Computer program]. Atlanta: Centers for Disease Control and Prevention, The Division of Surveillance and Epidemiology, Epidemiology Program Office, in collaboration with the Global Programme on AIDS, World Health Organization, Geneva, Switzerland.

Dibley, M.J., Goldsby, J.B., Staehling, N.W., & Trowbridge, F.L. (1987). Development of normalized curves for the international growth reference: Historical and technical considerations. *American Journal of Clinical Nutrition, 46,* 736–748.

Drotar, D. (1990). Sampling issues in research with nonorganic failure-to-thrive children. *Journal of Pediatric Psychology, 15,* 255–272.

Elias-Jones, A.C., Larcher, V.F., & Price, E.H. (1987). AIDS in an infant causing severe failure to thrive. *Journal of Infection, 15,* 69–72.

Federation of American Societies for Experimental Biology, Life Sciences Research Office. (1995a). *Third report on nutrition monitoring in the United States* (Vol. 1). Washington, DC: U.S. Government Printing Office. (Prepared for the Interagency Board for Nutrition Monitoring and Related Research.)

Federation of American Societies for Experimental Biology, Life Sciences Research Office. (1995b). *Third report on nutrition monitoring in the United States* (Vol. 2). Washington, DC: U.S. Government Printing Office. (Prepared for the Interagency Board for Nutrition Monitoring and Related Research.)

Food Research and Action Center. (1995). *Community Childhood Hunger Identification Project: A survey of childhood hunger in the United States.* Washington, DC: Author.

Frank, D.A., Silva, M., & Needlman, R. (1993). Failure to thrive: Mystery, myth, and method. *Contemporary Pediatrics, 10,* 114–133.

Gayle, H.D., Dibley, M.J., Marks, J.S., & Trowbridge, F.L. (1987). Malnutrition in the first two years of life. *American Journal of Diseases of Children, 141,* 531–534.

Goldson, E., & Hagerman, R.J. (1993). Fragile X syndrome and failure to thrive. *American Journal of Diseases of Children, 147,* 605–607.

Gorstein, J., Sullivan, K., Yip, R., deOnis, M., Trowbridge, F., Fajans, P., & Clugston, G. (1994). Issues in the assessment of nutritional status using anthropometry. *Bulletin of the World Health Organization, 72,* 273–283.

Granot, E., Matoth, I., & Feinmesser, R. (1990). Chronic middle ear effusion—A possible cause of protracted vomiting and failure to thrive in infancy. *Clinical Pediatrics, 29,* 722–724.

Guo, S., Roche, A.F., Fomon, S.J., Nelson, S.E., Chumlea, W.C., Rogers, R.R., Baumgartner, R.N., Ziegler, E.E., & Siervogel, R.M. (1991). Reference data on gains in weight and length during the first two years of life. *Journal of Pediatrics, 119,* 355–362.

Hamill, P.V.V., Drizd, T.A., Johnson, C.L., Reed, R.B., Roche, A.F., & Moore, W.M. (1979). Physical growth: National Center for Health Statistics percentiles. *American Journal of Clinical Nutrition, 32,* 607–629.

Hamilton, W.L., Cook, J.T., Thompson, W.W., Buron, L.F., Frongillo, E.A., Olson, C.M., & Wehler, C.A. (1997). *Household food security in the United States in 1995: Summary report of the food security measurement project.* Alexandria, VA: U.S. Department of Agriculture, Food and Consumer Service.

Herman-Staab, B. (1992). Antecedents of nonorganic failure-to-thrive. *Pediatric Nursing, 18,* 579–590.

Hill, P.D. (1992). Insufficient milk supply syndrome. *Clinical Issues in Perinatal and Women's Health Nursing, 3,* 605–612.

Jain, R., Isaac, R.M., Gottschalk, M.E., & Myers, T.F. (1994). Transient central hypothyroidism as a cause of failure to thrive in newborns and infants. *Journal of Endocrinological Investigation, 17,* 631–634.

Janner, D. (1990). Failure to thrive and anasarca in a young infant. *Pediatric Infectious Disease Journal, 9,* 519, 531–532.

Kelleher, K.J., Casey, P.H., Bradley, R.H., Pope, S.K., Whiteside, L., Barrett, K.W., Swanson, M.E., & Kirby, R.S. (1993). Risk factors and outcomes for failure to thrive in low birth weight preterm infants. *Pediatrics, 91,* 941–948.

Klerman, L.V., & Parker, M.B. (1990). *Alive and well? A review of health policies and programs for poor young children.* New York: Columbia University, School of Public Health, National Center for Children in Poverty.

Kotch, J., & Shackelford, J. (1989). *The nutritional status of low-income preschool children in the United States: A review of the literature.* Washington, DC: Food Research and Action Center.

Kotelchuck, M., & Newberger, E.H. (1983). Failure to thrive: A controlled study of familial characteristics. *Journal of the American Academy of Child Psychiatry, 22,* 322–328.

Lax, D., Butto, F., Leonard, S.A., Ring, W.S., & Dunnigan, A. (1989). Occult pulmonary artery associated with failure to thrive and recurrent pneumonia—A case report. *Angiology, 40,* 849–853.

Listernick, R., Christoffel, K., Pace, J., & Chiaramonte, J. (1985). Severe primary malnutrition in U.S. children. *American Journal of Diseases of Children, 139,* 1157–1160.

Livingstone, V.H. (1990). Problem-solving formula for failure to thrive in breast-fed infants. *Canadian Family Physician, 36,* 1541–1545.

Marcus, C.L., Carroll, J.L., Koerner, C.B., Horner, A., Lutz, J., & Louphlin, G.M. (1994). Determinants of growth in children with the obstructive sleep apnea syndrome. *Journal of Pediatrics, 125,* 556–562.

Mcdowell, A., Engel, A., Massey, J., & Maurer, K. (1981). *Plan and operation of the second National Health and Nutrition Examination Survey, United States, 1976–1980* (Series 1, 15, No. 15). Hyattsville, MD: National Center for Health Statistics.

Mitchell, W.G., Gorrell, R.W., & Greenberg, R.A. (1980). Failure-to-thrive: A study in a primary care setting—Epidemiology and follow-up. *Pediatrics, 65,* 971–977.

Morris, C.S., Lough, L.R., & Weinberger, E. (1990). Infant with lethargy, failure to thrive, and abnormal blood smear. *Investigative Radiology, 25,* 1054–1057.

Morton, J.A. (1992). Ineffective suckling: A possible consequence of obstructive positioning. *Journal of Human Lactation, 8,* 83–85.

Motil, K.J., Sheng, H.-P., & Montandon, C.M. (1994). Case report: Failure to thrive in a breast-fed infant is associated with maternal dietary protein and energy restriction. *Journal of the American College of Nutrition, 13,* 203–208.

National Center for Children in Poverty. (1996). *One in four: America's youngest poor.* New York: Columbia University, School of Public Health.

National Center for Health Statistics. (1977). *NCHS growth curves for children birth–18 years, United States: Vital and health statistics* (Series 11, No. 165). Washington, DC: U.S. Government Printing Office. (DHEW Publication No. PHS 78-1650)

National Center for Health Statistics, Centers for Disease Control. (1973). *Plan and operation of the National Health and Nutrition Examination Survey, United States, 1971–1973* (Series 1, 11, No. 10). Hyattsville, MD: National Center for Health Statistics.

National Center for Health Statistics, Centers for Disease Control and Prevention. (1994). *Plan and operation of the third National Health and Nutrition Examination Survey, United States, 1988–1994.* Hyattsville, MD: National Center for Health Statistics.

Peterson, K.E., & Chen, L.C. (1990). Defining undernutrition for public health purposes in the United States. *Journal of Nutrition, 120,* 933–942.

Pollitt, E., & Eichler, A. (1976). Behavioral disturbances among failure-to-thrive children. *American Journal of Diseases of Children, 130,* 24–29.

Poskitt, E.M.E. (1993). Failure to thrive in congenital heart disease. *Archives of Disease in Childhood, 68,* 158–160.

Powell, G.F., & Low, J. (1983). Behavior in nonorganic failure to thrive. *Journal of Developmental and Behavioral Pediatrics, 4,* 26–33.

Pugliese, M.T., Weyman-Daum, M., Moses, N., & Lifshitz, F. (1987). Parental health beliefs as a cause of nonorganic failure to thrive. *Pediatrics, 80,* 175–182.

Rapisarda, R., Muntoni, F., Gobbi, P., & Dubowitz, V. (1995). Duchenne muscular dystrophy presenting with failure to thrive. *Archives of Disease in Childhood, 72,* 437–438.

Roche, A.F. (1994, February). *Executive summary of the growth chart workshop sponsored by: National Center for Health Statistics, Division of Health Examination Statistics, December 1992.* Hyattsville, MD: National Center for Health Statistics.

Roche, A.F., & Himes, J.H. (1980). Incremental growth charts. *American Journal of Clinical Nutrition, 91,* 2041–2052.

Smith, M.M., & Lifshitz, F. (1994). Excess fruit juice consumption as a contributing factor in nonorganic failure to thrive. *Pediatrics, 93,* 438–443.

Society for Research in Child Development; Society for Research on Adolescence; International Society for Infant Studies; & American Psychological Association, Division 7. (1994). *Research briefs: Adolescent nonmarital childbearing and welfare; Childcare; Child nutrition; Consequences of poverty for children and families; Violence prevention.* Chicago: Society for Research in Child Development.

Stier, D.M., Leventhal, J.M., Berg, A.T., Johnson, L., & Mezger, J. (1993). Are children born to young mothers at risk for maltreatment? *Pediatrics, 91,* 642–648.

Sullivan, K.M., & Gorstein, J. (1990). Anthro (Version 1.01): Software for calculating pediatric anthropometry [Computer program]. Atlanta: Centers for Disease Control and Prevention, Division of Surveillance and Epidemiology, Epidemiology Program Office, in collaboration with the Global Programme on AIDS, World Health Organization, Geneva, Switzerland.

Swanson, H. (1994). Case 3 presentation. *Pediatrics in Review, 15,* 39–40.

Taitz, L.S., & King, J.M. (1988). Growth patterns in child abuse. *Acta Paediatrica Scandinavica, 343*(Suppl.), 62–72.

Tuchman, M., Berry, S.A., Thuy, L.P., & Nyhan, W.L. (1993). Partial methyl crotonyl-coenzyme A carboxylase deficiency in an infant with failure to thrive, gastrointestinal dysfunction and hypertonia. *Pediatrics, 91,* 664–666.

Waterlow, J.C., Buzina, R., Keller, W., Lane, J.M., Nichaman, M.Z., & Tanner, J.M. (1977). The presentation and use of height and weight data for comparing the nutritional status of groups of children under the age of 10 years. *Bulletin of the World Health Organization, 55,* 489–498.

Weston, J.A., Stage, A.F., Hathaway, P., Andrews, D.L., Stonington, J.A., & McCabe, E.B. (1987). Prolonged breast-feeding and nonorganic failure to thrive. *American Journal of Diseases of Children, 141,* 242–243.

Wilcox, W.D., Nieburg, P., & Miller, D.S. (1989). Failure to thrive: A continuing problem of definition. *Clinical Pediatrics, 28,* 391–394.

Willis, C.E., & Livingstone, V. (1995). Infant insufficient milk syndrome associated with maternal postpartum hemorrhage. *Journal of Human Lactation, 11,* 123–126.

Woolridge, M.W., & Fisher, C. (1988). Colic, "overfeeding," and symptoms of lactose malabsorption in the breast-fed baby: A possible artifact of feed management? *The Lancet, 2,* 382–384.

World Health Organization Expert Committee on Physical Status. (1995). *Physical status: The use and interpretation of anthropometry* (World Health Organization Technical Report Series, 854). Geneva, Switzerland: World Health Organization.

World Health Organization Working Group. (1986). Use and interpretation of anthropometric indicators of nutritional status. *Bulletin of the World Health Organization, 64,* 929–941.

Yip, R., & Mei, Z. (1996). Variation of infant and childhood growth: Observations from the U.S. nutrition surveillance systems. In F. Battaglia, C. Pedraz, G. Sawatzki, F. Falkner, E. Doménech, J. Morán, C. Garza, J. Monleón, B. Salle, M. Moya, J. Rey, R. Jiménez, B. Lönnerdal, & A. Martínez-Valverde (Eds.), *Maternal and extrauterine nutritional factors: Their influence on fetal and infant growth* (pp. 77–84). Madrid, Spain: Ediciones Ergon, S.A.

Yip, R., Scanlon, K., & Trowbridge, F. (1992). Improving growth status of Asian refugee children in the United States. *Journal of the American Medical Association, 267,* 937–940.

SUGGESTED READINGS ON EPIDEMIOLOGICAL METHODS

Hulley, S.B., & Cummings, S.R. (1988). *Designing clinical research: An epidemiologic approach.* Baltimore: Williams & Wilkins.

Sackett, D.L., Haynes, R.B., & Tugwell, P. (1991). *Clinical epidemiology: A basic science for clinical medicine* (2nd ed.). Boston: Little, Brown.

Sherry, B. (1992). Descriptive epidemiologic research. In E.R. Monsen (Ed.), *Research: Successful approaches* (pp. 100–110). Chicago: The American Dietetic Association.

Sherry, B. (1992). Epidemiologic analytic research. In E.R. Monsen (Ed.), *Research: Successful approaches* (pp. 133–150). Chicago: The American Dietetic Association.

Chapter 3

Effects of Undernutrition on Growth and Development

Elizabeth Metallinos-Katsaras
and Kathleen S. Gorman

This chapter reviews and interprets the current research regarding the effects of undernutrition on physical growth and development and assesses the implications of this research for the treatment of pediatric undernutrition, also known as *failure to thrive* (FTT). The chapter begins with a definition of terms and a discussion of the importance of growth and development. Evidence that undernutrition can account for physical growth delay and behavioral alterations in undernourished populations is presented. In addition, proposed mechanisms of these effects are discussed. Although most of the research in this area has been conducted in low-income countries in which undernutrition is endemic, the implications of results found in such populations for children presenting with undernutrition in industrialized countries are addressed.

This chapter uses the term *malnutrition* intentionally to refer to the study of nutritional deficiencies in low-income countries. In contrast, *failure to thrive* is conceptualized primarily as pediatric undernutrition diagnosed in industrialized countries. Although some may argue against these definitions, the authors believe that they accurately reflect the state of the research on these populations. In particular, the data that are reviewed on malnutrition come primarily from population-based studies in low-income countries, whereas the data on pediatric undernutrition come most often from clinical populations among generally well-nourished populations. These distinctions provide a framework for a discussion of the similarities and differences between these two groups.

DEFINITION OF *UNDERNUTRITION*

In general terms, *undernutrition* refers to an inadequate supply of nutrients in relation to the biological needs for optimal function of an organism. Inadequate nutrient supply at the cellular level can stem from dietary inadequacies, inadequate absorption (including intestinal losses), and/or increased metabolic requirements. These can occur in isolation or in combination with one another to affect the presence and degree of undernutrition. Optimal function can be viewed as optimum growth, development, and maintenance of organ systems. The presence of undernutrition is inferred in the presence of delays in growth or organ maintenance. Although dietary nutrient intake has been used to represent supply of nutrients, this does not directly measure cellular supply. In the study of undernutrition, various indicators are frequently used. For example, in studying the effects of **protein-energy malnutrition** (PEM) on physical growth, indices of intake are frequently used (e.g., dietary intakes and/or supplementation intakes). In the case of **micronutrient** deficiencies, however, biochemical indicators of nutrient levels are most commonly used. Furthermore, it is important to note that, in many studies, physical growth indicators are commonly used as indicators of undernutrition. In this case, the growth delay is used as an indicator rather than a consequence of undernutrition.

EFFECTS OF UNDERNUTRITION ON PHYSICAL GROWTH

This section reviews the literature on the impact of undernutrition on physical growth. The effects of PEM and micronutrient deficiencies are reviewed separately. Although the results of some correlational studies are presented, the focus is on intervention studies, whenever available, because these studies provide the most direct evidence for a causal relationship between malnutrition and growth.

Significance of Poor Growth

It is widely accepted that in well-nourished populations, variations in growth are due to genetic rather than environmental factors (United Nations Administrative Committee on Coordination/Subcommittee on Nutrition [ACC/SCN], 1990); however, in lower-income countries where malnutrition is endemic, differences in growth velocity and size, particularly in those younger than 5 years, are primarily the result of dietary insufficiencies and infectious disease (R.E. Black, 1991; United Nations ACC/SCN, 1990).

Attained size and lean muscle mass have direct implications for reproductive capacity in women. For example, in low-income countries, maternal size has been found to be related to birth weight: Taller women have heavier babies, a lower rate of low birth weight, and lower infant mortality (James, 1994; Martorell, Delgado, Valverde, & Klein, 1981). There also is evidence that size is associated with work capacity and economic productivity (Haas et al., 1995; Kennedy & Garcia, 1994).

More important than the direct effects of stature, however, are potential adverse effects that are associated with the process of becoming small (United Nations ACC/SCN, 1990). Physical growth delay is a surrogate for other physiological processes (Hambidge, 1997) that also have been affected by undernutrition but that are not as easily measured as growth (e.g., host defense mechanisms, organ development, hormonal function, brain development). Thus, physical growth is used as a proxy for effects of undernutrition on these other physiological processes; therefore, when examining effects of specific nutrients or dietary quality on physical growth, one is assessing risk of effects on physiological processes that are more difficult to detect.

A Conceptual Framework

Figure 1 provides a framework that depicts the factors that affect the development of undernutrition and the pathway(s) through which undernutrition can affect physical growth and other biological processes. It is intended to provide a guide for the interpretation of the research in this area and to depict the complex nature of these relationships.

As depicted, dietary intake, morbidity, appetite, and physical activity all can affect the development of undernutrition. In turn, undernutrition can affect physical growth either directly or through its influence on biological processes such as immune function, hormonal function, and organ development.

These relationships are not unilateral, however. Dietary intake is affected by morbidity, appetite, and physical activity (Black, Brown, & Becker, 1984; Martorell et al., 1975). In addition, effects on biological processes presumably can be reflected in overt effects of undernutrition on morbidity, appetite, and activity. This is supported by studies that show a causal relationship between deficiencies in iron or zinc and immune function and morbidity (Castillo-Duran, Heresi, Fisberg, & Uauy, 1987; Chwang, Soemantri, & Pollitt, 1988; Ninh et al., 1996; Rosado, Lopez, Munoz, Martinez, & Allen, 1997; Schlesinger et al., 1992). There also is some limited support for effects of iron or zinc supplementation on the energy intake or appetite of children with such deficiencies (Lawless, Latham, Stephenson, Kinoti, & Pertet, 1994; Nakamura, Nishiyama, Futagoishi-Suginohara, Matsuda, & Higashi, 1993).

Figure 1 also illustrates that the effects of the infection–malnutrition cycle often are intertwined with the effects of dietary inadequacies (R.E. Black, 1991). Consequently, it is virtually impossible to examine them in isolation. The strength of the association between the various factors that affect growth will likely depend on the age of the child, the phase of **linear growth** of the child (Karlberg, Jahil, Lam, Low, & Yeung, 1994), and the environmental conditions under which the child lives. For example, there is evidence that raising animals under unsanitary conditions results in a diversion of nutrients from growth to the immune response; in animals, this has been called *immunologic stress*. It has been hypothesized that this may also occur in children who live under very unsanitary conditions (Solomons, Mazariegos, Brown, & Klasing, 1993) such that, independent of whether a child is overtly ill, continuous exposure to an unhygienic environment may stimulate an immune response, which affects growth negatively (Solomons et al., 1993).

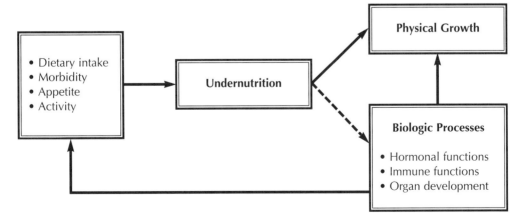

Figure 1.   Conceptual framework: Antecedents and biologic consequences of undernutrition.

Physical Growth Indicators

Comprehensive reviews of anthropometric assessment of growth and nutritional status have been written (Gibson 1990; United Nations ACC/SCN, 1990) and are summarized only briefly here. Indicators of physical growth include static standard deviation scores (also known as z-scores) or percentiles for height-for-age, weight-for-age, and weight-for-height, using the National Center of Health Statistics age- and gender-specific reference data (Hamill et al., 1979). Another indicator of physical growth status has been weight or height velocity. One diagnostic characteristic of poor growth velocity is when a child's growth crosses two major percentiles in the downward direction (Frank & Zeisel, 1988). Although growth implies a change in weight or height over time, the most commonly used indicators and cutoffs[1] of undernutrition in the literature utilize static measurements (e.g., height-for-age). As a result, the diagnosis of the timing and duration of the growth faltering is often impossible to ascertain. Anthropometric indicators of body composition are also used and include triceps (TSF) and subscapular (SSF) skinfold thicknesses (as indicators of fat stores), mid–upper-arm circumference (MUAC), and mid-arm muscle area (indicator of muscle) (Gibson, 1990).

Protein-Energy Malnutrition

PEM is the most prevalent form of malnutrition. It is estimated that PEM affects up to 40% of children younger than 5 years and living in low-income countries (Ricci & Becker, 1996). Correlational data have established a relationship between such deficiencies in energy and/or protein and physical growth delays (Allen, 1994; Neumann & Harrison, 1994). Supplementation studies have demonstrated quite clearly that improvements in energy intake in populations that are likely to have inadequate dietary calories available improved linear growth (Allen, 1994; Gopalan, Swaminathan, Kumari, Rao, & Vijayaraghavan, 1973; Kusin, Kardjati, Houtkooper, & Renquist, 1992; Martorell, 1995; Perez-Escamilla & Pollitt, 1995; Super, Herrera, & Mora, 1990; Walker, Powell, Grantham-McGregor, Himes, & Chang, 1991), including bone mineralization and skeletal maturation (Caulfield, Himes, & Rivera, 1995; Pickett, Haas, Murdoch, Rivera, & Martorell, 1995).

Early studies demonstrated that physical growth is affected by dietary protein or energy. Supplementation of protein-rich foods was shown to significantly improve linear growth or weight gain of stunted children (Beaton & Ghassemi, 1982; Lampl, Johnston, & Malcolm, 1978). Research in which the energy content of infant formula was manipulated in infants between 8 and 41 days of age and between 112 and 167 days of age showed that, although infants compensated to some extent by consuming a higher volume of formula, the lower energy intake (Fomon, Filer, Thomas, Anderson, & Nelson, 1975; Fomon, Filer, Ziegler, Bergmann, & Bergmann, 1977) resulted in significantly lower weight gain ($p < .01$) in comparison with those infants on a higher-energy formula, although length gain was not affected.

Supplementation studies generally have shown that supplementation with protein and energy positively affects attained size. Two examples that are illustrative are derived from

---

[1]In terms of cutoffs used to identify infants and children who are at risk for undernutrition, the Centers for Disease Control and Prevention use the cutoff of less than the fifth percentile (standard deviation score less than -1.65) (Yip et al., 1992). The World Health Organization describes the prevalence of wasting (low weight-for-height), stunting (low height-for-age), and underweight (low weight-for-age) by using two different cutoffs: 1) standard deviation scores that are less than -2 (the 2.3rd percentile) and 2) standard deviation scores that are less than -3.0 (0.1 percentile) (de Onis, Monteiro, Akre, & Clugston, 1993). In general, moderate to severe undernutrition is inferred when the standard deviation score is less than -3.

research in Guatemala and Colombia. These studies demonstrated that energy supplementation during gestation and during the first 3 years of life can result in significantly higher linear growth and greater height-for-age at 3 years (Martorell, 1995; Super et al., 1990). In Colombia, children who were supplemented with dry skim milk, enriched bread, and vegetable oil providing an average of 623 kilocalories (kcals) per day per child were significantly taller than those who received medical care alone (Super et al., 1990). At 6 years of age, improvements in height persisted. Supplementation included additional micronutrients, so some of the effects observed also may have been a result of the micronutrients supplemented.

The second study, carried out in Guatemala, was one of the largest and most comprehensive studies of the effects of supplementary feeding on early growth and development (Martorell, 1995). In this study, a high-protein, high-calorie gruel (Atole) or a low-calorie, no-protein drink (Fresco) was made available to all inhabitants of randomly assigned villages. Subsequent growth was examined in early life (ages birth–7) and at a follow-up, carried out when the supplemented infants and children were adolescents or adults (ages 11–26). At 3 years of age, children who were supplemented with Atole were taller than those given Fresco. In addition, the effects of the supplement on physical growth continued into adolescence and adulthood; adolescents and adults who had been supplemented with Atole prenatally and during the first 2 years of life were significantly taller, weighed more, and had greater fat-free mass than those who received Fresco (Martorell, 1995). Not only were these parameters affected, but also children who consumed more cumulative energy from either supplement had more bone mineral content, bone width, and bone mineral density during adolescence than those who consumed less energy (Caulfield et al., 1995).

In summary, supplementation studies provide the strongest evidence that energy and/or protein deficiency can affect physical growth. Supplementation of populations that are likely to be deficient in these macronutrients improves linear growth. Some of these studies also provided support for long-term benefits of supplementation on growth, which are reflected in adolescence and adulthood.

Micronutrients

It has been noted that despite adequate intakes of protein and energy, growth faltering continues to occur in certain populations (Allen, 1994; Beaton, Calloway, & Murphy, 1992). One explanation for this finding is that diets may be deficient in either one or a number of micronutrients. Many clinical trials have examined the effects of supplementation with a single micronutrient on physical growth. Implicit in such research is that it is that specific nutrient that is growth limiting. From a scientific perspective, single-nutrient supplementation studies allow for the effects to be attributed to a specific nutritional cause; however, micronutrient deficiencies commonly coexist so that single nutrient supplementation studies may not remedy all of the nutritional causes of growth faltering.

An alternative approach to single-nutrient studies has been to study overall dietary adequacy, including dietary quality (Allen, 1994; Allen et al., 1991; Neumann & Harrison, 1994). Whereas dietary quality studies do not allow for pinpointing specific nutrients, they have the benefit of being more ecologically sound because they examine the diets that are commonly consumed in specific populations. There have been attempts to examine how overall dietary quality affects physical growth. Findings suggest that the overall adequacy of the diet in energy and in macro- and micronutrients as represented by particular food patterns is predictive of physical growth (Allen, 1994; Neumann & Harrison, 1994).

The research on specific micronutrients focuses mostly on zinc and iron and less on copper and vitamin A. This emphasis reflects knowledge about the specific role that these micronutrients play in growth and the evidence that they frequently are limiting in the diets of malnourished populations.

Iron Deficiency Anemia

Iron deficiency anemia (IDA) continues to be a public health problem for between 500 million and 600 million people in the world (Hunt, Zito, Erjavec, & Johnson, 1994). It is one of the few nutritional deficiencies that is not only prevalent in the undernourished populations of low-income countries but also is common in generally well-nourished populations. Unlike many other micronutrients, the presence and degree of IDA can be assessed with relative certainty because of the multiple biochemical measures of iron status that are available. These include **hemoglobin, hematocrit, transferrin saturation, ferritin, free erythrocyte protoporphyrin,** and the newly utilized transferrin receptor (Cook, Baynes, & Skikne, 1994). In the clinical setting, hemoglobin and hematocrit continue to be the most widely utilized screening tools for IDA. The National Academy of Sciences, Institute of Medicine, Food and Nutrition Board (1993) has recommended that all children with anemia be reevaluated after 4 weeks of iron treatment. If there is a response to treatment of an increase in hemoglobin level greater than 1 gram per deciliter or greater than or equal to a rise of 3 units in hematocrit or a value within the normal range, then iron should be continued for 2 more months. If no hemoglobin or hematocrit response to treatment is observed, then this can be due to one of two reasons: 1) there has been poor compliance, or 2) iron deficiency is not the cause of the anemia. Testing of serum ferritin may shed light on whether iron deficiency is the cause of the anemia; a serum ferritin concentration of greater than 15 µg/liter suggests that the anemia is not caused by iron deficiency (National Academy of Sciences, Institute of Medicine, Food and Nutrition Board, 1993). (See Chapter 17.)

Clinical trials of iron supplementation in iron deficient anemic (IDAn) infants and children have shown positive effects of iron on either weight gain (Aukett, Parks, Scott, & Wharton, 1986; Judisch, Naiman, & Oski, 1966; Latham, Stephenson, Kinoti, Zaman, & Kurz, 1990) or linear growth (Angeles, Schutnick, Matulessi, Gross, & Sastroamidjojo, 1993) or both (Chwang et al., 1988; Lawless et al., 1994).

In infants, toddlers, and preschoolers, randomized clinical trials of iron supplementation have consistently shown that 2–3 months of iron supplementation of those who were IDAn resulted in a significantly greater improvement in growth (weight gain or linear growth) than those who were given a placebo (Angeles et al., 1993; Aukett et al., 1986). In one of these studies, positive effects of iron on weight gain but not on linear growth were found (Aukett et al., 1986). In another study, effects on height-for-age but not on weight gain were noted (Angeles et al., 1993). Furthermore, none of the aforementioned studies supported any effect of iron in those who were not IDAn. In addition, there is evidence from one study that supplementation of infants who were iron replete (i.e., all indicators of iron status, including iron stores, were normal) may have had an adverse effect on weight gain in this group (Idjradinata, Watkins, & Pollitt, 1994); however, these findings have not been replicated.

In school-age children, double-blind, randomized, placebo-controlled clinical trials also have shown that 3–4 months of iron supplementation positively affected weight, body composition, and/or height of IDAn children (Chwang et al., 1988; Latham et al., 1990; Lawless et al., 1994). In Indonesian school children, iron supplementation positively affected weight and height z-scores and MUAC in IDAn children (but not in "normal" children). Latham et al. (1990) showed that iron supplementation of Kenyan children resulted in significantly greater weight gain and triceps and subscapular skinfolds in those given iron than placebo. No effect on linear growth was observed. Lawless et al. (1994) also reported similar effects of an iron supplement on weight-for-age and weight-for-height z-scores. In this study, iron appeared to prevent some of the decline in height-for-age z-scores with age that was observed in children who were given a placebo.

Zinc Deficiency

Research on effects of zinc deficiency in humans has been limited by the lack of a good indicator of zinc status, although both plasma zinc and hair zinc have been utilized (Gibson, 1990). Correlational studies established an association between poor zinc status and anthropometry (Cavan et al., 1993; Chakar et al., 1993; Ferguson et al., 1993; Fons et al., 1992; Golden & Golden, 1981; Neumann & Harrison, 1994; Scholl, Hediger, Schall, Fischer, & Khoo, 1993). Several double-blind, randomized, clinical trials on infants and children younger than 5 years, with evidence of either compromised zinc status or moderate malnutrition (diagnosis of PEM, **marasmus,** undernutrition), demonstrated that zinc supplementation improved weight gain (Castillo-Duran et al., 1987; Walravens, Hambidge, & Koepfer, 1989) or linear growth (Schlesinger et al., 1992) or both weight gain and linear growth (Dirren et al., 1994; Ninh et al., 1996). The duration of zinc supplementation for each of these studies varied between 2 and 6 months.

Other studies have not shown effects of zinc supplementation on growth (Bates et al., 1993; Rosado et al., 1997), but children in these studies did not have evidence of zinc deficiency and/or were only mildly undernourished. In one 12-month clinical trial of zinc supplementation in 18- to 36-month-old Mexican children who were mildly malnourished, there was no effect of zinc on weight, stature, or other anthropometric indices (Rosado et al., 1997). Similarly, a 15-month zinc intervention trial in children with high plasma and hair zinc levels (i.e., good zinc status) showed no effects of zinc on height or weight, although a significant effect on mid-upper arm circumference was noted (Bates et al., 1993).

Research with older children (older than 5 years) has shown mixed results depending somewhat on the children's baseline zinc status. Among children with no evidence of poor zinc status, double-blind clinical trials of zinc supplementation either did not affect any of the growth indicators (Gibson et al., 1989) or affected triceps skinfold thicknesses (an indicator of body fat) but not weight or height (Cavan et al., 1993). In contrast, interventions in children who had evidence of poor zinc status (i.e., low dietary intake or low hair zinc) resulted in better linear growth in those given zinc than placebo (Castillo-Duran et al., 1994; Gibson et al., 1989; Walravens, Chakar, Mokni, Denise, & Lemonnier, 1992). Weight gain was not affected by zinc in these studies. In some studies, the beneficial effect of zinc on linear growth was evident among boys but not girls (Castillo-Duran et al., 1994; Walravens et al., 1992).

Other Micronutrients

Vitamin A and copper have also been studied in conjunction with physical growth; however, the number of intervention studies is limited (Castillo-Duran, Fisberg, Valenzuela, Egana, & Uauy, 1983; Castillo-Duran & Uauy, 1988; Muhilal, Permeisih, Idjradinata, Muherdiyantiningsih, & Karyadi, 1988; Rahmathullah, Underwood, Thulasiraj, & Milton, 1991; West et al., 1988).

Copper intervention trials that were conducted on infants during rehabilitation from marasmus have produced varied results with respect to physical growth. One intervention on infants who had marasmus showed no effects (Castillo-Duran et al., 1983) of copper supplementation on physical growth (neither weight gain nor linear growth). Another, also on infants who had marasmus, indicated that copper supplementation of infants who had evidence of copper deficiency was associated with a significant increase in weight gain, whereas copper supplementation in those who had no evidence of copper deficiency (i.e., the control group) resulted in no significant increase in weight gain (Castillo-Duran & Uauy, 1988). Unfortunately, there were differences in baseline weight-for-age between these two groups, which may account for the differences in weight gain observed.

Clinical trials of vitamin A supplementation have not consistently shown effects of vitamin A supplementation on physical growth. Although some have shown that vitamin A (through either fortification or supplementation) is associated with improvements in linear growth (Muhilal et al., 1988) or weight gain (West et al., 1988), the effects were not consistent across ages (1–5 years) or genders (effects limited to males only). One large-scale, double-blind, placebo-controlled intervention trial conducted in India among infants and children younger than 5 years did not demonstrate any effect of weekly doses of vitamin A on linear growth or weight gain after 1 year of the intervention, although effects on mortality were observed (Rahmathullah et al., 1991).

Interpretation of Effects

The research on PEM suggests that supplementation of populations at risk for PEM improves linear growth (i.e., height) and body composition. Not only can growth be positively affected in early life, but also improvements in attained stature can be sustained in adolescence and adulthood.

The micronutrient research reviewed also suggests that when infants or children have evidence of iron or zinc deficiency, supplementation is likely to improve physical growth. Whether effects of zinc or iron supplementation are seen in linear growth (i.e., height) or weight gain seems to depend on the children's baseline status. Supplementation generally improved height of children who were moderately to severely stunted (i.e., height-for-age z-score less than 1.5–2 below the median) but not of those who were only mildly stunted; however, there is no evidence that there is an effect of supplementing children with either of these nutrients when there are no signs of deficiency (i.e., status is good) and the infants or children are only mildly malnourished. The evidence also suggests that iron or zinc interventions are more likely to improve physical growth in younger malnourished children than in older (school age) malnourished children, although part of this effect may be because younger children were more likely to be more severely malnourished than the school-age children in the studies that were reviewed.

Although limited research on copper and vitamin A supplementation suggests that supplementation may improve physical growth of malnourished infants or children, ongoing research is needed to better determine effects of these and other micronutrients.

Summary

In summary, the research supports the contention that malnutrition affects physical growth. In particular, there is evidence that PEM, zinc deficiency, and iron deficiency affect physical growth. Although some studies demonstrate an impact of supplementation of these nutrients, the strength of the effect and the parameter (height or weight) affected varies. Some considerations in explaining lack of effects or differential effects are 1) ability to identify those who have deficiencies, 2) detection of significant growth differences in a short period of time (i.e., when either duration of supplementation or follow-up is short),

3) the degree and chronicity of undernutrition, 4) coexistence of other nutritional deficiencies, and 5) age of the individuals under study.

EFFECTS OF UNDERNUTRITION ON BEHAVIORAL DEVELOPMENT

One of the goals of this chapter is to examine the evidence for the causal effects of malnutrition on behavioral outcomes in children. *Behavior* as discussed in this chapter refers to a variety of outcomes that have been studied in association with malnutrition, including motor development, cognition, achievement, and activity.

Context of Malnutrition

Any discussion of the effects of malnutrition on cognitive development must be framed within the broader context. The difficulties of examining nutritional effects on behavior are constrained by the ability to isolate specific nutritional deficiencies (Golden, 1991). For example, children rarely experience a single nutritional deficiency; poor diets often result in multiple nutrient deficiencies concurrently. Similarly, nutritional risk almost always covaries with a wide range of other psychosocial risk factors that put children at risk for poor developmental outcomes. These psychosocial risk factors include more stressful living environments, increased risk of other health problems (e.g., morbidity, infection), and decreased opportunities for psychosocial stimulation.

In low-income countries, mild to moderate malnutrition affects large numbers of the population, with women, infants, and children at highest risk. In such environments, children and families live under conditions of limited water supply, contaminated water, inadequate hygiene and sanitation, few opportunities for health care, poor or nonexistent schools, and restricted access to other types of information and services (e.g., employment). For example, data from four rural villages in Guatemala that had participated in a nutritional supplementation study indicate that fewer than half of the village families had homes with a well or a direct connection to water, and little more than half had any means of human waste disposal (e.g., latrines) (Engle, Carmichael, Gorman, & Pollitt, 1993). There is little doubt that living under such conditions poses a number of serious health risks, in addition to malnutrition, that may further jeopardize the developmental process.

The study of malnutrition among human populations is limited both in its ability to experimentally manipulate critical nutritional variables and in its ability to isolate nutrition from social and environmental variables (Dobbing, 1984; Smart, 1993; Stein & Susser, 1985). In fact, some researchers have argued that isolating the nutritional effects within the complexity of human behavior may be a futile endeavor (Dobbing, 1990). Still others have hypothesized a number of environmental pathways through which malnutrition may operate (Pollitt, 1994; Pollitt, Gorman, Engle, Martorell, & Rivera, 1993; Riccuiti, 1979, 1991; Wachs, 1995; Wachs et al., 1995). Although none of these theories discount the possibility of direct effects on brain function, research has focused on identifying the environmental factors that interact with or confound the nutritional effects. In the study of malnutrition, as well as its implications for understanding FTT, an emphasis on models that integrate nutritional variables within a contextual framework is essential (Lozoff, 1989b; Wachs et al., 1995).

Evidence

The data on malnutrition come primarily from low-income countries and provide evidence of the effects of nutrient restrictions on infant and child development. A large body of evidence attests to positive associations between indicators of nutritional status (e.g., growth and dietary intake data) and cognitive and behavioral outcomes.

Correlational Data

Measures of length and weight positively correlated with both concurrent and predictive measures of infant motor and mental development on the Composite Infant Scales at 6, 15, and 24 months of age (Lasky, Klein, Yarbrough, Engle, et al., 1981); preschool cognitive scores (Freeman, Klein, Townsend, & Lechtig, 1980); and later school performance (Gorman & Pollitt, 1996; Martorell, Rivera, Kaplowitz, & Pollitt, 1992) in Guatemala. Stunted children in Jamaica were found to be less active and to engage in less-vigorous activities than nonstunted children (Meeks Gardner, Grantham-McGregor, Chang, & Powell, 1990). In Kenya, height and weight significantly correlated with cognitive measures in toddlers (Sigman, McDonald, Neumann, & Bwibo, 1991; Sigman, Neumann, Baksh, Bwibo, & McDonald, 1989). Nutritional status indicators (height, weight, hemoglobin) in childhood predicted school performance and attendance in nutritionally at-risk Jamaican children (Clarke, Grantham-McGregor, & Powell, 1991), whereas concurrent measures of nutritional status of school-age children correlated significantly with school achievement measures in the Philippines (Popkin & Lim-Ybanez, 1982).

Studies of dietary intakes also have established correlations between the amounts and types of specific nutrients and cognitive and behavioral outcomes. A three-country study from Egypt, Kenya, and Mexico provides detailed information on the associations between quantities of specific nutrients (e.g., animal fat, protein, animal protein) and cognitive and behavioral outcomes (Sigman, Newmann, Baksh, et al., 1989; Wachs et al., 1993). In Egyptian toddlers, performance on tests of cognitive development was predicted by intakes of calories, protein, and fat (Wachs et al., 1993). Similarly, animal protein consumption between 18 and 30 months of age was associated with cognitive performance at 5 years of age in Kenyan children (Sigman et al., 1991), and fat intake was predictive of performance among school-age children (Sigman, Neumann, Jensen, & Bwibo, 1989). Furthermore, consumption of animal source foods among Egyptian youth was correlated with verbal abilities and classroom involvement among females and with classroom behavior and activity levels among males (Wachs et al., 1995). In addition, maternal vitamin B_6 status was associated with performance on neonatal assessments, maternal responsiveness, and infant development between 3 and 6 months of age (McCullough et al., 1990).

Despite a wide range of associations between nutritional status indicators and cognitive outcomes, limitations of correlational data restrict the ability to make inferences regarding the causal nature of such associations. Although anthropometry may be an indicator of nutritional status, it also is known to covary with a number of other variables that may confound the association with cognitive development (Barrett, 1984; Pollitt, 1988a). Maternal education, socioeconomic status, school exposure, and psychosocial rearing environment are only a few of a wide number of variables that account for variation in cognitive development and covary with nutritional status indicators as well (see, e.g., Gorman & Pollitt, 1996). Furthermore, both macro- and micronutrient deficiencies are associated with other outcomes, such as poor growth (Rivera, Martorell, Ruel, Habicht, & Haas, 1995; Schroeder, Martorell, Rivera, Ruel, & Habicht, 1995), increased morbidity (Neumann, McDonald, Sigman, Bwibo, & Marquardt, 1991; Pollitt, 1990), and decreased immune function (Buzina et al., 1989), which may result in indirect effects on cognitive and behavioral outcomes.

Supplementation Data

The strongest evidence for establishing the relation between nutrition and behavior comes primarily from supplementation studies that allow for specifically testing between-group differences on supplementary intakes. During the 1960s and 1970s, several large field studies were conducted in low-income countries to test the hypothesis that improved nutrition among nutritionally at-risk populations was associated with improved cognitive performance (Chavez, Martinez, & Yaschine, 1975; Freeman et al., 1980; Joos, Pollitt, Mueller, & Albright, 1983; McKay, Sinisterra, McKay, Gomez, & Lloreda, 1978; Rush, Stein, & Susser, 1980; Waber et al., 1981). In each of these studies, pregnant women and/or their children received some form of nutritional supplementation and the cognitive performance of the children was compared with an unsupplemented control group. Despite differences between studies on a number of critical characteristics (e.g., type of supplement, recipient of supplement, timing and duration of supplement), the results suggest small yet statistically significant findings on a variety of outcomes (e.g., mental and motor development, preschool cognitive function) (Pollitt, 1988b). Subsequently, better-designed studies and the use of improved statistical analyses have strengthened the conclusions of a causal relationship between nutrition and behavior and furthered the understanding of the mechanisms that account for such effects (Gorman, 1995; Husaini et al., 1991; Pollitt & Oh, 1994). The following sections briefly review some of the most important evidence for the effects of malnutrition on motor development, activity, and cognitive function.

Motor Development

Despite variation in the measures of motor development across studies (e.g., the Psychomotor Development Index [PDI] of the Bayley Scales of Infant Development [BSID], Griffiths Subscales), one of the strongest and most consistent findings from supplementation studies has been in this area (Grantham-McGregor, Powell, Walker, & Himes, 1991; Husaini et al., 1991; Joos et al., 1983; Pollitt et al., 1993; Waber et al., 1981). In a study in Taiwan conducted by Chow and his colleagues (Joos et al., 1983), mothers were supplemented beginning after their first pregnancy, through a second pregnancy, and through the lactation of the second birth. Infants born to mothers who were supplemented with a high-calorie, high-protein drink as compared with those born to mothers who received a placebo scored significantly higher on the PDI of the BSID; there were no differences on the Mental Development Index (MDI) of the BSID. In Indonesia, nutritionally at-risk infants were randomly assigned to a short-term dietary supplementation or to a control group for 3 months (Husaini et al., 1991). As compared with nonsupplemented infants, supplemented Indonesian infants scored significantly higher on the PDI. Finally, meta-analysis of six supplementation studies (Engle, Gorman, Martorell, & Pollitt, 1993; Grantham-McGregor et al., 1991; Husaini et al., 1991; Joos et al., 1983; Rush et al., 1980; Waber et al., 1981) that included measures of motor development during infancy supports this conclusion. The results indicate that supplementary feeding of nutritionally at-risk infants results in beneficial effects on motor development among younger (8–15 months) as well as older infants (18–24 months) (Pollitt & Oh, 1994).

Cognitive Function

Almost all supplementation studies have assessed some aspect of cognitive function. As noted previously, despite variations in methodology, the results of these studies consistently have reported significant effects of supplementation on cognitive outcomes. Some of the most comprehensive and convincing data on the effects of supplementary feeding on cognition and psychoeducational outcomes come from a 20-year longitudinal study of infant feeding in Guatemala (Pollitt et al., 1993). The study began in 1969 in four rural villages in Guatemala. All pregnant and lactating women, all infants and children up to the age of 7 years, and all infants born in the villages until 1977 were enrolled in the study. Villages were randomly assigned to either a high-calorie, high-protein drink (Atole) or a low-calorie, no-protein drink (Fresco). Beverages were provided from a central locale in each village and were available on a daily basis, twice per day, to all villagers. In addition, health care and medical services were provided to all villagers, independent of their participation in the study.

Over the course of 7 years (1969–1977), data were collected on growth and morbidity, sociodemographic factors, income and economic productivity, developmental assessments, and cognitive functioning from more than 2,000 participants and their families. Participating infants and young children were tested on the Composite Infant Scale at 6, 15, and 24 months and the Preschool Battery annually between the ages of 3 and 7. The Composite Infant Scale was designed to assess mental and motor development and adapted items from a number of traditional infant assessments (e.g., Bayley, Gesell, Psyche-Cattell) (Lasky, Klein, Yarbrough, Engle, et al., 1981; Lasky, Klein, Yarbrough, & Kallio, 1981). The Preschool Battery consisted of 10 tests administered at ages 3–7 and an additional 12 tests at ages 5–7. The battery was designed to test a wide range of traditional cognitive behaviors as well as Piagetian tasks.

Analyses of the intervention yielded statistically significant findings on the Composite Infant Scale (Klein et al., 1976) and the Preschool Battery (Townsend et al., 1982) between the children who were receiving Fresco and the children who were receiving Atole. Although in most cases of significant differences children who were receiving Atole scored significantly higher on the outcome than did the children who were receiving Fresco, the magnitude of such differences was modest, at best (Pollitt, 1988a).

To assess the long-term effects of the intervention, a study team returned to the villages in 1988–1989. Approximately 70% of the original subjects were located and recruited for participation. At the time of the follow-up, subjects ranged in age from 11 to 26 years. All were given a medical exam, an anthropometric exam, and two psychological test batteries. The first test of cognitive functioning consisted of a series of computerized tests to assess information-processing capabilities (e.g., memory, attention). The other was a psychoeducational battery that included tests of reading, **numeracy,** general knowledge, comprehension, vocabulary, and nonverbal intelligence (Raven's Progressive Matrices [Pollitt et al., 1993]). Complete school records for all children in all villages dating back to 1965 also were obtained as were data on family background, income, education, and socioeconomic status (SES).

The analyses of the hypothesis that early supplementary feeding of infants and children would result in significant effects on adolescent psychoeducational test performance as compared with nonsupplemented children yielded remarkably consistent results. On tests of numeracy, reading comprehension, vocabulary, and general knowledge, subjects from the Atole villages scored significantly higher than subjects from the Fresco villages. These differences were observed after controlling for SES (mother's education, father's occupation, and house quality factor score), school experience (age at school entry and maximum grade attained), age, gender, and attendance at the feeding centers. On tests of information processing, subjects who had received Atole performed faster and more efficiently on a memory test than did subjects who had received Fresco; there were no treatment differences on tests of simple or choice reaction time.

More important, analyses of the interactions between treatment and SES indicated that subjects from the lowest ends of the socioeconomic continuum benefited the most from the supplementation. That is, although Atole and Fresco subjects from families at the upper end of the SES continuum performed similarly, Atole subjects from lower-SES families performed significantly above low-SES Fresco subjects and more similarly to children from families who were relatively advantaged in terms of parental education, occupation, and house quality. These findings were consistent across the range of outcomes: numeracy, knowledge, reading comprehension, and vocabulary.

In addition, when the infant and preschool data were reanalyzed following the same analytic procedure, a similar pattern of results emerged. As compared with the controls (Fresco), Atole infants performed significantly higher on the motor scale at 24 months. In the early preschool period, Atole children performed significantly above Fresco children on factor scores representing general verbal and cognitive abilities at 4 and 5 years of age. Furthermore, significant interactions at these same ages indicated that among Atole subjects, those at highest environmental or psychosocial risk—that is, children from families with poor-quality homes, fathers with low-status occupations, and mothers with low levels of education—benefited most from the supplementation.

In summary, data from this study, in conjunction with other, more recent data, provide evidence that nutritional supplementation is associated with improvements in cognitive functioning among nutritionally at-risk populations. Furthermore, the effects of supplementation vary as a function of other characteristics of the environment, and, specifically, children from families with limited socioeconomic resources may benefit more than those from higher levels of SES.

Activity

Finally, it also has been hypothesized that among malnourished children, activity levels may be reduced as an adaptive mechanism to maintain energy balance (Beaton, 1984). Behavioral descriptions of malnourished children typically note lethargic and listless behavior, suggesting relatively low levels of activity (see Barrett, 1986). Correlations between nutritional status indicators and measures of activity are inconclusive. Nutritional intakes in Egyptian children predicted activity levels among school-age males (Wachs et al., 1995). In Jamaica, stunted children engaged in less overall activity and spent less time in activities that required more strenuous activity than nonstunted peers (Meeks Gardner et al., 1990); however, in a separate study in Jamaica, activity levels were not related to supplementation or to subsequent developmental assessments (Meeks Gardner, Grantham-McGregor, Chang, Himes, & Powell, 1995). Differences in the measurement of activity (e.g., play and exploration versus energy expenditure) as well as differences in the age of the subjects may account for the apparent discrepancies in the findings.

In one of the few supplementation studies that included measures of activity (Chavez et al., 1975), Mexican infants whose mothers were supplemented prenatally and then received supplements during the latter part of their infant's first year were reportedly more active, showed enhanced mother–infant interaction, and showed more positive interactions with both parents as compared with nonsupplemented controls. Although suggestive, these findings must be interpreted with caution given lack of random assignment to treatment groups and that subjects, parents, and investigators were not blind to the treatment.

Micronutrient Effects

Research on malnutrition has increasingly focused on the effects of micronutrient deficiencies on cognitive development. This shift in attention may be in part due to an increased awareness of and knowledge about the prevalence of micronutrient deficiencies. One of the most highly studied micronutrient deficiencies, which clearly is linked to adverse cognitive development, is IDA. In contrast to the literature on malnutrition, the data on IDA come from studies of low-income populations as well as from U.S. and other industrialized samples.

It is well established that IDAn infants score lower on the BSID in comparison with nonanemic infants (Deinard, List, Lindgren, Hunt, & Chang, 1986; Driva, Kafatos, & Solman, 1985; Idjradinata & Pollitt, 1993; Lozoff, Brittenham, Viteri, Wolf, & Urrutia, 1982a, 1982b; Oski & Honig, 1978; Palti, Meijer, & Alder, 1985; Walter, Andraca, Chadud, & Perales, 1989; Walter, Kovalskys, & Stekel, 1983). Further data from randomized clinical trials provide convincing evidence that the relationship is causal; IDAn infants who were treated with iron show significant gains in developmental scores (Idjradinata & Pollitt, 1993; Walter et al., 1983), whereas those receiving placebo do not. Other investigations have focused on the reversibility of the effects of IDA, which have been reported by some (Ekins & Harding, 1984; Idjradinata & Pollitt, 1993; Walter et al., 1983) but not all investigators (Lozoff et al., 1982a; Walter et al., 1989). Although these findings have been interpreted by some to suggest that IDA results in a permanent and irreversible alteration in the developmental trajectory of the infant (Lozoff, 1989a; Walter et al., 1989), this conclusion may be premature. For example, in some studies, IDA was not successfully eliminated, despite treatment. Similarly, confounding factors that are associated with greater severity and chronicity of IDA (e.g., poorer home stimulation, lower parental IQ scores, socioeconomic factors) (Lozoff, 1989a) have often not been accounted for in these studies.

A clinical trial of iron supplementation in Indonesian infants (Idjradinata & Pollitt, 1993) resulted in reversal of IDA and improvements in developmental indicators. At baseline, infants between the ages of 12 and 18 months were classified into three groups based on an extensive hematological assessment: IDAn, iron deficient nonanemic (IDNAn), and iron replete. Within each iron status group, infants were randomly assigned to either 3 mg/kg ferrous sulfate or placebo. After 4 months of supplementation, iron-treated IDAn and IDNAn infants became similar to iron-replete infants in all hematological parameters (hemoglobin, transferrin saturation, ferritin). At baseline, IDAn infants scored significantly lower on both the MDI and the PDI than did infants who were either iron replete or IDNAn. After supplementation, there were no significant differences among the three groups on either the MDI or the PDI. Conversely, the IDAn, placebo-treated infants continued to score significantly lower than all other groups on both the MDI and the PDI.

In contrast, work in Costa Rica showed that IDAn infants scored significantly lower on the MDI and the PDI than did infants who were iron replete and that, on average, these differences persisted even after 3 months of iron therapy (Lozoff et al., 1987). Further analyses revealed that the effect of iron supplementation was dependent on the degree to which the anemia was reversed (Lozoff, 1989a). Specifically, infants whose IDA was reversed completely scored similarly on the MDI and the PDI to the infants who were iron sufficient, whereas infants whose deficiency was not corrected completely continued to score significantly lower than the infants who were iron sufficient. It should be noted that significant treatment effects were the result of an observed decline in performance in the iron-sufficient children, which was not evident in children who were treated successfully with iron (Lozoff, 1989a). Such a decline in the latter part of infancy has been reported elsewhere in disadvantaged populations (Lozoff, 1989a; Saco-Pollitt, Pollitt, & Greenfield, 1985). It is possible that the successful iron treatment of these infants prevented a further decline in this group; however, without a comparable placebo group, this hypothesis could not be tested (Lozoff, 1989a).

At a 5-year follow-up of these children, despite excellent current hematology, children who had had moderate to severe anemia during infancy but had not become iron replete performed significantly poorer on the Wechsler Preschool Primary Scale of Intelligence (WPPSI) than all other children (Lozoff, Jimenez, & Wolf, 1991). At issue is whether to attribute these differences to the irreversibility of the effects of IDA. Although the data are inconclusive, the fact that most of these formerly IDAn infants still exhibited some biochemical signs of iron deficiency suggests that other factors (e.g., other nutrient deficiencies, parasitic infection) may have limited the efficacy of the iron treatment. Further differences between the IDAn and the iron-sufficient infants at the end of the study on a number of other parameters (e.g., home stimulation, mother's IQ score, proportion who were male, duration of breast-feeding) may also account for between-group differences (Lozoff et al., 1991).

Although fewer in number, studies on preschool- and school-age children show an effect of IDA on measures of intelligence and other cognitive processes (e.g., discrimination learning tasks, visual recall) (Pollitt, Leibel, & Greenfield, 1983; Pollitt, Saco-Pollitt, Leibel, & Viteri, 1986; Seshadri & Gopaldas, 1989; Soewondo, Husaini, & Pollitt, 1989). These studies generally provide support for the notion that brain function is vulnerable to the effects of iron deficiency even after the brain growth spurt has been completed.

In summary, the evidence from numerous studies supports the contention that IDA has an adverse impact on cognitive development. The effects of iron supplementation have been observed on a wide range of outcomes from performance on global tests of intelligence to very specific cognitive processes (Pollitt, 1993). Theories hypothesize that IDA has an effect on affective and motivational processes, which indirectly influence a child's performance by modifying his or her ability to attend to relevant information. It is not yet clear whether and to what extent the effects of chronic anemia in infancy are irreversible.

In addition to the fairly conclusive evidence on IDA, it has been well established that maternal iodine deficiency during pregnancy causes severe mental retardation (e.g., cretinism) as well as serious neuromotor and hearing impairments in offspring (Bautista, Barker, Dunn, Sanchez, & Kaiser, 1982; Bleichrodt, Garcia, Rubio, Morreale de Escobar, & Escobar del Rey, 1987; Boyages et al., 1989; Fierro-Benitez, 1986; Hetzel, 1993; Pharoah, Connolly, Ekins, & Harding, 1984; Stanbury, 1987). Although the evidence is convincing for populations in which iodine deficiency is severe—that is, among populations in which infants with cretinism continue to be born and palpable goiter rates are greater than 20% among the school-age population—much less is known about areas where iodine deficiency is mild. Very little evidence is available to establish a link between iodine deficiency and mental development in areas where cretinism has been eliminated and goiter prevalence is low (e.g., less than 15% of school-age children).

In contrast, the data on the effects of most other micronutrient deficiencies are not well documented (Pollitt, 1990). For example, recent interest in the effects of zinc deficiency on growth has led researchers to hypothesize its effects on cognitive and behavioral development as well. Zinc deficiency is characterized by lethargy, apathy, and slow movement—behaviors that closely parallel those described in other malnourished groups. In the laboratory, zinc-deprived rhesus monkeys had lower activity levels, longer response times, and impaired success at learning tasks as compared with control-group monkeys (Golub, Gershwin, Hurley, Hendrickx, & Saito, 1985; Golub, Keen, Gershwin, & Hendrickx, 1995). The available evidence among human populations has not supported such an association. For example, comparisons between school-age children with and without zinc deficiency showed no differences in school performance, and no effects of zinc supplementation were noted (Gibson et al., 1989).

Despite the brief attention to other micronutrients, it is important to note that the number of nutrients with the potential to affect behavior is vast; knowledge of the roles of specific nutrients is constantly being revised. For example, evidence from correlational data has suggested that maternal vitamin B_6 status is associated with performance on neonatal assessments, maternal responsiveness, and infant development between 3 and 6 months (McCullough et al., 1990).

IMPLICATIONS OF THE RESEARCH ON MALNUTRITION FOR UNDERSTANDING PEDIATRIC UNDERNUTRITION IN DEVELOPED COUNTRIES

The purpose of this chapter is to review the research on the effects of malnutrition on physical growth and development and to discuss the implications of these data for a population of children with pediatric undernutrition, traditionally known as *failure to thrive*. To do this, it is essential to address the extent to which these two populations can be compared. This chapter has used the term *malnutrition* intentionally to refer to the study of nutritional deficiencies in low-income countries where malnutrition is endemic. In contrast, *failure to thrive* has been conceptualized primarily as pediatric undernutrition diagnosed in industrialized countries. The following discussion of the similarities and differences between these two groups is based on this distinction.

The question addressed here is whether it is reasonable to draw inferences regarding children who typically are diagnosed with undernutrition in industrialized countries from the research on malnourished children in low-income countries. What, then, are the factors that predict pediatric undernutrition in industrialized countries, and are these factors similar to those that are associated with malnutrition in low-income countries?

A comparison of the theoretical models that predict poor nutritional status in these two populations may shed some light on the extent to which they are comparable. Figure 2 depicts the theoretical model of pediatric undernutrition in industrialized countries, whereas Figure 3 shows the model predicting malnutrition in low-income countries. First,

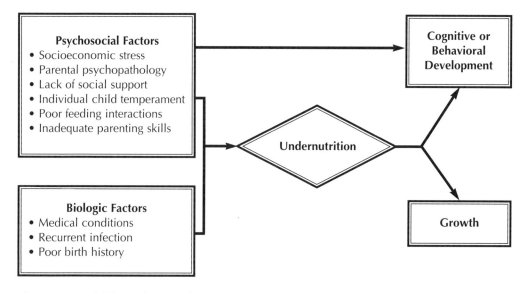

Figure 2.   Model for pediatric undernutrition.

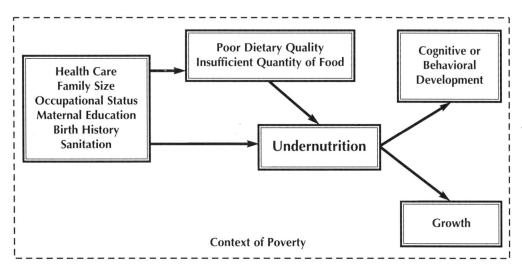

Figure 3.   Model for malnutrition in low-income countries.

it is noteworthy that although both growth and cognitive delays may stem from nutritional deficiencies, it is the distal causes of the resultant pediatric undernutrition or malnutrition that are different. At the same time, it is important to acknowledge that irrespective of the underlying causes, the proximal cause of undernutrition in both low-income countries and industrialized countries is an inadequate supply of nutrients to meet the needs of the organism (Heffer & Kelley, 1994), likely a result of the factors that are described in Figure 1.

The emphasis in the model describing pediatric undernutrition (Figure 2) is on the psychosocial factors that represent various nonoptimal behaviors or interactions that occur within the context of familial, psychological, and social stressors (Drotar, 1989, 1991; Drotar, Eckerle, Salota, Pallotta, & Wyatt, 1990; Phelps, 1991; Rathbun & Peterson, 1987). In the case of the child with undernutrition, growth failure is caused by a combination of psychosocial stressors including parental psychopathology (Whiffen & Gotlib, 1989), socioeconomic stress (M. Black, 1991, as cited in Heffer & Kelley, 1994), and lack of social support (Gorman, Leifer, & Grossman, 1993), in combination with individual child factors (e.g., temperament) (Wolke, Skuse, & Mathisen, 1990) and inappropriate parental feeding practices (Chatoor & Egan, 1983; Woolston, 1983). Furthermore, organic factors (e.g., recurrent infections, specific medical conditions, oral-motor dysfunction) also may contribute to the development of pediatric undernutrition and, in many cases, may interact with nonorganic risk factors. It is when growth is compromised that children are identified and diagnosed with undernutrition. The actual "growth failure" then serves as a crucial indicator of a problem (Drotar & Sturm, 1991).

In contrast, the model for malnutrition (Figure 3) in low-income countries places the focus on the context in which food quality and quantity are constrained. With few exceptions, a major and uniform causal factor of malnutrition is poverty. Within the context of poverty, undernutrition coexists with a wide range of other factors: inadequate health care, poor-quality education, unemployment, large family size, unclean water, and poor sanitation. As a result, the challenge for much of the research on malnutrition has been to identify the unique contribution of nutrition to cognitive development. Although research has provided evidence for a causal link (see Pollitt et al., 1993), the overriding evidence suggests that nutritional variables interact with contextual variables (e.g., occupation, education) to determine outcomes.

Although the discussion of causal factors emphasizes differences between pediatric undernutrition and malnutrition, there are similarities across the two models as well. For example, as with families in low-income countries, it is not uncommon that families of children with undernutrition are also economically at risk (Massachusetts Department of Public Health, 1997). Many of these high-risk families live under conditions of poverty, low maternal education, inadequate employment, and other stressors. At the same time, although the research on malnutrition has emphasized community-level risk factors (e.g., sanitation, health care, endemic poverty), family stress and child factors are likely contributors to the ongoing developmental processes that also contribute to malnutrition as well as its concomitant outcomes (Gorman, 1998).

Similarly, factors that are known to interact with poor nutritional status (e.g., morbidity) are common problems that children in both low-income and developed countries face. For example, it has been estimated that recurrent infections (e.g., upper respiratory, otitis media) contribute to pediatric undernutrition in more than 27% of those with this diagnosis (Massachusetts Department of Public Health, 1997), and there is evidence for the role of infection in low-income countries as well (Waterlow & Tomkins, 1992).

Before drawing conclusions regarding the implications of the research on malnutrition for pediatric undernutrition, one final distinction must be made. The topic of this chapter is the effects of malnutrition on growth and development, and the research in relation to these two sets of outcomes has been discussed separately. Theoretically, it is also important to distinguish between the outcomes. Physical growth is primarily dependent on dietary adequacy to meet nutritional needs irrespective of the underlying causes. Consequently, different underlying causes of undernutrition (e.g., lack of food, inadequate consumption of food secondary to psychosocial factors) lead to the same end: growth failure. Thus, the research from low-income countries indicating that energy, protein, and micronutrient deficiencies limit growth has direct implications for populations with pediatric undernutrition.

In contrast, the same assumptions cannot be made about the independence of etiology on outcomes in the study of human behavior and cognition. Research in the psychological literature attests to a complex relationship between psychosocial risk factors and adverse developmental outcomes (Rutter, 1988; Sameroff, 1993; Sameroff & Chandler, 1975) such that increased exposure to risk factors increases the likelihood of negative outcomes. Furthermore, unidirectional models have been replaced by transactional models in which behaviors interact with responses from the environment to create subsequent behaviors. In thinking about the effects of malnutrition on cognitive and behavioral development, one must understand the interactions among the context, the individual, and the individual's environment to predict long-term consequences of undernutrition.

The concept of interactions between nutrition and environmental factors provides an important framework for interpreting the research on malnutrition for populations with pediatric undernutrition and for drawing inferences regarding the implications of such research. In low-income populations, intervention strategies require an understanding that the obstacles to optimal development are not limited to malnutrition. To observe improvements among populations, attention to structural obstacles (e.g., income, education, health care) as well as individual-level variables is considered essential.

Among populations with pediatric undernutrition, there is also an understanding that nutritional intervention, without attention to psychosocial risk factors, may be ineffective. Although improved feeding and, hence, improved growth are obvious components of any intervention with pediatric undernutrition, there is a recognition that the causal factors that led to the feeding disorder (e.g., psychosocial risk factors) need to be addressed before substantial improvements in cognitive or behavioral development will be evident. This has two implications: 1) Workers who are addressing undernutrition should broaden their programs or collaborate with ones that address broader needs, and 2) programs that serve children at risk (e.g., foster care) should address undernutrition when it occurs (see, e.g., Chapter 25).

The research reviewed in this chapter supports intervention for the treatment of pediatric undernutrition at an early age (the earlier the better). The reasoning for this is twofold: 1) There is a large degree of physical growth and development that occurs at an early age; and 2) the younger the child is at initiation of treatment, the less time he or she has spent at a disadvantage; consequently, chronicity and severity of the undernutrition are minimized. This implies that earlier treatment of the pediatric undernutrition maximizes the potential for optimal growth and development thereafter. There is no evidence, however, that it ever is too late to intervene to improve the growth and development of children.

Whether data from research designs described in this chapter are directly applicable to government policies also is a question that merits consideration. Although the data reviewed here do not explicitly support or refute any specific policy or program, they do attest to the elevated risks that are associated with the effects of poor nutrition on the cognitive development of infants and young children. With this in mind, it is noteworthy that many federal- and state-funded programs (e.g., Special Supplemental Nutrition Program for Women, Infants and Children [WIC]) are concerned specifically with the effects of poor nutrition on infants and young children. WIC has been shown to provide direct benefits to low-income children at risk (Rush, Leighton, Sloan, Alvir, & Garbowski, 1988; Rush, Leighton, Sloan, Alvir, Horvitz, et al., 1988; Rush, Sloan, et al., 1988). Similarly, successful early intervention programs include integrated curricula that target social, cognitive, and health factors that are related to children (see, e.g., Barnett, 1995). Elements of such programs are based on the assumption that adequate nutrition is essential to a child's ability to actively participate in the learning process. Finally, school feeding programs (breakfast and lunch) are funded on the assumption that children who are hungry are not in an optimal position to learn (Pollitt, 1995). Funding for such programs should be evaluated in relation to what is known about the importance of both quality and quantity of diets for the optimal growth and development of young children.

In summary, intervention strategies may vary as a function of the goal of the intervention. The question remains whether interventions are aimed at remedying the "undernutrition" per se or the consequent effects of the undernutrition. In the case of pediatric undernutrition, nutritional status is not likely to improve unless the psychosocial factors that contribute to the undernutrition are addressed. In contrast, among low-income countries, nutritional status could potentially be improved independent of other potential psychosocial risk factors (e.g., food fortification).

Despite what may be subtle differences, if the goal is to prevent cognitive delay or behavior disorders, then an approach that fails to address the complexity of the context in which the undernourished child lives will be insufficient. Although improved nutrition among chronically undernourished populations may lead to increases in some outcomes, such as physical growth, optimal development will occur only under conditions that target a variety of risk factors and build skills and competencies within populations. Similarly, in the case of pediatric undernutrition, the psychosocial risk factors, in conjunction with nutritional deficiencies, put the child at elevated risk for developmental sequelae. Attention to these factors will be required to promote optimal development. In addition, because of

the complexity with which the context interacts with undernutrition in affecting development, there is no established threshold of undernutrition that could be used as a cutoff to
predict effects of undernutrition on development. In clinical practice, the degree of undernutrition should be evaluated in conjunction with the other risk factors present.

Finally, it would be remiss to end this chapter without acknowledging the difficulties
that are inherent in discussing the pediatric undernutrition population as an identifiable
entity. The obvious caveat is that not all children with undernutrition are the same. As such,
broad generalizations can be misleading. For example, some with pediatric undernutrition
come from families in which none of these psychosocial risk factors has been identified
and would not fit clearly into the proposed model. At the same time, however, it is likely
that these children will be less likely to evidence the same degree of developmental delay
as their more highly stressed peers. Further research on such hypotheses is warranted.

REFERENCES

Allen, L.H. (1994). Nutritional influences on linear growth: A general review. *European Journal of
Clinical Nutrition, 48*(Suppl. 1), S75–S89.

Allen, L.H., Black, A.K., Backstrand, J.R., Pelto, G.H., Ely, R.D., Molina, E., & Chávez, A. (1991).
An analytical approach for exploring the importance of dietary quality versus quantity in the
growth of Mexican children. *Food and Nutrition Bulletin, 13*(2), 95–104.

Angeles, I.T., Schutnick, W.J., Matulessi, P., Gross, R., & Sastroamidjojo, S. (1993). Decreased rate
of stunting among anemic Indonesian preschool children through iron supplementation. *American
Journal of Clinical Nutrition, 58,* 339–342.

Aukett, M.A., Parks, Y.A., Scott, P.H., & Wharton, B.A. (1986). Treatment with iron increases
weight gain and psychomotor development. *Archives of Disease in Childhood, 61,* 849–857.

Barnett, W.S. (1995). Long-term effects of early childhood programs on cognitive and school outcomes. *The Future of Children, 5*(3), 25–50.

Barrett, D.E. (1984). Malnutrition and child behavior: Conceptualization, assessment and an empirical study of social-emotional functioning. In J. Broek & B. Schürch (Eds.), *Malnutrition and
behavior: Critical assessment of key issues* (pp. 280–306). Lausanne, Switzerland: Nestlé
Foundation.

Barrett, D.E. (1986). Nutrition and social behavior. In H.E. Fitzgerald, B.M. Lester, & M.W. Yogman
(Eds.), *Theory and research in behavioral pediatrics* (pp. 147–198). New York: Plenum.

Bates, C.J., Evans, P.H., Dardenne, M., Prentice, A., Lunn, P.G., Northrop-Clewes, C.A., Hoare, S.,
Cole, T.J., Horan, S.J., Longman, S.C., Stirling, D., & Aggett, P.J. (1993). A trial of zinc supplementation in young rural Gambian children. *British Journal of Nutrition, 69,* 243–255.

Bautista, A., Barker, P.A., Dunn, J.T., Sanchez, M., & Kaiser, D.L. (1982). The effects of oral iodized
oil on intelligence, thyroid status, and somatic growth in school-age children from an area of
endemic goiter. *American Journal of Clinical Nutrition, 35,* 127–134.

Beaton, G.H. (1984). Adaptation to an accommodation of long term low energy intake: A commentary on the conference of energy intake and activity. In E. Pollitt & P. Amante (Eds.), *Intake and
activity* (pp. 395–403). New York: Alan R. Liss.

Beaton, G.H., Calloway, D.H., & Murphy, S.P. (1992). Estimated protein intakes of toddlers:
Predicted prevalence of inadequate intakes in village populations in Egypt, Kenya, and Mexico.
American Journal of Clinical Nutrition, 55, 902–911.

Beaton, G.H., & Ghassemi, H. (1982). Supplementary feeding programs for young children in developing countries. *American Journal of Clinical Nutrition, 35,* 864–916.

Black, M. (1991, April). *Family characteristics of infants with failure to thrive.* Paper presented at
the meeting of the Florida Conference on Child Health Psychology, Gainesville.

Black, R.E. (1991). Would control of childhood infectious diseases reduce malnutrition? *Acta
Paediatrica Scandinavica, 374*(Suppl.), 133–140.

Black, R.E., Brown, K.H., & Becker, S. (1984). Effects of diarrhea associated with specific
enteropathogens on growth of children in rural Bangladesh. *Pediatrics, 73,* 799–805.

Bleichrodt, N., Garcia, I., Rubio, C., Morreale de Escobar, G., & Escobar del Rey, F. (1987). Developmental disorders associated with severe iodine deficiency. In B.S. Hetzel, J.T. Dunn, & J.B.

Stanbury (Eds.), *The prevention and control of iodine deficiency disorders* (pp. 65–84). Amsterdam: Elsevier Science Publishers.

Boyages, S.C., Collins, J.K., Maberly, G.F., Jupp, J.J., Morris, J., & Eastman, C.J. (1989). Iodine deficiency impairs intellectual and neuromotor development in apparently normal persons: A study of rural inhabitants of north-central China. *The Medical Journal of Australia, 150,* 676–682.

Buzina, R., Bates, C.J., van der Beek, J., Brubacher, G., Chandra, R.K., Hallberg, L., Heseker, J., Mertz, W., Pietrzik, K., Pollitt, E., Pradilla, A., Suboticanec, K., Sandstead, H.H., Schalch, W., Spurr, G.B., & Westenhöfer, J. (1989). Workshop on functional significance of mild-to-moderate malnutrition. *American Journal of Clinical Nutrition, 50,* 172–176.

Castillo-Duran, C., Fisberg, M., Valenzuela, A., Egana, J.I., & Uauy, R. (1983). Controlled trial of copper supplementation during the recovery from marasmus. *American Journal of Clinical Nutrition, 37,* 898–903.

Castillo-Duran, C., Garcia, H., Venegas, P., Torrealba, I., Panteon, E., Concha, N., & Perez, P. (1994). Zinc supplementation increases growth velocity in male children and adolescents with short stature. *Acta Paediatrica, 83,* 833–837.

Castillo-Duran, C., Heresi, G., Fisberg, M., & Uauy, R. (1987). Controlled trial of zinc supplementation during recovery from malnutrition: Effect on growth and immune function. *American Journal of Clinical Nutrition, 45,* 602–608.

Castillo-Duran, C., & Uauy, R. (1988). Copper deficiency impairs growth of infants recovering from malnutrition. *American Journal of Clinical Nutrition, 47,* 710–714.

Caulfield, L.E., Himes, J.H., & Rivera, J.A. (1995). Nutritional supplementation during early childhood and bone mineralization during adolescence. *Journal of Nutrition, 125,* 1104S–1110S.

Cavan, K.R., Gibson, R.S., Grazioso, C.F., Isalgue, A.M., Ruz, M., & Solomons, N.W. (1993). Growth and body composition of periurban Guatemalan children in relation to zinc status: A cross-sectional study. *American Journal of Clinical Nutrition, 57,* 334–352.

Chakar, A., Mokni, R., Walravens, P.A., Chappuis, P., Bleiberg-Daniel, F., Mahu, J.L., & Lemonnier, D. (1993). Plasma zinc and copper in Paris area preschool children with growth impairment. *Biological Trace Element Research, 38,* 97–106.

Chatoor, I., & Egan, J. (1983). Non-organic failure to thrive and dwarfism due to food refusal: A separate disorder. *Journal of the American Academy of Child Psychiatry, 22,* 294–301.

Chavez, A., Martinez, C., & Yaschine, T. (1975). Nutrition, behavioral development, and mother–child interaction in young rural children. *Federation Proceedings, 34*(7), 1574–1582.

Chwang, L., Soemantri, A.G., & Pollitt, E. (1988). Iron supplementation and physical growth of rural Indonesian children. *American Journal of Clinical Nutrition, 47,* 496–501.

Clarke, N., Grantham-McGregor, S.M., & Powell, C. (1991). Nutrition and health predictors of school failure in Jamaican children. *Ecology of Food and Nutrition, 26,* 47–57.

Cook, J.D., Baynes, R.D., & Skikne, B.S. (1994). The physiological significance of circulating transferrin receptors. *Advances in Experimental Medicine and Biology, 352,* 119–126.

de Onis, M., Monteiro, C., Akre, J., & Clugston, G. (1993). The worldwide magnitude of protein-energy malnutrition: An overview from the WHO Global Database on Child Growth. *WHO Bulletin, 71,* 703–712.

Deinard, A.S., List, A., Lindgren, B., Hunt, J.V., & Chang, P.N. (1986). Cognitive deficits in iron-deficient and iron-deficient anemic children. *Journal of Pediatrics, 108*(5, pt. 1), 681–689.

Dirren, H., Barclay, D., Ramos, J.G., Lozano, R., Montalvo, M.M., Davila, N., & Mora, J.O. (1994). Zinc supplementation and child growth in Ecuador. In L. Allen, J. King, & B. Lonnerdal (Eds.), *Nutrient regulation during pregnancy, lactation, and infant growth* (pp. 215–222). New York: Plenum.

Dobbing, J. (1984). Infant nutrition and later achievement. *Nutrition Reviews, 42*(1), 1–7.

Dobbing, J. (1990). Vulnerable periods in developing brain. In J. Dobbing (Ed.), *Brain, behavior and iron in the infant diet.* New York: Springer-Verlag.

Driva, A., Kafatos, A., & Solman, M. (1985). Iron deficiency and the cognitive and psychomotor development of children: A pilot study with institutionalized children. *Early Child Development Care, 22,* 73–82.

Drotar, D. (1989). Behavioral diagnosis in nonorganic failure to thrive: A critique and suggested approach to psychological assessment. *Journal of Developmental and Behavioral Pediatrics, 10,* 48–55.

Drotar, D. (1991). The family context of non-organic failure to thrive. *American Journal of Orthopsychiatry, 61,* 23–34.

Drotar, D., Eckerle, D., Satola, J., Pallotta, J., & Wyatt, B. (1990). Maternal interactional behavior with nonorganic failure-to-thrive infants: A case comparison study. *Child Abuse and Neglect, 14,* 41–51.

Drotar, D., & Sturm, L. (1991). Psychosocial influences in the etiology, diagnosis, and prognosis of non-organic failure to thrive. In H.E. Fitzgerald, B.M. Lester, & M.W. Yogman (Eds.), *Theory and research in behavioral pediatrics* (Vol. 5, pp. 19–59). New York: Plenum.

Engle, P.L., Carmichael, S.L., Gorman, K., & Pollitt, E. (1993). Demographic and socio-economic changes in families in four Guatemalan villages, 1967–1987. *Food and Nutrition Bulletin, 14*(3), 237–245.

Engle, P.L., Gorman, K., Martorell, R., & Pollitt, E. (1993). Infant and preschool psychological development. *Food and Nutrition Bulletin, 14*(3), 201–214.

Ferguson, E.L., Gibson, R.S., Opare-Obisaw, C., Ounpuu, S., Thompson, L.U., & Lehrfeld, J. (1993). The zinc nutriture of preschool children living in two African countries. *Journal of Nutrition, 123,* 1487–1496.

Fierro-Benitez, R. (1986). Long term effects of correction of iodine deficiency on psychomotor and intellectual development. In J.T. Dunn, E.A. Pretell, C.H. Daza, & F.E. Viteri (Eds.), *Towards the eradication of endemic goiter, cretinism, and iodine deficiency* (pp. 182–200). Washington, DC: Pan American Health Organization. (PAHO Publication No. 502)

Fomon, S.J., Filer, L.J., Jr., Thomas, L.N., Anderson, T.A., & Nelson, E. (1975). Influence of formula concentration on caloric intake and growth of normal infants. *Acta Paediatrica Scandinavica, 64,* 172–181.

Fomon, S.J., Filer, L.J., Jr., Ziegler, E.E., Bergmann, K.E., & Bergmann, R.L. (1977). Skim milk in infant feeding. *Acta Paediatrica Scandinavica, 66,* 17–30.

Fons, C., Brun, J.F., Fussellier, M., Cassanas, G., Bardet, L., & Orsetti, A. (1992). Serum zinc and somatic growth in children with growth retardation. *Biological Trace Element Research, 32,* 399–404.

Frank, D.A., & Zeisel, S.H. (1988). Failure to thrive. *Pediatric Clinics of North America, 35,* 1187–1206.

Freeman, E., Klein, R.E., Townsend, J.W., & Lechtig, A. (1980). Nutrition and cognitive development among rural Guatemalan children. *American Journal of Public Health, 70,* 1277–1285.

Gibson, R.S. (1990). *Principles of nutritional assessment.* New York: Oxford University Press.

Gibson, R.S., Smit Vanderkooy, P.D., MacDonald, A.C., Goldman, A., Ryan, B.A., & Berry, M. (1989). A growth-limiting, mild zinc-deficiency syndrome in some Southern Ontario boys with low height percentiles. *American Journal of Clinical Nutrition, 49,* 1266–1273.

Golden, M.H.N. (1991). The nature of nutritional deficiency in relation to growth failure and poverty. *Acta Paediatrica Scandinavica, 374*(Suppl. 374), 95–110.

Golden, M.H.N., & Golden, B.E. (1981). Effect of zinc supplementation on the dietary intake, rate of weight gain, and energy cost of tissue deposition in children recovering from severe malnutrition. *American Journal of Clinical Nutrition, 34,* 900–908.

Golub, M.S., Gershwin, M.E., Hurley, L.S., Hendrickx, A.G., & Saito, W.Y. (1985). Studies of marginal zinc deprivation in rhesus monkeys: Infant behavior. *American Journal of Clinical Nutrition, 42,* 1229–1239.

Golub, M., Keen, C., Gershwin, M.E., & Hendrickx, A. (1995). Developmental zinc deficiency and behavior. *Journal of Nutrition, 125*(8S), 2263S–2271S.

Gopalan, C., Swaminathan, M.C., Kumari, V.K.K., Rao, D.H., & Vijayaraghavan, K. (1973). Effect of calorie supplementation on growth of undernourished chidren. *American Journal of Clinical Nutrition, 26,* 563–566.

Gorman, J., Leifer, M., & Grossman, G. (1993). Non-organic failure to thrive: Maternal history and current maternal functioning. *Journal of Clinical Child Psychology, 22,* 327–336.

Gorman, K.S. (1995). Malnutrition and cognitive development: Evidence from experimental/quasi-experimental studies among the mild-to-moderately malnourished. *Journal of Nutrition, 125*(8S), 2239S–2244S.

Gorman, K.S. (1998). Malnutrition and mother–infant interaction: Expanding the model of nutritional effects on development. In C. Rovee-Collier & L. Lipsitt (Eds.), *Advances in infancy research, 12,* 1–41. Greenwich, CT: Ablex.

Gorman, K.S., & Pollitt, E. (1996). Does schooling buffer the effects of early risk? *Child Development, 67,* 314–326.

Grantham-McGregor, S.M., Powell, C.M., Walker, S.P., & Himes, J.H. (1991). Nutritional supplementation, psychosocial stimulation, and mental development of stunted children: The Jamaican study. *The Lancet, 338*(8758), 1–5.

Haas, J.D., Martinez, E.J., Murdoch, S., Conlisk, E., Rivera, J.A., & Martorell, R. (1995). Nutritional supplementation during the preschool years and physical work capacity in adolescent and young adult Guatemalans. *Journal of Nutrition, 125,* 1078S–1089S.

Hambidge, K.M. (1997). Zinc deficiency in young children. *American Journal of Clinical Nutrition, 65,* 160–161.

Hamill, P.V.V., Drizd, T.A., Johnson, C.L., Reed, R.B., Roche, A.F., & Moore, W.M. (1979). Physical growth: National Center for Health Statistics percentiles. *American Journal of Clinical Nutrition, 32,* 607–629.

Heffer, R.W., & Kelley, M.L. (1994). Non-organic failure to thrive: Developmental outcomes and psychosocial assessment and intervention issues. *Research in Developmental Disabilities, 15,* 247–268.

Hetzel, B.S. (1993). The control of iodine deficiency. *American Journal of Public Health, 83*(4), 494–495.

Hunt, J.R., Zito, C.A., Erjavec, J., & Johnson, L.K. (1994). Severe or marginal iron deficiency affects spontaneous physical activity in rats. *American Journal of Clinical Nutrition, 59,* 413–418.

Husaini, M.A., Karyadi, L., Husaini, Y.K., Sandjaja, B., Karyadi, D., & Pollitt, E. (1991). Developmental effects of short-term supplementary feeding in nutritionally-at-risk Indonesian infants. *American Journal of Clinical Nutrition, 54,* 799–804.

Idjradinata, P., & Pollitt, E. (1993). Reversal of developmental delays in iron-deficient anemic infants treated with iron. *The Lancet, 341,* 1–4.

Idjradinata, P., Watkins, W.E., & Pollitt, E. (1994, May 21). Adverse effect of iron supplementation on weight gain of iron-replete young children. *The Lancet, 343,* 1252–1254.

James, W.P.T. (1994). Introduction: The challenge of adult chronic energy deficiency. *European Journal of Clinical Nutrition, 48,* S1–S9.

Joos, S.K., Pollitt, E., Mueller, W.H., & Albright, D.L. (1983). The Bacon Chow Study: Maternal nutritional supplementation and infant behavioral development. *Child Development, 54,* 669–676.

Judisch, J.M., Naiman, J.L., & Oski, F.A. (1966). The fallacy of the fat iron-deficient child. *Pediatrics, 37,* 987–990.

Karlberg, J., Jahil, F., Lam, L., Low, L., & Yeung, C.Y. (1994). Linear growth retardation in relation to the three phases of growth. *European Journal of Clinical Nutrition, 48,* S25–S44.

Kennedy, E., & Garcia, M. (1994). Body mass index and economic productivity. *European Journal of Clinical Nutrition, 48,* S45–S55.

Klein, R.E., Arenales, P., Delgado, H., Engle, P., Guzman, G., Irwin, M., Lasky, R., Lechtig, A., Martorell, R., Mejfa Pivaral, V., Russell, P., & Yarbrough, C. (1976). Effects of maternal nutrition on fetal growth and infant development. *Bulletin of the Pan American Health Organization, 10,* 301–316.

Kusin, J.A., Kardjati, S., Houtkooper, J.M., & Renquist, U.H. (1992). Energy supplementation during pregnancy and postnatal growth. *The Lancet, 340,* 623–626.

Lampl, M., Johnston, F.E., & Malcolm, L.A. (1978). The effects of protein supplementation on the growth and skeletal maturation of New Guinean school children. *Annals of Human Biology, 5*(3), 219–227.

Lasky, R.E., Klein, R.E., Yarbrough, C., Engle, P.L., Lechtig, A., & Martorell, R. (1981). The relationship between physical growth and infant behavioral development in rural Guatemala. *Child Development, 52,* 219–226.

Lasky, R.E., Klein, R.E., Yarbrough, C., & Kallio, K.D. (1981). The predictive validity of infant assessments in rural Guatemala. *Child Development, 52,* 847–856.

Latham, M.C., Stephenson, L.S., Kinoti, S.N., Zaman, M.S., & Kurz, K.M. (1990, March/April). Improvements in growth following iron supplementation in young Kenyan school children. *Nutrition, 6*(2), 159–165.

Lawless, J.W., Latham, M.C., Stephenson, L.S., Kinoti, S.N., & Pertet, A.M. (1994). Iron supplementation improves appetite and growth in anemic Kenyan primary school children. *Journal of Nutrition, 124*(5), 645–654.

Lozoff, B. (1989a). Methodological issues in studying behavioral effects of infant iron-deficiency anemia. *American Journal of Clinical Nutrition, 50,* 641–654.

Lozoff, B. (1989b). Nutrition and behavior. *American Psychologist, 44*(2), 231–236.

Lozoff, B., Brittenham, G.M., Viteri, F.E., Wolf, A.W., & Urrutia, J.J. (1982a). Developmental deficits in iron-deficient infants: Effects of age and severity of iron lack. *Journal of Pediatrics, 101,* 948–951.

Lozoff, B., Brittenham, G.M., Viteri, F.E., Wolf, A.W., & Urrutia, J.J. (1982b). The effects of short-term oral iron therapy on developmental deficits in iron-deficient anemic infants. *Journal of Pediatrics, 100,* 351–357.

Lozoff, B., Brittenham, G.M., Wolf, A.W., McClish, D.K., Kuhnert, P.M., Jiminez, R., Mora, L.A., Gomez, I., & Krauskoph, D. (1987). Iron deficiency anemia and iron therapy effects on infant developmental test performance. *Pediatrics, 79,* 981–995.

Lozoff, B., Jimenez, E., & Wolf, A.W. (1991). Long-term developmental outcome of infants with iron deficiency. *New England Journal of Medicine, 325,* 687–694.

Martorell, R. (1995). Results and implications of the INCAP follow-up study. *Journal of Nutrition, 125,* 1127S–1138S.

Martorell, R., Delgado, H., Valverde, V., & Klein, R.E. (1981). Maternal stature, fertility, and infant mortality. *Human Biology, 53,* 303–312.

Martorell, R., Habicht, J.-P., Yarbrough, C., Leitig, T.A., Klein, R., & Western, K. (1975). Acute morbidity and physical growth in rural Guatemalan children. *American Journal of Diseases in Children, 129,* 1296–1301.

Martorell, R., Rivera, J., Kaplowitz, H., & Pollitt, E. (1992). Long-term consequences of growth retardation during early childhood. In M. Hernández & J. Argente (Eds.), *Human growth: Basic and clinical aspects* (pp. 143–149). Amsterdam: Elsevier Science Publishers.

Massachusetts Department of Public Health. (1997). *Report on the Massachusetts Growth and Nutrition Program FY 1993–FY 1995.* Boston: Author.

McCullough, A.L., Kirksey, A., Wachs, T.D., McCabe, G.P., Bassily, N.S., Bishry, Z., Galal, O.M., Harrison, G.G., & Jerome, N.W. (1990). Vitamin B-6 status of Egyptian mothers: Relation to infant behavior and maternal–infant interactions. *American Journal of Clinical Nutrition, 51,* 1067–1074.

McKay, H., Sinisterra, L., McKay, A., Gomez, H., & Lloreda, P. (1978). Improving cognitive ability in chronically deprived children. *Science, 200,* 270–278.

Meeks Gardner, J.M., Grantham-McGregor, S.M., Chang, S.M., Himes, J.H., & Powell, C.A. (1995). Activity and behavioral development in stunted and nonstunted children and response to nutritional supplementation. *Child Development, 66*(6), 1785–1797.

Meeks Gardner, J.M., Grantham-McGregor, S.M., Chang, S.M., & Powell, C.A. (1990). Dietary intake and observed activity of stunted and non-stunted children in Kingston, Jamaica: Part II. Observed activity. *European Journal of Clinical Nutrition, 44,* 585–593.

Muhilal, Permeisih, Idjradinata, Muherdiyantiningsih, & Karyadi. (1988). Vitamin A–fortified monosodium glutamate and health, growth, and survival of children: A controlled field trial. *American Journal of Clinical Nutrition, 48,* 1271–1276.

Nakamura, T., Nishiyama, S., Futagoishi-Suginohara, Y., Matsuda, I., & Higashi, A. (1993). Mild to moderate zinc deficiency in short children: Effect of zinc supplementation on linear growth velocity. *Journal of Pediatrics, 123,* 65–69.

National Academy of Sciences, Institute of Medicine, Food and Nutrition Board. (1993). *Recommended guidelines for the prevention, detection and management of iron deficiency anemia.* Washington, DC: National Academy Press.

Neumann, C.G., & Harrison, G.G. (1994). Onset and evolution of stunting in infants and children: Examples from the Human Collaborative Research Support Program—Kenya and Egypt studies. *European Journal of Clinical Nutrition, 48*(Suppl. 1), S90–S102.

Neumann, C., McDonald, M.A., Sigman, M., Bwibo, N., & Marquardt, M. (1991). Relationships between morbidity and development in mild-to-moderately malnourished Kenyan toddlers. *Pediatrics, 88,* 934–942.

Ninh, N.X., Thissen, J.P., Collette, L., Gerard, G., Khoi, H.H., & Ketelslegers, J.M. (1996). Zinc supplementation increases growth and circulating insulin-like growth factor I (IGF-I) in growth-retarded Vietnamese children. *American Journal of Clinical Nutrition, 63,* 514–519.

Oski, F.A., & Honig, A.S. (1978). The effects of therapy on the developmental scores of iron-deficient infants. *Journal of Pediatrics, 92,* 21–25.

Palti, H., Meijer, A., & Alder, B. (1985). Learning, achievement and behavior at school of anemic and non-anemic infants. *Early Human Development, 10,* 217–223.

Perez-Escamilla, R., & Pollitt, E. (1995). Growth improvements in children above 3 years of age: The Cali study. *Journal of Nutrition, 25,* 885–893.

Pharoah, P., Connolly, K., Ekins, R.P., & Harding, A.G. (1984). Maternal thyroid hormone levels in pregnancy and the subsequent cognitive and motor performance of children. *Clinical Endocrinology, 21,* 265–270.

Phelps, L. (1991). Non-organic failure-to-thrive: Origins and psychoeducational implications. *School Psychology Review, 20,* 417–427.

Pickett, K.E., Haas, J.D., Murdoch, S., Rivera, J.A., & Martorell, R. (1995). Early nutritional supplementation and skeletal maturation in Guatemalan adolescents. *Journal of Nutrition, 125,* 1097S–1103S.

Pollitt, E. (1988a). A critical view of three decades of research on the effects of chronic energy malnutrition on behavioral development. In B. Schurch & N.S. Scrimshaw (Eds.), *Chronic energy deficiency: Consequences and related issues* (pp. 79–93). Lausanne, Switzerland: Nestlé Foundation.

Pollitt, E. (1988b). Developmental impact of nutrition on pregnancy, infancy, and childhood: Public health issues in the United States. *International Review of Research in Mental Retardation, 15,* 33–80.

Pollitt, E. (1990). *Malnutrition in the classroom.* Lausanne, Switzerland: Unesco.

Pollitt, E. (1993). Iron deficiency and cognitive function. *Annual Review of Nutrition, 13,* 521–537.

Pollitt, E. (1994). A developmental view of cognition in the undernourished child. *Nestlé Foundation for the Study of the Problems of Nutrition in the World, Annual Report 1994,* 88–104.

Pollitt, E. (1995). Does breakfast make a difference in school? *Journal of the American Dietetic Association, 95*(10), 1134–1139.

Pollitt, E., Gorman, K.S., Engle, P., Martorell, R., & Rivera, J. (1993). Early supplementary feeding and cognition: Effect over two decades. *Monographs of the Society for Research in Child Development, 58*(7, Serial No. 235).

Pollitt, E., Leibel, R.L., & Greenfield, D.B. (1983). Iron deficiency and cognitive test performance in preschool children. *Nutrition and Behavior, 1,* 137–146.

Pollitt, E., & Oh, S. (1994). Early supplementary feeding, child development, and health policy. *Food and Nutrition Bulletin, 15*(3), 208–214.

Pollitt, E., Saco-Pollitt, C., Leibel, R.L., & Viteri, F.E. (1986). Iron deficiency and behavioral development in infants and preschool children. *American Journal of Clinical Nutrition, 43,* 555–565.

Popkin, B.M., & Lim-Ybanez, M. (1982). Nutrition and school achievement. *Social Science & Medicine, 16,* 53–61.

Rahmathullah, L., Underwood, B.A., Thulasiraj, R.D., & Milton, R.C. (1991). Diarrhea, respiratory infections, and growth are not affected by a weekly low-dose vitamin A supplement: A masked, controlled field trial in children in southern India. *American Journal of Clinical Nutrition, 54,* 568–577.

Rathbun, J.M., & Peterson, K.E. (1987). Nutrition in failure to thrive. In R.J. Grand, J.L. Sutphen, & W.H. Dietz (Eds.), *Pediatric nutrition: Theory and practice* (pp. 627–643). Boston: Butterworth-Heinemann.

Ricci, J.A., & Becker, S. (1996). Risk factors for wasting and stunting among children in Metro Cebu, Philippines. *American Journal of Clinical Nutrition, 63,* 966–975.

Ricciuti, H.N. (1979). Malnutrition and cognitive development: Research issues and priorities. In J. Brozek (Ed.), *Behavioral effects of energy and protein deficits* (pp. 297–313). Washington, DC: National Institute of Health. (NIH Publication No. 79-1906)

Ricciuti, H.N. (1991). Malnutrition and cognitive development: Research–policy linkages and current research directions. In R.J. Sternberg & L. Okagaki (Eds.), *Directors of development: Influences on the development of children's thinking* (pp. 59–80). Mahwah, NJ: Lawrence Erlbaum Associates.

Rivera, J.A., Martorell, R., Ruel, M.T., Habicht, J.-P., & Haas, J.D. (1995). Nutritional supplementation during the preschool years influences body size and composition of Guatemalan adolescents. *The Journal of Nutrition, 125*(4S), 1068S–1077S.

Rosado, J.L., Lopez, P., Munoz, E., Martinez, H., & Allen, L.H. (1997). Zinc supplementation reduced morbidity, but neither zinc nor iron supplementation affected growth or body composition of Mexican preschoolers. *American Journal of Clinical Nutrition, 65,* 13–19.

Rush, D., Leighton, J., Sloan, N.L., Alvir, J.M., & Garbowski, G.C. (1988). The National WIC Evaluation: Evaluation of the Special Supplemental Food Program for Women, Infants and Children. II: Review of past studies of WIC. *American Journal of Clinical Nutrition, 48*(2 Suppl.), 394–411.

Rush, D., Leighton, J., Sloan, N.L., Alvir, J.M., Horvitz, D.G., Seaver, W.B., Garbowski, G.C., Johnson, S.S., Kulka, R.A., Devore, J.W., Holt, M., Lynch, J.T., Virag, T.G., Woodside, M.B., & Shanklin, D.S. (1988). Study of infants and children. *American Journal of Clinical Nutrition, 48,* 484–511.

Rush, D., Sloan, N.L., Leighton, J., Alvir, J.M., Horvitz, D.G., Seaver, W.B., Garbowski, G.C., Johnson, S.S., Kulka, R.A., Holt, M., Devore, J.W., Lynch, J.T., Woodside, M.B., & Shanklin, D.S. (1988). Longitudinal study of pregnant women. *American Journal of Clinical Nutrition, 48,* 439–483.

Rush, D., Stein, Z., & Susser, M. (1980). *Diet in pregnancy: A randomized controlled trial of nutritional supplements.* New York: Alan R. Liss.

Rutter, M. (Ed.). (1988). *Studies of psychosocial risk: The power of longitudinal data.* Cambridge, England: Cambridge University Press.

Saco-Pollitt, C., Pollitt, E., & Greenfield, D.B. (1985). The Cumulative Deficit Hypothesis in the light of cross-cultural evidence. *International Journal of Behavioral Development, 8,* 75–94.

Sameroff, A.J. (1993). Models of development and developmental risk. In C.H. Zeanah, Jr. (Ed.), *Handbook of infant mental health* (pp. 3–13). New York: Guilford Press.

Sameroff, A.J., & Chandler, M.J. (1975). Reproductive risk and the continuum of caretaking casualty. In F.D. Horowitz, E.M. Hetherington, S. Scarr-Salapatek, & G. Siegel (Eds.), *Review of child development research, 4,* 187–244. Chicago: University of Chicago Press.

Schlesinger, L., Arevalo, M., Arredondo, S., Diaz, M., Lonnerdal, B., & Stekel, A. (1992). Effect of a zinc-fortified formula on immunocompetence and growth of malnourished infants. *American Journal of Clinical Nutrition, 56,* 491–498.

Scholl, T.O., Hediger, M.L., Schall, J.I., Fischer, R.L., & Khoo, C.S. (1993). Low zinc intake during pregnancy: Its association with preterm and very preterm delivery. *American Journal of Epidemiology, 137,* 1115–1124.

Schroeder, D.G., Martorell, R., Rivera, J.A., Ruel, M.T., & Habicht, J.-P. (1995). Age differences in the impact of nutritional supplementation on growth. *The Journal of Nutrition, 125*(4S), 1051S–1059S.

Seshadri, S., & Gopaldas, T. (1989). Impact of iron supplementation on cognitive functions in preschool and school-aged children: The Indian experience. *American Journal of Clinical Nutrition, 50*(Suppl.), 675–681.

Sigman, M., McDonald, M.A., Neumann, C., & Bwibo, N. (1991). Prediction of cognitive competence in Kenyan children from toddler nutrition, family characteristics and abilities. *Journal of Child Psychology and Psychiatry and Allied Disciplines, 32,* 307–320.

Sigman, M., Neumann, C., Baksh, M., Bwibo, N., & McDonald, M. (1989). Relationship between nutrition and development in Kenyan toddlers. *Journal of Pediatrics, 115,* 357–364.

Sigman, M., Neumann, C., Jensen, A., & Bwibo, N. (1989). Cognitive abilities of Kenyan children in relation to nutrition, family characteristics, and education. *Child Development, 60,* 1463–1474.

Smart, J.L. (1993). Malnutrition, learning and behavior: 25 years on from the MIT symposium. *Proceedings of the Nutrition Society, 52,* 189–199.

Soewondo, W., Husaini, M., & Pollitt, E. (1989). Effects of iron deficiency on attention and learning processes in preschool children: Bangdung, Indonesia. *American Journal of Clinical Nutrition, 50*(Suppl.), 667–673.

Solomons, N.W., Mazariegos, M., Brown, K.H., & Klasing, K. (1993). The underprivileged, developing country child: Environmental contamination and growth failure revisited. *Nutrition Reviews, 51*(11), 327–332.

Stanbury, J.B. (1987). The iodine deficiency disorders: Introduction and general aspects. In B.S. Hetzel, J.T. Dunn, & J.B. Stanbury (Eds.), *The prevention and control of iodine deficiency disorders* (pp. 35–47). Amsterdam: Elsevier Science Publishers.

Stein, Z., & Susser, M. (1985). Effects of early nutrition on neurological and mental competence in human beings. *Psychological Medicine, 15,* 717–726.

Super, C.M., Herrera, M.G., & Mora, J.O. (1990). Long-term effects of food supplementation and psychosocial intervention on the physical growth of Colombian infants at risk of malnutrition. *Child Development, 61,* 29–49.

Townsend, J.W., Klein, R.E., Irwin, M.H., Owens, W., Yarbrough, C., & Engle, P.L. (1982). Nutrition and preschool mental development. In D.A. Wagner & H.W. Stevenson (Eds.), *Cross-cultural perspectives on child development* (pp. 124–145). San Francisco: W.H. Freeman.

United Nations Administrative Committee on Coordination/Subcommittee on Nutrition. (1990). *Appropriate uses of anthropometric indices in children.* New York: Author.

Waber, D.P., Vuori-Christiansen, L., Ortiz, N., Clement, J.R., Christiansen, N.E., Mora, J.O., Reed, R.B., & Herrera, M.G. (1981). Nutritional supplementation, maternal education, and cognitive development of infants at risk of malnutrition. *American Journal of Clinical Nutrition, 34,* 807–813.

Wachs, T.D. (1995). Relation of mild-to-moderate malnutrition to human development: Correlational studies. *Journal of Nutrition, 125*(8 Suppl.), 2245S–2254S.

Wachs, T.D., Bishry, Z., Moussa, W., Yunis, F., McCabe, G., Harrison, G., Swefi, I., Kirksey, A., Galal, O., Jerome, N., & Shaheen, F. (1995). Nutritional intake and context as predictors of cognition and adaptive behavior of Egyptian school age children. *International Journal of Behavioral Development, 18*(3), 425–450.

Wachs, T.D., Moussa, W., Bishry, Z., Yunis, F., Sobhy, A., McCabe, G., Jerome, N., Galal, O., Harrison, G., & Kirksey, A. (1993). Relations between nutrition and cognitive performance in Egyptian toddlers. *Intelligence, 17,* 151–172.

Walker, S., Powell, A., Grantham-McGregor, S., Himes, J., & Chang, S. (1991). Nutritional supplementation, psychosocial stimulation, and growth of stunted children: The Jamaican study. *American Journal of Clinical Nutrition, 54,* 642–648.

Walravens, P.A., Chakar, A., Mokni, R., Denise, J., & Lemonnier, D. (1992). Zinc supplements in breastfed infants. *The Lancet, 340,* 683–685.

Walravens, P.A., Hambidge, K.M., & Koepfer, D.M. (1989). Zinc supplementation in infants with a nutritional pattern of failure to thrive: A double-blind, controlled study. *Pediatrics, 83,* 532–538.

Walter, T., Andraca, I.D., Chadud, P., & Perales, C. (1989). Iron deficiency anemia: Adverse effects on infant psychomotor development. *Pediatrics, 84,* 7–17.

Walter, T., Kovalskys, J., & Stekel, A. (1983). Effect of mild iron deficiency on infant mental development scores. *Journal of Pediatrics, 102,* 519–522.

Waterlow, J.C., & Tomkins, A.M. (1992). Nutrition and infection. In J.C. Waterlow (Ed.), *Protein-energy malnutrition* (pp. 290–324). London: Edward Arnold.

West, K.P., Djunaedi, E., Pandji, A., Kusdiono, M.D., Tarwotjo, I., Sommer, A., & Aceh Study Group. (1988). Vitamin A supplementation and growth: A randomized community trial. *American Journal of Clinical Nutrition, 48,* 1257–1264.

Whiffen, V.E., & Gotlib, I.H. (1989). Infants of post partum depressed mothers: Temperament and cognitive status. *Journal of Abnormal Psychology, 98,* 274–279.

Wolke, D., Skuse, D., & Mathisen, B. (1990). Behavioral styles in failure to thrive infants: A preliminary communication. *Journal of Pediatric Psychology, 15,* 237–254.

Woolston, J.L. (1983). Eating disorders in infancy and early childhood. *Journal of the American Academy of Child Psychiatry, 22,* 114–121.

Yip, R., Parvanta, I., Scanlon, K., Borland, E.W., Russell, C.M., & Trowbridge, F.L. (1992). Pediatric Nutrition Surveillance System—United States, 1980–1991. *CDC Morbidity and Mortality Weekly Report, 41*(SS-7), 1–24.

Chapter 4

Working with Families
An Overview for Providers

Lynne Sturm and Peter Dawson

Undernourished children and their families receive diagnostic and treatment services in a variety of settings, including pediatric inpatient wards and outpatient clinics; early intervention centers; Special Supplemental Nutrition Program for Women, Infants and Children (WIC) nutrition clinics; and social services agencies. This chapter describes strategies that providers can employ to develop collaborative relationships with parents of undernourished children.

All stages of evaluation and treatment of undernutrition call for a collaboration, or "working alliance," between key family members and professionals (Kalmanson & Seligman, 1992). Professionals depend on parents to provide accurate historical information, cooperate with diagnostic procedures, be receptive to staff's impressions and recommendations, and enter actively into the process of helping their child recover from compromised nutritional status. Developing such relationships can be a challenge, and it requires commitment by staff to the time-intensive process of developing effective communication and building trust.

WORKING WITH PARENTS

The pattern of open, respectful communication between staff and parents can be set during the very first visit with a family. During this visit, the main emphasis should be on building a relationship rather than on completing the details of a medical or nutritional history. Even when the degree of undernutrition calls for prompt medical intervention, it is important to take some time to support the parents in their adult caregiver role by inquiring about and listening carefully to their concerns about their child. Providers should make special efforts to adopt a respectful attitude toward parents of undernourished children. Parents should sometimes be asked how they would like to be addressed (e.g., Ms., Mrs., Mr., first name). Respect should extend to how providers communicate with one another about the family as well. When documenting in written form (e.g., medical charts, agency contact records), it is preferable to refer to parents by name than by such generic terms as "the mother" or "MOC" (mother of the child).

Start Where the Parents Are

The language that professionals use to refer to a child's condition sets the tone for the provider–parent relationship. The term *failure to thrive* should be avoided because of its negative implications (e.g., the parents have failed, the child does not thrive in their care). Instead, more neutral terms such as *growth problem, difficulty with gaining weight,* or *undernutrition* can be employed.

Take time to understand in depth the parents' concerns about their child's condition. It is important to find out how concerned the parents are about their child's undernutrition. To do so, providers can ask about their understanding of the child's problem; causal explanations (etiology of the condition); optimum treatment approaches; consequences of the problem if untreated (short term and long term); and reactions of significant others in their social network, including advice that they have received (Drotar & Sturm, 1988; Sturm & Drotar, 1992). These beliefs, when considered as a whole, serve as a window to the parental concern or worry about the child and may provide information about priorities for intervention.

When providers are unaware of how parents understand their child's undernutrition and any concurrent developmental or behavior problems, communication problems are more likely to occur. Predictable problems in achieving shared understanding may result from the cultural differences between professionals and parents that can stem from education, language, class, ethnicity, or many other factors (Sharf & Kahler, 1996).

Starting where the parents are, a hallmark of family-centered early intervention (Part H of the Education of the Handicapped Act Amendments of 1986 [PL 99-457], now Part C of the Individuals with Disabilities Education Act Amendments of 1997 [PL 105-17]), can foster rapport with a family who does not yet appreciate the seriousness of undernutrition. Sometimes, parents may not be able to join with care providers around the issue of undernutrition until their concerns and priorities for intervention receive serious consideration. If the parents are concerned about something (e.g., weaning, a need for vitamins), then it may be best to start with that issue. For example, Drotar and Sturm (1988) described a family in which the mother did not appreciate the seriousness of her toddler's growth and feeding problems. She was able to ally with health care staff when she redefined her son's difficult behavior as a discipline problem that she wanted to change. Only after her priority for intervention was respected and addressed by staff could she begin to attend to her son's nutritional status.

Expect the parents to voice a medical explanation for their child's undernutrition. There are a range of parental explanations for growth problems, the most typical involving an illness, condition, or structural problem that prevents weight gain (e.g., food allergies, low immunity to colds, stomach problems). Medical causes probably are the least personally threatening explanation for parents when they are faced with the anxiety-arousing condition of poor growth. It is useful to determine whether a particular child has had prior physical illnesses that reinforce parental perceptions of the child as more sickly than other children and might have impaired the child's weight gain.

When suggesting changes in caregiving practices (e.g., dietary routines, interactions during feeding), the provider should evaluate the factors that would need to change for the family to carry out the provider's recommendations. One entry to discovering potential barriers is to discuss directly with parents what might make it difficult for members of their household to carry out a suggestion. These include tangible obstacles (e.g., availability of food, money for transportation, dietary preferences of other family members) and attitudes that clash with those of the provider (e.g., a parent believes that disengaging from control struggles about food intake with a toddler will spoil him or her).

Deal with the Parents' Degree of Concern

It is important to be sensitive to the fact that undernutrition may pose a significant threat to a parent's feelings of competence. Many parents will worry or feel guilty if they cannot feed their infants or toddlers adequately. Their anxiety may cause them to push food on their children and make feeding interactions worse. Parents may fear that they will be blamed for their child's condition or even that their child might be removed from their care for neglect. Such fears may prevent parents from sharing important information with providers and result in missed appointments or arguments with staff. If parents are worried, then provide realistic reassurance, do not overemphasize weight, and do not give general advice to increase caloric intake without specific guidance on how to do it. For example, it may be tempting to have a child visit a clinic just for a weight check; but this practice may increase the parents' anxiety, especially if helpful advice does not follow.

Conversely, some parents are unconcerned about the child's undernutrition and/or behavior and developmental problems. It is helpful to conceptualize "lack of worry" about a pediatric condition in terms of a threshold for parental concern. Some parents quickly become overly alarmed by very mild pediatric symptoms, whereas other parents underreact to significant symptoms that require prompt action. Care providers need to understand that for some parents growth may not be a cause for concern. Instead, parents may focus on behavioral dimensions such as alertness or locomotor development (Worthman, 1995). Parents often define "ill health" on the basis of acute sickness symptoms such as fever, listlessness, or vomiting. To such a parent, the undernourished child may appear to be developing as expected and not to be exhibiting acute illness; thus, the threshold for parental concern and cue for action (e.g., taking the child to the doctor) may not be reached.

It often is helpful to empathize with the confusion that a parent may experience but not feel safe to express as he or she negotiates the service delivery system. An example is,

> Many parents have told me that they find it confusing or upsetting to hear from a doctor that something is wrong with their child's growth when their child may not show symptoms of illness. You see your child running around, playing without problems that would lead you to suspect there might be a problem. (Drotar & Sturm, 1988, pp. 309–310)

When children have behavioral feeding problems, recognize that it is confusing when professionals tell parents that their child needs more food and yet they have to let the child do the eating.

It may be necessary to warn parents that undernutrition can impair their child's physical growth and mental development. With one family, staff's use of the phrase "not growing well" was less effective than the term "malnutrition" in tapping a mother's concern for her child's well-being (Drotar & Sturm, 1988). Even with warnings and explanations, some parents may choose not to become involved, and, unless there are other grounds for involving child protective services, it may be best to let them be.

Work with the Whole Family

Effective assessment and intervention require that the professional understand the roles of important people in the child's caregiving. Medical charts and registration forms that include a household roster (i.e., a list of who lives in the household, including names, ages, and position within the family) allow providers to enter into initial conversations with families with some *a priori* sense of the family composition. As a matter of course, parents should be asked for the name, address, and telephone number (if available) of someone who will know where they are if they move during the course of intervention. It often is enlightening to ask parents what other significant relatives (e.g., a grandmother, mother's sister) and family friends have said to them about their child's condition and what advice they have received. One mother acknowledged that she did not become concerned about her 9-month-old baby's weight until an old and trusted friend, also a mother, voiced concern about how thin the baby looked.

A family genogram (Rauch & Curtiss, 1992) is a family tree that includes multiple generations of family members. Creating this diagram with the child's parents can be an efficient way to learn about the structure of the family and family history and to identify family members with whom the professional needs to work on the child's behalf. The genogram and other techniques of "family mapping" (Kertesz, 1987) cast a wide net in contrast to the more traditional pediatric focus on the mother–child relationship. The provider–parent relationship can be strengthened by using the genogram as an interview format. The process of creating a family genogram can actively unite the parents and the professional with a joint focus, allowing side-by-side exploration that reduces the parents' sense of threat. Staff with medical or social services backgrounds often are familiar with this technique and feel comfortable using it to ask parents for information about medical history, long-term family relationships, and sensitive psychosocial topics (e.g., intergenerational patterns of alcohol and substance abuse or mental illness).

Of particular relevance to cases of undernutrition is the mapping of the larger household family (Kahler & Sharf, 1996). This involves *all* significant people who come and go in a child's immediate environment rather than only the people to whom the child is biologically related or with whom the child currently lives. It is useful to include in these household maps child care settings where the child receives snacks and meals. The provider should ask who feeds the child or otherwise cares for him or her for even brief periods of time during the week and on weekends.

For example, a 2-year-old Latino boy presented with significant undernutrition that was not recognized by his parents. His parents were separated and kept separate households but continued to interact around the care of the boy. The child lived part of each week at each parent's house. At the father's house were other family members, including several grown children from a previous relationship. In addition, the mother often was present at the father's house. The child was reported to eat more at the father's house than at the mother's. The understanding of the complex family structure was aided by the use of a household family map (see Figure 1). Learning with whom the child ate in each home was instrumental to developing an effective intervention plan.

Give Parents Credit

Prior to making suggestions for changes in parenting around nutrition, it is advisable to praise parents for what they already are doing well. For example, identifying a strength in the child's development that reflects parental input or commenting on how well the parent remains calm during the child's protest at meals will reassure the parent that the profes-

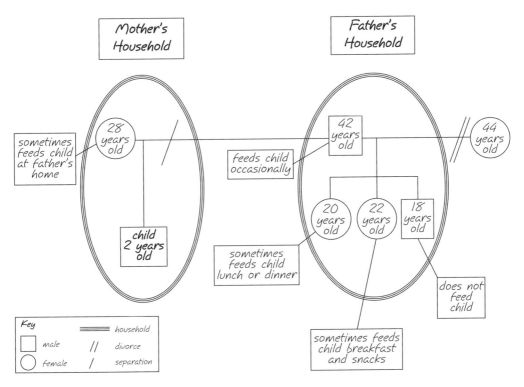

Figure 1.   Household map.

sional thinks that he or she is doing a good job as a parent. This will help the parent to be
open to suggestions to try something new. It also is important to gather thorough information about what the parents are doing before rushing in with information or instructions.
For example, automatically presenting the food pyramid before it is clear that it is needed
is likely to be counterproductive. When discussing the child's condition and treatment
options, the provider should focus on the future and be concerned with how staff and parents can work together to improve the child's growth and development. Avoiding a blaming stance and focusing on active steps that parents can take to help their child works well
with families of undernourished children. Parental guilt sometimes presents as withdrawal
from, avoidance of, mistrust of, or anger toward providers. By adopting a positive, proactive approach, providers can promote parental feelings of control and efficacy while con-
veying respect for the parent as a crucial member of the treatment team.

At the time of diagnosis, professionals should be prepared for some degree of disagreement and conflict with parents. Differences of opinion may arise around whether the
child has an undernutrition problem, which factors play a role in the problem, and/or the
steps to take to improve the undernutrition. In general, it is useful to adopt a model of clinical negotiation in treatment planning (Katon & Kleinman, 1981; Kleinman, Eisenberg, &
Good, 1978). This model transforms the traditional "treatment recommendations" from a
set of tasks prescribed to the parent by the expert into a mutual problem-solving activity
within the provider–parent partnership. This attitude also is consistent with the strength-
based approach to human services programs (Powell, Batsche, Ferro, Fox, & Dunlap,
1997). (Strategies for negotiating treatment approaches with parents are discussed in
Chapter 26.)

Allowing parents as many choices as possible both increases their sense of control and conveys respect for their joint roles as parents and treatment team members. For example, if the initial evaluation indicates the need for diagnostic procedures such as a 3-day food record with a visit to the dietitian and a medical visit with a questionnaire and physical examination, then one can ask the parent with which he or she would prefer to start. With families from nonmainstream cultures, however, it is important to be aware of cultural expectations for authority behavior on behalf of the physician so as not to undermine a family's confidence in their physician (see Chapter 26).

Organize Services to Address Families' Preferences

Continuity of care by professionals (i.e., a family meets with the same physician, nutritionist, or social worker across visits) fosters a working alliance and should be a cornerstone of all service programs. Parents should not have to tell their story anew to different providers each time they attend an outpatient visit. Appointments that can be scheduled at the parents' convenience (e.g., early evening hours for working parents) are more likely to be kept than those that are imposed without consideration of the family's needs.

Providers should take special steps to assess the parents' individual learning styles. Rather than rely on oral instructions, providers should determine the parents' comfort with written versus visual materials and routinely write out their instructions in a format that is understandable to the family (e.g., step-by-step picture sequences of preparing formula). Staff also should plan to remain available by telephone after face-to-face contacts to provide support and problem solving when parents attempt to carry out their suggestions.

Professionals should review missed appointments with care by quickly reaching out to parents by means of telephone calls, written notes, or home visits. Missed appointments may serve as a form of communication by the parent that something is awry in the relationship with the provider. It is always important to try to find out which practical obstacles (e.g., financial, time) or interpersonal barriers (e.g., confusion about different advice from the professional and family members, domestic violence) have prevented the family from attending a scheduled visit.

To improve service delivery in general, it is invaluable to obtain the parents' feedback about which aspects of a program's services they have found to be helpful and which they have not. This can be accomplished by using a brief questionnaire near the end of intervention services. A simple set of questions can ask for parent feedback in order to help the program providers to better serve undernourished infants and toddlers and their parents. The parents' subjective experience of specific procedures such as home visiting and videotaping of feeding interactions as well as more subjective impressions of provider–parent relationships can be obtained. Program evaluation procedures should routinely include consumer (i.e., parent) satisfaction with services.

Terminate Relationships with Care

The provider–parent relationship requires special consideration as parents prepare to move on from intervention services for undernutrition. The importance to the family of the provider–parent relationship, particularly in cases of socially isolated families, never should be underestimated by busy professionals. The termination phase of program delivery must be handled sensitively. It is advisable to identify clearly in advance a time line for termination of services, to say good-bye clearly to the parents and the child, and to allow them to say good-bye as well. Families often find it meaningful to review the course of treatment with the professional, to celebrate jointly any progress, and to build in plans for subsequent contacts with the provider in several months. It is important to arrange specific appointments for follow-up services. For example, it may be necessary to reduce the use of fat in the child's diet if it is no longer needed. Children may later become overweight or develop high-fat dietary habits unless the parents change back to an ordinary diet.

Bright Futures

Bright Futures: Guidelines for Health Supervision of Infants, Children, and Adolescents (Green, 1994)[1] is a book of guidelines for health care providers to use in well-child care. It was developed over the course of 4 years by task forces of experts in collaboration with 16 national organizations. Its chapters correspond to the usual ages for well-child visits. Each chapter contains suggested questions for the practitioner to ask about health, child development, and family function, followed by developmental milestones and suggestions about physical examination and anticipatory guidance (Green, 1994). A special project, Building Bright Futures, is developing further materials. A guide on oral health (Casamassimo, 1997) was published, and future guides are to address nutrition, mental health, and child health and development. Content of the series also is being published in pocket guides and reference cards. The special project has provided training at professional meetings and offers a slide series and a newsletter.

APPROACHES OUTSIDE THE OFFICE OR THE CLINIC

A number of service delivery models can serve as useful alternatives or adjuncts to more traditional center-based programs. These include home visiting, parent support groups, and a variety of family resource programs.

Home Visiting

Home visiting in a variety of service programs has a long history in the United States, and interest continues (Behrman, 1993). Home visits have been made by public-health nurses, although more rarely now than in the past, and by early intervention programs. Approaches to treatment of pediatric undernutrition in the home have been described by public-health nurses (Klein, 1990; Sullivan, 1991; Yoos, 1984). Many multidisciplinary growth clinics use home visiting (Bithoney et al., 1991; Black, Dubowitz, Hutcheson, Berenson-Howard, & Starr, 1995; Drotar, 1991). The advantages and disadvantages of home visiting are discussed thoroughly by Drotar and Crawford (1987).

Home visiting has important advantages in working with pediatric undernutrition. It often strengthens relationships between home visitors and families (Klass, 1997). It also allows the intervenor to meet other family members, which is very important when issues about food selection, feeding, discipline, child behavior, or family relationships are key to improving the child's undernutrition (Figure 2). It also allows one to follow up with families who are unable or not motivated to come into a clinic or an office yet may be willing to accept advice.

During evaluation of undernutrition, home visiting enables a more complete and rapid assessment of the many influences on the child's nutritional intake and overall development. The professional has the opportunity to see specific aspects of the feeding interaction and family interactions that parents would not think to report during a clinic visit. In their own home, parents may bring out their baby book, and one can ask valuable ques-

---

[1]For further information or to receive a Bright Futures Resource Catalog of all publications and related materials, write to 2000 15th Street North, Suite 701, Arlington, VA 22201-2617, call (703) 524-7802, fax (703) 524-9335, or e-mail: BrightFutures@ncemch.org.

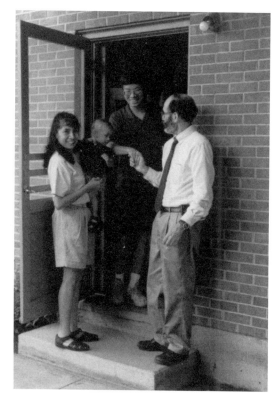

Figure 2.   On a home visit, one can get to know
all of the members of the family.

tions. One may see that a teenage mother feeds her child in the basement to avoid her
mother's supervision and advice and thus have an important clue about family interactions
(Black & Bentley, 1995). Or one may see parents using the television to distract their child
during feeding, anxiously changing channels when the child slows down in eating. One
may see both parents drinking sugary soft drinks and the child going to the refrigerator to
get some. The professional also is exposed to neighborhood and community characteristics
(e.g., violence, social support networks, isolation) that may have an impact on the child as
well. Often, providers develop a sense of empathy for the family's unique circumstances.

Many aspects of intervention with undernutrition lend themselves to intervention via
home visiting. For example, helping parents with difficult feeding interactions, improving
dietary habits, and addressing family communication problems often can be done more
effectively in the naturally occurring environment of the home than in a clinic setting.
Home visiting enables the professional to fit recommendations to changing family needs.
For example, when the professional witnesses improvement in feeding behavior, he or
she can devote time to other family issues. Parents also may put greater credence in advice
that they know is founded on direct knowledge of the child's environment. Observations
of child behavior gathered in clinic settings may be perceived as artificial and not truly
representative.

Disadvantages of home visiting should be considered in program planning. Because of
travel time for professionals, a home visit may take more time than center-based contacts,

although time may be saved in clinic visits. Home visits are expensive and seldom reimbursed in medical settings; however, many early intervention programs for child development routinely employ home visits, and physicians, social services staff, or dietitians may be able to collaborate with others who already are visiting a family. For the professional, home visiting often is more challenging than center-based intervention. There are more people with whom to relate at one time, and the sheer amount of observational information that needs to be processed can be confusing. Professionals may become discouraged when faced with the sobering realities with which families must cope. Families of undernourished children often are multirisk and require interventions in many areas of their functioning.

Because the clinical challenges of intervening in community settings differ from those in center-based programs, all home visitors need support, supervision, or consultation with colleagues to intervene most effectively. New skills, such as how to focus on a limited set of goals in the face of multiple family problems, will need to be acquired by the intervenor. The home visitor also must become well versed in the cultural norms of the family (Slaughter-Defoe, 1993; Wayman, Lynch, & Hanson, 1990). For example, he or she should be ready to be offered not just beverages but actual meals. In some cultural groups, it is important to accept the meals because they are a cultural norm with anyone visiting the home. If the professional or paraprofessional will be visiting a parent of the opposite sex, then he or she should meet the first time with both parents, dress professionally, and ask the parents how they would like to proceed with subsequent visits. In Mexican American and other cultures, it is questionable for a man to visit a mother alone.

In some programs, home visits are assigned to paraprofessionals in the belief that their time is less expensive than that of professionals and that they relate better to parents; however, paraprofessionals actually may be time intensive for programs because they need substantial guidance and support from professionals. As a general guideline, parents whom professionals experience as challenging should be assigned to professional rather than paraprofessional staff.

Although some families may be cautious initially, many families welcome home visits by the child's care provider. Parents often feel more comfortable dealing with professionals when they are on familiar ground rather than in intimidating medical settings. It is important to discuss an upcoming home visit with parents in advance. One way to explain home visiting is the following introduction:

> To understand how we can help you with your child's growth, we'll need a few visits. In the clinic, you'll see the dietitian and the physician (for example). We'll ask you to write down what your child eats. We also find it very helpful to see how children eat at home, so I would like to visit you during a meal. It works best if I come at a time when your child is likely to be interested in eating.

(Further discussion of practical and clinical issues related to home visiting is provided by Klass, 1996, and Wasik, Bryant, & Lyons, 1990.)

Parent Groups and Family Resource Programs

Families benefit from contact with other parents who also are experiencing the stress of coping with an undernourished child and with the medical establishment. Some growth and nutrition service programs organize parent group meetings on a regular basis. They find that the parents learn from one another and benefit from sharing emotional burdens (Figure 3). It can be very supportive, for example, to hear from other parents that they are going through the same worries about feeding their children. A parent volunteer may be able to call other parents and set up meetings; other parents may wish to bring snacks to

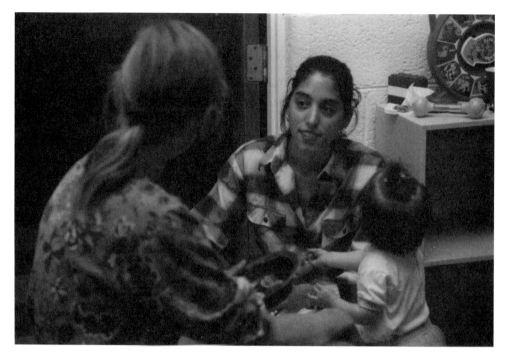

Figure 3.   Parents can gain ideas and support from one another at group meetings.

share. Planning a support group may require arranging for transportation and babysitting. Holding group meetings in the community in a nonclinic setting that can provide a kitchen, easy chairs, and toys goes a long way toward nurturing parents.

Some parents will not feel comfortable with participating in a group, however. In these cases, parents can be referred by providers to Parent to Parent programs (Santelli, Turnbull, Maruis, & Lerner, 1995), which connect parents whose children have similar problems. A newly referred parent is paired with a trained veteran parent of an under-nourished child and/or of a child with developmental delay.

When appropriate, care providers should identify appropriate family resource pro-grams in a family's community and offer the option of referrals. These are community-based programs that provide parent education and support groups, parent–child activities, family drop-in centers, parent-to-parent programs, home-visiting programs, and informa-tion and referral to community agencies (Dunst, 1995). The strength-based philosophy of building on pre-existing family competencies and resources for problem solving is useful for all families. Family resource programs support the parents' sense of personal efficacy and control. Families are encouraged to be active participants in setting personal goals for change, choosing options, and devising action plans.

To identify family support programs, contact local social services agencies. The United Way funds many such programs and can be a valuable referral source. Religious institutions and mental health agencies also are good starting contacts. Many programs for families also are run by cooperative extension specialists. Check local bulletin boards on the Internet for support groups, and tune in to the local access station on cable television. Parenting newspapers, distributed free in many metropolitan areas, are another useful referral source. The Family Resource Coalition of America[2] in Chicago is a national clearinghouse of information on family support programs and can provide resources for families who want to start their own support group.

Programs for families of infants and toddlers can be compared on a continuum of provider role, with traditional expert models at one end and strength-based family support models at the other. Service programs for undernourished children often include medical and human services providers who have been trained in the "expert" advice-giving model. This model tends to view families from the perspectives of disease and therapy and employs the language of medical and nutritional interventions. This approach contrasts with the strength-based model of family support that increasingly characterizes the field of early intervention services.

It would be useful for undernutrition services programs to conduct a self-assessment with staff about the program's philosophy with respect to expert-advice versus strength-based principles. Specifically, to what extent do providers actualize the principles of strength-based family support? When describing families to colleagues, do staff highlight strengths or do they characterize the family as broken and needing to be fixed by focusing on family deficits? Are parents treated as members of the multidisciplinary team and encouraged to participate in decision making about goals for their child and family? What is the nature of professionals' hesitation about implementing a family-centered model of early intervention in pediatric settings? As Dunst stated, "The goal of intervention must be viewed not as 'doing for people' but rather as strengthening the functioning of families to help them become less dependent upon professionals for help" (1995, p. 23).

REFERENCES

Behrman, R. (Ed.). (1993). Home visiting [Special issue]. *The Future of Children, 3*(3).

Bithoney, W.G., McJunkin, J., Michalek, J., Snyder, J., Egan, H., & Epstein, D. (1991). The effect of a multidisciplinary team approach on weight gain in nonorganic failure to thrive children. *Developmental and Behavioral Pediatrics, 12,* 254–258.

Black, M.M., & Bentley, M.E. (1995). Adolescent parenthood: A family-centered, culturally-based perspective. *Pediatric Basics, 73,* 2–9.

Black, M.M., Dubowitz, H., Hutcheson, J., Berenson-Howard, J., & Starr, R.H. (1995). A randomized clinical trial of home intervention for children with failure to thrive. *Pediatrics, 95,* 807–814.

Casamassimo, P. (1997). Bright Futures in practice: Oral health. *The Future of Children, 3,* 172–183.

Drotar, D. (1991). The family context of nonorganic failure to thrive. *American Journal of Orthopsychiatry, 61,* 23–34.

Drotar, D., & Crawford, P. (1987). Using home observation in the clinical assessment of children. *Journal of Clinical Child Psychology, 16,* 342–349.

Drotar, D., & Sturm, L. (1988). Parent–practitioner communication in the management of nonorganic failure to thrive. *Family Systems Medicine, 6,* 304–316.

Dunst, C. (1995). *Key characteristics and features of community-based family support programs.* Chicago: Family Resource Coalition.

Education of the Handicapped Act Amendments of 1986, PL 99-457, 20 U.S.C. §§ 1400 *et seq.*

Green, M. (Ed.). (1994). *Bright futures: Guidelines for health supervision of infants, children, and adolescents.* Arlington, VA: National Center for Education in Maternal and Child Health.

Individuals with Disabilities Education Act Amendments of 1997, PL 105-17, 20 U.S.C. §§ 1400 *et seq.*

Kahler, J., & Sharf, B.F. (1996). From pedagogy to praxis: Affecting communication in an inner city AIDS clinic. In E.B. Ray (Ed.), *Case studies in communication and disenfranchisement* (pp. 31–43). Mahwah, NJ: Lawrence Erlbaum Associates.

---

[2]For information, call (312) 338-0900; write 20 N. Wacker Drive, Suite 1100, Chicago, IL 60606; or visit the World Wide Web site at http//:www.frca.org.

Kalmanson, B., & Seligman, S. (1992). Family–provider relationships: The basis of all interventions. *Infants and Young Children, 4,* 46–52.

Katon, W., & Kleinman, A. (1981). Doctor–patient negotiation and other social science strategies in patient care. In L. Eisenberg & A. Kleinman (Eds.), *The relevance of social science for medicine* (pp. 253–279). Boston: D. Reidel.

Kertesz, J. (1987). Urban family mapping. In R.B. Birrer (Ed.), *Urban family medicine* (pp. 72–81). New York: Springer-Verlag.

Klass, C.S. (1996). *Home visiting: Promoting healthy parent and child development.* Baltimore: Paul H. Brookes Publishing Co.

Klass, C.S. (1997). The home visitor–parent relationship: The linchpin of home visiting. *Zero to Three, 17,* 1–9.

Klein, M.J. (1990). The home health nurse clinician's role in the prevention of nonorganic failure to thrive. *Journal of Pediatric Nursing, 5,* 129–135.

Kleinman, A., Eisenberg, L., & Good, B. (1978). Culture, illness, and care: Clinical lessons from anthropologic and cross-cultural research. *Annals of Internal Medicine, 88,* 251–258.

Powell, D., Batsche, C., Ferro, J., Fox, L., & Dunlap, G. (1997). A strength-based approach in support of multi-risk families: Principles and issues. *Topics in Early Childhood Special Education, 17,* 1–26.

Rauch, J.B., & Curtiss, C.R. (1992). *Taking a family health/genetic history: An ethnocultural learning guide and handbook.* Baltimore: University of Maryland at Baltimore, School of Social Work.

Santelli, B., Turnbull, A.P., Maruis, G., & Lerner, E.P. (1995). Parent to Parent programs: A unique form of mutual support. *Infants and Young Children, 8,* 48–57.

Sharf, B.F., & Kahler, J. (1996). Victims of the franchise: A culturally sensitive model of teaching patient–doctor communication in the inner city. In E.B. Ray (Ed.), *Case studies in communication and disenfranchisement* (pp. 95–115). Mahwah, NJ: Lawrence Erlbaum Associates.

Slaughter-Defoe, D.T. (1993). Home visiting with families in poverty: Introducing the concept of culture. *The Future of Children, 3,* 172–183.

Sturm, L., & Drotar, D. (1992). Communication strategies for working with parents of infants who fail to thrive. *Zero to Three, 12,* 25–28.

Sullivan, B. (1991). Growth-enhancing interventions for nonorganic failure to thrive. *Journal of Pediatric Nursing, 6,* 236–242.

Wasik, B.H., Bryant, D.M., & Lyons, C.M. (1990). *Home visiting: Procedures for helping families.* Thousand Oaks, CA: Sage Publications.

Wayman, K.L., Lynch, E.W., & Hanson, M.J. (1990). Home-based early childhood services: Cultural sensitivity in a family systems approach. *Topics in Early Childhood Special Education, 10,* 56–75.

Worthman, C. (1995). Ethnopediatrics: An outline. *Items, 49,* 6–10.

Yoos, L. (1984). Taking another look at failure to thrive. *American Journal of Maternal–Child Nursing, 9,* 32–36.

Chapter 5

Researching Failure to Thrive Progress, Problems, and Recommendations

Dennis Drotar and Jane Robinson

The importance of psychosocial research concerning failure to thrive (FTT), or pediatric undernutrition, stems from FTT's high incidence and prevalence, significant psychological and medical comorbidity, difficulties of clinical management, risk for long-term health and psychological deficits, and costs to society for medical and psychological intervention (Drotar, 1995; Frank & Drotar, 1994). Continuing research concerning the psychosocial aspects of this complex disorder is very much needed to develop more effective methods of clinical management; however, the significant methodological and logistical challenges of conducting such research with this population have limited the development of scientific knowledge and, ultimately, the quality of care (Boddy & Skuse, 1994; Drotar, 1988). To develop effective strategies to manage the difficulties that are encountered in research with children who experience impaired growth, researchers need to be aware of the characteristic problems and pitfalls that are involved in this work. Accordingly, based on the lessons learned in years of research, this chapter has a threefold purpose: 1) to describe areas of psychosocial research with undernourished children, historically and hereafter referred to simply as *FTT*, and their families, including areas of progress; 2) to describe common methodological, pragmatic, and ethical problems that are encountered in research on FTT; and 3) to recommend approaches to manage these problems in future research.

The assistance of Claudia Weier in the processing of this manuscript is gratefully acknowledged.

SUMMARY OF RESEARCH PROGRESS

Research on FTT has included four basic kinds of studies: 1) description and epidemiology, which is discussed elsewhere in this volume; 2) etiology and risk for FTT; 3) description of associated psychological and family risk factors and impact on children's psychological development; and 4) studies of efficacy of intervention. Researchers have utilized a range of designs to address these topics. Uncontrolled retrospective studies, case reports, and subjective methods predominated in early research on FTT. Although later work has been characterized by more rigorous designs that have included objective measures and more appropriate comparison groups (Drotar, 1988), experimental designs that allow the strongest inferences concerning cause and effect have been infrequent.

The purpose of this section is to give readers a brief summary of progress in major areas of research on FTT. Readers who are interested in more detailed information should consult other research reviews (e.g., Boddy & Skuse, 1994; Casey, 1992; Drotar, 1988, 1995; Frank & Drotar, 1994; Frank & Zeisel, 1988; Lachenmeyer & Davidovicz, 1987; Skuse, 1993).

Etiological Factors

Scientific understanding of the etiology of FTT has been limited by the practical difficulties of identifying and studying children prior to the onset of their growth problems. Because most children generally come to the attention of researchers and practitioners only after growth delay and, in some instances, after the problem has become chronic, scientific knowledge of etiological factors is very limited. Data from the few available prospective studies suggest multifactorial influences on the development of FTT. For example, the Nashville prospective study (Altemeier, O'Connor, Sherrod, & Vietze, 1985) followed mothers from low-income families from the time of their pregnancies to 1 year after the child's birth and identified two sets of risk factors that predicted FTT: 1) mothers' own child-rearing histories, especially reports that their own parents did not give them adequate care when they were children, and 2) current family influences, especially a conflictive relationship with the child's father. In a survey of children in inner-city clinics in London, England, Mathisen, Skuse, Wolke, and Reilly (1989) found that specific physical characteristics such as oral-motor difficulties discriminated children with problematic growth from those who grew normally. Although these few prospective studies have identified potential risk factors, the specific ways in which various risk factors combine to disrupt the child's caloric intake and eventually produce deficient physical growth have yet to be clarified.

Physical and Psychological Problems that Accompany Delayed Growth

Researchers consistently have found that, compared with their physically healthy peers from comparable socioeconomic backgrounds, children with FTT present with a wide range of psychological impairments including cognitive and/or motor developmental problems (Singer & Fagan, 1984); affective disturbances such as social withdrawal (Benoit, 1993a, 1993b; Polan et al., 1991); feeding problems (Benoit, 1993a, 1993b); fussy, demanding behavior (Wolke, Skuse, & Mathisen, 1990); and insecure attachments (Ward, Kessler, & Altman, 1993). These group differences, however, mask considerable variation in type and severity of associated psychological impairments. Some children with FTT have relatively few behavior or psychological problems, whereas others demonstrate multiple and severe difficulties. The origins of such variation largely are unknown. Moreover, the incidence and prevalence of patterns of comorbid behavior and developmental impairments among children who experience growth delays have yet to be identified systematically.

Longer-Term Psychological Outcomes of Failure to Thrive

Several studies have suggested that infants who present with FTT are at risk for behavior problems (Drotar & Sturm, 1992, 1994; Oates, Peacock, & Forrest, 1985), impairments in behavioral organization and control (Drotar & Sturm, 1992, 1994), cognitive impairments (Dowdney, Skuse, Heptinstall, Puckering, & Zur-Szpiro, 1987; Singer & Fagan, 1984), and/or academic difficulties as preschool- and school-age children (Oates et al., 1985); however, the prevalence of behavior and cognitive impairments, especially among school-age children and adolescents with early histories of FTT or undernutrition, has not been well articulated. Moreover, very little is known about early factors that predict individual variations in longer-term psychological outcomes. Follow-up studies of preschoolers who originally were identified as growing poorly at an average of 5 months indicated that less-adaptive family relationships (e.g., more conflict) (Drotar & Sturm, 1992) and insecure attachments at age 12 months (Brinich, Drotar, & Brinich, 1989) predicted the frequency of behavior problems at 4 years of age; however, the factors that predict psychological outcomes among school-age children with early histories of FTT have not been identified.

Studies of Treatment Efficacy

A wide range of interventions have been proposed to manage FTT and accompanying psychological impairments (e.g., hospitalization, comprehensive team management [Berkowitz, 1985; Frank & Drotar, 1994; Peterson, Washington, & Rathbun, 1984], supportive outreach [Drotar, Wilson, & Sturm, 1989], and specialized interventions to enhance feeding and nutrition [Chatoor, Dickson, Schaefer, & Egan, 1985]). Although controlled studies of treatment efficacy have been rare, case reports and series have documented the efficacy of behavioral interventions (Iwata, Riordan, Wohl, & Finney, 1982) as well as parent education to enhance nutrition and physical growth (Pugliese, Weyman-Daum, Moses, & Lifshitz, 1987). A meta-analysis of published studies indicated that children who were hospitalized for FTT generally demonstrated improved physical growth (Fryer, 1988); however, such data are not applicable to current managed care settings in which fewer and fewer children are hospitalized for shorter lengths of stay.

The efficacy of alternative approaches to ambulatory management of FTT has not been evaluated extensively. Bithoney and his colleagues (Bithoney et al., 1989; Bithoney et al., 1991) have documented improved physical growth outcomes among children with FTT who received a comprehensive ambulatory multidisciplinary approach to care compared with those who did not.

Only two randomized controlled trials have assessed the impact of intervention on cognitive development and behavior of children with FTT. Research has indicated that alternative approaches to home visitation that varied in focus (parent versus family centered) and frequency of contact (once per week versus less frequently) did not have differential effects on the physical growth or psychological development of preschool-age children with early histories of FTT ($N = 68$), with one exception: Parent-centered intervention was associated with a lower frequency of behavior problems in 4-year-olds (Drotar & Sturm, 1994). A small sample size, however, may have limited the detection of intervention effects.

Black, Dubowitz, Hutcheson, Berenson-Howard, and Starr (1995) evaluated the effects of family-focused, home-based intervention that was tailored to the typical presenting problems (attachment, feeding, and parenting) in a large sample ($N = 130$) of infants with FTT. Compared with standard pediatric care, family-focused outreach intervention was associated with better developmental outcomes, such as receptive language development, but only among younger children.

GENERAL LIMITATIONS OF AVAILABLE
RESEARCH ON FAILURE TO THRIVE IN CHILDREN

Despite the progress that has been made, considerable gaps remain in scientific understanding of FTT. Moreover, the conclusions that can be drawn from available research
have been limited by several key methodological problems in areas such as sampling,
assessment, and interpretation. This section considers these methodological and practical
problems that typically are encountered in research on FTT and ways of managing them.

Sampling

Sampling issues present significant challenges in research on FTT. Table 1 outlines major
sources of variation in sampling characteristics in studies of FTT, their impact on findings,
and suggested approaches for management. These variations, described in more detail
next, include issues in definition and assessment, influence of settings from which samples
are drawn, referral practices and biases, sample heterogeneity, additional criteria, impact
of parent refusal to participate and sample attrition, and difficulties with obtaining access
to participants.

Issues in Definition and Assessment

Ambiguities in the definition and concept of FTT (Casey, 1992; Smith & Berenberg, 1970)
coupled with varied operational definitions have made comparability of samples and,
hence, generalizability of findings across different sites a recurrent problem (Drotar, 1989).
Moreover, the large number of environmental and organic factors that can influence physical growth limit reliable categorization of FTT into organic and nonorganic factors
(Bithoney & Dubowitz, 1985). In addition, specific criteria that have been proposed to
identify nonorganic FTT (NFTT), such as weight gain with improved nutrition (Bell &
Woolston, 1985) or behavior impairments (Powell, Low, & Speers, 1987; Rosenn, Loeb, &
Jura, 1980) cannot be regarded as definitive. Finally, experienced clinicians and researchers
have questioned the validity of a hard and fast dichotomy between organic and nonorganic
FTT because many children who have growth deficiencies have at least one "organic" problem: nutritional deficiency, which has well-documented effects on children's physical status and behavior (Bithoney & Dubowitz, 1985; Casey, 1992; Frank & Drotar, 1994).

Influence of Settings from Which Samples Are Drawn

Over and beyond the problems that are related to reliable definition and identification of
FTT, several other sampling factors have important effects. For example, the type of clinical setting from which children and families are recruited can influence sample selection
and, hence, findings. For example, compared with children who are recruited from ambulatory care settings (Drotar, 1990), hospitalized children are more likely to have severe
FTT that has not responded to treatment. Children who are recruited from clinics in areas
that are at an economic disadvantage would be expected to have higher frequencies of family risk factors and, hence, associated psychological problems than those who are recruited
from private pediatric practices.

Because most infants with FTT receive some form of medical, psychological, or
nutritional treatment, it is very difficult to study this problem apart from the influence of
pediatric diagnostic and treatment practices. The content, structure, intensity, and frequency of treatments given to children and their families, which vary considerably as a
function of accompanying problems, treatment resources, and so forth, may influence family members' participation in research and/or the child's health and psychological outcome

Table 1. Sources of variation in sampling characteristics in FTT

	Source of variation	Possible impact	Suggested approach
I.	Definition of growth deficiency	Growth norms Variations in criteria for growth deficiency (type and severity)	Variations in incidence and severity of FTT limit generalizability of findings	Use National Center for Health Statistics growth norms and weight-for-age to define FTT; growth deceleration and weight-for-height are useful supplementary criteria
II.	Diagnostic procedures used to identify NFTT	Number and type of physical diagnostic tests Psychosocial assessment Weight gain in controlled environment	Variations in application of criteria and level of ascertainment limit generalizability of findings; psychosocial factors are unreliable	Use comprehensive diagnostic approach, specify diagnostic procedures, apply criteria uniformly, use pediatric case review
III.	Additional exclusionary/ inclusionary criteria	Sample restrictions (e.g., prematurity, child abuse, age)	Helpful way to reduce variation in risk factors; limit generalizability of findings	Provide detailed rationale and description of criteria, consider impact on findings
IV.	Population from which sample is drawn	Type of pediatric setting Type of clinical population	Influences biological and environmental risk factors and psychological outcomes	Describe population from which samples are drawn, consider effect of sample characteristics on findings, recruit samples from multiple settings, utilize comparison groups
V.	Self-selection and attrition	Refusals and/or dropouts	Introduces sampling bias; limit generalizability and validity of findings	Obtain information concerning characteristics of refusals and attrition and compare with study group
VI.	Treatment services	Differences in duration, intensity, and type of medical or psychosocial treatment	Can obscure group differences; limit detectability of treatment effects and comparability of findings across settings	Carefully describe treatment services in local setting
VII.	Sample heterogeneity	Biological, family, and psychological characteristics	Influences findings concerning outcomes; factors may be difficult to control	Include comprehensive description of sampling characteristics, study subgroups of NFTT, utilize control groups, recruit large samples,

81

(Drotar, 1990). The pediatric and supportive care received by children with FTT and their families poses a special problem in evaluating treatment outcome studies because it may obscure the effects of the specific psychosocial treatment under investigation.

Referral Practices and Biases

Referral practices exert another set of important but little-recognized influences on research findings. Some practitioners have their own implicit criteria for the definition of a child with growth deficiency. Moreover, research has found that, in an attempt to be helpful to investigators, some practitioners may attempt to screen out parents with severe psychopathology or identify the most highly motivated patients (Drotar & Sturm, 1994). Another problem is that pediatricians may underidentify the incidence of children with FTT in families of higher socioeconomic status (SES). Potential problems with referral bias are not restricted to children with FTT but can involve the recruitment of comparison groups. For example, parents of physically healthy, normally growing children may be selected because they are viewed as having exemplary parenting skills or as being especially cooperative. Selective recruitment of such children and families in comparison groups erroneously can inflate differences on psychosocial characteristics between the children with FTT and controls.

Sample Heterogeneity

Depending on the setting in which they are recruited, samples of children who have growth deficiencies will differ on a wide range of clinically relevant variables, such as 1) psychosocial etiology (e.g., parental underfeeding based on misinformation and serious attachment problems), 2) history of growth deficiency (e.g., age of onset, duration, rate of growth deceleration), 3) prior or concurrent family environmental risk factors (e.g., level of family stability and/or conflict), 4) prior or concurrent biologic risk factors (e.g., prematurity, birth complications), 5) severity of growth and nutritional deficiency, and 6) demographic factors (e.g., child's gender, race, family income, parental age, education). Risk factors and associated characteristics influence the nature and interpretation of findings, especially in studies that compare children who have FTT with physically healthy children. Because the levels of psychological morbidity (e.g., behavior and developmental problems) that are found to be associated with FTT vary dramatically as a function of associated risk factors in the specific population from which children are selected, associated morbidity can be attributed erroneously to the child's FTT alone.

Additional Criteria

Some investigators have utilized other inclusionary or exclusionary criteria (e.g., age, presence of child abuse) to reduce the considerable variation in samples of children who have FTT. Although this generally is a useful practice, in some studies, the nature of the criteria that are used and the specific rationale for them are not specified clearly. Moreover, investigators do not always consider the impact of these secondary criteria on the generalizability of their findings.

Impact of Parent Refusal to Participate and Sample Attrition

Researchers who conduct research with the parents of children who have FTT face considerable challenges in engaging and maintaining families in their studies. Many parents of children who have FTT are highly stressed by financial and family problems that limit their availability and readiness to participate in research protocols. Some parents prove to be very difficult to contact to discuss their participation in research. Others may be threatened by potential involvement in psychological research and refuse to participate. Such parents may believe that if they participate, then their parenting skills will be criticized or they will be viewed as neglecting their child.

As is the case for other populations of children who participate in research (Beck, Collins, Overholser, & Terry, 1984), it is very possible that parents who are not available for their consent or who refuse to participate may have more psychological problems than those who participate. Unfortunately, most studies of children who have FTT have not reported rates of subject refusal or the characteristics of participants versus nonparticipants, let alone considered the potential impact of sample self-selection on their findings (Drotar, 1990).

Other problems are raised by sample attrition. Children who have FTT often come from families who are highly stressed and at an economic disadvantage and who move a great deal, do not have consistent access to transportation, and have difficulty attending scheduled visits; thus, even when parents of children who have FTT have consented to research, they may have difficulty participating, especially in prospective studies. Consequently, rates of sample attrition in prospective studies of children who have FTT tend to be high, in some cases 50% or more (Fitch et al., 1976), which clearly can threaten the validity of findings. Similar to other high-risk populations (Aylward, Hatcher, Stripp, Gustafson, & Leavitt, 1985), families of infants with FTT who cannot be located for follow-up would be expected to have greater frequencies of associated psychosocial problems than those for whom complete data can be obtained.

Difficulties Obtaining Access to Participants

Researchers who do not provide care to children who have FTT may have difficulty obtaining access to such children and their families for several reasons. First, practitioners are very busy and may not have time to identify potential participants. Second, the prospect of identifying children who have FTT from one's practice may be threatening to practitioners. Third, practitioners may not believe that the research is relevant to their practice. Consequently, investigators have an important challenge in developing collaborations with practitioners who work with children with FTT.

Assessment

Researchers who work with children with FTT need to contend with special problems in assessment. These include problems in selecting measures that are appropriate for this population and difficulties that arise from assessing parents and other family members.

Problems in Selecting Appropriate Measures

Researchers who evaluate psychosocial outcomes of children with FTT and their families face difficult challenges in selecting measures that test their research questions effectively and have adequate reliability and validity. The problems of measurement selection are magnified because researchers often are interested in assessing a broad range of domains that are related to the psychological development, parent–child interaction and relationships, and family of the child with FTT. As shown in Table 2, a broad range of measures are available; however, very few of them have been developed for and standardized on children with FTT. Consequently, researchers cannot be certain that measures are applicable directly to or feasible for use in research with children who have FTT or their families. Moreover, some available measures have limited reliability or validity for any population.

Special Problems in Assessing Parents and Family Members

Data from assessments of parents of children who have FTT may prove to be difficult to obtain or interpret for various reasons. For example, parents who are especially threat-

Table 2. Assessment of psychosocial factors in failure to thrive

Domain of assessment	Sample assessment methods	Information obtained
Child's Psychological Status		
Cognitive development	Bayley Scale of Mental Development (Bayley, 1993); Fagan Test (Fagan, Singer, Montie, & Shepherd, 1986)	Cognitive strengths and deficits
Social and affective responsiveness	Bayley Infant Behavior Record (Wolf & Lozoff, 1985); Rating Scales (Wolke et al., 1990)	Child's degree of social withdrawal; adaptive response to objects
Behavior during feeding	Observations and rating scales (Linscheid & Rasnake, 1985); mealtime behavior (Heptinstall et al., 1987); parent–child interaction (Clark, 1985)	Presence of behavioral feeding problems and skill deficits
Parent–Child Relationship	Ratings of mother–child interaction (Ainsworth, Blehar, Waters, & Wall, 1978; Barnard, 1987; Clark, 1985; Wolke et al., 1990)	Strengths and deficits in parent–child relationship
Family Environment		
Stimulation provided to child	HOME scale (Caldwell & Bradley, 1984)	Level of stimulation provided by family members
Family structure	Interview, family tree (Hartman, 1979)	Family structure
Family resources	Interview concerning finances and food (Frank & Drotar, 1994)	Level of family resources and depletion
Family stress	Interview, Parenting Stress Inventory (Abidin, 1985); Family Inventory of Life Events (McCubbin & Patterson, 1988); CRISYS (Shalowitz, Berry, Rasinski, & Dannhausen-Braun, in press)	Level of family stress
Family relationships and support	Family Environment Scale (Moos & Moos, 1976); FACES (Olson, 1986); Social Support (Heitzman & Kaplan, 1988)	Family functioning and relationships
Parental beliefs about FTT	Parent Interview (Drotar & Sturm, 1988; Sturm & Drotar, 1991)	Parental beliefs about causes and consequences of FTT

ened by participation in research and concerned about how the information from their responses will be used may give defensive, minimal answers that are misleading and, hence, inconclusive.

Another set of problems concerns the application of measures that have been standardized on populations that are very different from the families of children with FTT. For example, measures of life stresses that were standardized on middle-class families may not capture adequately the life events that are applicable to families of many children with FTT who are seen in clinical settings. Moreover, family members who are at an educational disadvantage or who are from different cultural backgrounds may have difficulty reading and understanding questionnaires that have been standardized on different populations. Other parents may have difficulty responding to certain items in measures because of emotional problems, such as depression (Singer, Song, Hill, & Jaffe, 1990).

Observer Bias

One of the most important problems in measurement of children with FTT is the potential for observer bias. Observers who are aware of the child's growth deficit may assess the child's psychological status in a biased manner, especially when they are aware of the study hypotheses. This is a special problem in studies that compare children who have FTT with normally growing children.

Interpreting Data

Growth delay is a broad, descriptive term that does not in and of itself provide any information concerning specific etiological factors or influences on the child's behavior or development. Consequently, when investigators obtain differences between children with growth delays (or their families) on behavior or developmental measures, it is very difficult to know what accounts for them. One of the most common misinterpretations of data is to attribute to the child's FTT findings (e.g., presence of behavior problems) that may be accounted for by other risk factors (e.g., low SES) that commonly are associated with FTT. This is a special problem in uncontrolled studies or in research in which potentially relevant cofactors, such as SES, are not controlled for carefully.

Another common misinterpretation of data is to attribute findings to psychological or family risk factors rather than to associated physical or nutritional problems. This is a special problem in FTT research because chronic mild malnutrition, which, by definition, is associated with FTT, usually is related to other biological and environmental risk factors (Wachs, 1995). Moreover, physical symptoms and nutritional deficits, which can affect the child's development and behavior, commonly are associated with FTT (Black & Dubowitz, 1991).

Special Ethical Issues

Although FTT clearly is not synonymous with neglect or abuse, very difficult clinical and ethical challenges can arise when these problems do overlap (Frank & Drotar, 1994). Researchers may encounter situations in which they may ascertain levels of neglect or abuse among children with FTT that warrant reporting to child protective services agencies. When such reports are made, investigators no longer can keep research data confidential and thereby enter into a very different relationship with the family than was described in the initial consent procedures. In such instances, it is appropriate to drop child and family from the research.

A related problem is raised by the fact that a subset of families of children who have FTT may, in fact, expose themselves to greater scrutiny concerning neglect by participating in a study than they would by not participating. Investigators face a significant dilemma in such cases. If they inform families about the potential for ascertainment of neglect, then they may have difficulty recruiting families to participate in research. If they do not inform families of the potential for ascertainment of neglect, then the consent procedure is not truly informed. Informing families about investigators' legal obligation to report instances of abuse and neglect in the consent form provides the necessary information without causing major difficulties in recruitment (D. Kessler, personal communication, January 1997).

Another type of ethical problem may arise when families are coerced in some way to participate in research. For example, in the course of conducting a treatment outcome study (Drotar et al., 1985), some house staff informed families that they needed to participate in our research; otherwise, they could risk reports to child protective services. Clearly, this was coercion rather than informed consent. In this instance, the relevant physicians needed to be informed about this problem and implement standardized procedures to present the study to families in such a way as to preserve their right to refuse.

The conduct of treatment outcome studies with children who have FTT poses special ethical problems. Because it is not ethical to withhold interventions from children with FTT, true no-treatment control groups cannot be utilized.

RECOMMENDATIONS TO ENHANCE THE QUALITY OF RESEARCH ON FAILURE TO THRIVE

The methodological, practical, and ethical problems that are involved with research of children who are undernourished or who have FTT are difficult but not insurmountable. Experience suggests that investigators can either avoid or minimize the influence of these problems by planning carefully and anticipating potential problems. This section offers suggestions for such planning.

Carefully Select Sampling Criteria

Various strategies can be used to evaluate and manage the sampling problems that typically are encountered in research with children who have FTT (see Table 1). Researchers should consider carefully the rationale for each criterion that they use to select children who have FTT and state these clearly in the method. For example, is the criterion used to reduce heterogeneity of the sample? Is it to limit the influence of specific confounding influences on growth (e.g., exclusion of infants who are born small for gestational age)?

Investigators should differentiate between primary criteria that are used to describe the child's FTT (e.g., weight-for-age below the 5th percentile) and secondary criteria that are used to identify the specific population of interest (e.g., FTT or growth delay that is not attributable to chronic disease). Depending on the purpose of their study, investigators may employ other criteria (e.g., selecting children of selected ages) to increase the homogeneity of their samples and to improve the clarity of interpretation of findings; however, in selecting their criteria, researchers should consider carefully sample size. Researchers need to have access to a large sample size to be most selective in setting criteria.

Define Organic Problems Clearly and Independently

It is unlikely that any available classification system can distinguish reliably between organic and nonorganic FTT (Skuse, 1993); however, depending on the purpose of the study, samples can be selected to minimize the impact of various acute and chronic physical conditions on children's growth (Frank & Drotar, 1994). For example, to answer many questions concerning FTT, it is appropriate to exclude children who have chronic physical conditions (e.g., heart disease, renal problems), which clearly affect physical growth. Conversely, investigators who primarily are interested in identifying how environmental or family influences affect physical growth of children with specific organic conditions might want to include these children. Irrespective of the specific focus of the study, defining physical or organic factors that may relate to physical growth is difficult. Woolston's (1985) scoring system, which assesses the degree of organicity that is associated with FTT, should be considered as a method to describe physical status.

Carefully Consider the Effects of Risk Factors on Growth

Investigators who are interested primarily in psychosocial influence or outcomes in FTT also will need to define and control for physical factors. Dowdney et al. (1987) noted that it is important to control for birth weight and genetic potential for growth in evaluating the extent of FTT. Consequently, depending on the purpose of the study, it may be necessary to exclude children who had low birth weight or who were small for gestational age.

Employ Population-Based or Multisite Samples When Possible

The overwhelming majority of studies of children who have FTT have gathered data from children at only one site. Such data have limited generalizability. Population-based studies (see Skuse, 1993) and multisite studies clearly are needed to enhance the generalizability of findings in FTT (Drotar, 1994). Although large multisite studies are beyond the resources of most researchers, it often is possible to collect data at more than one clinical site in the same geographical location.

Ensure that Sampling Criteria Are Applied Uniformly

Investigators need to ensure that their criteria are applied uniformly on the sample of interest. This can be done by defining criteria clearly prior to the study and implementing uniform recruitment procedures throughout the study. Investigators also should develop strategies to limit the potential biases that are involved in having practitioners identify and select their samples. Practitioners are very busy and may underidentify or refer FTT in highly selective ways. Consequently, identification of patients from clinic records, databases, and charts provides a more effective way than referral to ensure that all patients who fit the investigator's criteria for FTT have an equal chance of being identified and included in the study. Researchers who have no other choice except to rely heavily on practitioners' referrals as the sole source of identifying subjects should work closely with their colleagues to inform them of their criteria and to impress upon them the need to use objective criteria. For ease of explanation of the study and to reduce variation in how the study is presented to families, researchers should standardize the language and information that is used by the project staff and practitioners to describe the study to families.

Carefully Describe Procedures for Criteria, Sampling, and Sample Recruitment

Investigators should describe the specific criteria for FTT and procedures that were used to recruit their sample in sufficient detail to allow others to replicate them. Such information should include which patients were included and how they were identified (by referral, chart review, or both) and recruited (e.g., who approached parents to obtain their consent, specific methods that were used).

Describe the Characteristics of Nonparticipants and Dropouts

Most investigators will not be able to prevent dropouts from their studies or to ensure 100% participation rate; however, they can provide a careful description of their samples, including the number and characteristics of children and families (e.g., ages, gender, SES, severity of growth delay) who participated and those who chose not to participate (Drotar, 1990), as well as information from parents concerning why they did not participate (e.g., lack of time). A careful description of those families who chose to participate initially but then could not be reached or dropped out of the study, together with a description of the reasons for attrition (e.g., refused to continue, unable to locate family), also should be provided. Finally, investigators should compare participants versus nonparticipants, and dropouts versus nondropouts, on demographic characteristics to document whether there are any obvious differences in these groups that could bias or otherwise influence their findings (Aylward et al., 1985).

Use Comparison Groups to Facilitate Stronger Inferences

Investigators should design their studies carefully to include comparison groups to control for factors that could generate competing or alternative interpretations of their data. Depending on the study question, these comparison groups could involve normally growing children or children with a clear organic basis to their FTT and growth delay. Designing studies to assess the outcomes of subgroups of children who have FTT that differ on clinically relevant characteristics of interest (e.g., family dysfunction, presence of clinically significant parent–child relationship problems) provides a useful but little-used approach, albeit one that requires large numbers of children.

STRATEGIES FOR IMPLEMENTING DATA COLLECTION

As in research with other clinical populations, a well-conceived study design and data analysis are necessary but not sufficient ingredients of a successful study. Investigators need to implement the data collection effectively. The considerable obstacles that limit recruitment and maintenance of samples require researchers to plan ways to implement their study and anticipate problems that could arise. The following sections suggest ways to accomplish this.

Enhance Collaboration with Practitioners

Researchers need to work very hard to ensure that pediatricians, nurse practitioners, and other health care providers who are in a position to identify and recruit families to participate in research understand the purpose of their study and want to help recruit families for the study. Even when they are interested, most practitioners are extremely busy and find it difficult, if not impossible, to invest very much additional time in research. For this reason, for maximum effectiveness, researchers should develop the resources to support additional staff (e.g., research assistants) to reduce the time that is required from practitioners in implementing the study. Such resources can be developed by recruiting student volunteers and/or by funding small research grants.

Researchers also should maximize the incentives to their colleagues to participate in research. Most clinicians will want to know how this research will benefit their patients. It may be helpful to have practitioners participate as actively as possible by soliciting their ideas concerning strategies of recruitment, study design, and logistics and informing them in detail about all procedures.

Develop Strategies to Enhance Family Participation and Reduce Attrition

Several strategies can increase the likelihood that parents of children who have FTT will participate in research. First, it is very important to have the child's primary health practitioner (physician or nurse) make the initial contact with the families to inform them of the general purpose of the study. Second, investigators should make sure that they spend a good deal of time with the family to discuss the purpose of the study and the nature of their participation. Parents often are confused and frustrated that no one has found a cause for their child's growth delays or concerned that they will be blamed for their child's problem. For this reason, parents should be given ample opportunity to express their concerns about their child's condition and about participating in the study. The opportunity for dialogue between families and investigators also is necessary to ensure that families understand what is expected of them in the research and that their consent truly is informed.

To reduce sample attrition, it is necessary to address practical barriers that may limit parents' participation. For example, increasing parents' access to transportation by reimbursing for bus fare, providing coupons for taxis, and paying for parking may increase participation. Similarly, it may be necessary to provide supervision for siblings during the research, thus relieving parents of the burden of finding child care while they participate. Offering families payment for their time also can enhance their participation as can offering copies of videotaped interactions of their child's performance on tasks (Black et al., 1995).

Several steps can be taken prior to the scheduled appointment to maximize participation rates. For example, once the research appointment is scheduled, send a letter with the pertinent information and reconfirm with a telephone call 1 day prior to the appointment. For the purpose of contacting parents, obtain several telephone numbers and additional addresses. Parents usually are willing to give a telephone number and address where messages can be left (e.g., their mother's, sister's, or friend's home), which is important, given the potential for moves and telephone disconnections and so forth. Information about the family network also can be critical in maintaining contact during prospective studies.

Once parents have agreed to participate, it is very important to maintain close contact with them over the course of the study in as many ways as are feasible. For example, a thank-you letter serves as an expression of appreciation for their participation and provides families with a staff member's telephone number should questions and concerns arise. Birthday cards (for the child or the mother), holiday greetings, and/or regular telephone contact to inquire about the child's progress are other helpful vehicles to keep families aware of the study and motivated to participate.

Carefully Consider Choice of Measures

As shown in Table 2, researchers have many choices concerning measures that are suitable for children who have FTT and their families. To avoid overburdening parents of children with FTT, who often are highly stressed, investigators should be very selective in their choice of measures. Just because a measure is available does not mean that it should be used. The focus should be on measures that are most central to study hypotheses and that have adequate reliability and validity. Special caution should be observed in using measures for research on FTT that have not been used in similar populations. If investigators choose to use such measures, then they should test the feasibility of the measures in pilot work and document psychometric properties (i.e., reliability and validity) in their research.

Reduce Observer Bias

Investigators should anticipate and take steps to reduce the bias that can be involved in data collection. Several strategies may be helpful in this regard. For example, all staff who conduct assessments should not be aware of the study hypotheses and should have no or little information about the children (including their growth or physical status) who are enrolled in the study. Biases can be limited by giving to staff who collect data very specific instructions that clarify the need for objective information and by structuring the data-collection task as much as possible.

To provide a check on observer bias, it is useful for investigators to ask staff who are conducting assessments and observations whether they were aware of the study hypotheses and children's growth status. When it is not possible to keep observers blind or when researchers ascertain that their assessments were not conducted in a blind manner, they should consider how this bias might affect interpretation of their findings.

Enhance Quality Control of Data

Investigators should take several steps to ensure that their protocols are carried out in a standardized fashion, which is very difficult to accomplish in clinical settings. For example, to reduce the inherent threats to the validity of research that is conducted in clinical settings (e.g., practitioners' biases, inconsistent records), investigators should develop forms to help ensure that data are gathered in a standardized fashion and that criteria are applied uniformly for each subject. Research staff such as project coordinators are invaluable for ensuring that the protocol's procedures are applied uniformly within the same site but are most critical for research that takes place across different sites. Investigators should meet periodically with their staff to review and structure procedures for recruitment and data collection, including forms to monitor the quality of data. Assessment of interrater reliability, including assessment of potential changes in reliability, across the period of data collection is critical, especially in observational studies.

Enhance Quality of Assessment

The quality of data that are obtained from families can be enhanced by taking time to ensure that parents understand the questions that are asked of them and by choosing measures that are appropriate for the cultural backgrounds and literacy levels of families that participate in research. In some instances, modification of procedures, such as reading items to family members, may be necessary. Investigators also should employ measures that are appropriate to the specific cultural characteristics and stresses that are experienced by families of children who present with FTT in various settings. Shalowitz, Berry, Rasinski, & Dannhausen-Braun (in press) developed a measure of life events, the Crisis in Family Systems Scale, which was derived from the experiences of inner-city families, that is applicable to families of children with FTT who would be expected to have similar experiences.

Manage Ethical Issues

Investigators who conduct research with children who have FTT or undernutrition and their families should be especially sensitive to issues that are related to informed consent. It is important that families understand clearly the essentials of what is expected of them and are not coerced to participate. To help ensure that families understand what is expected of them, researchers should ask them to repeat their understanding of the procedures before they sign consent. Moreover, investigators need to monitor carefully how the study is presented to families by various practitioners to ensure that the study is presented clearly in a noncoercive manner. Investigators who conduct treatment studies can avoid the ethical problems involved in withholding treatment to families of children who have FTT by comparing alternative types of treatment or by comparing a new treatment with traditional care that reaches an acceptable clinical standard (see Bithoney et al., 1989; Bithoney et al., 1991). State-level reporting requirements for child abuse and neglect that occurs among research participants should be reviewed carefully (Liss, 1994).

EVALUATING PUBLISHED RESEARCH ON FAILURE TO THRIVE

Given the problems that are inherent in research on FTT, consumers of published research should read past, current, and future literature in this area with a critical eye and ask the following questions:

- From which setting and population is the study sample recruited?
- Is the sample size adequate in terms of statistical power?
- Is this sample generalizable to the children whom I see in my setting?
- Are the criteria for the sample defined and rationalized clearly?
- Did the investigator describe families who refused to participate and sample attrition? (See Drotar, 1989, for a more detailed discussion of sampling considerations.)
- Are the research questions and hypotheses defined clearly?
- Did the investigator include controls that are appropriate to the study question?
- Have risk factors that would affect outcomes been considered in the design?
- Are the measures that were chosen appropriate to the design in question?
- Are the measures reliable and valid?
- Have they been used previously in a sample of children who have FTT?
- Are the measures appropriate for this population in terms of SES and so forth?
- Are the conclusions that are drawn warranted by the data?
- Do the data have clinical implications for management of FTT? If so, then are these implications justified?
- Are informed consent procedures described?
- Does the investigator consider relevant ethical issues?

RESEARCH QUESTIONS AND PRIORITIES

Despite progress (e.g., Black et al., 1995; Drotar, 1995), research concerning the psychosocial aspects of FTT is very much in its infancy. Consequently, the field is wide open for researchers who are sufficiently knowledgeable and persistent to take up the challenges. A review of the literature suggests several priorities for future research. One important set of questions concerns individual differences in psychological risk and prognosis. For example, it will be important to determine whether infants who have growth deficiencies with particular clusters of behavior and family characteristics at point of diagnosis demonstrate differential prognosis and/or responsiveness to intervention (Ayoub & Milner, 1985).

The impact of developmental factors such as age of onset on the expression of FTT and psychological outcomes also is not well understood. Do age and developmental stage make a difference in the types of presenting problems and, hence, in the nature of intervention that is needed? In an instructive example of the kind of research that is needed, Black et al. (1995) observed that mothers of toddlers with NFTT (ages 13–26 months) experienced more difficulty in feeding interactions than did mothers of 8- to 13-month-old infants with NFTT.

Description of the longer-term psychological and family outcomes of children with early histories of undernutrition is another high-priority research area, especially given Galler, Ramsey, Solimano, and Lowell's (1985) finding that school-age children with early histories of malnutrition demonstrated significant behavior and attention problems. Given the considerable variation in the quality of psychological outcomes that has been observed among children with FTT, longer-term outcome studies also should focus on identifying factors that predict psychological risk versus resilience.

Studies also are needed to document the factors that account for the higher rates of behavior and developmental problems and parent–child relationship difficulties that have been observed in children who have FTT compared with normally growing children of comparable SES. In this regard, testing specific models of how parental behaviors (e.g., emotional responsiveness) affect the psychological development of children who have FTT is of particular importance. Empirical studies of family contextual variables, especially family relationships and parental competence (Belsky, 1984), also would help to clarify the processes that contribute to risk versus resilience among children who fail to thrive. Fathers of infants with FTT or undernutrition thus far have received remarkably little empirical scrutiny and should be studied in future research (Drotar & Sturm, 1987).

A final set of critical research questions concerns evaluation of services and treatment programs for children with FTT. Although all pediatric hospitals manage FTT, only some have specialized treatment programs for infants who have this condition. Little systematic information is available, however, about which families participate in these programs, the quality of their participation, or the outcomes of children and families (Drotar, 1995). Information from case reports that assess the efficacy of treatment approaches that are tailored to subgroups of children who have FTT, using detailed baseline and follow-up data, also is needed.

Close integration of research and clinical practice will be needed to advance scientific knowledge concerning how best to manage the complex spectrum of problems that are subsumed under the general label of *FTT,* or *pediatric undernutrition,* a term preferred by the editors of this volume. To enhance such integration, practitioners who see large numbers of children should either team up with researchers or develop research skills that are necessary for conducting clinical research of undernourished children who present in clinical settings. Studies of morbidity and service utilization, including the costs and benefits of various approaches to diagnosis and/or intervention, very much are needed. In some instances, studies of the efficacy of intervention also can be used to convince health care planners and administrators concerning the necessity of services for this population. Black and her colleagues have noted that the findings from their intervention studies were highly influential in convincing the Maryland Department of Health and Mental Hygiene to provide resources to develop a comprehensive pediatric clinic for children with FTT (M. Black, personal communication, December 1993). Black and her colleagues' work provides an excellent example of how research findings can be used to enhance the services that are provided to children who have FTT. It is hoped that her experience and the information presented here encourage others to take on the challenges of research with children who have FTT and their families.

REFERENCES

Abidin, R. (1985). *Parenting Stress Index.* Charlottesville, VA: Pediatric Psychology Press.

Ainsworth, M.D.S., Blehar, M.D., Waters, E., & Wall, S. (1978). *Patterns of attachment.* Mahwah, NJ: Lawrence Erlbaum Associates.

Altemeier, W.A., O'Connor, S., Sherrod, K., & Vietze, P. (1985). Prospective study of antecedents for non-organic failure to thrive. *Journal of Pediatrics, 106,* 360–365.

Aylward, G.P., Hatcher, R.P., Stripp, B., Gustafson, N.F., & Leavitt, C.P. (1985). Who goes and who stays: Subject loss in a multicenter longitudinal follow-up study. *Journal of Developmental and Behavioral Pediatrics, 6,* 3–8.

Ayoub, C.C., & Milner, J.S. (1985). Failure to thrive: Parental indicators, types and outcomes. *Child Abuse & Neglect, 9,* 491–499.

Barnard, K. (1987). *The Nursing Child Assessment Satellite Training.* Seattle: University of Washington.

Bayley, N. (1993). *Bayley Scales of Infant Development* (2nd ed.). San Antonio, TX: The Psychological Corporation.

Beck, S., Collins, L., Overholser, J., & Terry, K. (1984). A comparison of children who receive and who do not receive permission to participate in research. *Journal of Abnormal Child Psychology, 12,* 575–580.

Bell, L.S., & Woolston, J.L. (1985). The relationship of weight gain and caloric intake in infants with organic and nonorganic failure to thrive syndrome. *Journal of the American Academy of Child Psychiatry, 24,* 447–452.

Belsky, J. (1984). The determinants of parenting: A process model. *Child Development, 55,* 83–96.

Benoit, D. (1993a). Failure to thrive and feeding disorders. In C.H. Zeanah, Jr. (Ed.), *Handbook of infant mental health* (pp. 317–331). New York: Guilford Press.

Benoit, D. (1993b). Phenomenology and treatment of failure to thrive. *Child and Adolescent Psychiatric Clinics of North America, 2,* 61–73.

Berkowitz, C. (1985). Comprehensive pediatric management of failure to thrive: An interdisciplinary approach. In D. Drotar (Ed.), *New directions in failure to thrive: Implications for research and practice* (pp. 193–211). New York: Plenum.

Bithoney, W.G., & Dubowitz, H. (1985). Organic concomitants of nonorganic failure to thrive: Implications for research. In D. Drotar (Ed.), *New directions in failure to thrive: Implications for research and practice* (pp. 47–68). New York: Plenum.

Bithoney, W.G., McJunkin, J., Michalek, J., Egan, H., Snyder, J., & Munier, A. (1989). Prospective evaluation of weight gain in both nonorganic and organic failure-to-thrive children: An outpatient trial of a multidisciplinary team intervention strategy. *Journal of Developmental and Behavioral Pediatrics, 10,* 27–31.

Bithoney, W.G., McJunkin, J., Michalek, J., Snyder, J., Egan, H., & Epstein, M. (1991). The effect of a multidisciplinary team approach on weight gain in nonorganic failure-to-thrive children. *Journal of Developmental and Behavioral Pediatrics, 12,* 254–258.

Black, M., & Dubowitz, H. (1991). Failure-to-thrive: Lessons from animal models and developing countries. *Journal of Developmental and Behavioral Pediatrics, 12,* 259–267.

Black, M., Dubowitz, H., Hutcheson, J., Berenson-Howard, J., & Starr, R.H. (1995). A randomized clinical trial of home intervention for children with failure to thrive. *Pediatrics, 95,* 807–814.

Black, M.M., Hutcheson, J.J., Dubowitz, H., & Berenson-Howard, J. (1994). Parenting style and developmental status among children with nonorganic failure to thrive. *Journal of Pediatric Psychology, 19,* 689–707.

Boddy, J.M., & Skuse, D.H. (1994). Annotation: The process of parenting in failure to thrive. *Journal of Child Psychology and Psychiatry, 35,* 491–524.

Brinich, L., Drotar, D., & Brinich, P. (1989). Security of attachment and outcome of preschoolers with histories of nonorganic failure to thrive. *Journal of Clinical Child Psychology, 18,* 142–152.

Caldwell, B.M., & Bradley, R.H. (1984). *Home Observation for the Measurement of the Environment.* Little Rock: University of Arkansas, Center for Child Development and Education.

Casey, P.H. (1992). Failure to thrive. In M.D. Levine, W.B. Carey, & A.C. Crocker (Eds.), *Developmental-behavioral pediatrics* (2nd ed., pp. 375–383). Philadelphia: W.B. Saunders.

Chatoor, I., Dickson, L., Schaefer, S., & Egan, J. (1985). A developmental classification of feeding disorders associated with failure to thrive: Diagnosis and treatment. In D. Drotar (Ed.), *New directions in failure to thrive: Implications for research and practice* (pp. 235–258). New York: Plenum.

Clark, R. (1985). *The Parent–Child Early Relational Assessment: Instrument and manual.* Madison: University of Wisconsin Medical School.

Dowdney, L., Skuse, D., Heptinstall, E., Puckering, C., & Zur-Szpiro, S. (1987). Growth retardation and developmental delay amongst inner city children. *Journal of Child Psychology and Psychiatry, 28,* 529–541.

Drotar, D. (1988). Failure to thrive. In D.K. Routh (Ed.), *Handbook of pediatric psychology* (pp. 71–107). New York: Guilford Press.

Drotar, D. (1989). Behavioral diagnosis in nonorganic failure to thrive: A critique and suggested approach to psychological assessment. *Journal of Developmental and Behavioral Pediatrics, 10,* 48–55.

Drotar, D. (1990). Sampling issues in research with nonorganic failure-to-thrive children. *Journal of Pediatric Psychology, 15,* 255–272.

Drotar, D. (1994). Psychological research with pediatric conditions: If we specialize can we generalize? *Journal of Pediatric Psychology, 19,* 403–414.

Drotar, D. (1995). Failure to thrive (growth deficiency). In M.C. Roberts (Ed.), *Handbook of pediatric psychology* (2nd ed., pp. 516–536). New York: Guilford Press.

Drotar, D., Malone, C.A., Devost, L., Brickell, C., Mantz-Clumper, C., Negray, L., Wallace, M., Woychik, J., Wyatt, B., Eckerle, D., Bush, M., Finion, M.A., El-Amin, D., Nowak, M., Satola, J., & Palotta, J. (1985). Early preventive intervention in failure to thrive: Methods and early outcome. In D. Drotar (Ed.), *New directions in failure to thrive: Implications for research and practice* (pp. 119–138). New York: Plenum.

Drotar, D., & Sturm, L. (1987). Paternal influences in nonorganic failure to thrive: Implications for clinical management. *Infant Mental Health Journal, 8,* 37–50.

Drotar, D., & Sturm, L. (1988). Parent–practitioner communication in the management of nonorganic failure to thrive. *Family Systems Medicine, 6,* 304–316.

Drotar, D., & Sturm, L. (1992). Personality development, personality solving and behavioral problems among preschool children with early histories of nonorganic failure to thrive: A controlled study. *Journal of Developmental and Behavioral Pediatrics, 13,* 266–273.

Drotar, D., & Sturm, L. (1994). Psychological outcomes of preschool children with early histories of failure to thrive. In B. Stabler & L. Underwood (Eds.), *Growth, stature and adaptation: Behavioral, social, and cognitive aspects of growth delay* (pp. 221–232). Chapel Hill: University of North Carolina, School of Medicine, Office of Continuing Education.

Drotar, D., Wilson, F., & Sturm, L. (1989). Parent intervention in the management of failure to thrive. In C.E. Schaefer & J.M. Bruesmeister (Eds.), *Handbook of parent training* (pp. 314–391). New York: John Wiley & Sons.

Fagan, J.F., Singer, L.T., Montie, J.E., & Shepherd, D.A. (1986). Selective screening device for the early detection of normal or delayed cognitive development in infants at risk for later mental retardation. *Pediatrics, 78,* 1021–1026.

Fitch, M.J., Cadol, R.V., Goldson, E., Wendel, T., Swartz, D., & Jackson, E. (1976). Cognitive development of abused and failure to thrive children. *Pediatric Psychology, 1,* 32–37.

Frank, D.A., & Drotar, D. (1994). Failure to thrive. In R.M. Reece (Ed.), *Child abuse: Medical diagnosis and management* (pp. 298–325). Philadelphia: Lea & Febiger.

Frank, D.A., & Zeisel, S.H. (1988). Failure to thrive. *Pediatric Clinics of North America, 35,* 1187–1206.

Fryer, G.E. (1988). The efficacy of hospitalization of nonorganic failure to thrive children: A meta-analysis. *Child Abuse & Neglect, 12,* 375–381.

Galler, J.R., Ramsey, F., Solimano, G., & Lowell, W. (1985). The influences of early malnutrition on subsequent behavioral development: The child's behavior at home. *Journal of the American Academy of Child Psychiatry, 24,* 58–64.

Hartman, A. (1979). *Finding families: An ecological approach to family assessment in adoption.* Thousand Oaks, CA: Sage Publications.

Heitzman, C.A., & Kaplan, R.M. (1988). Assessment of methods for measuring social support. *Health Psychology, 7,* 75–109.

Heptinstall, E., Puckering, C., Skuse, D., Start, K., Zur-Szpiro, S., & Dowdney, L. (1987). Nutrition and mealtime behaviour in families of growth retarded children. *Human Nutrition: Applied Nutrition, 41A,* 390–402.

Iwata, S., Riordan, M.M., Wohl, M.K., & Finney, J.W. (1982). Pediatric feeding disorders: Behavioral analysis and treatment. In P.J. Accardo (Ed.), *Failure to thrive in infancy and early childhood: A multidisciplinary team approach* (pp. 297–325). Baltimore: University Park Press.

Lachenmeyer, J.R., & Davidovicz, H. (1987). Failure to thrive: A critical review. In B. Lahey & A. Kazdin (Eds.), *Advances in clinical child psychology* (pp. 335–358). New York: Plenum.

Linscheid, T., & Rasnake, L.K. (1985). Behavioral approaches to the treatment of failure to thrive. In D. Drotar (Ed.), *New directions in failure to thrive: Implications for research and practice* (pp. 259–284). New York: Plenum.

Liss, M.D. (1994). Child abuse: Is there a mandate for researchers to report? *Ethics and Behavior, 4,* 133–146.

Mathisen, B., Skuse, D., Wolke, D., & Reilly, S. (1989). Oral-motor dysfunction and failure to thrive among inner-city infants. *Developmental Medicine and Child Neurology, 31,* 293–302.

McCubbin, H.L., & Patterson, J.M. (1988). *Systematic assessment of family stress, resources, and coping.* Minneapolis: University of Minnesota, Family Social Science.

Moos, R., & Moos, B. (1976). A typology of family social environments. *Family Process, 15,* 237–351.

Oates, R.K., Peacock, A., & Forrest, D. (1985). Long-term effects of nonorganic failure to thrive. *Pediatrics, 75,* 36–40.

Olson, D.H. (1986). Circumplex model VII: Validation studies and FACES III. *Family Process, 25,* 337–351.

Peterson, K.E., Washington, J., & Rathbun, J.M. (1984). Team management of failure to thrive. *Journal of the American Dietetic Association, 84,* 810–815.

Polan, H.J., Kaplan, M., Kessler, D.B., Shindeldecker, R., Newmark, M., Stern, D., & Ward, M.J. (1991). Psychopathology in mothers of children with failure to thrive. *Infant Mental Health Journal, 12,* 55–64.

Powell, G.F., Low, J., & Speers, M.A. (1987). Behavior as a diagnostic aid in failure to thrive. *Journal of Developmental and Behavioral Pediatrics, 8,* 18–24.

Pugliese, M.T., Weyman-Daum, M., Moses, N., & Lifshitz, F. (1987). Parental health beliefs as a cause of non-organic failure to thrive. *Pediatrics, 80,* 175–182.

Rosenn, D.W., Loeb, L.S., & Jura, M.B. (1980). Differentiation of organic from nonorganic failure to thrive syndrome in infancy. *Pediatrics, 66,* 698–704.

Shalowitz, M.U., & Berry, C.A., Rasinski, K.A., & Dannhausen-Braun, C.A. (in press). A new measure of contemporary sources of life stress: Development, validity and reliability of the CRISYS (Crisis in Family Systems). *Health Services Research.*

Singer, L., & Fagan, J. (1984). Cognitive development in the failure to thrive infant: A three year longitudinal study. *Journal of Pediatric Psychology, 9,* 363–383.

Singer, L.T., Song, I., Hill, B.P., & Jaffe, A.C. (1990). Stress and depression in mothers of failure to thrive children. *Journal of Pediatric Psychology, 15,* 711–720.

Skuse, D.A. (1993). Epidemiologic and definitional issues in failure to thrive. *Child and Adolescent Psychiatric Clinics of North America, 2,* 37–59.

Smith, L.A., & Berenberg, W. (1970). The concept of failure to thrive. *Pediatrics, 46,* 661–663.

Sturm, L., & Drotar, D. (1991). Maternal perceptions of the etiology of nonorganic failure to thrive. *Family Systems Medicine, 9,* 53–63.

Wachs, J.D. (1995). Relation of mild-to-moderate malnutrition to human development: Correlational studies. *Journal of Nutrition, 125*(8 Suppl.), 2445S–2454S.

Ward, M.J., Kessler, D.B., & Altman, S.C. (1993). Infant–mother attachment in children with failure to thrive. *Infant Mental Health Journal, 14,* 208–220.

Wolf, A.W., & Lozoff, B. (1985). A clinically interpretable method for analyzing the Bayley Infant Behavior Record. *Journal of Pediatric Psychology, 10,* 199–214.

Wolke, D., Skuse, D., & Mathisen, B. (1990). Behavioral style in failure to thrive infants: A preliminary communication. *Journal of Pediatric Psychology, 15,* 237–243.

Woolston, J. (1985). Diagnostic classification: The current challenge in failure to thrive syndrome research. In D. Drotar (Ed.), *New directions in failure to thrive: Implications for research and practice* (pp. 225–234). New York: Plenum.

Section II

Nutrition

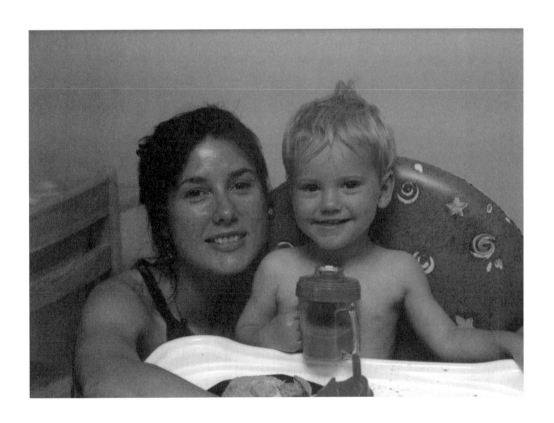

Chapter 6

Nutrition

Kathy F. Cunningham and Mary McLaughlin

A child's dietary intake should meet individual needs for adequate growth, metabolism, utilization of food, and activity. Basic guidelines exist and serve as a framework for providing age-appropriate calories and **nutrients.** These guidelines assist not only in planning suitable intakes but also in assessing dietary or nutritional adequacy of individuals throughout the life cycle. Appropriate growth, especially in infants and young children, traditionally has been used as the major criterion for assessing nutritional adequacy. To develop and implement a treatment plan for undernourished infants and young children, it first is necessary to understand normal growth.

During the first 2 years of life, rapid physical growth and development characterize infants' and toddlers' nutritional needs. Infants usually double their birth weight by 5 months of age and triple it by 1 year. Infants increase their length by 50% during the first year of life and double it by 4 years of age (Suskind, 1981). Healthy, well-nourished infants and toddlers require adequate energy, often referred to as *calories*. In addition, nutrients for growth are needed by infants so that they can respond to and learn from stimuli in their environment and interact with their parents in a manner that encourages a positive feeding relationship (see Chapter 7).

The need for certain vitamins and minerals (calcium, vitamin D, and zinc) is greater during periods of rapid growth and development. Growth velocity decreases after the first year of life until the adolescent growth spurt occurs. Calorie and protein needs per kilogram of body weight decrease as growth is less rapid.

NORMAL NUTRITION REQUIREMENTS

The recommended dietary allowances (RDAs), published by the National Research Council, contain the standards against which nutrient intake of normal, healthy children in the United States can be measured (National Academy of Sciences, 1989). These standards are based on average daily amounts of nutrients that healthy population groups should consume over time. The Committee on Dietary Allowances has estimated ranges of intake for calories, protein, vitamins, and minerals (National Academy of Sciences, 1989). The RDAs for infants ages birth to 6 months are based primarily on the nutritional composition of breast milk. The allowances for infants who are 6–12 months of age are based on consumption of formula and progressive intake of solids (National Academy of Sciences, 1989).

Energy

Energy needs of infants reflect calories required for basic body functions and those needed for activity and growth. Studies have defined the minimum acceptable levels for energy. The RDA for energy is based on predicting how to meet these needs; it is expressed in kilocalories needed per kilogram of body weight (kcal/kg). RDAs for infants and toddlers are as follows:

> birth to 5 months—108 kcal/kg
> 6 months to 1 year—98 kcal/kg
> 1 year to 3 years—102 kcal/kg

During the first few months of life, infants have very high energy needs. These needs are 1½ times that of children ages 7–10 years based on body weight. To meet basic energy requirements, infants and toddlers need food that is calorically dense (high in calories), that is absorbed easily, and that contains appropriate levels of the protein, carbohydrates, fats, vitamins, and minerals that are necessary to maintain normal bodily functions and growth. Breast milk unquestionably is the food of choice for the first 4–6 months. Its composition is designed to provide the necessary energy and nutrients, as well as provide protection against acute infection. Many infants who are at risk for developing allergic reactions may show a reduced incidence and reduced severity of symptoms early in life when breast-fed for 4 months or longer (Lawrence, 1997). Breast milk is, however, low in the fat-soluble vitamin D, which is important for preventing rickets, or demineralization of bone. Sufficient amounts of vitamin D can be obtained through adequate exposure to sunlight; however, studies have indicated that it is safest to support routine supplementation of 400 international units (IU) per day of vitamin D in solely breast-fed infants for the first 6 months (National Academy of Sciences, 1989). Nutritional inadequacy of vitamin D and iron may occur in cases of prolonged breast-feeding without age-appropriate introduction of a variety of solid baby foods and without appropriate use of **supplements.**

For infants whose mothers are unable to breast-feed, infant formula provides the same nutrient composition as breast milk. Formulas are milk or soy based and contain high-quality protein, readily digestible sugars and fats, and an appropriate mix of vitamins and minerals to sustain growth (Kraus & Mahank, 1984). Vitamin D and iron supplementation also would be indicated for formula-fed infants if the formula does not contain sufficient amounts of iron and vitamin D. As energy needs increase between the ages of 6 and 12 months, intakes should include iron-fortified formulas, iron-fortified cereals, and an iron supplement to maintain iron stores.

Protein

In the United States and other industrialized countries, infants and young children generally have an abundance of protein, and deficiency is uncommon, although the intake of protein and essential amino acids by infants and young children in developing countries often is insufficient to promote normal growth. Dietary protein provides energy, but its most important function in growth is to provide the amino acids that are necessary for synthesis of body proteins and the hormones and enzymes that regulate metabolism. Protein requirements are high during the first year of life because of rapid synthesis of protein into tissues, enzymes, and hormones. During the first 6 months of life, protein requirements usually are met through the infant's intake of breast milk or commercial infant formula that contains a quality of protein that is equivalent to breast milk. Breast milk and formula contain the essential amino acids that are needed to support such rapid growth and to meet protein needs of 2.2 grams per kilogram (g/kg) of body weight. During the second 6 months, an infant's growth rate slows and protein needs decrease to 2.0 g/kg (American Academy of Pediatrics, 1993). Breast milk and formula contain less protein than is needed for the second 6 months; therefore, infants should begin to consume additional sources of protein, such as infant cereal, pasteurized or cooked egg yolks, and strained meats. Children who have not gained weight appropriately may need a diet that is calorically dense and high in protein to promote increased growth.

Fats

Restricted-fat diets and low-fat milks are not recommended for infants under the age of 2. Restricting fats limits the essential fatty acids that are needed for growth. Nutrition priorities during infancy and for children younger than 2 years should promote growth and development rather than prevention of degenerative disease in later life (Glinsmann, Bartholmey, & Coletta, 1996). The routine advice often given to limit foods that are high in fat and sugars (those items at the peak of the Food Guide Pyramid [see Figures 1–3 on pages 105–107]) may not be appropriate for undernourished children. These children require energy-dense foods with good nutritional value to help meet their growth requirements.

Fats, or lipids, serve several functions in an infant's diet. They supply a significant source of energy with 9 calories per gram (cal/g) as compared with 4 cal/g for protein and carbohydrates. Because infants have a limited capacity to consume foods, they require energy-dense foods to support their rapid metabolic and growth rates. Fats are an excellent source for these essential, energy-dense calories. Fats also supply essential fatty acids, transport fat-soluble vitamins, and aid in the development of the brain and the nervous system (Glinsmann et al., 1996).

Fats account for approximately half of the calories that are provided in breast milk. The fat content of breast milk may vary depending on the mother's diet and time of feeding. Standard infant formula provides 30%–54% of the total calories from fats as recommended by the American Academy of Pediatrics (1993). Linoleic acid is the primary fatty acid in breast milk. Deficiency of this fatty acid may result in inadequate growth and skin lesions (Howard & Winter, 1984). Approximately 8%–10% of breast milk's fat calories is linoleic acid, compared with 4% of most formulas. When linoleic acid and other **polyunsaturated** fats are present in the infant's diet, there also is an increased need for the antioxidant vitamin E. Standard formulas, which are rich in the polyunsaturated oils, contain sufficient essential fatty acids and vitamin E; however, for premature infants who may not absorb vitamin E effectively and have low vitamin E stores, it is recommended that they be supplemented with vitamin E and given special formulas with an adequate amount of polyunsaturates (Groh-Wargo, Thompson, & Cox, 1994; Howard & Winter, 1984).

Fiber

As the infant grows, gradual introduction of cereals, fruits, and vegetables aids in the transition from an all-milk diet to acceptance of complex carbohydrates in the form of solids.

Recommendations for when to introduce infants to solid foods should be based on infants' developmental progress (American Academy of Pediatrics, 1993; see also Chapter 7).

Fruits, vegetables, and grains such as breads and cereals are important during the second year of life when growth slows and demand for energy-dense foods decreases. To help balance the infant's dietary intake, foods that contain simple and complex carbohydrates, vitamins, minerals, and a mixture of fiber should be selected. It is important to introduce fruits, vegetables, and grains into the infant's diet, but do not exceed 3 g of fiber per serving (Glinsmann et al., 1996).

Infants have a small stomach capacity, and the caloric density of high-fiber foods is low; therefore, if an undernourished child consumes a high-fiber diet, then the caloric density of intake may be compromised. The bulking effect of high-fiber foods such as fruits with skins, whole-kernel corn, peas, and whole grains may yield a feeling of fullness and result in decreased intake of calories and nutrients. Conversely, increased intake of dietary fiber may influence absorption of certain minerals, such as calcium, iron, copper, and zinc (American Academy of Pediatrics, 1993). Infants and young children who are offered a varied diet of fruits, vegetables, and grains should receive adequate fiber. Moderation of fiber should be maintained with children who have been diagnosed as undernourished.

Iron

Iron is needed to maintain hemoglobin concentration and increase total body iron stores. To ensure adequate iron stores and prevent anemia, the RDA for iron is set at an adequate level of 10 milligrams (mg) per day from 6 months to 3 years of age. The American Academy of Pediatrics (1993) has recommended 1 mg/kg of body weight per day for full-term infants and 2 mg/kg of body weight per day for low birth weight (LBW) infants. Supplementation of iron for normal or LBW infants should not exceed 15 mg per day.

Healthy, full-term infants have sufficient iron stores to provide growth for the first 4 months of life. A premature infant's iron stores may become depleted much earlier depending on the birth weight, rate of growth, and transfusion history. Because iron stores are accumulated in the last trimester of pregnancy, premature infants are at a higher risk for iron deficiency. Regardless of the birth weight or gestational age, all infants should receive iron supplementation to meet growth needs and replace normal loss (Groh-Wargo et al., 1994). Iron supplementation should take place after 4 months of age (see Chapter 17). Infants with a **hematocrit** of less than 34% should be considered anemic and treated with iron drops.

Breast milk and cow milk are poor sources of iron; however, iron from breast milk is better absorbed, and iron deficiency is rare. Commercial formulas are fortified with iron to meet infants' growth needs. Cow milk is low in iron and may cause intestinal irritation; therefore, it is recommended that infants remain on breast milk or iron-fortified formula through the first year of life (American Academy of Pediatrics, 1993).

To supplement iron needs when infants begin consuming solid foods, items such as iron-fortified cereals, strained meats, and dark green vegetables such as strained peas, spinach, and green beans should be encouraged. Foods that are high in vitamin C also should be encouraged to increase iron absorption and protein utilization. There have been improvements in the iron status of low-income children, and it has been suggested that participation in the Special Supplemental Nutrition Program for Women, Infants and Children (WIC) may be a primary factor (Oski, 1989).

Zinc

Zinc is involved with several **metabolic pathways** and is a requirement for cell synthesis. Full-term infants who consume breast milk show no signs of deficiency in the first 6 months of life because the absorption of zinc from breast milk is greater than the absorption from commercial formulas. Commercial formula contains 3.7–6.0 mg of zinc per liter. Infants from birth to age 6 months will show adequate growth and have adequate zinc intakes from breast milk or formula to meet the RDA of 1 mg/kg of body weight. At 6 months, solid foods should help satisfy the need to reach the RDA of 3–5 mg per day (American Academy of Pediatrics, 1993; National Academy of Sciences, 1989).

Meats, seafood, whole grains, and to a lesser extent legumes all are high in zinc. Children who do not receive a varied diet that contains foods that are high in zinc may not be receiving adequate amounts of zinc. Supplementary zinc may be given to undernourished children if analysis of their average food intake indicates inadequate zinc for age and weight. Some clinicians recommend giving zinc routinely for 3–6 months in cases of pediatric undernutrition. Inadequate zinc has been associated with decreased appetite; therefore, the use of zinc supplements may result in increased appetite for undernourished children (Krebs, Hambridge, & Walravens, 1984; see also Chapter 3). Zinc also may play an important role in taste perception (Fomon, 1974). Children with malabsorption or growth problems may show signs of zinc deficiency, which may result in a syndrome of growth retardation, loss of appetite, dermatitis, and impaired wound healing, although clinical zinc deficiency is rare. The RDA for zinc provided as sulfate, gluconate, or acetate is 5 mg per day for children up to 1 year of age and 10 mg per day for children 1–10 years of age. The pharmacist should mix it as a solution of 10 mg of zinc per 5 ml flavored water for children. Zinc also is available in chewable, "complete" vitamins for children.

CLINICAL ASSESSMENT

The purpose of a feeding interview, often referred to as a diet history, is to obtain baseline data that are necessary for implementing a plan of nutritional intervention. A detailed history of present and past feeding practices is essential to accurately determine nutritional status. Information that is gleaned from the feeding history will help health care providers and families develop and implement realistic goals for dietary changes.

To begin a nutritional assessment, a 24-hour dietary recall is used at the time of the first visit. Although the 24-hour recall is a useful tool, it has its limitations. It relies on the parents' recalling foods that the child has eaten within the previous 24 hours. An example of this would be to recall foods that were eaten at breakfast, lunch, and dinner from the previous day. Care should be taken to encourage the parents (or individuals serving in this role) to recall any snacks and/or circumstances that would be out of the usual daily pattern (see Chapter 27). Diet recall may be more successful if the interviewer uses open-ended questions such as, "When your child gets up in the morning, what does he or she have to eat or drink?" versus "What does your child have for breakfast?" Do not phrase questions that imply a specific meal pattern or time, and avoid questions that suggest a specific response. (For a brief list of questions to ask about nutrition and feeding, see Table 1 in Chapter 9.) Further evaluation of caloric intake can be performed by obtaining a 3-day food intake record or food frequency report. This report is helpful for identifying consistency of meal scheduling and foods that might be in excess or avoided in the child's diet. With an undernourished child, it is important to keep in mind that a 3-day record or a 24-hour recall may contain overreporting because of concerns that the meals or snacks offered will appear inappropriate as judged by the health care provider.

To determine feeding patterns, the interviewer should ask questions that relate to breast milk or formula intake, age at which solid foods were introduced, or when the diet changed from breast milk or formula to whole milk. The use of vitamin or mineral supplementation and any unusual dietary habits or pica should be noted. An example of a food diary is included in Appendix F. Once a 24-hour recall or a 3-day food diary is obtained and family resources are determined, an assessment can be made of whether the present dietary conditions are adequate to promote appropriate growth.

The child's behavior around feeding also should be assessed (see Chapters 7 and 8). The interviewer should ask the caregiver questions that are related to any difficulty with sucking, chewing, or swallowing (see Chapter 23). The interviewer should ascertain the frequency of feedings and who the primary feeders are to determine who should be the main target of intervention. Information may need to be shared with more than one individual if a child has multiple people involved in feeding. Other information that should not be overlooked includes safety conditions around feeding: Where does the child sit for a meal? Does the child have an appropriate highchair or booster seat that promotes good posture for feeding?

Along with assessing the nutritional needs of the child, it is necessary to evaluate the caregivers' or family's resources that influence their ability to feed the child effectively. Identification of resources includes financial and material resources for food purchases, preparation, and storage. Identification of resources is necessary for determining intervention or referrals to nutrition programs or social services for assistance such as WIC and food stamps (see Chapter 33). It is helpful to gather information about the level of the nutrition knowledge of the parents. Do they have language or literacy difficulties that will determine the types of educational materials offered? Does the family have different dietary habits or beliefs, such as religious or food constraints, that would influence food selection (see Chapter 26)? Possible contributions to inadequate intake for the child may be discovered during a dietary history that explores feeding interactions, nutritional misinformation, and/or parental expectations. For example, it is important to determine how food refusal and length of mealtimes are handled by the parent (see Chapter 8). In addition, observing feeding behavior and caregiver interactions yields valuable information that helps in formulating care plans.

INTERVENTION

Once information has been obtained regarding current feeding practices and behaviors, the information should be reviewed, evaluated, and used as a basis for developing strategies for nutritional intervention. Recommendations should be based on realistic actions that caregivers can perform with guidance and support from the multidisciplinary team.

Nutritional Intervention

To provide nutritional counseling, the basic guidelines from the United States Department of Agriculture (USDA) Food Guide Pyramid can be used for consistency (see Figures 1–3). The Food Guide Pyramid is a useful tool for guidance in providing adequate variety and sufficient numbers of servings of appropriate foods. Educational materials that provide instructions on feeding practices also can be used. These materials should include essential practices of meal scheduling (see Chapter 27). Appropriate foods and snacks should be discussed in detail. Food and snack selections should be culturally appropriate to enhance consumption (see Chapter 26). Offer solids before liquids, and limit low-calorie liquids. During counseling sessions, discuss the feeding environment. This discussion should include adequate seating and positioning of the child during feeding. To ensure that the total environment is pleasant, address issues of food presentation. Base your advice on what parents are already doing (see Chapter 4). Look for ways to build on current prac-

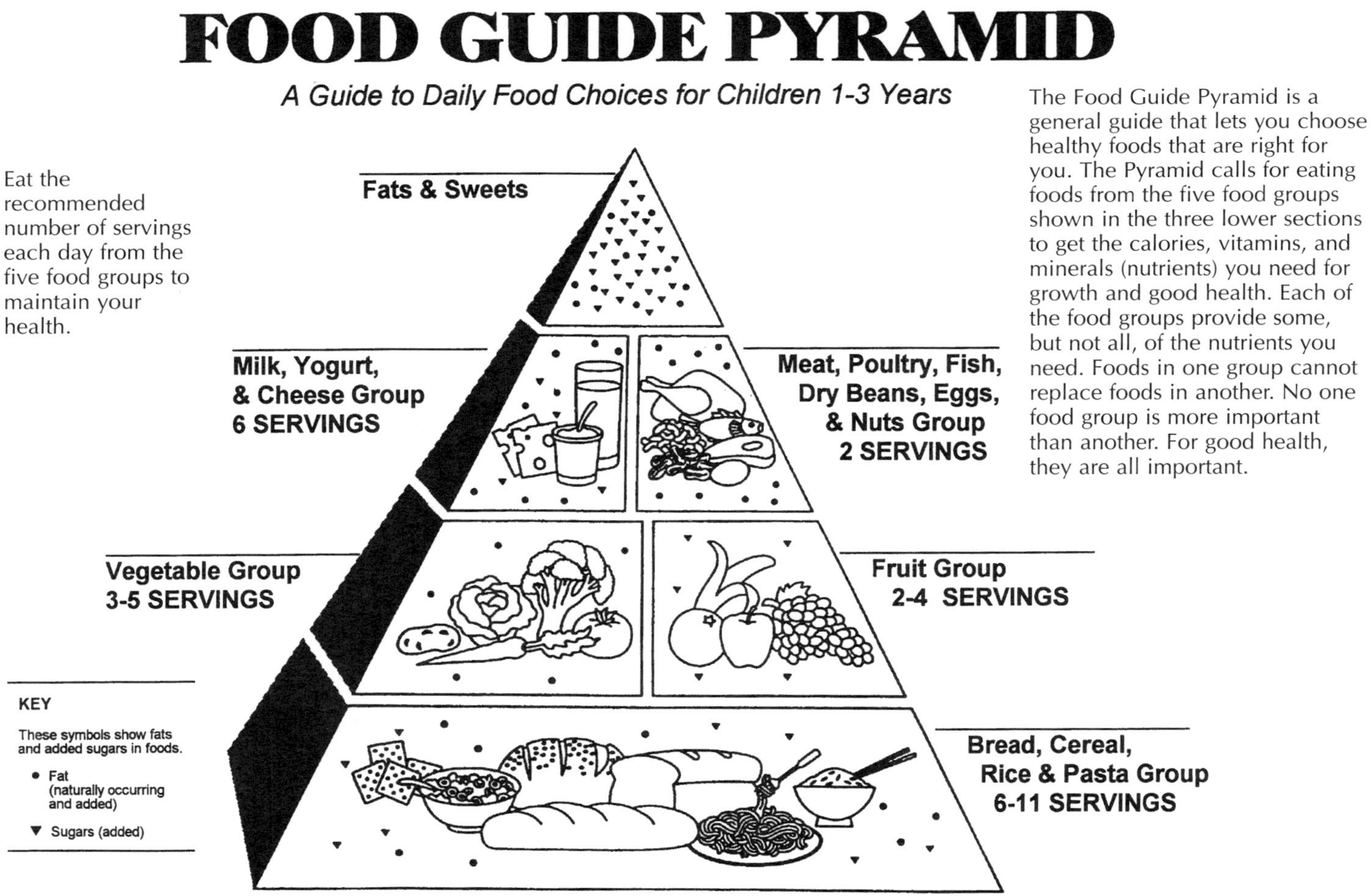

FOOD GUIDE PYRAMID

A Guide to Daily Food Choices for Children 1-3 Years

The Food Guide Pyramid is a general guide that lets you choose healthy foods that are right for you. The Pyramid calls for eating foods from the five food groups shown in the three lower sections to get the calories, vitamins, and minerals (nutrients) you need for growth and good health. Each of the food groups provide some, but not all, of the nutrients you need. Foods in one group cannot replace foods in another. No one food group is more important than another. For good health, they are all important.

Eat the recommended number of servings each day from the five food groups to maintain your health.

Fats & Sweets

Meat, Poultry, Fish, Dry Beans, Eggs, & Nuts Group
2 SERVINGS

Milk, Yogurt, & Cheese Group
6 SERVINGS

Fruit Group
2-4 SERVINGS

Vegetable Group
3-5 SERVINGS

Bread, Cereal, Rice & Pasta Group
6-11 SERVINGS

KEY

These symbols show fats and added sugars in foods.

• Fat (naturally occurring and added)
▼ Sugars (added)

Figure 1. Food guide pyramid for children 1–3 years (English). (From Colorado Department of Public Health & Environment, Nutrition Services [n.d.a]; reprinted by permission. Adapted from the United States Department of Agriculture and the United States Department of Health and Human Services.)

LA PIRÁMIDE, GUÍA DE COMIDA

Guía Diaria de Comidas para Niños de 1 a 3 Años de Edad

Alimente a su pequeño/a diariamente con el número de raciones/porciones recomendadas en cada uno de los cinco grupos de alimentos, para mantenerlo sano.

La Pirámide, Guía de Comidas es una lista general que le permite elegir alimentos sanos que son buenos para su salud. La Pirámide nos sugiere comer los alimentos que encontramos en cinco grupos de comidas que se muestran en las tres secciones inferiores, para obtener todas las calorías, vitaminas y minerales (nutrientes) que necesita para crecer y tener buena salud. Cada uno de estos grupos de alimentos proporciona algunos, pero no todos, los nutrientes que necesita. Los alimentos de un grupo no pueden reemplazar a los que están en otro. Ningún grupo es más importante que el otro. Para tener una buena salud, todos son muy importantes.

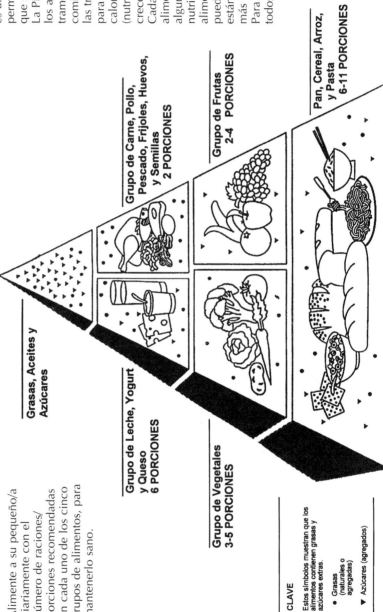

Grasas, Aceites y Azúcares

Grupo de Carne, Pollo, Pescado, Frijoles, Huevos, y Semillas 2 PORCIONES

Grupo de Frutas 2-4 PORCIONES

Grupo de Leche, Yogurt y Queso 6 PORCIONES

Grupo de Vegetales 3-5 PORCIONES

Pan, Cereal, Arroz, y Pasta 6-11 PORCIONES

CLAVE

Estos símbolos muestran que los alimentos contienen grasas y azúcares extras.

● Grasas (naturales o agregadas)

▶ Azúcares (agregados)

Figure 2. Food guide pyramid for children 1–3 years (Spanish). (From Colorado Department of Public Health & Environment, Nutrition Services [n.d.b]; reprinted by permission. Adapted from the United States Department of Agriculture and the United States Department of Health and Human Services.)

106

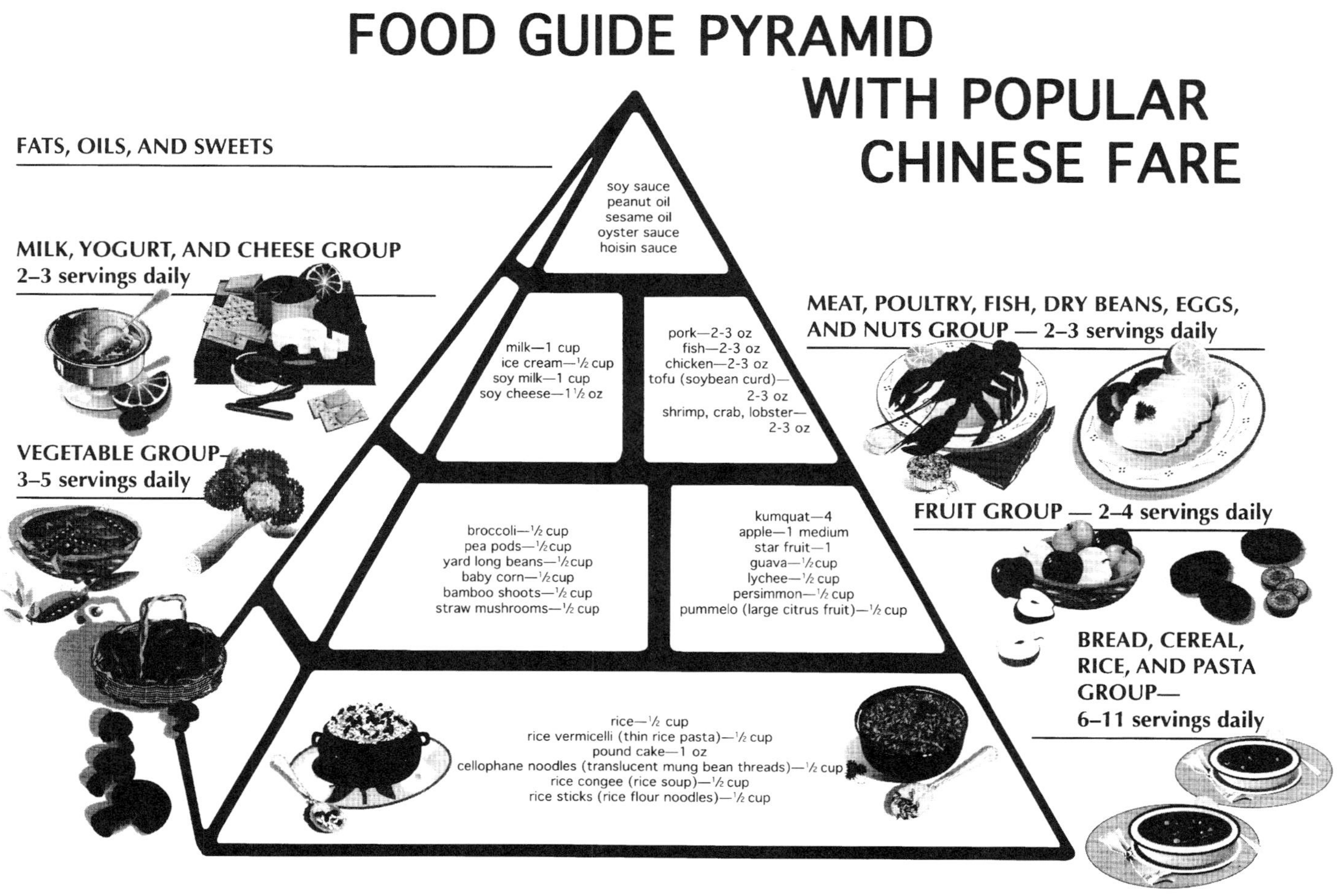

FOOD GUIDE PYRAMID WITH POPULAR CHINESE FARE

FATS, OILS, AND SWEETS

soy sauce
peanut oil
sesame oil
oyster sauce
hoisin sauce

MILK, YOGURT, AND CHEESE GROUP
2–3 servings daily

milk—1 cup
ice cream—½ cup
soy milk—1 cup
soy cheese—1½ oz

MEAT, POULTRY, FISH, DRY BEANS, EGGS, AND NUTS GROUP — 2–3 servings daily

pork—2–3 oz
fish—2–3 oz
chicken—2–3 oz
tofu (soybean curd)—2–3 oz
shrimp, crab, lobster—2–3 oz

FRUIT GROUP—2–4 servings daily

kumquat—4
apple—1 medium
star fruit—1
guava—½ cup
lychee—½ cup
persimmon—½ cup
pummelo (large citrus fruit)—½ cup

VEGETABLE GROUP
3–5 servings daily

broccoli—½ cup
pea pods—½ cup
yard long beans—½ cup
baby corn—½ cup
bamboo shoots—½ cup
straw mushrooms—½ cup

BREAD, CEREAL, RICE, AND PASTA GROUP—6–11 servings daily

rice—½ cup
rice vermicelli (thin rice pasta)—½ cup
pound cake—1 oz
cellophane noodles (translucent mung bean threads)—½ cup
rice congee (rice soup)—½ cup
rice sticks (rice flour noodles)—½ cup

Figure 3. Food guide pyramid with popular Chinese fare. (*Source:* National Center for Nutrition and Dietetics, The American Dietetic Association. Based on the USDA Food Guide Pyramid. © 1996, The American Dietetic Association Foundation. *Food Guide Pyramid with Popular Chinese Fare.* Used by permission. Reproduction of this fact sheet is permitted for educational purposes. Reproduction for sales purposes is not permitted.)

tices. Give positive reinforcement to practices that are appropriate. Make suggestions for improvements in habits that do not promote growth.

The dietitian should calculate the reported intake for calories, protein, and other nutrients and compare the intake with the appropriate RDA needs for normal growth of the child based on age. A food diary can be used for rapid assessment of general adequacy (see Appendix F). Comparison of reported intake with the RDA will allow the areas of appropriate intake or deficits to become an educational tool for developing interventions. Requirements for an individual infant or child will vary according to degree of illness, chronic disease, genetic syndromes, family's pattern of growth (see Chapter 10), and physical activity. If a comprehensive diet interview and feeding evaluation reveal an intake that should result in adequate growth, then a further look at possible organic causes for inadequate growth should be taken.

Nutritional intervention should be based on the positive nutritional needs to achieve catch-up growth. It is important to reinforce the positive components of the diet plan that the caregiver is fulfilling. It would be most helpful to determine one or two areas of change and focus on those methods of intervention that can be incorporated into the family structure. This will help to develop trust and enhance the family's ability to achieve the desired recommendations.

Requirements for Catch-Up Growth

The term *catch-up growth* refers to the increase in growth velocity following a period of impaired growth that is due to primary or secondary undernutrition (see Chapter 10). Children who have experienced delays in growth, regardless of cause, require extra calories, protein, and other nutrients above normal requirements. This is necessary to catch up to appropriate growth patterns based on family and medical histories. These needs can be up to 1½–2 times the RDA for age (Ashworth & Millward, 1986). If not given extra calories and nutrients, then the child may grow at a rate that fails to allow him or her to catch up to his or her growth potential. For children who are mildly undernourished, intake should be ad libitum initially and advanced to meet catch-up needs once they have been assessed fully. For the severely malnourished child, it is important to restrict intake to the child's usual amount, encouraging frequent, small meals for 7–10 days and then increasing gradually to catch-up needs. This will prevent the possibility of refeeding diarrhea (McLean, 1987).

In clinical practice, one uses standard calculations of minimum and maximum caloric requirements for catch-up growth. To do this, one first plots the child's length (or height, with an older child), weight, and weight-for-length on the appropriate National Center for Health Statistics (NCHS) growth chart. Then one determines weight-age, ideal (median) weight-for-age, and ideal (median) weight-for-length as follows:

1. Weight-age is the age at which a child's actual weight would be at the 50th percentile (see Figure 4a). On the weight-for-age graph, one draws a horizontal line from the child's weight to the 50th percentile, then a vertical line down to the age axis.
2. Ideal (median) weight (IBW) for age is found on the weight-for-age graph. Starting at the child's age, one draws a vertical line to the 50th percentile, then a horizontal line to the right to the weight axis (see Figure 4a).
3. Ideal (median) weight for actual length (or height) is found on the weight-for-length graph. Starting at the child's actual length, one draws a vertical line to the 50th percentile, then a horizontal line to the weight axis (see Figure 4b).

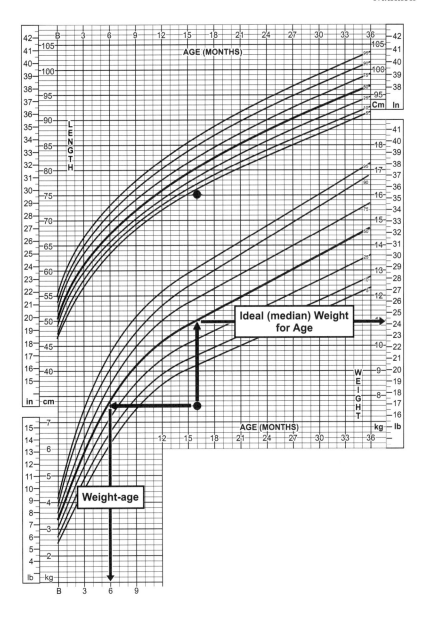

Patient	DB	Weight	Weight-Age	IBW/Age	Wt/Lt	IBW/Lt
Male	16 months	7.6 kg <5th percentile	5½ months	11 kg	<5th percentile	9.5 kg
Z-score		−3.11			−2.77	

Figure 4a.   Weight-age, ideal (median) weight-for-age, actual weight, and actual length.

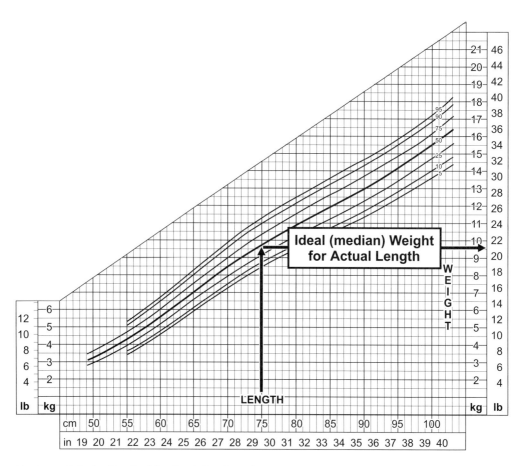

Maximum Calories Required for Catch-Up Growth:

$$\frac{\text{RDA Kcal/Kg Weight-age} \times \text{Ideal (median) Weight-for-Age in Kilograms}}{\text{Actual Weight}}$$

$$= \text{kcal/kg} \; \frac{108 \times 11}{7.6} = 156 \text{ kcal/kg or } 1186 \text{ kcal/day}$$

Minimum Calories Required for Catch-Up Growth:

$$\frac{\text{RDA Kcal/Kg Weight-age} \times \text{Ideal (median) Weight for Actual Height in Kilograms}}{\text{Actual Weight}}$$

$$= \text{kcal/kg} \; \frac{108 \times 9.5}{7.6} = 135 \text{ kcal/kg or } 1026 \text{ kcal/day}$$

Figure 4b.   Ideal (median) weight for actual length.

The clinician then determines the recommended calories for the child's weight-age and uses these amounts in the formulas in Figure 4b. To determine the total calories needed for catch-up growth, simply eliminate the actual weight in the formula. This will provide the number of calories that are required per day for catch-up. These calculations are shown in Figure 4b. Protein needs for catch-up growth are calculated using a similar formula for calories (Peterson, 1993).

An alternative method for determining the minimum number of calories that are necessary for catch-up is to use the weight that the child would be if he or she were to reach the 5th percentile for age on the NCHS growth charts rather than the ideal weight-for-height as indicated in the formula in Figure 4b (for minimum number of calories) or ideal (median) weight-for-age (in the calculation of maximum number of calories). In the case of DB (calculation as in Figure 4b), his growth at 16 months is below the 5th percentile for weight, height, and weight-for-height; his weight-age is 33% of his chronological age. Expressed in z-scores (see Chapter 2), these are -3.11 (weight-for-age), -1.88 (length-for-age), and -2.77 (weight-for-length). When evaluating a child with inadequate growth, it is desirable to have a series of growth measurements, over a period of time, to better assess growth patterns. The calculations of 135 kilocalories (kcal)/kg needed for minimum catch-up growth and 156 kcal/kg needed for maximum catch-up growth need to be reviewed in terms of current reported intake and the number of kcal/kg that the reported intake supplies. The caloric deficit then can be determined. Taking into account a child's feeding patterns, medical condition, developmental readiness, and family resources, a realistic plan can be developed to increase caloric density to a desired level. The appropriate plan may involve a number of visits and may need to be done gradually.

A number of postnatal growth charts are available; they have been developed from extrauterine growth data (see Chapter 10). There also are intrauterine growth charts available, which are useful for determining expected growth (weight, length, and head circumference) at various gestational ages. Preterm infants who have reached a corrected age of 40 weeks can be plotted on NCHS growth charts (Groh-Wargo et al., 1994).

Adjustments for prematurity can be made on the NCHS growth charts and are considered in the calculations (Peterson, Washington, & Rathbun, 1984). For the premature child, weight is adjusted up to 24 months, height up to 40 months, and head circumference up to 36 months (Frank, Needlman, & Silva, 1993; Kraus & Mahank, 1984) when using standard NCHS growth charts. Another option is to use growth charts that adjust for prematurity (Hamill et al., 1992; see Appendix F). These charts are based on a large cohort of infants with LBW who weigh between 1,501 and 2,500 g with gestational ages less than or equal to 37 weeks (Casey, Kraemer, Bernbaum, Yogman, & Sells, 1991). Charts for infants born below 1,500 g are also available (Ross Products Division, Abbott Laboratories).

Rapid rates of catch-up growth have been observed in some children; however, the average expected weight gain is 1 g/kg of body weight per day for every 5–7 kcal consumed above 80 kcal/kg (Ashworth & Millward, 1986). Rapid weight gain can be expected when children are wasted (i.e., greater deficit in weight-for-age than in height). Children who merely are stunted (i.e., greater deficit in height than in weight-for-age) do not gain as rapidly as wasted children (see Chapters 2 and 10). This occurs because the peak velocity for catch-up in linear growth occurs 1–3 months later than weight; thus, during the rehabilitation of children with both wasting and stunting, weight gain can be rapid until the child attains a weight that is appropriate for height. It may take up to 2 weeks of increased intake to see any weight gain, and increased requirements can persist for several months. It is important to note that conditions of poverty affect catch-up growth outcomes. Studies have shown that children who live in poverty may have little opportunity to achieve catch-up growth because of continuous nutritional deprivation (Ashworth & Millward, 1986); therefore, all opportunities for increased support should be explored.

Although some children could eat and tolerate twice as much as they consume currently, many require foods with increased caloric density to meet increased caloric needs. Total calories and protein rather than variety are important at this stage. As a base, it is important to use foods that the child likes to eat. Infants may require more than the standard 20 calories per ounce of formula for a variety of reasons including presence of a medically prescribed fluid restriction (e.g., because of heart failure), decreased ability to take adequate formula (e.g., because of energy, strength, or suck factors), increased **energy expenditure** (e.g., because of seizures or respiratory problems), or malabsorption of carbohydrate or fat (e.g., because of cystic fibrosis). The simplest, least expensive method should be used to increase caloric density, taking into consideration the age of the child, the child's and family's present dietary practices, financial constraints, scheduling, and home, child care, or baby-sitter feeding environment.

In clinical practice, it is helpful to focus on one problem area at a time and to suggest that changes be made gradually. Concrete instructions (written and verbal) should be provided, and progress in meeting goals should be monitored in a nonthreatening way. Liquids of low caloric density should be limited, the frequency of feeding should be evaluated, and the caloric density of solid foods should be assessed. If supplements are recommended, then their tolerance should be monitored and appropriate adjustments should be made when indicated. Following are intervention strategies for achieving catch-up weight gain:

Food Choices

1. With a child who is taking solid foods, monitor for appropriate texture for age and developmental ability. Discuss portion sizes, quantities, variety, and texture diversity to enhance the development and enjoyment of foods offered to children.
    Intervention: Review the age at which solid foods and appropriate texture should be introduced. For caregivers who have limited knowledge of portion sizes, use food models and visual demonstrations. Review the child's current feeding schedule and food selections for age appropriateness and timing. The goal is six small meals.
2. Are labels of baby foods checked so that higher-calorie ones are chosen?
    Intervention: This should be done to offer foods of higher caloric density. Home-prepared baby foods may have more calories than commercially prepared foods and be less expensive.
3. Address the process of how to obtain formulas or necessary food items.
    Intervention: Discuss supply to the home and child care environment. Review food assistance as needed (e.g., WIC, food stamps, food pantries; see Chapter 33).

Calorie Boosters

1. Calculate the volume of formula, milk, or juice reported. Is the child perhaps receiving too much low-calorie fluid, such as juice (or soda), and insufficient formula or milk? An appropriate amount of milk for a child is 16–24 ounces per day.
    Intervention: Increase the volume of milk or formula to meet growth needs, and limit juice intake. If the volume of formula or milk is adequate for normal growth, then one may increase caloric concentration to achieve catch-up growth. Dry cereal should be mixed with formula rather than with water for infants or half and half (cream and milk) for older children.
2. Discuss high-quality, nutrient-dense foods that promote increased growth. Increase caloric density of food that usually is consumed by using common additives.
    Intervention: Foods that provide few calories should be limited. Snacks should provide some protein but be high in fat. Utilize margarine, oil, cheese, or peanut butter as tolerated. Try adding 1 teaspoon of oil, butter, or margarine to vegetables and meats. Also try adding a little whole-milk yogurt to fruits. These tips can be used with infant

foods as well as foods for an older child. Caloric value of meats, potatoes, rice, and pastas can be increased by adding gravies and sauces.

3. Are extra calories added to vegetables?

    Intervention: Adding cream sauce, cheese sauce, salad dressings, butter, margarine, mayonnaise, or oil to vegetables or using these foods as a dip for vegetables increases caloric content and adds flavor. Many children like to dip finger foods into something (see Table 6 in Chapter 9).

4. Are fruits served plain, or are extra calories added?

    Intervention: The use of puddings, whole-milk yogurts, and sour cream as dips or sauces for fruit will increase calorie intake (see Table 6 in Chapter 9).

5. Is anything added to whole milk to increase calorie content?

    Intervention: Use whole milk that is fortified with cream (three parts milk to one part cream) as a beverage, in cooking, and on foods such as cereal and puddings for children who are older than 18 months and who can tolerate whole-milk products.

Feeding Behavior, Snacking, and Scheduling

1. Discuss the feeding environment. Mealtimes should be pleasant and should include modeling of mealtime behaviors by adults as well as by peers or older children.

    Intervention: Children should be provided meals in a safe and secure seating position. Infants should be held in a cradle position for breast- or bottle-feeding to enhance social interaction. Older infants or toddlers should be fed in infant seats or highchairs to promote an adequate feeding position and to increase self-feeding skills.

2. Do the parents offer the child solids before liquids at meals?

    Intervention: If so, then the practice should be encouraged. If not, then explain that solids offer more nutrition for the same volume.

3. Is the child allowed to fill up on water, soda, or juice, especially before meals?

    Intervention: Juice (and soda) intake should be limited, and calorically dense liquids should be used instead. When preparing juices from concentrate, use less water. You may add 1 tablespoon of **polycose** to 2–3 ounces of juice. Explain that the more calorically dense liquids should be used, except within 30–60 minutes prior to mealtime so that the liquids will not interfere with solid food intake.

4. Does the child have a feeding schedule?

    Intervention: Establish a feeding schedule that includes meals and snacks. Allow at least 2 hours between meals and snacks (see Chapter 27).

Some infants who are exclusively breast-fed may not achieve appropriate growth velocity. Nutritional status of breast-fed infants is affected by several factors: nutritional stores at birth (related to length of gestation and maternal nutrition during pregnancy), amount of nutrients that are supplied by breast milk (influenced by extent and duration of breast-feeding), and certain genetic factors that affect the way in which nutrients are absorbed and used. When assessing the growth of breast-fed infants, the standard by which one evaluates the adequacy of growth is critical and can influence one's definition of normal and how one responds to deviations from the norm.

Several studies have indicated that the pattern of growth demonstrated by breast-fed infants differs from that of NCHS reference data (1977), which were based on the Fels longitudinal study conducted between 1929 and 1975 (Dewey et al., 1995). At that time, very few infants were breast-fed for longer than 3 months. Most of these studies indicated that breast-fed infants grew as rapidly or more rapidly than the reference population for the first 2–3 months of life and less rapidly (especially in weight) from 3 to 12 months. As a result, their growth often gave the appearance of growth faltering beyond the first few months even if the infants were obviously healthy and thriving. Because of this, parents often were counseled either to wean their infants from the breast or to add supplemental foods or formula, often resulting in premature weaning. Such advice creates a significant barrier to efforts to promote exclusive breast-feeding, a recommendation of the American Academy of Pediatrics and the World Health Organization. This is problem enough in developed countries; in developing countries, the hazards of early weaning from breast milk and the introduction of other foods, generally under unsanitary conditions, is even more significant.

Given the pattern of more rapid growth in breast-fed infants during the first 2–3 months of life, the infant who is faltering during this period deserves a careful assessment. It is important to pay careful attention to the adequacy of the milk supply, infant intake and elimination, and the infant's feeding pattern (Lawrence, 1997). If necessary, in the breast-fed infant who has been found to be undernourished, supplemental feedings (with either expressed breast milk or formula) can be used to increase the caloric density of breast milk and formulas (see Table 1). However, in the latter part of the first year of life, when breast-fed infants may show some decline in weight percentiles, this deviation from historical growth standards should not be construed as pathological growth faltering and used as an indication for weaning. Each mother–infant pair deserves to be treated supportively if the infant is healthy and otherwise thriving. A revision of the 1977 NCHS growth standards includes a more representative sample of breast-fed infants (see Chapter 2). (For additional information on managing breast-feeding, see Lawrence, 1994; Powers & Slusser, 1997; and Riordan & Auerbach, 1993.)

Supplementation

It is appropriate in some cases to increase the caloric density of infants' milk. This is especially true when infants cannot take in enough formula, as with congenital heart disease (see Chapter 12) or cerebral palsy (see Chapter 14). Unless medically indicated, special formulas should not replace meals but should be used to supplement intake at a time when they will not interfere with meals. Although their use has become increasingly common, they should not be viewed as a replacement for a healthful, developmentally appropriate diet. Increasing caloric density is not a substitute for understanding the reasons that a child is not taking in adequate calories for growth. Special formulas are expensive, and they may mask or delay more appropriate understanding and intervention.

Caloric density can be increased by using special formula, by concentrating ordinary formula, and by adding special products (see Table 1). Commercially available special products can be used. Pediasure (Ross Laboratories) and Kindercal (Mead-Johnson) have 30 calories per ounce as opposed to the 20 calories per ounce in milk or standard formulas. These formulas are appropriate for children ages 1–10 years. MCT oil is a specially formulated oil that contains medium-chain triglycerides, which are digested easily. One can also use liquid corn oil if MCT oil is unavailable or too costly. Enfamil Human Milk Fortifier (Ross Laboratories) can be added to breast milk. Polycose, made from cornstarch, adds calories but is not high in **renal solute load.**

When concentrating an infant's milk, one must be careful not to go too far. This may occur when one increases the renal solute load too much. Renal solute load consists of excess nitrogen (the metabolic end product of protein metabolism), sodium, chloride, and potassium that are excreted in the urine with water. Because of the way the kidney functions, an excessive solute load may draw water into the urine, depleting the body of water

Table 1. Tips for increasing caloric density of breast milk and infant formulas

Formula type	Amount formula	Water	Concentrated formula	Powder formula	Breast milk fortifier	Polycose powder (23 kcal/tbs)	Polycose liquid (30 kcal/tbs)	Vegetable oil or MCT oil
20 kcal/oz								
Breast milk	variable							
Ready to use	1 can							
Concentrate	13 oz	13 oz						
Powder	1 scoop	2 oz						
24 kcal/oz								
Breast milk	4 oz		1 oz					
Breast milk	4 oz			1 scoop				
Breast milk	4 oz				4 packets			
Ready to use	4 oz		1 oz					
Ready to use	4 oz		1 oz	1 scoop				
Concentrate	13 oz	8 oz						
Powder	5 scoops	8 oz						
28 kcal/oz								
Breast milk	4 oz		1 oz			2½ tsp		
Breast milk	4 oz		1 oz				2 tsp	
Breast milk	4 oz			1 scoop		2 tsp		
Breast milk	4 oz			1 scoop			1½ tsp	
Breast milk	4 oz				4 packets	2 tsp		
Breast milk	4 oz				4 packets		1½ tsp	
Ready to use	4 oz		1 oz			2½ tsp		
Ready to use	4 oz		1 oz				2 tsp	
Ready to use	4 oz			1 scoop		2 tsp		
Ready to use	4 oz			1 scoop			1½ tsp	
Concentrate	13 oz	8 oz				3 tbs + 2 tsp		
Concentrate	13 oz	8 oz					2 tbs + 2½ tsp	
Powder	5 scoops	8 oz				1 tbs + 1½ tsp		
Powder	5 scoops	8 oz					1 tbs	

(continued)

115

Table 1. (*continued*)

Formula type	Amount formula	Water	Concentrated formula	Powder formula	Breast milk fortifier	Polycose powder (23 kcal/tbs)	Polycose liquid (30 kcal/tbs)	Vegetable oil or MCT oil
30 kcal/oz								
Breast milk	4 oz		1 oz			2½ tsp		¼ tsp
Breast milk	4 oz		1 oz				2 tsp	¼ tsp
Breast milk	4 oz			1 scoop		2 tsp		¼ tsp
Breast milk	4 oz			1 scoop			1½ tsp	¼ tsp
Breast milk	4 oz				4 packets	2 tsp		¼ tsp
Breast milk	4 oz				4 packets		1½ tsp	¼ tsp
Ready to use	4 oz		1 oz			2½ tsp		¼ tsp
Ready to use	4 oz		1 oz				2 tsp	¼ tsp
Ready to use	4 oz			1 scoop		2 tsp		¼ tsp
Ready to use	4 oz			1 scoop			1½ tsp	¼ tsp
Concentrate	13 oz	8 oz				3 tbs + 2 tsp		1 tsp
Concentrate	13 oz	8 oz					2 tbs + 2½ tsp	1 tsp
Powder	5 scoops	8 oz				1 tbs + 1½ tsp		1 tsp
Powder	5 scoops	8 oz					1 tbs	1 tsp

and causing dehydration. This is most likely to occur when the infant's diet includes too much salt or protein. (The metabolism of protein produces a higher solute load than does the metabolism of carbohydrate or fat.) The solute concentration of liquid is measured in osmolality (Osm). The average Osm of standard infant formula (20 cal/oz) and breast milk is 300 milliosmoles (mOsm) per liter. The American Academy of Pediatrics recommends that osmolality not exceed 400 mOsm/liter water (Packard, 1982). It is possible to exceed this figure when concentrating infant formula (American Academy of Pediatrics, Committee on Nutrition, 1976).

Dehydration is more likely to occur in an infant's first 6 months of life, when the kidneys are less able to retain water despite a high solute load. It is also more likely to occur when infants do not have enough water in their diet, sweat in hot weather, or are ill, especially with diarrhea (Fomon, 1993). It is best to prevent solute overload by carefully monitoring an infant's diet for adequate water rather than detect it after it occurs.

Based on food record analysis and on medical and laboratory indices, it may be advisable for an infant or a child to have a vitamin and/or a mineral supplement prescribed to further enhance his or her nutritional status, although isolated vitamin deficiencies are rare. Unless medically prescribed, any vitamin supplement given should not contain any individual nutrient that exceeds 100% of the RDA for age. The use of vitamin supplementation always should be discussed with the physician; however, infants or children with inadequate intakes, decreased absorption, increased requirements, or increased losses should be considered for vitamin and/or mineral supplementation. Low iron or zinc levels in many cases serve as indicators for provision of supplementation.

Home and Child Care Observations

Observation in the home provides the dietitian, nurse, or home visitor with the opportunity to see feeding interactions between parent and child as well as to assess the feeding environment (see Chapter 32). The home or child care visit also is the time to review with providers dietary instructions and answer any misconceptions that may have arisen during their clinic visit. This is the time that dietary instructions can be given to all care providers, and one can form a relationship with other family members and understand their ideas and concerns about food and feeding.

When observing a meal, check that food selection, preparation, and presentation are adequate to encourage a pleasurable feeding experience for the child. Within the feeding experience, look for cues that engage the child in readiness to eat and food exploration to increase interest in food offered. Observe feeding dynamics. Support habits that foster positive feeding, and provide alternative methods to decrease feeding struggles.

The home and child care environments should be assessed for sanitation, safe seating, and the ability of the caregiver to measure formulas or prepare supplements appropriately. Assess whether meals can be prepared and stored adequately within the home and child care environments. The food and feeding utensils should be correct for the child's developmental abilities. Keep outside distraction to a minimum so that the child's attention is not taken away from feeding.

During observations, the home or child care environment often is the place where the caregivers will offer more information as to the child's habits and lifestyles, contributing more detailed insights into possible reasons or clues for the child's growth delay. Use the home or child care visit to offer instructions regarding improvements in food preparation, feeding skills, and enhancements of environment, as well as provide information on other services that can assist the family.

CONCLUSION

Through nutritional and multidisciplinary intervention, positive growth velocity in infants and children can be achieved. The nutritional goals to achieve positive outcomes are to assist the caregiver with understanding the relationship between appropriate caloric and nutrient intake and its effect on the child's growth and development. The dietitian and the caregiver will develop strategies to increase the caloric density of foods that are available to the family. This will promote catch-up weight gain as well as develop a feeding plan that fosters the development of positive relationships involving food.

The dietitian and other team members will assist the family with resources to cope with the many social and economic issues that are involved in feeding. They also will provide positive developmental stimulation to improve the health and well-being of a growing child.

REFERENCES

American Academy of Pediatrics. (1993). *Pediatric nutrition handbook.* Elk Grove Village, IL: Author.

American Academy of Pediatrics, Committee on Nutrition. (1976). Commentary on breast feeding and infant formulas, including proposed standards for formulas. *Pediatrics, 58,* 276.

Ashworth, A., & Millward, D.J. (1986). Catch-up growth in children. *Nutrition Reviews, 44,* 157–163.

Casey, P.H., Kraemer, H.C., Bernbaum, J., Yogman, M.W., & Sells, J.C. (1991). Growth status and growth rates of a varied sample of low birth weight, preterm infants: A longitudinal cohort from birth to three years. *Journal of Pediatrics, 119,* 599–605.

Colorado Department of Public Health & Environment, Nutrition Services. (n.d.a). *Food guide pyramid: A guide to daily food choices for children 1–3 years.* Denver: Author.

Colorado Department of Public Health & Environment, Nutrition Services. (n.d.b). *La pirámide, guía de comida: Guía diaria de comidas para niños de 1 a 3 años de edad.* Denver: Author.

Dewey, K.G., Peerson, J.M., Brown, K.H., Krebs, N.F., Michaelsen, K.F., Persson, L.A., Salmenpera, L., Whitehead, R.G., Yeund, D.L., & World Health Organization Working Group on Infant Growth. (1995). Growth of breast-fed infants deviates from current reference data: A pooled analysis of US, Canadian and European data sets. *Pediatrics, 95,* 495–503.

Fomon, S.J. (1974). *Infant nutrition* (2nd ed.). Philadelphia: W.B. Saunders.

Fomon, S.J. (1993). *Nutrition of normal infants.* St. Louis: Mosby.

Frank, D., Needlman, R., & Silva, M. (1993, February). Failure to thrive: Mystery, myth and method. *Contemporary Pediatrics,* 114–133.

Glinsmann, W.H., Bartholmey, S.J., & Coletta, F. (1996). Dietary guidelines for infants: A timely reminder. *Nutrition Reviews, 54,* 2–6.

Groh-Wargo, S., Thompson, W., & Cox, J. (Eds.). (1994). *Nutritional care for high risk newborns* (rev. ed.). Chicago: Precept Press.

Howard, R., & Winter, H. (1984). *Nutrition and feeding of infants and toddlers.* Boston: Little, Brown.

Kraus, M., & Mahank, L.H. (1984). *Food nutrition and diet therapy.* Philadelphia: W.B. Saunders.

Krebs, N.F., Hambridge, K.M., & Walravens, P.A. (1984). Increased food intake of young children receiving a zinc supplement. *American Journal of Diseases of Children, 138,* 270–273.

Lawrence, R.A. (1994). *Breastfeeding: A guide for the medical profession.* St. Louis: Mosby-Year Book.

Lawrence, R.A. (1997). *A review of medical benefits and contraindications to breastfeeding in the United States* (Maternal and Child Health Technical Information Bulletin). Arlington, VA: National Education in Maternal and Child Health.

McLean, W.C. (1987). Protein-energy malnutrition. In R.J. Grand, J.L. Sutphen, & W. Dietz (Eds.), *Pediatric nutrition: Theory and practice* (pp. 421–450). Boston: Butterworth Publishers.

National Academy of Sciences. (1989). *Recommended dietary allowances* (9th ed.). Washington, DC: National Research Council, Food and Nutrition Board.

National Academy of Sciences, Subcommittee on Nutrition During Lactation, Committee on Nutritional Status During Pregnancy and Lactating, Food and Nutrition Board. (1991). *Nutrition during lactation.* Washington, DC: National Academy Press.

Oski, F.A. (1989). *The causes of iron deficiency in infants' dietary iron: Birth to two years.* New York: Raven Press.

Packard, V.S. (1982). *Human milk and infant formula.* New York: Academic Press.

Peterson, K.E. (1993). Failure to thrive. In S.P. Queen & C.E. Lang (Eds.), *Handbook for pediatric nutrition* (pp. 366–383). Gaithersburg, MD: Aspen Publishers.

Peterson, K.E., Washington, J., & Rathbun, J. (1984). Team management of failure to thrive. *Journal of the American Dietetic Association, 84,* 810–815.

Powers, N.G., & Slusser, W. (1997). Breastfeeding update 2: Clinical lactation management. *Pediatrics in Review, 18,* 147–161.

Riordan, J., & Auerbach, K.G. (1993). *Breastfeeding and human lactation.* Boston: Jones and Bartlett Publishers.

Ross Products Division, Abbott Laboratories. (1992). *IHDP growth percentiles: VLBW premature boys and girls.* Columbus, OH: Author.

Suskind, R.M. (1981). *Textbook of pediatric nutrition.* New York: Raven Press.

The American Dietetic Association. (1996). *Food guide pyramid with popular Chinese fare.* Chicago: Author.

Chapter 7

The Feeding Relationship

Ellyn Satter

Eating is a complex set of skills that children learn gradually and over time. As children grow, their nervous system settles down, they slowly gain more and more control over their body, and they can eat more and more challenging food. At each stage of development, children master particular eating competencies and use those achievements as a basis for moving on to the next stage. Whether children develop and retain these capabilities with eating depends on parental behavior.

To allow children to do well with eating, the feeding environment must be positive and their food must be appropriate both nutritionally and developmentally. Unless they are having physical problems, children do well with eating when they are given a positive and supportive environment and realistic limits. They eat the right amount of food to grow in a way that is biologically appropriate for them, and they learn gradually to like a variety of nutritious foods.

In some situations, however, children get too little support or too much pressure to grow well. Parents might give too little support by failing to respond to children's bids for feeding or by offering nipple-feeds or solid foods that are poorly digestible, developmentally inappropriate, or distorted in caloric density. At the other extreme, parents might be overly controlling, restricting the children's food intake because of misplaced health or weight concerns. Or parents might try to coerce children to eat more than they are hungry for, leading children to recoil by undereating or to comply by overeating.

Often, children's temperamental or physical characteristics contribute to parents' tendencies to be overcontrolling or undersupportive. For instance, the ill, passive, or sleepy infant who does not ask to be cared for may be underfed. The aggressive or exceptionally combative toddler may pull parents into struggles for control over feeding.

The author thanks Paulette Bochnig Sharkey for editorial assistance in the preparation of this chapter.

Positive associations and experiences between parents and children around food depend on children's being offered food that is appropriate for their neuromuscular capability. For most of the first year, children depend on nipple-feeding. The cuddling and touching of nipple-feeding during the early months helps them establish **homeostasis** and develop attachment. Sometime around 6 months of age, children who are developing normally have the neuromuscular skills to sit up, see food coming, maintain visual and verbal connection with parents, and start eating from a spoon. Spoon-feeding and the transition to table food, then, reflect children's separation and individuation process as they move from the primary one-to-one feeding relationship to the broader social world of the family table. Eventually, they learn to eat with people outside the family and to cope with unfamiliar foods.

INTRODUCTION

Effective feeding requires a give-and-take exchange between parent and child with the behavior of each depending on what the other does (Satter, 1986). The parent must acknowledge and respect the child's capability and autonomy but also provide the proper food, in a form that the child can manage and in a social environment that is loving and accepting.

The focus of feeding should not be to get food into the child. Such an emphasis puts pressure on both the feeder and the child, often resulting in disrespectful feeding tactics that preempt the child's initiative. Such pressure tactics limit the child's possibility for success and instill long-term negative eating attitudes and behaviors.

Instead, the focus should be on the achievable goal of helping the child learn eating skills and positive eating attitudes and behaviors. If the feeding relationship is smooth and congenial and appropriate for the child's nutritional needs and neuromuscular development, then the child will do well with eating.

THE FEEDING RELATIONSHIP

The feeding relationship is the complex of interactions that takes place between parent (or primary caregiver) and child as they engage in food selection, ingestion, and regulation. Feeding is an interactive process that depends on the abilities and characteristics of both parent and child. The child indicates an interest in being fed, with more or less clarity; the parent responds to that interest readily, reluctantly, or by ignoring it completely.

Once feeding starts, parent and child work on the process with more or less flexibility and skill. Some parents, at times, are very skillful and resourceful; some, at times, are awkward or impatient. Children respond to their parents' efforts in a similar variety of ways. They may react cheerfully and with resourcefulness of their own, or they may display bewilderment and impatience.

Parents may be accepting and supportive of a child's constitutional endowment for growth and body shape or be dissatisfied and controlling. And, of course, the child may grow and develop in a way that is pleasing to the parent or may do the opposite.

An appropriate feeding relationship supports a child's developmental tasks at every age, allowing the child to be well nourished and to achieve optimum, genetically determined growth as well as positive development in other areas. High-quality feeding interactions during the first years of life are linked positively to a child's subsequent cognitive and linguistic competence and to more secure attachments to major caregivers (Barnard et al., 1989). At all stages, optimum interaction between parent and child depends on emotionally healthy, sensitive, and responsive parents as well as on a child who is able to achieve an adequate level of communication and stability (Satter, 1990).

Optimum feeding at every stage—from the newborn to the older baby to the toddler—depends on negotiating successfully the balance of communication and control in the stage before. From birth, parents optimally see the child as an individual who is able to play an active role in feeding. In deferring to the infant and depending on his or her cues to guide feeding, parents recognize and support the child's autonomy well before autonomy becomes a primary developmental issue. Although parents and providers are most aware of feeding problems among toddlers, prevention of these problems lies in the early feeding relationship.

DIVISION OF RESPONSIBILITY IN FEEDING CHILDREN

Feeding children depends on a division of responsibility between parent and child. This division integrates a developmental understanding of the child with clinical observations and the research on feeding dynamics. During the first 6 months, the division of responsibility in feeding is simple: Parents are responsible for *what* infants are offered to eat; and infants are responsible for everything else about eating, including *how much* they eat (Satter, 1987).

To feed the infant well, parents dedicate themselves to understanding information that comes from the child and work to keep the child happy and comfortable. If, however, parents try to keep their toddler (the child between 6 and 36 months) happy and comfortable, then they will fail him or her utterly. Securely attached toddlers need to discover that they are separate from their parents. To do this, they need structure and limits; therefore, for toddlers and older children, the division of responsibility becomes more complex: Parents are responsible for the what, when, and where of *feeding*; and, given the support and limits provided by parents, children become responsible for the how much and whether of *eating*.

Embedded in the division of responsibility are some assumptions about parents' responsibilities with feeding and children's capabilities with eating. Parents are responsible for choosing and preparing food, providing regularly scheduled meals and snacks, making eating times pleasant, and providing mastery expectations for the child. Given the reasonably effective execution of these responsibilities, children are able to manifest their capabilities with eating. Children, for the most part, *will* eat, they *want* to eat, they know how much to eat, they automatically will eat a variety of foods, they will grow predictably, and they will mature with their eating.

ENERGY REGULATION AND FEEDING DYNAMICS

To establish a positive feeding relationship, the parent must trust in the child's capabilities with eating. If the child is extreme in eating or growth, however, then parents have difficulty sustaining that trust. If a child eats a relatively small amount of food or grows relatively slowly, then parents are likely to try to overrule his or her feeding cues and get him or her to eat more or grow faster. Such tactics backfire: Children who are urged or coerced to eat consume less, not more, and grow more slowly. Because parents' tendency to compensate is so common as to be predictable, teaching positive feeding is essential for parents of the small or small-eating child. Children eat best when parents do their part in feeding, provide children with the appropriate support for their developmental stage, and avoid putting pressure on feeding.

To support parents in establishing a positive feeding relationship with their child, health care providers must be exceptionally careful not to impose outside expectations on how much a child should eat. Such expectations put pressure on feeding and, in turn, are likely to make the child eat less, not more. Infants often are discharged from the newborn intensive care unit (NICU) or sent home from growth workups with such prescriptions. In reality, it is not possible to predict with any accuracy a child's energy requirements, and attempts to do so will only distort feeding.

Given a supportive feeding relationship, infants and young children have the innate ability to regulate how much they eat. It is impossible to calculate precisely how much children need to eat in order to grow well. Children's energy requirements vary depending on gender, size, growth rate, physical activity, and metabolic efficiency. Two children who look and seemingly behave identically can vary greatly from one another in calorie requirement. Some children are extremely efficient metabolically and grow along the 50th percentile or even higher on relatively small amounts of calories. Other small or lean children appear to expend considerably more calories in daily activity and require relatively high food intake. In their observational work with 4- to 6-month-olds, Rose and Mayer (1968) found that the fattest infants ate the least and were the least active, and the leanest infants ate the most and were the most active. Children require energy for growing, and they grow inconsistently. Children's height increases in spurts, then stabilizes (Lampl, Veldhuis, & Johnson, 1992).

Energy intake figures can vary from child to child by as much as 20% over or under the average daily calorie requirements based on body weight (National Research Council, 1989). In addition, it is not unusual for children to vary from day to day by 25% over or under their average caloric intake. As a consequence, extremes in food intake on a given day may be entirely normal. Despite this considerable fluctuation, children are able to maintain stable growth. Children know how much they need to eat, and they can make up for their errors in feeding. If they are underfed inadvertently, then they get hungry sooner and eat more at the next feeding.

Disrupting children's natural capabilities in food regulation requires considerable and continuous efforts, efforts that often are well intentioned. Parents might underfeed consistently because of some imposed expectation about amount or timing of feedings or because they are so distracted that they do not respond to infant cues. The child may contribute to the underfeeding by becoming anxious or revolted by unpleasant feeding interactions and resist the feeding. The emotional static in the interaction between parent and child may become so salient that it drowns out the child's ability to distinguish and respond to feeding cues.

In contrast, parents are less stressed and can do better with feeding when they understand the child's natural variation in food intake. Parents who are concerned about poor growth or are trying to get a child ready nutritionally for surgery scrutinize the amounts that a child eats. When the child eats a lot, the parents' hopes soar; when the child compensates by eating less, the parents' hopes are dashed.

Manipulating Calories in Food

To support and preserve the feeding relationship, the child's food must be appropriate not only nutritionally and developmentally but also with respect to caloric density (calories per unit volume). Formula must be properly diluted, and, for the older child, foods of a variety of caloric densities must be offered. Manipulating caloric density, however, does not substitute in any way for attending to feeding dynamics. Such manipulations may or may not be helpful. Once they are past the age of 6 weeks, children are such resilient and resourceful regulators that they compensate by consuming more of a dilute formula or less of a concentrated, high-calorie formula or high-calorie semisolid or table food (Fomon, Filer, Thomas, Anderson, & Nelson, 1975).

With older children, the issue of caloric density of the diet often is synonymous with fat content. Ideally, at a given meal, children will be offered foods of a variety of fat contents. On a given day, they eat more or less of foods that they have found to be high in energy, depending on how hungry they are (Kern, McPhee, Fisher, Johnson, & Birch, 1993). From year to year, they show similar variations. Children followed from one year to the next varied widely in their fat intake (Beal, 1961), apparently shifting their food preferences depending on energy needs.

Given the current wellness emphasis in public health nutrition policy, it is important to be sure that poorly growing children are offered adequate fat in their diets. Some children have shown compromised growth when nutrition-conscious parents were overzealous about restricting dietary fat (Pugliese, Weyman-Daum, Moses, & Lifshitz, 1987) and imposing vegetarian diets (Dwyer, Andrew, Valadian, & Reed, 1980) or other alternative diets (Dagnelie, Van-Staveren, & Hautvast, 1991). Unless a particular effort is made to include good fat sources, the vegetarian diet is so high in bulk and low in caloric density that children are unable to consume enough energy to grow properly.

In selected cases, to preserve the feeding relationship as well as to allow the child to achieve appropriate growth, it is helpful to manipulate caloric density. This would be as an adjunct, not as a substitute, for working with feeding and a strategy that would be intended to help parent and child be successful with oral feeding.[1] Children who have physical or neuromuscular limitations may benefit from a higher-calorie formula and only moderate use of relatively low-calorie food. Children who have heart defects may not have the strength to take in enough food to sustain growth. Children who have cerebral palsy may be so disorganized in their sucking and swallowing that they are unable to sustain optimum nutritional status and growth with a formula of standard dilution. Ashworth and Millward (1986) found that children who are wasted (low weight-for-height) but not stunted (low height-for-age) can experience catch-up growth in weight at a rate of up to 20 times the normal rate. Such children may be willing and able to consume up to double their usual energy intake and need to be offered routinely foods of relatively high caloric density; however, extremes of caloric densities may precipitate other health problems, which, in turn, can distort the child's growth. A child on highly concentrated formula may experience dehydration; a child on a highly dilute formula may experience water intoxication. Because these risks exist, it is essential to vary the concentration of an infant's formula only under careful supervision of a physician.

PRIMARY PREVENTION OF FEEDING PROBLEMS

Most problems concerning feeding can be prevented by routine support and education about feeding and parenting in health supervision and/or nutrition counseling sessions (Satter & Sharkey, 1995). Parents need to learn how to observe, understand, and respond to their child's feeding cues; how to select appropriate food; and how to establish comfortable feeding styles. They should be alerted to the natural progression that children go through as their chewing, swallowing, and manual dexterity mature (see Table 1). Parents who are prone to precipitating feeding problems and parents of children who are prone to

---

[1]For some children, supplemental tube feedings may be helpful in preserving oral feeding and a positive feeding relationship (see Chapter 11).

Table 1.   Eating competence

HOMEOSTASIS—Birth to three months
- Can root, suck and swallow
- Shows readable, moderate feeding cues
- Remains calm and alert during feeding
- Is generally positive during feeding
- Can eat enough to get full
- Shows readable, positive signs of fullness
- Grows in a predictable way
- Can tolerate the available food

ATTACHMENT—Three to six months
- Maintains competencies of earlier stage
- When hungry, opens mouth for nipple
- Shows non-anxious arousal when hungry
- "Talks" and gestures with feeder
- Is generally positive during feeding
- Looks and smiles at feeder
- Shows clear, positive signs of fullness
- Sustains predictable growth
- Toward end of period, may be ready for solids
- Can tolerate the available food

SEPARATION/INDIVIDUATION—Six months to three years

Six to twelve months
- Maintains competencies of earlier stage
- Shows readable, moderate, varied hunger cues
- Is generally positive during feeding
- Progressively develops eating skills
- Will experiment with cup
- Shows a positive interest in the food, feeder
- Has a range of communications about eating
- Will experiment with new tastes
- Can eat and tolerate available food
- Will explore increasingly difficult textures
- Shows clear, varied and positive satiety cues
- Maintains consistent growth

Twelve to eighteen months
- Maintains competencies of earlier stage
- Shows interest in eating
- Is generally positive about eating
- Can tolerate hunger briefly, wait to eat
- Participates in family meals, eats soft solid food

- Feeds self with hands or utensils
- Drinks from a cup
- Solid food is primary source of nutrients
- Starts to eat at reasonably predictable times
- Generally eats to satiety, stops when full
- Eats enough to be comfortable between feedings
- Indicates satiety in positive ways
- Maintains consistent growth

Eighteen months to three years
- Maintains competencies of earlier stage
- Shows interest in eating
- Is generally positive about eating
- Can wait briefly to eat when hungry
- Participates in family meals
- Tastes new foods repeatedly, masters many
- Refuses food without becoming upset
- Eats and tolerates the available food
- Takes pleasure in eating
- Can accept limits in feeding
- Maintains nutritional adequacy
- Eats to satiety, stops when full
- Expresses satiety in positive ways
- Maintains consistent growth

INITIATIVE—Three years to six years
- Maintains competencies of earlier stage
- Is generally positive around feeding
- Is interested in food and eating
- Can eat in unfamiliar surroundings with unfamiliar people
- Is calm when offered new or disliked food
- Can refuse food politely
- Can "make do" with less-favorite foods
- Accommodates to feeding limits
- Can tolerate hunger, wait to eat
- Takes initiative, pride in mastery with foods
- Uses learning about food to aid in mastery
- Is influenced by peers in food preference
- Eats variety, amount for nutritional adequacy
- Shows reasonably civilized table manners
- Experiences and expresses pleasure in eating
- Eats to satiety, stops when full
- Maintains consistent growth
- Is comfortable with and accepting of body

From Satter, E.M. (1996). *Feeding with love and good sense: Training manual for the VISIONS workshop* (pp. 49–51). Madison, WI: Ellyn Satter Associates; reprinted by permission.

developing feeding problems (see Table 2) require careful anticipatory guidance and follow-up (Satter, 1995). For instance, parents whose children have been identified as "at risk" or "at nutritional risk" (designations that are used routinely by public health programs such as the Special Supplemental Nutrition Program for Women, Infants and Children [WIC] and the Early Intervention Programs) have a strong tendency to put pressure on feeding (Field, 1977).

Parents may be offered verbal and written information on choosing food that is appropriate for their child's stage of development; on identifying and understanding mouth, hand, and body development as it relates to feeding; and on ways of feeding that allow children to be successful and safe with eating (see *How to Feed Your Toddler* in the appendix at the end of this chapter).

Any food selection or feeding information that is given to parents must support rather than interfere with sensitivity to the child's feeding cues. For instance, a parent who is advised to feed an infant on demand will be supported in seeking and responding to the child's cues in feeding, whereas a parent who is advised to feed on a schedule will be trained to ignore the child's feeding cues. Dictating amounts of formulas or insisting on slavish adherence to growth charts can make a parent focus on getting food into the child rather than on the child's messages about how hungry or how full he or she is.

In routine health supervision, minor growth divergences generally are ignored and the parent is reassured; however, these minor divergences should be attended to as part of routine care because they may be a sign of difficulty in the feeding relationship. In the primary care setting, the provider can matter-of-factly inquire about the quality of the feeding relationship and the parents' attitudes, concerns, or satisfaction with the child's eating and growth. Children who diverge slightly downward on their growth curve may be showing a normal growth adjustment; however, this downward divergence also may signal dif-

Table 2.   Characteristics that impair feeding

Children prone to developing feeding problems:
1. Children who are temperamentally negative or slow to warm up
2. Children "at risk" or "at nutritional risk"
3. The exceptionally large or small child
4. The exceptionally large or small eater
5. The child who has been ill
6. Children who were prematurely born
7. Children with neuromuscular and/or cognitive limitations
8. Children on modified diets; for example, children with diabetes

Parents prone to precipitating feeding problems:
1. Parents who are overactive and too stimulating
2. Parents who are underactive or not engaging
3. Parents who are unusually rigid or controlling
4. Parents who are unusually chaotic or disorganized
5. Parents who are excessively concerned about their child's diet and weight
6. Parents who are excessively concerned about their own diet and weight
7. Parents who have a particular agenda with growth

From Satter, E.M. (1994, October 25). *Preventing childhood obesity: A new paradigm.* Paper presented at the Wisconsin Special Supplemental Food Program for Women, Infants and Children (WIC) and Maternal Child Health (MCH) conference: "Uniting Communities for Mothers and Children," Wisconsin Dells, WI; reprinted by permission.

ficulties in feeding. Catching these feeding problems early may allow their resolution in the primary care setting.

Moderate growth decreases could indicate that a parent is restricting food because he or she is reluctant to gratify fully the large child's appetite for fear that the child will become fat. Or the parent of the NICU graduate may be following early directions to get a certain amount of food into the child but the child fights back and refuses to eat.[2] Or the parent of the toddler who is eating and growing poorly may be having trouble with establishing structure and limits with feeding and the toddler begs for—and gets—enough juice to spoil his or her appetite for meals (Smith & Lifshitz, 1994).

Secondary Intervention

Because feeding is such a familiar and seemingly accessible process, established or entrenched feeding problems may be overlooked or underestimated. Careful evaluation and treatment are required when parents and children with an established feeding problem cannot change in response to the primary intervention. Parents may be too afraid, too chaotic, or too rigid. A child may have a neuromuscular problem that first presents itself as a difficulty with eating. Parents of a child who was born prematurely or was ill may be unable to stop pushing food because they are so afraid that the child will not survive. Or parents may be restricting the child's food intake because they are vehement about preventing fatness and alarmed about the child's robust appetite.

In contrast to primary problems, secondary problems are well established and the feelings about them are stronger. There is likely to be a secondary problem when

- The child's growth continues to be erratic or to diverge from the growth curve
- The parent continues to complain about feeding, even if growth is all right
- The child continues to have trouble with eating

Children's growth normally is resilient. It takes a major or prolonged insult to disrupt a child's growth. As a consequence, when growth diverges significantly and the problem is distortion in feeding dynamics, the feeding disruption is an established one. Intervention with an established problem requires careful evaluation to identify the problem concretely and distinguish its source, to develop a behavioral treatment plan, and to institute that plan progressively over several sessions.[3]

Tertiary Intervention

Seemingly familiar and accessible feeding problems that are presented in the primary care setting may require tertiary intervention. Because eating is such a sensitive barometer of emotional state and parent–child interaction, psychosocial distortions often appear first to the health care worker as distortions in feeding. Parents who require tertiary intervention are those who are entrenched in their way of doing things to the extent that they cannot respond to the child's distress or bids for attention. These parents may be very disorganized or overwhelmed by life's demands, or they may be rigidly controlling from fear of being defeated by their feelings or their life circumstances.

---

[2]It is not uncommon for parents of NICU graduates to be warned not to feed too much for fear that the child's "stomach will blow up." This probably is a reference to **necrotizing enterocolitis** and the erroneous conviction that it is caused by overloading the gastrointestinal tract.

[3]The Feeding with Love and Good Sense intensive workshop by Ellyn Satter trains professionals in secondary intervention with child-feeding problems. For information, call Ellyn Satter Associates, (800) 808-7976, or visit her World Wide Web site at www.ellynsatter.com.

The need for tertiary intervention becomes apparent to the provider because parents are too rigid or disorganized to apply the systematic and sequential change of the secondary intervention. Parents may be unconcerned about serious divergences in growth or vehement about getting the child to behave in certain ways. To be able to learn and change their feeding behaviors, such families require not only secondary feeding intervention but also psychotherapy or social casework to bring them to the point at which they can respond to that intervention.

HOMEOSTASIS: BIRTH TO THREE MONTHS

During the first 2–3 months of life, the infant's primary developmental task is to regulate sleep and awake states and achieve the quiet, alert state of homeostasis. Achieving self-regulation is necessary for infants to be able to interact with what goes on around them. Conversely, interacting with what goes on around them and taking an interest in outside events help infants remain self-regulated. Infants work instinctively to remain organized, calm, and interested. Increasingly during the first several months, infants master the ability to be calm and alert when they are awake, to be soundly asleep when they are asleep, to go smoothly from one state to another, and to be tolerant enough of what goes on outside or inside them that they can remain composed.

The parents' task is to discover, through trial and error, what helps their infant to stay organized and, conversely, what makes their infant overstimulated or upset. An infant may calm down when he or she is rocked during feeding, or the rocking may make him or her too stimulated to eat. A fretful infant may be captivated and settled by a gaudy toy or may be upset and further disorganized by it.

Feeding that Supports Homeostasis

Attitudes and behaviors that parents learn regarding feeding affect feeding and their relationship with their child throughout the growing-up years. If parents develop an early attitude of curiosity and trust toward their child, then they will be willing to guide feeding by information that comes from the child. Such an attitude and the behaviors that grow out of it actively support the infant's attempts to achieve and maintain homeostasis (and, later, attachment and separation-individuation). Early feeding is an important behavioral organizer to the newborn (Chatoor, Dickson, Schaefer, & Egan, 1985); most of the time that parent and infant are together during the early months is spent during feeding. Generally, feeding supports homeostasis when the infant is fed in a trusting and supportive fashion; feeding undermines homeostasis when the parent ignores input from the child, takes control, and imposes expectations on the child (see *Control of Feeding* in the appendix at the end of this chapter). Parents trust the infant and share control by feeding on demand, by feeding as much or as little as the infant wants to eat, by working to calm the infant, and by feeding in a smooth and continuous fashion in response to signs that come from the infant.

To do their part with breast- or bottle-feeding, infants need to cry or move around and let their parents know that they are hungry. They must be able to respond to their parents' efforts to feed without getting overstimulated (Mogan, 1987), and they need to stay awake during the feeding. The poorly growing, seemingly content breast-fed infant might have difficulties with waking up or staying awake during the feeding. At the other extreme, an infant might be so easily agitated that he or she can nurse for only short periods before getting too disorganized and upset to continue eating. Many infants who were born prematurely or ill are both sleepy and easily agitated. When parents try to wake them enough to feed them, it sends these infants off into irritable crying.

Responsive and attentive feeding helps the infant tolerate the arousal that goes along with being hungry. A hungry infant who is fed promptly and given enough to eat comes to pair hunger with positive and satisfying interactions. Over time, these experiences contribute to homeostasis. Conversely, domineering feeding undermines homeostasis; it is harder for an infant to stay organized when he or she is staved off to follow a schedule or forced to eat beyond satiety. In fact, it is quite possible that such tactics contribute to infantile colic—abdominal pain that is experienced by some infants during the early months and that is characterized by unexplained, strident crying. According to Taubman's (1988) clinical observations, many infants become colicky when parents chronically misinterpret crying. For instance, thinking their recently fed infant cannot possibly be hungry, parents will stave off a feeding until the child is so frantic and exhausted from crying that he cannot do a good job with eating, thus starting the cycle all over again.

Errors in Feeding that Disrupt Homeostasis

Certain parental behaviors appear to disrupt homeostasis and undermine the child's ability to eat the right amount of food to grow well. Based on their observations of children who gained weight poorly in the first month, Pollitt and Wirtz (1981) observed that mothers worked against a smooth feeding with such activities as frequently taking the nipple from the infant's mouth, continuously rotating or moving the nipple, and grooming the infant's body. Infants whose mothers were too active ate less than infants whose mothers provided a smooth, continuous feeding.

Crow, Fawcett, and Wright (1980) found a marked difference in the manner in which parents fed small infants compared with average-size infants. Parents who bottle-fed small infants were relatively active in feeding, and infants grew less well. Parents who bottle-fed average-size infants remained appropriately active in feeding as did parents who breast-fed both small and average-size infants. All infants of the appropriately active parents grew well. Ainsworth and Bell (1969) observed that parents who terminated feeding at pauses rather than gave the infant time to finish the feeding were more likely to underfeed. Such parents interpreted infant fussiness as satiety rather than soothed the fussiness and checked back with the infant to determine whether he or she still was hungry. In many cases, the observed mothers claimed to be feeding on demand but seemed eager to finish caring for their infants and put them down when the infants stopped to smile or fuss. In many cases, nipple holes were too big and when infants interrupted the feeding to gag, feedings were terminated. Field (1977) found that feeders tended to be more active with both premature and postmature babies. She surmised that the "at risk" designation and parental perception of it acted as stimuli to parents to increase their attempts to promote food intake, using pressure tactics such as jiggling the nipple (and the infant).

Although feeding is intensely comforting and calming to a hungry infant, attempting to feed the satiated infant is likely to disrupt homeostasis. Ainsworth and Bell (1969) observed that some mothers fed well past satiety, some to gratify infants who appeared to enjoy eating, others so that infants would sleep longer between feedings. The infants were tense and unhappy, and feedings "had to be seen to be believed" (Ainsworth & Bell, 1969, p. 148).

Parents may put their infants to bed with bottles as a way of putting them to sleep or prop bottles to cut down on feeding time. Babies need the stimulation and stabilizing of cuddling while they nipple-feed. Infants who feed themselves may have trouble staying awake to eat or may get so disorganized that they cannot sustain the feeding. Although young breast- or bottle-fed infants do go to sleep while they are being fed, it generally is best to work toward having them be awake when they finish eating. Being able to put themselves to sleep is part of the homeostatic rhythm that they need to develop during the early months.

Changing the infant's food or switching mechanics of feeding can interfere with homeostasis and impair the infant's ability to eat. Infants' relationships with the world are mediated through their mouths. Although differences in nipples or taste and texture of foods may seem slight to us, they are major and upsetting changes to infants. Changes may include switching formulas or nipples abruptly (including introducing the breast-fed infant to an artificial nipple), putting semisolids in the infant's bottle, and introducing solid foods too early. Beal (1957) found that when mothers tried to introduce solids before age 3–4 months, they had significant and upsetting conflicts with their infants over feeding. These same children accepted solid foods readily when they were older.

ATTACHMENT: THREE TO SIX MONTHS

By age 2–3 months, infants who can sustain a reasonable level of calmness and focused attention can direct their interest outside themselves. During the time from 3 to 6 months, when attachment is the child's primary emotional task, the child begins learning to love and to actively engage the interest of the people around him or her. He or she begins to reach out, smile, make noises, and develop an increasing variety of ways to attract and hold the parents' attention.

To continue to generate ways of actively engaging the interest and involvement of their parents, infants need to get a reasonably frequent answering response. To preserve their child's interest and delight in being sociable, parents need to maintain an active state of give and take, responding when the infant smiles, talks, or reaches out but being careful not to overwhelm the infant with the energy of the interaction. If parents do not respond or if they act in contradictory or confusing ways, then children compensate. They may give up and become listless and apathetic, they may exaggerate their efforts to connect by being demanding and aggressive, or they may guard against negative interactions by becoming watchful and hypervigilant. **Rumination** has been hypothesized to be the attention-getting or self-stimulating response of a poorly attached infant.

Feeding that Supports Attachment

During the second 6 months, feeding continues to be the focus of much of the time that infants and parents spend together. As a consequence, eating competence is correlated closely with emotional attachment. The sensitive and responsive feeding behaviors that support homeostasis are equally important in supporting attachment. In fact, even though attachment has become primary, the work with homeostasis continues. Optimum nipple-feeding from ages 2 to 6 months keeps the child firmly in control. Supportive parents modulate arousal when they attend promptly to the infant's crying, comfort the infant, and feed in a smooth and continuous fashion, paying attention to signals from the child to guide the feeding process. Parents help their child feel loved when they time feedings in response to the child's signs of hunger and let the routine of feeding evolve from the child's increased regularity of eating and sleeping.

The 2- to 6-month-old child is easier for parents to manage because his or her nervous system is more mature, he or she is better at keeping calm, and his or her feeding cues are more readable. Parents mature as well: They get better at following the child's lead and become increasingly skillful in identifying feeding cues—although infants support their parents' skill by signaling their needs more clearly. Affect-laden interactions become more apparent: The parent smiles, speaks pleasantly and encouragingly, and appears to enjoy the infant. The infant, in turn, smiles, cuddles, takes the initiative in indicating hunger, and appears to enjoy the parent and the feeding process.

The pause in feeding becomes important social time (Pridham, 1989). When the parent interprets the pause correctly, the infant socializes, rests, or looks around, then returns to feeding; however, parents often interpret the pause incorrectly and respond with behaviors that intrude on feeding. They may perceive the pause as discomfort and a sign for burping. Unnecessary burping arouses the infant and disrupts the rhythm of the feeding. The parent may interpret the pause as a sign of satiety and may stop feeding. This pattern has been observed frequently in poorly growing infants (Whitten, Pettit, & Fischoff, 1969).

As infants approach 6 months of age, feeding gets complicated by the addition of solid foods. When parents introduce solid foods, not only do they need to tune in to the infant's feeding cues, emotional overtures, and sleep states; but they also need to understand the child's neuromuscular development relative to feeding (Table 3).

During the early months, infants can only root for the nipple and suck. In sucking, they keep their mouth fastened on the nipple (partially by suction) and their tongue goes backward and forward as they stroke the milk from the nipple and swallow. If solid foods are offered by spoon at this stage, then the sucking motion becomes an extrusion reflex, which pushes the food back out of the mouth.

Usually, some time between 5 and 7 months of age, the extrusion reflex gets toned down and children begin to show developmental signs of readiness for the more mature feeding style of solid foods (see Table 3). Children who are ready to begin solid foods sit up (with or without support), are able to see food approaching, and open their mouth for it. They have developed enough control of their mouth muscles so that they can learn (sometimes immediately) to close their lips over a spoon, scrape the food from the spoon with their lips, and transfer the food from the tip of their tongue to the back where they swallow it. Sitting up straight enhances their ability to manage food in their mouth and to swallow it safely and properly (see Table 4).

As mentioned previously, children do best in feeding when they feel that they have control. The infant who can sit up and hold up his or her head can give a variety of messages to feeders about the way in which he or she wants to be fed. He or she can open his or her mouth and move forward, can close his or her mouth and turn away, and can swipe the food toward his or her mouth or bat it away.

Errors in Feeding: Three to Six Months

At the same time as eating competence is associated with emotional attachment, so, too, do emotional difficulties between parents and children play themselves out in feeding and may be reflected in the infant's growth. When parents are depressed and unresponsive, infants may demand extra food as a way of getting attention, substituting food for the emotional gratification that they miss (Satter, 1990); or they may lose interest in feeding altogether. If parents are overly aggressive, then children may become agitated or withdrawn. Poorly attached children may fail to signal their hunger and may sink into a profound state of undernourishment (Chatoor et al., 1985).

Introducing solid food too early can cause poor food acceptance as well as disrupt attachment. Not until infants approach the age of 6 months can most of them sit up, manage the mechanics of spoon-feeding, and maintain a sense of involvement with the parent over a greater physical distance (American Academy of Pediatrics, Committee on Nutrition, 1980). When parents introduce solids too early, before the child shows signs of developmental readiness, children accept the foods reluctantly and struggle with parents about feeding (Beal, 1957). When parents fail to allow a child time to experiment and get used

Table 3.   Feeding capabilities and food selection for infants and toddlers

Age	Feeding capabilities	Manner of feeding	Suggested foods
Birth to 6 months	Cuddles Roots for nipple Sucks Swallows	Nipple-feeding	Breast milk or iron-fortified formula
5 to 7 months	Begins to sit Follows food with eyes Opens for spoon Closes lips over spoon Moves semi-solids to back of tongue Swallows semi-solids	Spoon-feeding of semi-solid food	Iron-fortified baby rice or barley cereal mixed with formula or breast milk
6 to 8 months	Moves tongue to sides Positions food in mouth Delays swallow Munches: chews up and down Palms food Scrapes food into mouth	Spoon-feeding and finger-feeding of thicker, lumpier food	Mashed potatoes Well-cooked, mashed vegetables and beans Soft, diced fruits Sticky rice Chopped noodles and other pasta
7 to 10 months	Bites off food Chews with rotary movement Moves food side-to-side in mouth, pausing in the middle Curves lips around cup Uses thumb and forefinger to finger-feed	Finger-feeding of lumpy food, pieces of soft food Drinking from the cup	Cut-up vegetables Diced fruits Tender chopped meats Casseroles Tortillas
12 months and beyond	Becomes more skillful with hands Finger-feeds Improves chewing Improves cup-drinking Is interested in food Becomes more sociable at family table	Finger-feeding of table foods	Pieces of soft, cooked foods Pieces of soft, raw food (like bananas or peaches) Dry cereal Toast and crackers Cheese and eggs Anything that sticks together

From Satter, E.M., & Sharkey, P.B. (1997). *Montana feeding relationship training package.* Madison, WI: Ellyn Satter Associates; adapted by permission.

Table 4.   How to feed solid foods

- Feed your baby when she is hungry and wants to eat, but work toward regular feeding times.
- Put her in the highchair, perhaps propped up with a couple of pillows.
- Have her sit up straight and face you: She'll be able to swallow better and be less likely to choke.
- Sit right in front of her.
- Hold the spoonful of food about 12 inches away from her face. (It's easiest to start out with a long-handled baby spoon.)
- Wait for her to pay attention and open her mouth before you try to feed her.
- Feed as slowly or as fast as she wants to eat.
- Let her touch her food.
- Respect her caution. It will take a while for her to get used to the spoon and the flavors of the foods.
- Talk to her, keep her company, but don't be exciting or entertaining.
- Let her eat as much as she wants.
- Stop feeding as soon as she shows you she's done.

From Satter, E.M., & Sharkey, P.B. (1995). *Ellyn Satter's nutrition and feeding for infants and children: Handout masters* (p. 61). Madison, WI: Ellyn Satter Associates; adapted by permission.

to the radically different textures and mechanics of the new feeding style, the child may feel overwhelmed and try to get away or he or she may submit and lose an important sense of connectedness with self and with parent. Although breast-fed infants are more receptive to new foods than formula-fed infants, all infants need to taste new foods a number of times before they accept them readily (Sullivan & Birch, 1994). Spoon-feeding does not make feeding skills mature any faster (Morris, 1989).

Finally, the distress that grows out of children's struggles with parents over solid foods may interfere with children's ability to regulate food intake. Children become so upset that they cannot tune in to their internal regulators of hunger, appetite, and satiety and, therefore, may underfeed or overfeed themselves. In any case, if children's needs are ignored consistently, then they will develop, on a preverbal level, negative feelings about self and other people.

SEPARATION-INDIVIDUATION: SIX TO THIRTY-SIX MONTHS

Beginning at about 6 months of age and continuing until age 3 years, children move from being infants to being toddlers. Toddlers have grave—and appropriate—difficulty being amenable to suggestion. Toddlers' primary task is to discover autonomy, to establish that autonomy in their own minds and those of other people, and to experience themselves as separate from the important people in their lives. Toddlers *must* move and manipulate to give themselves experiences of separateness and scope. Toddlers are without internal limits in their cognitive immaturity, their drive to establish territory, and their enthusiasm for discovering how the world works.

Toddlers can roam and explore and come back and check in because they have learned to deal with physical separation and to maintain emotional contact over distance. They depend absolutely on their parents to keep them safe enough to strike out on their own. At all times, they are ambivalent. This ambivalence was captured richly by writer Roberta Israeloff:

Just up from his nap, my son sits on my lap and softly cries, "I want my mommy." He tries to push his way into my very body, to crawl back inside. He is seeking some abstract mother, some enfolding presence from which he can never be taken. I kiss him gently. "Don't kiss me, Mom," he says, indignantly wriggling out of my arms, trying to wipe the kiss off his cheek. (1991, p. 84)

To be helpful to a toddler with his or her struggle for autonomy, parents need to hold steady. They need to remain present without taking over and to give freedom without abandoning. The toddler challenges authority strongly at the same time that he or she is profoundly afraid of getting the upper hand with his or her parents. Ideally, a parent will be secure enough to be accepting of the toddler's aggression and ambivalence and firm enough to set limits when the toddler goes too far. The role of limits is to reduce the toddler's world to the size that he or she can handle safely; however, instead of matter-of-factly setting limits, parents may react angrily or be intimidated by the toddler's aggression. Then the toddler, rather than feel comfortable about his or her aggression and learn to channel it as assertiveness, experiences shame and doubt.

The control issues that become primary in feeding the toddler are important in feeding from birth. Parents who were willing to learn to share control with their infant (see *Control of Feeding* in the appendix at the end of this chapter) are less likely to get into control battles with their toddler. Children whose parents have shared control all along do better with the challenges of separation-individuation because they already have a beginning sense of themselves as separate and of their parents as willing to support their separateness. As Stayton, Hogan, and Ainsworth (1971) observed with 9- to 12-month-olds, infant compliance to maternal limits was correlated strongly with sensitivity of maternal responsiveness to infant signals.

Toddlers explore and struggle for control with eating the same as in all of the other areas of their lives. In fact, it is with eating that the developmental task of **somatopsychological differentiation** is enacted most concretely.

In distinguishing among feelings and sensations, the task for both infants and parents becomes sorting out inner arousal and identifying correctly causes and solutions. Infants help with this task by signaling clearly their physiological or emotional needs; parents help by reading infants' signals correctly and responding appropriately—at least much of the time. If somatopsychological differentiation goes well, then the child learns, for instance, to distinguish hunger from anger and anger from being cold—and to apply the correct solution.

If somatopsychological differentiation goes poorly, then the child may learn to use food for emotional reasons—or may be unable to identify hunger and distinguish it from other states of arousal. In their observations of mothers and children during feeding, Ainsworth and Bell (1969) identified behaviors that would contribute to poor differentiation. Some mothers fed arbitrarily, putting down their infants for long periods and not seeming to notice when the infants cried. At other times, they picked up the infants and fed them, although children's bids for attention were not clear.

Those infants who were fed arbitrarily would not have had a clear sense that the discomfort that they were feeling was hunger, nor would they have known what to do about it. Infants who are tube-fed set amounts of formula at set times are fed equally arbitrarily and have similar difficulties. For the child to learn to differentiate appropriately and make the connection between oral and stomach sensations, tube-feedings need to be conducted in response to infant cues of hunger and satiety and the child needs to be provided with pleasant oral stimulation during the tube-feeding.

Feeding that Supports Separation-Individuation

During the toddler stage, feeding gradually broadens from an intimate relationship with the parent to participation in the social event of the family meal. To do well with feeding the toddler, parents must both follow the child's developmental lead and provide him or her with opportunities to learn as they offer him or her increasingly lumpy and textured food and soft pieces of table food (Table 3). Such opportunities help children develop their oral-motor skills with eating.

As noted previously, the division of responsibility in feeding the toddler becomes more complex. Now, in addition to the primary responsibility of choosing *what* the child shall be offered to eat, the parent begins to take responsibility and put limits on the *when* and *where* of eating. Within those limits, however, toddlers continue to be responsible for *how much* and *whether* they eat. Toward the end of the first year, the parent appropriately begins to move the child away from demand feeding and toward the meals-plus-snacks routine of the older child.

Parents often become alarmed about toddlers' eating because it changes so much and, often, so abruptly from the way that they ate as infants. As with younger children, toddlers are *neophobic:* They do not like new food (Birch & Marlin, 1982). Their neophobia becomes more pronounced than earlier because they have developed cognitively to the point that they know by looking at a food that it is new—and they refuse to eat it. Toddlers have not developed cognitively enough to be reassured by discussing or manipulating the food. They have to taste the food, take it back out of their mouth, and taste it again—perhaps as many as 10 or 20 times before they like it (Birch & Marlin, 1982). And they usually will.

Toddlers are *erratic:* What they like one day, they do not like the next. They may eat a lot one day and hardly anything the next. They do not eat some of everything at a meal as adults do—they eat only one or two foods. Despite their erratic patterns of eating, over time they tend to eat a variety and consume a nutritionally adequate diet if parents continue to have regular meals and snacks and offer a variety of wholesome food. Children continue to be reluctant to experiment and eat only a few preferred foods if parents limit the menu to what the child accepts readily or provide substitute foods when children will not eat what is offered (Pelchat & Pliner, 1986).

Not only are toddlers erratic and neophobic about eating, but also their growth rate decreases, their comparative energy requirement decreases, and their food intake falls off. In response to this sudden change, parents often become alarmed and entice, urge, or even force their toddlers to eat. Such tactics are counterproductive.

Putting pressure on toddlers to eat simply does not work. Toddlers are passionate about being separate, and they show that passion by being oppositional. As a consequence, pushing toddlers along to increase food intake or to hurry food acceptance is likely to slow it instead. In the choice between a struggle with a parent and eating, the toddler cannot help but choose the struggle. In fact, if older toddlers sense that the parent is invested in their eating, then they may refuse to eat as a way of trying to engage the parent in struggles for control. Parents can stop toddlers from doing what they *do not* want—like causing a ruckus at mealtime—but they cannot get them to do what they *do* want—like eat.

Six to Twelve Months

Generally, when parents and professionals think about separation-individuation, they visualize the aggressive and mobile toddler: the 15- to 18-month-old "demon explorer" or the legendary "terrible two." It comes as a surprise to many that the separation-individuation process starts as early as ages 6–9 months. As Chatoor et al. (1985) pointed out, the time of peak incidence of failure to thrive comes at age 9 months. Although young children are not as resourceful or as aggressive as older children about exerting their will, they already have begun to care deeply about doing things themselves and in their own way (Figure 1)— so deeply, in fact, that they may choose the struggle over the eating. The parent who continues to feed an infant who wants to feed him- or herself may precipitate a struggle for control that makes the child seem as though he or she does not want to eat.

Parents may miss the early signs of separation-individuation and fail to move their child along with eating skills because they continue to think of him or her as being an infant. They may be reluctant to give up the intense intimacy of earlier cuddling and nipple-feeding and move to a more grown-up feeding style, particularly when the child's infancy has been made more difficult by challenges with homeostasis or by illness.

Feeding the Six- to Twelve-Month-Old

To support this early stage of separation and individuation, it is critical for parents to provide a feeding context that both gives structure and limits and allows children to take the initiative with eating. Early on, part of that context is building toward structured meals and snacks by gradually substituting solid foods for nipple-feedings.

To begin making the transition from feeding the child as an infant to feeding the child as a toddler, the parent can begin offering food at regular times rather than feed on demand. For instance, after a nap and before a shopping trip, rather than wait for the child to ask for a between-meal nipple-feeding (Satter, 1984), the parent can take the initiative to offer a snack. The child can sit in the highchair and be offered nutritious food, such as graham crackers or arrowroot biscuits and milk from a cup (or formula, for the child who is not yet

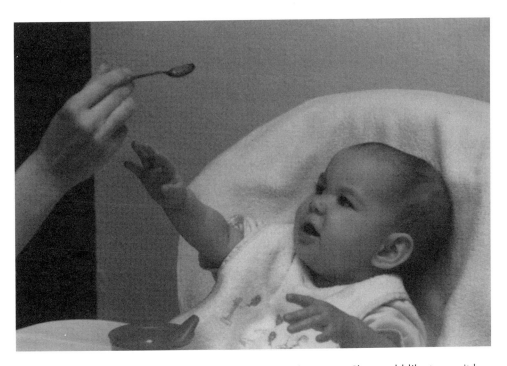

Figure 1.   At 10 months of age, this child reaches for the spoon. She would like to use it herself. Finger foods would be a good idea now.

well established on table food). Juice from a cup also can be used as part of snacks, but it should not exceed 3–4 ounces per day. Most developmentally ready 8- to 9-month-olds will be so captivated by the opportunity to manipulate and mouth that they forget all about their bottles.

Between 6 and 12 months, children are in constant transition as they develop the oral-motor skills that go along with eating. To enjoy and support their development as well as to keep them safe with eating, parents benefit greatly from being able to identify and understand the neuromuscular progression of feeding skills: the palmar to the pincer grasp; putting pieces of food in the mouth to being able to bite off; sending semisolid food straight down to being able to retain food in the mouth and mash or chew it before swallowing; developing judgment about bite size and mouth fill.

Gradually, the child moves through the major transition with eating, and the routine will be established as the parent sequentially substitutes solid foods and drinking milk or juice from the cup for nipple-feedings. Part of establishing the routine is making judicious use of snacks and adjusting timing of meals so that the child can come to the table hungry but not famished. By the time children are 1 year old, most will be ready for three meals and two or three snacks per day, or a planned feeding about every 2–3 hours. This routine should be maintained throughout the preschool years. As the child becomes established on the meals-plus-snacks routine, any food or caloric beverages should be included in these regular eating times.

Parents help children make the transition to table food by setting up feeding so that children can be successful. Parents can seat children in highchairs or other infant seats that keep them at a good height to the table with their feet well supported. Parents can give children small dishes, cups, and utensils (although children may not use them effectively for months) and modify the food in appropriate ways so that it is safe and easy to pick up, chew, and swallow. Throughout the toddler stage and even as preschoolers, children eat predominantly with their fingers (Figure 2). For the young child, a finger food is anything that hangs together long enough to get from table to mouth. Foods that more generally are thought of as finger foods are listed in Table 3. Most important, parents need to remain with children while they eat and slow their own tempo so that children have *time* to eat. Children always do more and dare more with eating in the presence of a trusted adult.

Parental supervision during feeding is critical at this early stage of learning to eat solid food. Choking on food presents an immediate danger throughout the growing-up years, but it is particularly pronounced for the child under age 2 years. Most parents treat this danger matter-of-factly by gradually progressing the texture, piece size, and firmness of their children's food as their abilities develop and by keeping an eye on children while they eat. This is appropriate. It is not appropriate, however, for parents to worry constantly or hover during the feeding or react so much to normal gagging that the child gets frightened.

Parents benefit from being able to distinguish between gagging and choking. Gagging is not dangerous; it is a normal part of the child's learning to eat. His or her awkward chewing lets pieces of food slip onto the back of his or her tongue, and he or she gags them up and tries again. Choking, however, *is* dangerous. A child chokes when he or she takes in a breath at the same time as food moves past the end of his or her windpipe. The food plugs up the windpipe, and he or she cannot breathe (see Table 5).

Twelve to Eighteen Months

As they become more mobile and physically capable, toddlers become aggressive explorers. During this early part of the second year, toddlers tend not to take the initiative with struggles; however, they respond to limits with upset and determination. As a consequence,

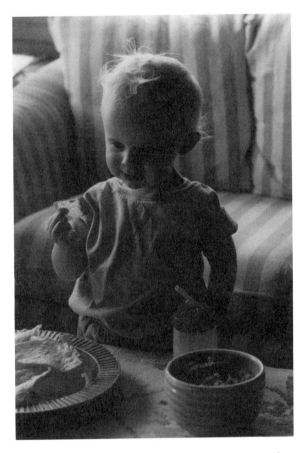

Figure 2.   Finger foods are the mainstay of eating during the toddler years.

it is important for parents to set clear limits but to give the child autonomy within those limits. For instance, a young toddler typically will get down from the table having eaten little or nothing of the food at the meal. A few minutes later, he or she will come back, begging the parents for a specific food or snack. The parent who sets a limit will say, "No," remind the child that snack is coming, and ignore the toddler's tantrum. Parents often try to manage this food begging (and avoid the outburst) by trying to get the child to eat more at mealtime. This is an undesirable tactic all around: The parent intrudes on the child's prerogative by trying to force eating, and the child misses out on an opportunity to test the parent's ability to withstand his or her rage and thereby increase his or her sense of separateness and safety.

For the 12- to 18-month-old, the division of responsibility in feeding becomes more important and well defined as the child finishes his or her transition to the family table and away from the nursing and demand feeding of the infant. Phasing out feeding in response to the child's random demands for food is important with food acceptance and social maturation. To be able to participate with the family in meals and to be able to take an interest in the food at the family table, the child needs to be hungry. Being allowed to panhandle for food or beverages between regular mealtimes interferes with food regulation. Children

Table 5.   Guidelines for feeding young children safely

1.   Build your child's eating skills, working up slowly to more difficult foods.
2.   Maintain an appropriate and positive feeding relationship with the focus on the child's capabilities.
3.   For children under age 3, avoid foods that are hard to control in the mouth, such as nuts, raw carrots, gum drops, hard candy and jelly beans.
4.   Modify some foods to reduce the risk of choking. Poultry and fish can be cooked tender and shredded, meat sliced finely across the grain, hot dogs cut lengthwise, carrots cooked, grapes quartered.
5.   Always provide adult supervision while children eat so you can see what they're doing. When children choke, they can't make noise to attract your attention.
6.   Insist that children sit down while they eat.
7.   Keep eating times free of intense feelings. Fighting, excitement, hilarity and conflict can cause children to catch their breath and inhale food.
8.   Have your health professional teach you first aid for choking.

From Satter, E.M., & Sharkey, P.B. (1995). *Ellyn Satter's nutrition and feeding for infants and children: Handout masters* (p. 12). Madison, WI: Ellyn Satter Associates; adapted by permission.

who were allowed to drink as much apple juice as they wanted grew poorly and resumed their growth only when the juice was restricted and a more varied diet offered (Smith & Lifshitz, 1994). Toddlers in a clinical setting who were allowed to graze for food ate only half as much as toddlers who were offered structured meals and snacks (Toomey, 1994).

Many parents will have missed the earlier opportunity to wean, and, for many young toddlers, breast- or bottle-feeding continues. Nipple-feeding (breast- or bottle-feeding) into the second year need not be a problem, as long as the child is not allowed to *misuse* it. Nipple-feedings should be separated from meals and made a part of snacks. Children should not be allowed to roam with a bottle, get a bottle- or a breast-feeding whenever they demand it, or nurse themselves to sleep. All of these tactics interfere with the child's growing up with eating, increase the likelihood of the child's learning to use the breast or the bottle for comfort or distraction, increase the risk of baby-bottle tooth decay, and may contribute to poor overall energy intake and growth.

Eighteen Months to Two Years

During the second half of the second year, toddlers start to take the initiative in testing their limits and trying out their ability to control. Once again, it is vital to help the toddler learn, on a preverbal level, to distinguish his or her own boundaries. That can happen only when he or she is neither controlling others nor being controlled. When parents offer the toddler limits, they are offering choices. He or she can battle about the limits—or he or she can discover the freedom that he or she has within those limits.

Toddlers cannot help but question and test the limits, but they depend on those limits, nonetheless, to be able to discover themselves as separate and to feel secure in their boldness. Toddlers are like the night watchman, checking all of the doors but not really wanting to find any open. Sometimes, however, they seem to be questioning and testing when they are simply behaving in developmentally predictable ways. Food acceptance is a case in point.

At around 18 months, children no longer have to taste a food to reject it. They begin to display the neophobia that goes along with looking at a food, recognizing that it is new, and refusing to eat it, often vigorously.

A parent who feels that the child must eat—or even taste—what is put before him or her can react to this neophobia by enticing, rewarding, playing games, or even getting into a full-blown battle with the toddler. In any battle for control, the toddler will win. In a battle for control of eating, the toddler can get a parent who is invested in getting food into him or her (or simply invested in being in control) to perform any number of humiliating and disgusting antics.

It is better to let time take care of the problem. Toddlers are neophobic, but they also are prone to experiment. On some level, they want to master food as much as they want to master everything else in their world. To master a food, toddlers first watch others eat it. Then they imitate by putting the food in their mouth—but they take it out again. Parents misinterpret this taking-out-again behavior as food rejection, but it actually is the toddler's way of getting accustomed to the taste and texture of the food. For the toddler, taking it out again counts as a taste; and after many tastes (at many meals), they are ready to swallow. Then they like it—and start the process all over again with another food.

When parents try to hurry the process, they slow it down. They should not force, reward, entice, play games, or withhold dessert to get children to eat. Neither should they limit the menu to foods that the child will accept readily because this prolongs and establishes their neophobia (Pelchat & Pliner, 1986). Toddlers typically find it easiest to learn to like sweets, fried foods, and starchy foods such as potatoes. Other foods—such as vegetables—take longer to master. Parents should continue to offer a well-balanced variety of nutritious foods, model good eating themselves, and wait. Eventually, unfamiliar foods become familiar, and toddlers incorporate them into their experience as acceptable foods. Children who are enticed with a reward to try a new food are *less* likely to go back to that food than those who simply are exposed to it and allowed to try it on their own (Birch, Marlin, & Rotter, 1984).

Two to Three Years

Just how terrible are the "terrible twos"? Much depends on how successful parents have been in distinguishing limits and safety from battles for control. Certainly, some children are far more aggressive than others and less amenable to suggestion in any form. At any point along the temperamental spectrum, however, parents who have a firm sense of the child as an individual and who have honored the child's autonomy consistently are likely to have fewer battles with their 2-year-old about control; nevertheless, those same parents must be capable of respecting their own rights and teaching the child that, to be a part of the social world of the family, he or she has to behave.

The necessary attitude is that the family table is a pleasant place to be and that the child is a valued member of the family. To make it pleasant for the child, parents need to understand and accept childish ways. Children will be sloppy because they are not yet skilled with their eating. They will be slow because feeding themselves is a new and wonderful challenge. They will eat oddly because they experiment with their food by touching it, squeezing it, and putting it in their mouth and taking it back out again; however, most parents can tell when exploring turns into messing around to get a reaction. Then it is time for the child to leave the table.

To make family meals pleasant for the parent, the child needs to be taught to behave appropriately at the table. He or she needs to come to the table willingly; deal with his or her own food; not whine, cry, or beg; and get down and play quietly if he or she finishes eating before his or her parents do. The family table provides a concrete metaphor for the child as he or she struggles with his or her **narcissistic resolution.** As a toddler, he or she is being asked to give up what he or she had as an infant: being the center of the universe.

The reward is sociability: joining the broader social world of the family. If all goes well, then the reward compensates for the loss. To help the child with this resolution, the parent must accomplish the tricky balance of both honoring the child as an individual and not letting him or her be a tyrant. In maintaining a division of responsibility with feeding, parents enact this balance.

The toddler's ability to eat the right amount of food to grow appropriately, as well as to learn to like a variety of foods, depends on maintaining this balance between autonomy and limits. If parents cannot withstand the child's begging for food, then a child could eat too little, do poorly with food acceptance, or learn to use food for emotional reasons.

A finicky toddler often is the product of parents who limit the menu to foods that their child will accept readily or who provide the child with special foods instead of expect him or her to learn to like what is on the table (Pelchat & Pliner, 1986). Parents hear that children go on "food jags," whereby they want and eat only a particular food for days at a time. Parents cater to the child's food preference, not realizing that they are promoting finicky eating. In addition, they are giving the child too much control with the family menu. Other typical negative food-related behaviors of parents with 2- to 5-year-old children include bargaining, bribing, and forcing; promising a special food, such as dessert, for eating a meal; withholding food as punishment; rewarding good behavior with food; persuading children to eat; playing a game to get children to eat; taking over and feeding children who refuse to eat; threatening punishment for not eating; and making children clean their plate (Stanek, Abbott, & Cramer, 1990). Such behaviors involve the parents' taking responsibility for the child's eating rather than expecting the child to take responsibility.

When parents fail to present mastery expectations, children do not grow up with eating and may even become more immature with eating. Patterns of food rejection that begin in the 2- to 3-year-old are likely to persist and get worse when the child is older. Finicky preschoolers often present with a history of a progressively shrinking list of acceptable foods.

Parents should not cater to the child, but neither should they be hard-nosed or sadistic about menu planning. The principle is to offer a broad enough variety of foods to give the child a chance to be successful with the meal. The Food Guide Pyramid (U.S. Department of Agriculture, Human Nutrition Information Service, 1992) helps define what constitutes a well-balanced meal: a main dish; fruit or vegetable or both; bread and one other good source of complex carbohydrate (children generally can eat bread when all else fails); milk; and butter, margarine, or salad dressing. Then children should be allowed to choose from what is available, eating as much or as little as they want. Parents should be reminded that, unlike adults, children usually do not eat some of everything on the table. They may eat a particular food with great enthusiasm one day and turn it down the next. Yet studies on sensory-specific satiety show that children's internal processes naturally promote variety in eating: They tire of even their favorite foods and will eat something else (Rolls, 1986). Parents should put their effort into what they prepare and serve rather than into getting their child to eat. For more detailed information about negotiating the feeding skirmishes of the toddler stage, consult the highly popular toddler chapter in *Child of Mine: Feeding with Love and Good Sense* (Satter, 1983/1986) or *How to Get Your Kid to Eat . . . But Not Too Much* (Satter, 1987).

CONCLUSION

If all has gone well with homeostasis, attachment, and separation-individuation, then children will emerge as preschoolers with a positive sense of self, wanting to learn about food and new eating situations. They are able to sit at the table with the rest of the family, handle utensils and cups reasonably well, accept most foods, try others repeatedly until they learn to like them, and politely refuse still others. Their aversion to new foods decreases as they develop cognitively and verbally. If parents continue to follow the division of responsibility in feeding, then preschoolers can carry on with their job of growing up to be competent eaters.

REFERENCES

Ainsworth, M.D.S., & Bell, S.M. (1969). Some contemporary patterns of mother–infant interaction in the feeding situation. In A. Ambrose (Ed.), *Stimulation in early infancy* (pp. 133–170). New York: Academic Press.

American Academy of Pediatrics, Committee on Nutrition. (1980). On the feeding of supplemental foods to infants. *Pediatrics, 65,* 1178–1181.

Ashworth, A., & Millward, D.J. (1986). Catch-up growth in children. *Nutrition Reviews, 44*(5), 157–163.

Barnard, K., Hammond, M.A., Booth, C.L., Bee, H.L., Mitchell, S.K., & Spieker, S.J. (1989). Measurement and meaning of parent–child interaction. In F. Morrison, C. Lord, & D. Keating (Eds.), *Applied developmental psychology* (Vol. 3, pp. 39–80). Orlando, FL: Academic Press.

Beal, V.A. (1957). On the acceptance of solid foods and other food patterns of infants and children. *Pediatrics, 20,* 448–456.

Beal, V.A. (1961). Dietary intake of individuals followed through infancy and childhood. *American Journal of Public Health, 51*(8), 1107–1117.

Birch, L.L., & Marlin, D.W. (1982). I don't like it; I never tried it: Effects of exposure on two-year-old children's food preferences. *Appetite, 3,* 353–360.

Birch, L.L., Marlin, D.W., & Rotter, J. (1984). Eating as the "means" activity in a contingency: Effects on young children's food preference. *Child Development, 55*(2), 431–439.

Chatoor, I., Dickson, L., Schaefer, S., & Egan, J. (1985). A developmental classification of feeding disorders associated with failure to thrive: Diagnosis and treatment. In D. Drotar (Ed.), *New directions in failure to thrive: Implications for research and practice* (pp. 235–258). New York: Plenum.

Crow, R.A., Fawcett, J.N., & Wright, P. (1980). Maternal behavior during breast- and bottle-feeding. *Journal of Behavioral Medicine, 3*(3), 259–277.

Dagnelie, P.C., Van-Staveren, W.A., & Hautvast, J.G. (1991). Stunting and nutrient deficiencies in children on alternative diets. *Acta Paediatrica Scandinavica, 374,* 111–118.

Dwyer, J.T., Andrew, E.M., Valadian, I., & Reed, R.B. (1980). Size, obesity, and leanness in vegetarian preschool children. *Journal of the American Dietetic Association, 77,* 434–439.

Field, T. (1977). Maternal stimulation during infant feeding. *Developmental Psychology, 13*(5), 539–540.

Fomon, S.J., Filer, L.J., Jr., Thomas, L.N., Anderson, T.A., & Nelson, S.E. (1975). Influence of formula concentration on caloric intake and growth of normal infants. *Acta Paediatrica Scandinavica, 64,* 172–181.

Israeloff, R. (1991, September). What it feels like to be two. *Parents Magazine,* 84–90.

Kern, D.L., McPhee, L., Fisher, J., Johnson, S., & Birch, L.L. (1993). The postingestive consequences of fat condition preferences for flavors associated with high dietary fat. *Physiology and Behavior, 54,* 71–76.

Lampl, M., Veldhuis, J.D., & Johnson, M.L. (1992). Saltation and stasis: A model of human growth. *Science, 258,* 801–803.

Mogan, J. (1987). What can nurses learn from structured observations of mother–infant interactions? *Issues in Comprehensive Pediatric Nursing, 10,* 67–73.

Morris, S.E. (1989). Development of oral-motor skills in the neurologically impaired child receiving non-oral feedings. *Dysphagia, 3,* 135–154.

National Research Council. (1989). *Recommended dietary allowances.* Washington, DC: National Academy Press.

Pelchat, M.L., & Pliner, P. (1986). Antecedents and correlates of feeding problems in young children. *Journal of Nutrition Education, 18*(1), 23–28.

Pollitt, E., & Wirtz, S. (1981). Mother–infant interaction and weight gain in the first month of life. *Journal of the American Dietetic Association, 78,* 596–602.

Pridham, K.F. (1989). Feeding behavior of 6- to 12-month-old infants: Assessment and sources of parental information. *Journal of Pediatrics, 117,* S174–S180.

Pugliese, M.T., Weyman-Daum, M., Moses, N., & Lifshitz, F. (1987). Parental health beliefs as a cause of nonorganic failure to thrive. *Pediatrics, 80*(2), 175–182.

Rolls, B.J. (1986). Sensory specific satiety. *Nutrition Reviews, 44,* 93–101.

Rose, H.E., & Mayer, J. (1968). Activity, calorie intake, fat storage, and the energy balance of infants. *Pediatrics, 41,* 18–29.

Satter, E. (1983/1986). *Child of mine: Feeding with love and good sense.* Palo Alto, CA: Bull Publishing.

Satter, E. (1984). Developmental guidelines for feeding infants and young children. *National Live Stock and Meat Board Food and Nutrition News, 56,* 21–28.

Satter, E.M. (1986). The feeding relationship. *Journal of the American Dietetic Association, 86,* 352–356.

Satter, E. (1987). *How to get your kid to eat . . . but not too much.* Palo Alto, CA: Bull Publishing.

Satter, E. (1990). The feeding relationship: Problems and interventions. *Journal of Pediatrics, 117,* S181–S189.

Satter, E.M. (1994, October 25). *Preventing childhood obesity: A new paradigm.* Paper presented at the Wisconsin Special Supplemental Food Program for Women, Infants and Children (WIC) and Maternal Child Health (MCH) conference: "Uniting Communities for Mothers and Children," Wisconsin Dells, WI.

Satter, E. (1995). Feeding dynamics: Helping children to eat well. *Journal of Pediatric Health Care, 9,* 178–184.

Satter, E.M. (1998). *Feeding with love and good sense: Training manual for the VISIONS workshop.* Madison, WI: Ellyn Satter Associates.

Satter, E., & Sharkey, P.B. (1995). *Ellyn Satter's nutrition and feeding for infants and children: Handout masters.* Madison, WI: Ellyn Satter Associates.

Satter, E.M., & Sharkey, P.B. (1997). *Montana feeding relationship training package.* Madison, WI: Ellyn Satter Associates.

Smith, M.M., & Lifshitz, F. (1994). Excess fruit juice consumption as a contributing factor in nonorganic failure to thrive. *Pediatrics, 93,* 438–443.

Stanek, K., Abbott, D., & Cramer, S. (1990). Diet quality and the eating environment of preschool children. *Journal of the American Dietetic Association, 90,* 1582–1584.

Stayton, D.J., Hogan, R., & Ainsworth, M.D.S. (1971). Infant obedience and maternal behavior: The origins of socialization reconsidered. *Child Development, 42,* 1057–1069.

Sullivan, S.A., & Birch, L.L. (1994). Infant dietary experience and acceptance of solid foods. *Pediatrics, 93,* 271–277.

Taubman, B. (1988). Parental counseling compared with elimination of cow's milk or soy milk protein for the treatment of infant colic syndrome: A randomized trial. *Pediatrics, 81*(6), 756–761.

Toomey, K.A. (1994). [Caloric intake of toddlers fed structured meals and snacks versus on demand]. Unpublished raw data.

U.S. Department of Agriculture, Human Nutrition Information Service. (1992, August). *The food guide pyramid* (Home and Garden Bulletin No. 252). Washington, DC: Author.

Whitten, C.F., Pettit, M.G., & Fischoff, J. (1969). Evidence that growth failure from maternal deprivation is secondary to undereating. *Journal of the American Medical Association, 209*(11), 1675–1682.

How to Feed Your Toddler and Control of Feeding

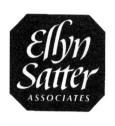

How To Feed
Your Toddler

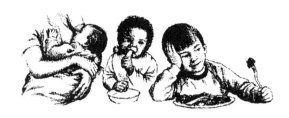

During the time from 12 months to 3 years, your child keeps getting taller and heavier, but his rapid growth rate slows down. He begins exploring with a vengeance, and he shows, at times, a fierce contrariness as he works at becoming a person separate from you.

He may eat less now. That's okay—he knows how much he needs to eat. If you pressure him to eat more, he's likely to resist and eat less. Toddlers would rather exert their independence than eat.

What a toddler is like

Toddlers are *neophobic*: They don't like new food. But they will learn to like it, if you just let them see it on the table and see you eating it. After a while, they will taste it—and take it back out of their mouth again. They'll do that many times, then eventually they will know it well enough so they swallow it—and like it.

Toddlers are *erratic*: What they like one day, they don't the next. They eat a lot one day and hardly anything the next. They don't eat some of everything at a meal like you do—they eat only one or two foods.

Toddlers are *opinionated*: They know what they do and don't want to do. You can stop them from doing what you don't want, like causing a ruckus at mealtime, but you can't get them to do what you *do* want—like eat.

Let your child control his eating

If you treat your toddler like you did when he was a baby, and try to constantly please him, it will drive you crazy and you will fail him utterly. He needs autonomy: control over his own life and his own world. He also needs limits, to reduce the size of his world to what he can handle.

With eating, that means you choose the menu that's safe and nutritious for him; you don't let him pick everything he wants from the supermarket shelves. You choose the times for eating. But once you have chosen the menu and the times, you must let your child decide what and how much he eats, even when he eats poorly.

Avoiding food battles

Eating gives your toddler lots of opportunities to test his limits. During this tricky time, remember the division of responsibility in feeding: You are responsible for *what* your child is presented to eat, he is responsible for *how much* and even *whether* he eats. As your child moves from being a baby to being a toddler, it's important that you also begin to take responsibility for the *when* and *where* of feeding and establish the structure of regular meals and snacks.

Your feeding responsibilities:

- Select and buy food.
- Make nutritious meals and snacks and offer them in a neutral fashion.
- Let your child eat as much as he wants.
- Don't press food on your child, or he'll play the toddler's favorite game of turning things down and watching you get desperate.

- Regulate timing of meals and snacks. Your toddler no longer benefits from being fed on demand, so begin scheduling meals and snacks now. His stomach is small and his energy needs are high, so he should have three meals a day with planned snacks in between. Don't allow panhandling for food or beverages (except water) at other times.
- Present foods in a form your child can handle. Your toddler can eat most food from the family table, but still depends on you to make minor changes in texture so he can be successful eating it. His chewing and swallowing are still somewhat immature. He can't chew tough, hard food. Smooth, round food can slide down his throat before he chews it, and dry food seems to get stuck in his mouth.
- Let him eat in his own way. If your child is allowed to look, feel, mash, and smell to explore food, he's more likely to accept it. However, when exploring becomes simply messing around to get you to react, it's time to let him get down from the table.
- Don't make your child clean his plate. Even adults have a hard time knowing how hungry they are. Encourage your child to take repeated small helpings—but at times his eyes *will* be bigger than his stomach and he'll waste food.
- Make family mealtimes pleasant. Don't argue, fight or scold at mealtimes. Talk and pay attention to your toddler, but don't make him the center of attention. Respect his slowness with eating.
- Sit down to eat with your toddler. Don't feed him separately so that you can have peace and quiet for your meal. He needs to be included at the family table. If he says he doesn't want to eat, tell him it's his choice, but that he's to stay at the table for a little while anyway and keep you company while you eat.
- Help your child pay attention to his eating. He needs to be calm, well-rested, and hungry to eat well. Turn the TV off: It distracts him from eating and interferes with family social time.

Getting enough of the right kind of food

If your child is growing well, he's eating the amount that's right for him. Toddlers often don't eat very much, but it turns out they don't *have* to eat so much to get what they need. Their helping size is only $1/4$ to $1/3$ the size of an adult's, or one tablespoon per year of age. Your child might eat a lot more than that, and that's okay. The point is that you should give children small helpings so they don't feel overwhelmed. If you're concerned, have a dietitian evaluate your child's diet.

What a meal should provide

Put a variety of foods on the table at mealtime: a meat or other protein source, milk, a fruit or vegetable or both, bread and other starchy food, butter or margarine, and let your child pick and choose from what's available.

Food waste

When your child is just learning to like new foods, you will have more food waste. He'll take food on his plate and eat just a bit, or not eat it at all. Or he won't be very good at estimating how much he'll eat, and will serve himself too much. You can remind him, gently, not to take so much, but you shouldn't make him clean up his plate.

In the long run, your child will waste less food if you don't get pushy. He'll learn to like more foods, and he'll take responsibility for his own eating.

Food jags

Planning meals out ahead of time helps you moderate your child's food jags. If you ask, he'll tell you he wants his favorite food. If you don't ask, he'll take his chances like the rest of the family—sometimes you get lucky, sometimes you don't.

Short-order cooking

When your toddler complains he doesn't like the food on the table, say, "Oh, okay," or ignore it. Don't jump up to short-order cook something else for him. Simply have his milk at his place when he arrives, put some bread on the table so he won't starve, give him some support in getting himself served, keep him company, and let him take care of his eating.

Feeding to quell the riot

Don't use food to solve problems like skinned knees, hurt feelings, or general crankiness. This teaches your child to eat whenever he gets upset. It's tempting to give him a cookie when you want some peace and quiet, but save this "self-defense" feeding for those times when you have *really* had it.

Safety

Children under age 3 have a higher risk of choking than older children. Always be there during feeding. Have your toddler sit down while he's eating, and keep things calm. When children scream or laugh they catch their breath and could inhale food.

Modify foods to reduce the risk of choking: Cut meat finely, quarter grapes, cook carrots, slice hot dogs lengthwise. Avoid nuts, gum drops, jelly beans, and other foods that are hard to control in the mouth.

Struggles for control

Since your toddler is working so hard right now at being his own person, you could get into struggles about control. Check yourself. You are being too controlling if you make your child: Stay at the table to eat his vegetables; clean his plate; eat everything before he can have dessert; get by on only three meals a day. You aren't being controlling enough if you: Give your child a snack whenever he wants one; let your child stay at the table when he behaves badly; short-order cook for your child; let your child have juice or milk whenever he wants it.

Struggles about control are a normal part of this age. But if the struggles are prolonged or continuous and you can't seem to get things to go right with your child, get professional help.

Ellyn Satter, author of *How to Get Your Kid to Eat . . . But Not Too Much.* Bull Publishing, Palo Alto, CA

CONTROL OF FEEDING

You and your baby need to share control of feeding. You help him wake up and stay calm. Then you pay attention to what he tells you about how he wants to be fed and how much he wants to eat. Babies eat better when they feel like you'll do what they want.

Check yourself. Do you and your baby share control of feeding?

PARENT AND BABY SHARE CONTROL	PARENT DOESN'T SHARE CONTROL
☐ Pay attention to what your baby tells you	☐ Go by how *you* want to feed your baby
☐ Let your baby eat as much or as little as he wants	☐ Make your baby eat a certain amount
	☐ Stop feeding before he is full
☐ Feed on demand	☐ Make your baby go by a schedule
☐ Sit still when you breastfeed or hold the bottle still	☐ Move around during feeding
	☐ Jiggle the bottle
☐ Touch your baby's lips to let him "open up" for the nipple	☐ Push the nipple into your baby's mouth
☐ Feed smoothly, don't interrupt	☐ Stop the feeding to check how much your baby eats
☐ Try to solve problems	☐ Jump to conclusions about why baby does what he does
☐ Let your baby slow down or stop sucking	☐ Keep on feeding when your baby turns away or shuts his mouth
☐ Let your baby go back to eating after he pauses	☐ Stop feeding when he slows down or stops sucking
☐ Help your baby settle down if he gets fussy, then offer more	☐ Stop feeding when he fusses

Chapter 8

Behavior Problems in Feeding
Individual, Family, and Cultural Influences

Maureen M. Black,
Pamela L. Cureton, and Julie Berenson-Howard

Feeding problems are very common during childhood, occurring in 25%–35% of all children (Linscheid, 1992). It is not uncommon for feeding problems to occur as children acquire new developmental skills and are challenged with new foods or mealtime expectations. Most feeding problems are temporary and resolved easily with little or no intervention. Feeding problems that persist can undermine children's growth, development, and relationships with their caregivers, which can lead to long-term health problems, including diabetes, heart disease, and complications of undernutrition or obesity. In addition, many serious emotional disorders may present initially as feeding problems during infancy (Rutter, 1987). Helping children learn to develop healthy eating habits by encouraging them to eat nutritious foods and to eat to satisfy hunger rather than to satisfy emotional needs can prevent subsequent health and developmental problems.

Feeding is a complex activity that reflects young children's emerging developmental skills (Rudolph, 1994; Skuse & Wolke, 1992). Not only is feeding a time for meeting infants' nutritional needs, but it also is an important opportunity for social interaction. Caregivers help their infants build expectations around food and mealtimes. Infants learn that

Partial support for this chapter was provided by grants from the Maternal and Child Health Research Program (Title V, Social Security Act), Health Resources and Services Administration, Department of Health and Human Services, and from Share Our Strength, Inc.

their cries for food will be answered and that feeding occurs according to a predictable schedule. Infants and caregivers establish a partnership in which they recognize and interpret communication signals from one another (Ainsworth & Bell, 1974; Satter, 1987; see Chapter 7). This reciprocal process forms a basis for the emotional bonding or attachment between infants and caregivers that is essential to healthy social functioning.

If there is a disruption in the communication between infants and caregivers, characterized by inconsistent, nonresponsive interactions, then the attachment bond may not be secure and feeding may become an occasion for unproductive, upsetting battles over food. When mealtimes become stressful or confrontational, infants may be denied both the nutrients that they require and healthy, responsive interactions with caregivers. Caregivers who are inexperienced or stressed and those who have poor eating habits themselves may be most in need of assistance to facilitate healthy, nutritious mealtime behavior with their children. Innovative strategies are needed to promote healthy eating habits and to prevent growth and developmental problems among young children.

CLASSIFICATION OF FEEDING PROBLEMS

Linscheid (1992) described a classification of feeding problems, based on the origin of the problem, that includes medical (e.g., gastroesophageal reflux, cystic fibrosis), oral-motor (e.g., cerebral palsy), and behavioral. These categories are not mutually exclusive and often overlap. For example, a child who has a medical disorder that disrupts feeding may develop feeding behavior problems, particularly if mealtimes are frustrating or if the caregiver attempts to force feed (Rudolph, 1994). Similarly, children who experience pain, vomiting, or choking while eating may become resistant to the foods or textures that are associated with the difficult experience. These problems can become so severe that children become physically ill or emotionally distressed in response to the sight, smell, or taste of specific foods.

Feeding problems may also be classified by the specific aspects of the behavior problem, including the developmental appropriateness of the food (e.g., reliance on limited textures or varieties), self-feeding skills (e.g., difficulty making the transition from bottle to cup, difficulty using utensils), the amount of food eaten (too much or not enough), and mealtime behaviors (e.g., gorging or refusing food, tantrums) (Linscheid, 1992). For example, some children will eat only a few restricted foods, others refuse to eat foods that vary in texture (e.g., only soft foods), and others do not progress to more advanced methods of feeding (e.g., difficulty moving from bottle to cup). Another common problem is the child who has a limited appetite and does not appear to be hungry even after long periods of not eating. These children eat small quantities of food, even preferred food. Finally, children develop a range of aversive behaviors to signal their refusal to eat. Children may reject food by throwing it, turning away, or refusing to open their mouths. Once food has been put into the mouth, children may reject it by holding it there, spitting, gagging, or regurgitating. Behavior problems during mealtime often co-occur and include temper tantrums, refusal to sit, and other disruptive behaviors.

At the other end of the spectrum, some children with feeding problems eat too much food. Overeating in infancy may result from a regulatory deficiency whereby the child does not recognize the signs of satiety, from a psychological problem that the child may attempt to resolve through eating, or from overfeeding by the caregiver. There also are children who hoard food and children who eat nonfood items (pica). (For a review of diagnostic coding, see Chapter 19.)

THEORETICAL BACKGROUND

Ecological theory provides a useful framework for examining the development of feeding because it uses systems theory to emphasize that developmental tasks, such as feeding, occur within an interactive social context (Bronfenbrenner, 1993). Children's behavior is influenced by factors that extend from direct interaction with family members to indirect influence from cultural traditions. Much of the research on feeding behavior has focused on the child and the primary caregiver, usually the mother. Attention should extend to other members of the child's family and should include the child's daily activities, roles, expectations, and interpersonal relationships within the family. Feeding is also influenced by children's interactions with other caregivers or in other settings (e.g., child care). At the broader levels, feeding may be influenced by systems that do not affect the child directly, including events that influence the family's financial, emotional, or physical status. For example, economic demands on women may limit the amount of time that is available for meal preparation and feeding (Engle, 1991). Likewise, influences from the community (e.g., religious practices, food prices, proximity of food stores) affect feeding practices and children's development (Wiecha & Palombo, 1989). For example, children who are raised in very low-income families are at an increased risk for feeding problems that are related to limited resources (Bronner, 1996; Wehler, 1991).

ECOLOGICAL PERSPECTIVES ON CHILDREN'S FEEDING PROBLEMS

In the past, feeding problems were sometimes conceptualized as child-related issues, with little attention directed to the role of the caregivers or to the social environment. In keeping with guidelines from ecological theory and with the recognition that feeding occurs within a social context. Most clinicians and investigators incorporate perspectives from the child, caregivers, caregiver–child interactions, and culture into the evaluation and treatment of feeding problems.

Child

From a child's perspective, feeding requires the integration of multiple systems, including physical development, temperament, psychosocial development, and food preferences. Problems in any one of these areas can undermine successful feeding.

Physical Development

Feeding progresses through increasingly complex stages as children acquire the skills to move food from the front of their mouth to the pharynx in preparation for swallowing (Rudolph, 1994; Skuse & Wolke, 1992). In the initial stage, liquid is drawn into the mouth by suckling and moved to the back of the mouth by extending and retracting the tongue. Many of the feeding problems in this stage are related to neurological or anatomical impairments, but behavior problems can emerge, especially when caregivers are not sensitive to their infant's needs. Caregivers can prevent feeding problems during the first few months of life by offering breast milk or formula frequently, at predictable intervals, and when the child exhibits signs of hunger; by holding the child during feeding in a comfortable, cradled position with the head and trunk well supported; and by responding to signals from the infant that indicate satiety, distress, or hunger (Wolf & Glass, 1996). For bottle-fed infants, ensuring that the nipple type and hole are providing an adequate supply of liquid helps the infant develop a rhythmic pattern of feeding without having to strain to get enough liquid or becoming overwhelmed by too much liquid.

Weaning occurs when children switch from a diet that is primarily breast milk or formula to solid food (Underwood, 1985). As children's neurological skills mature, their feeding skills become more sophisticated and they are able to handle a wider variety of textures and flavors (Morris, 1977). For example, children are unable to handle solids before they have achieved the oral-motor control that is necessary to move food to the back of their mouths in preparation for swallowing. When solid food is introduced too early, while feeding is still dominated by sucking, food is often pushed forward and out of the mouth. Caregivers may misinterpret this action as a signal that the child is rejecting the food or rejecting the caregiver rather than as a sign that the child is not ready for the feeding challenges of solid foods. If the caregiver responds to the perceived rejection with anger or by intensifying the pressure on the child to eat, then mealtime can become upsetting and stressful to both the child and the caregiver. To help caregivers avoid misinterpretations, clinicians should ask detailed questions about the feeding partnership with careful attention to the developmental challenges that the caregiver may be presenting to the child.

Conversely, delayed weaning may also be associated with feeding problems. Illingsworth and Lister (1964) have argued that there is a critical period (approximately 6 or 7 months of age) when children should be challenged with solid foods so that they learn to chew. They assert that children who are denied an opportunity to learn to chew are more likely to have feeding problems when solid foods are introduced at a later age. Although their claims have not been evaluated empirically, some children may become very comfortable with the ease of consuming liquids or soft foods and resist the challenges imposed by foods that require them to work harder by chewing.

Delayed weaning also is a concern because prolonged breast-feeding has been associated with malnutrition (Caulfield, Bentley, & Ahmed, 1996). Breast-feeding (or bottle-feeding) that persists into the second year of life *without adequate complementary feeding* may not provide children with the variety of nutrients that they require for healthy growth. In addition to taking time and energy away from acquiring a balanced diet, delayed weaning may interrupt the development of age-appropriate feeding skills by perpetuating an infantile behavior. Children who have become attached to the nurturant aspects of breast- or bottle-feeding may benefit from the security of an alternative transitional object, such as a blanket or a stuffed animal.

Once children learn to sit, they are more comfortable eating in a seated position than in a reclining position. Highchairs and booster seats provide support and enable children to achieve a body position that facilitates feeding, arm and hand control to pick up food, and coordinated hand-to-mouth control to bring food to the mouth (Wolf & Glass, 1996). Highchairs also restrain children, thus ensuring that they remain seated throughout the meal. Highchairs can also be aversive to children if they are introduced suddenly with little preparation, if children are confined for long periods, or if they are associated with negative aspects of feeding. To avoid behavior problems that involve highchairs, caregivers should ensure that children are seated comfortably with support, that they are not left unattended or for long periods of time, and that they associate sitting in a highchair with pleasant aspects of mealtime.

Temperament

Children who have feeding problems often display difficult behavior in other settings, measured through both observation and maternal report (Black, Hutcheson, Dubowitz, Berenson-Howard, & Starr, 1996). Among some children, the behavior problems that are associated with feeding are part of their overall temperament, including irritability, apathy, and generalized inactivity or overactivity (Polan et al., 1991; Powell, Low, & Speers, 1987; Singer, Song, Hill, & Jaffee, 1990; Wolke, Skuse, & Mathisen, 1990). *Temperament* refers to children's responses to their physical and social environment. A child with a passive temperament who does not demand food may be forgotten or neglected and not fed, particularly in a chaotic family. Conversely, a child who has a very active temperament may be very reactive to environmental events and have difficulty maintaining the attention and the focus that are necessary for successful feeding (Chatoor, Hirch, & Persinger, 1997). In either case, the relationship between feeding and the temperamental characteristics of the child cannot be understood without examining family dynamics and the relationship between the parent and the child.

Psychosocial Development

Chatoor and colleagues (Chatoor, Dickson, Schaefer, & Egan, 1985) have described a feeding classification system that is based on early psychosocial development (see Chapters 7, 19, and 29). The first stage is a regulatory phase that occurs early in life as infants establish patterns of wakefulness and sleep and adjust to the demands of their environments. Parents learn how to calm their infants and help them develop daily routines of eating, sleeping, and playing. During the first few months of life, feeding is an organizational task that requires reciprocal coordination between caregivers and infants. This reciprocity is evident among breast-fed infants who control the quantity of milk that the mother produces. Frequent sucking stimulates the release of prolactin, which controls the production of breast milk.

Caregivers learn to interpret their infants' cries for food, to prepare them for feeding, to hold them to facilitate feeding, and to interpret their signs of satiety. Infants who do not provide clear signals to their caregivers or who do not respond to their caregivers' efforts to help them establish predictable routines of eating, sleeping, and playing are at risk for a range of adjustment problems, including feeding disorders. For example, infants who are premature or ill may be less responsive than healthy, full-term infants and less able to communicate their feelings of hunger or satiety. These infants present special challenges to their caregivers. Conversely, caregivers who do not recognize their infants' satiety cues may overfeed them. This practice may lead infants to associate feelings of satiety with frustration and conflict because overfeeding is not pleasurable.

Attachment is the second stage of psychosocial development. It begins at approximately 3 months of life, extends through the first year, and is dominated by social explorations. Infants in the attachment stage signal pleasure and attract caregivers through smiles and coos. The social aspects of feeding become apparent as infants may interrupt their feeding for visual exploration or get distracted by external sights and sounds. If caregivers interpret these pauses as signals and stop feeding, then infants may not have met their nutritional requirements and may continue to be hungry. The hunger may lead to feelings of irritation because the infants have not reached satiety; thus, misinterpretation of cues may lead to feeding behavior problems. Conversely, if caregivers are persistent and force their infants to eat during their brief exploratory pauses, then infants may associate feeding with frustration and a loss of control.

The third psychosocial stage is separation-individuation. It begins at approximately 6 months and extends through toddlerhood until approximately 3 years of age. During this stage, not only are children acquiring the physical and oral-motor skills that enable them to handle a greater variety of textures and tastes, but they are also acquiring the verbal skills to express their pleasure or displeasure about food choices. Feeding also provides an ideal opportunity for young children to practice their increasing sense of autonomy and independence. Moreover, an important task of the separation-individuation period is the control that children are able to exercise over aspects of their environment. Because feeding is so central to the development of young children, it often becomes the central arena for young children to practice their emerging independence. Caregivers who do not understand their toddler's need for control may respond with harsh reprisals, almost ensuring that mealtimes will become a source of conflict (see Figure 1). Conversely, caregivers who provide opportunities for their toddler to exercise some control over the feeding situation are helping the toddler develop skills of autonomy. For example, caregivers can give children fixed choices about aspects of the meal, such as the food that is offered (e.g., type of cereal), the plates and utensils (e.g., pink or blue), or the bib or napkins to be used. Caregivers can also enhance children's sense of control and autonomy by encouraging them to feed themselves, first with their fingers, then with a spoon. Caregivers who prepare for messes by dressing their children in old clothes or a bib and placing paper on the floor are less likely to become upset when the inevitable mess occurs. Allowing children to help with meal preparation by stirring or setting the table is another way to help them feel invested by giving them control over aspects of the meal.

Food Preferences

Children accept or reject food based on intrinsic qualities of the food (e.g., taste, texture) and extrinsic factors that may be unrelated to the specific food (Rozin, 1990). Intrinsic qualities may be influenced by children's development. For example, infants are attracted to sweet tastes before salty tastes (Beauchamp, Cowart, & Moran, 1986). Extrinsic factors may include the anticipated consequences of eating or not eating. For example, con-

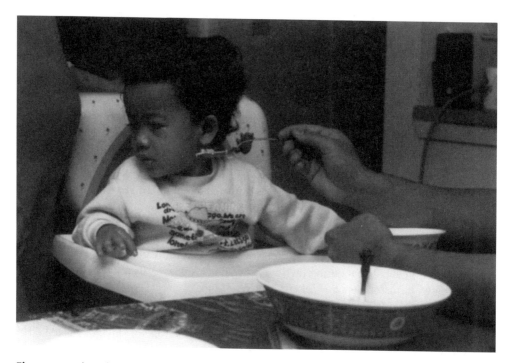

Figure 1.   This child averts his face rather than let his father feed him. Toddlers want to be independent and to eat on their own.

sequences of eating may include relief from hunger, participation in a social function, or praise from caregivers. Consequences of not eating may include additional time to play, becoming the focus of attention, or getting snack food instead of the regular meal. Often, both intrinsic and extrinsic factors influence food choices. For example, fat is an excellent source of energy and is an important component of many popular foods. Early in life, children learn that high-fat foods, such as ice cream and cake, signify festive or celebratory occasions (Birch, 1992). Thus, the preference for high-fat foods may be driven by both intrinsic qualities of the food and extrinsic factors that are influenced by cultural values.

Clara Davis's studies from the 1920s and 1930s on the food preferences of young children in orphanages (Davis, 1928, 1934) have formed the basis for the presumption that children will select a nutritious diet. In Davis's orginal studies, three infants (ages 6–12 months) were given a variety of fresh, unprocessed, unseasoned foods (e.g., oatmeal, wheat, beef, bone marrow, eggs, vegetables) and were permitted to select whichever foods they preferred. Basic techniques were used to prepare the foods, none of the foods were mixed or cooked together, and the children did not receive any sweets. After 6 months on their self-selected diet, the children were healthy and had grown well. Their food choices varied, but they displayed definite preferences, particularly for bone marrow, milk, eggs, fruit (bananas, apples, oranges), corn meal, whole wheat, and oatmeal. Although the infants in Davis's research were given a restricted choice of foods that did not include foods of inferior quality, such as potato chips or cookies, many clinicians have interpreted her findings to suggest that given a wide range of choices, infants will select a healthful, balanced diet (Story & Brown, 1987).

A similar methodology was used to study food preferences in preschool-age children during a period of 6 days (Birch, Johnson, Anderson, Peters, & Schulte, 1991). However, the food choices were expanded and represented foods that are typically eaten by preschoolers, including macaroni and cheese, sandwiches, potato chips, and cookies. The children's intake during individual meals varied significantly; high-energy intake in one meal often was followed by low-energy intake during the subsequent meal. The children's energy intake over a 24-hour period, however, was remarkably constant. These findings suggest that children are at least partially guided by an internal regulatory process that determines energy requirements.

Food preferences are also influenced by experience. Children often have an initial aversion to novel foods that may be reversed following repeated exposure (Sullivan & Birch, 1994). Increasing familiarity with the taste of a food increases the likelihood of acceptance. For example, young children may resist novel foods the first few times that they are presented. This hesitance may be biologically adaptive, as though children have to ensure the safety of the food prior to eating it (Sullivan & Birch, 1994). Caregivers can facilitate the introduction of novel foods by presenting the foods repeatedly so that they become familiar, pairing the novel food with preferred food, and eating the novel food themselves and signaling enjoyment.

Food preferences are also influenced by associated conditions. Foods that have been associated with unpleasant physical symptoms, such as nausea or pain, are subsequently avoided (Sullivan & Birch, 1990). Although most of the research has focused on the association among sensory cues, food, and subsequent food preferences (Ross & Zellner, 1985), it is also possible that repeated emotional feelings that are associated with feeding may become linked with food preferences through associative conditioning. For example, the anxiety or distress that often occurs with confrontational feeding may become associated with food and lead to subsequent avoidance.

Caregivers

Parents may contribute to feeding problems in their children by the foods that they provide and the feeding atmosphere (Birch & Johnson, 1994). For example, Johnson and Birch (1992) have shown that parents' mealtime behavior, especially harsh disciplinary practices, can be upsetting to children and affect the amount that they eat. A negative cycle can emerge in which children who refuse to eat have mothers who are harsh and rigid during feeding and rely on threats or physical intrusions to encourage eating. The negative cycle can be exacerbated by clinicians who either encourage mothers to get more calories into their children without addressing the problems that are associated with low weight gain or blame mothers when their children do not gain weight. Mothers whose competence is undermined by their children's low weight gain may feel anxious and react by becoming more rigid and controlling. It is not clear whether mothers react to their children's food refusal by increasing their rigidity and insistence that their child eat or children react to maternal harshness by resisting and refusing to eat (Black et al., 1996). In either case, unresponsive, rigid behavior by the parent is associated with unsuccessful feeding and a negative cycle of food refusal and parent rigidity. Effective feeding is dependent on sensitive, appropriate, and pleasant offers of food. Mealtimes that consist of battles, force feeding, and threats reinforce patterns of unpleasant struggles around food.

Caregivers influence the external aspects of mealtime through food choices, schedules, and the mealtime atmosphere. They also play an active role in their level of encouragement to the child. Although children are responsible for learning to regulate their internal food requirements, they benefit from caregivers who eat with them and provide encouragement through modeling (Bentley, Black, & Hurtado, 1995). When encouragement becomes manipulative or aversive (e.g., clapping after every bite, bribery, chasing the child around the room with food [Figure 2]), feeding is guided by external controls from the caregiver, rather than by the child's internal regulation. Parents should model appropriate feeding and respond to their child's cues but be respectful of their child's need to learn to regulate internal food requirements.

Some caregivers have misconceptions regarding the nutritional requirements for infants and young children and may contribute to their children's feeding problems by giving them inappropriate foods. For example, caregivers may not realize that many commercial products that are marketed for children, such as sweetened drinks, may satisfy hunger or thirst but provide minimal nutritional benefits (Smith & Lifshitz, 1994). Children who consume sweetened drinks may not be hungry at mealtimes. For other parents, an eagerness to eliminate fat and cholesterol from their children's diets can result in inadequate intake of required nutrients (Pugliese, Weyman-Daum, Moses, & Lifshitz, 1987).

Alternatively, caregivers may have unrealistic expectations about the amount that their children should eat at each meal. Children respond to internal cues by adjusting their intake at each meal so that their energy intake over 24 hours is relatively constant (Birch et al., 1991; Davis, 1928). In other words, children may have a limited intake at one meal but are likely to compensate at the next meal. Caregivers who do not realize this variability in intake may put unnecessary pressure on their children to eat whatever food they provide.

Early descriptive studies suggested that children's feeding problems and subsequent growth failure were related to maternal psychological factors, primarily depression (Elmer, 1960). However, controlled studies have reported no differences in psychopathology between mothers of children who have feeding problems and poor growth and mothers of adequately growing children from similar socioeconomic backgrounds (Singer et al.,

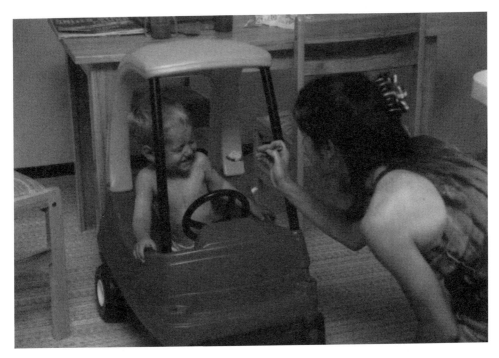

Figure 2.   This child does not like it when his mother follows him around with a spoon. He could eat better on his own and in a highchair.

1990). Thus, the emphasis has shifted from maternal psychopathology to interactions between the caregiver and the child.

Caregiver–Child Interactions

Interactions during mealtime between caregivers and children with feeding problems are often characterized by unclear messages, premature termination of feeding, inconsistent mealtimes, and limited food availability (Drotar, Eckerle, Satola, Pallotta, & Wyatt, 1990; Heptinstall et al., 1987; Hutcheson, Black, & Starr, 1993). There is a high rate of insecure attachment between children with feeding problems and their parents (Benoit, Zeanah, & Barton, 1989; Brinich, Drotar, & Brinich, 1989; Crittenden, 1987).

When parents do not structure mealtimes, children do not learn to anticipate when they will eat and may feel anxious and irritable. Children are more likely to develop an expectation and an appetite around mealtime when mealtimes are structured and children are not permitted to graze or eat throughout the day. Mealtimes should be pleasant and family oriented, with the goal of eating in a social context. When mealtimes are too brief (less than 10 minutes), children may not have enough time to eat, particularly when they are acquiring self-feeding skills and may eat slowly. Alternatively, sitting for more than 20 or 30 minutes often is difficult for a child and mealtime may become aversive.

Culture

In every family, there are cultural norms for when and how infants are fed (see Chapter 26). Cross-cultural studies of infant feeding document wide cultural variation in the timing, type, and amounts of food and in beliefs about the appropriate styles of feeding (Dettwyler, 1987, 1989). Each culture has a set of generalized traditions for feeding infants and for defining when more complex foods should be introduced. These cultural norms can change based on specific situations. However, they are passed down through subsequent generations and often retain at least some common features.

Although cultural traditions often favor a wide array of dietary options for young children, poverty may hinder a family's ability to comply with traditions. Children who are raised in low-income families are particularly vulnerable to growth deficiencies (Bronner, 1996), often because families are unable to provide them with adequate nutrients. Children who are limited to diets that lack diversity of food choices are more likely to experience nutrient deficiencies and malnutrition (Ross, 1989). A diet that is high in diversity results in a broad variety of tastes, flavors, aromas, and textures and provides a greater probability of meeting nutrient requirements, particularly **micronutrients** (Rozin, 1990).

ASSESSMENT OF FEEDING BEHAVIOR

Feeding problems are commonly assessed through a multidisciplinary approach that includes attention to the child's medical status (e.g., growth, gastrointestinal signs), development (e.g., oral-motor skills), behavior, feeding history, and relationship with the caregiver (Bithoney et al., 1991). In addition, family- and culture-level variables should be included in an assessment, including interviews about family growth patterns, mealtime expectations, and food-related behaviors (Black, 1995).

Family and Culture

At the family level, it is important to examine the cultural factors that influence nurturance, food selection, food offers, and mealtime behavior. Topics may include family stress, eligibility and access to public assistance programs, food availability, mealtime scheduling, and meal characteristics. These topics can be investigated through interviews and/or through observations of meals in the home. Tools such as the Home Observation for Measurement of the Environment (HOME) (Caldwell & Bradley, 1979) have been used to observe the child-centered quality of the home and could be supplemented by specific attention to mealtime settings and behavior. For example, child-oriented equipment, such as highchairs, bibs, and small utensils, may facilitate feeding and enable children to begin to acquire the skills of self-feeding.

Families who are experiencing stress that is related to poverty, housing, employment, or relationships may have little energy available to attend to the nutritional needs of their children, particularly when feeding itself may be stressful or unsatisfying. Parents who are well supported, however, often feel less isolated and may turn to supportive figures in times of stress. Stress and support can be assessed through interview questions about family responsibilities, life events that many families find stressful, and the supportive role of household or family members, with attention directed toward nurturance and feeding. There also are structured assessments for use in clinicians' offices to measure exposure to stressors in the family (Orr, James, & Charney, 1989) and emotional support and stimulation (Casey, Barrett, Bradley, & Spiker, 1993; see Appendix B).

Questions should also be directed to the availability of food. Low-income families may be eligible for food assistance programs, such as food stamps and the Special Supplemental Nutrition Program for Women, Infants and Children (WIC). However, barriers, such as lack of knowledge or difficulty complying with bureaucratic requirements, may interfere with access to available services (see Chapter 36). In addition, families' ability to buy food may be hampered by environmental constraints, such as lack of grocery stores in low-income neighborhoods, unavailability of transportation, or economic limitations (Wiecha & Palombo, 1989) (see Chapter 28). When families have to rely on convenience stores, they are often limited to expensive, prepared foods. Information should be collected on food purchasing patterns, including transportation and shopping frequency.

Regular scheduling of meals helps children establish patterns and develop expectations regarding mealtime (Satter, 1987). If children miss meals, then they lack nutrients and may experience irritability that is related to hunger. Similarly, if children snack or graze throughout the day, then they will not be hungry during meals. If meals are offered at different times each day, then children may become anxious and confused about when it is time to eat (Macht, 1990). Undependable mealtimes make it difficult for children to learn about hunger and satiety cues (see Chapter 27).

Questions should also be asked about competing activities during mealtimes and where meals are served. When meals are characterized by distractions from television, family arguments, or competing activities, children may have difficulty focusing on the feeding process and opportunities for modeling appropriate mealtime behavior may be minimized (Macht, 1990).

Parents

Evaluations of feeding problems should include a careful feeding history that includes parental beliefs about feeding and growth, eating habits, knowledge about nutritional requirements, response to children's feeding behavior, and social support. It is important to ask about parental beliefs about feeding and growth because beliefs form the basis of parental behavior (Harkness & Super, 1996; Pugliese et al., 1987). For example, parents who believe that children should be compliant and clean their plates may be less receptive to children's signals of satiety than parents who believe that children should regulate the amount of food that they eat.

Children's feeding habits are influenced strongly by patterns that are introduced by parents through their own dietary practices (Johnson & Birch, 1992). Thus, parents should be queried about their own dietary practices and nutritional concerns. For example, children of parents who do not eat regularly may have difficulty understanding why they should eat regularly. Similarly, when children observe parents eating snacks, they learn that snacks are desired foods and are more likely to prefer snacks over meals.

Children

Evaluations of children should include their growth and feeding history; cognitive, motor, language, and socioemotional development; temperament; oral-motor development; feeding behaviors; and parent–child interaction (Frank, Silva, & Needlman, 1993). Psychologists often administer standardized, norm-referenced assessments, such as the Bayley Scales of Infant Development, Second Edition (BSID-2) (Bayley, 1993) and the Receptive Expressive Emergent Language Scale (Bzoch & League, 1971), to collect information on children's cognitive, motor, language, and socioemotional development so that eligibility for early intervention services can be determined. In addition, scores on norm-referenced assessments can be used to track children's developmental progress through the intervention process. The Behavior Rating Scale on the BSID-2 is particularly useful because it provides norm-referenced data on children's behavior in a structured setting.

Children's temperament can be assessed directly through observations of the child during play or feeding and indirectly through questions to the mother regarding her perceptions. Standardized questionnaires, such as the Infant Characteristics Questionnaire (Bates, Freeland, & Lounsbury, 1979), may be useful.

Oral-motor problems may be present in children who have physical problems, such as cerebral palsy. If the parent provides a history that includes choking or difficulty with foods of varying texture, then the child's oral-motor development should be examined by an occupational therapist or another professional who has training in feeding disorders (Sullivan & Rosenbloom, 1996; see Chapter 23).

Behaviors that indicate food refusal, such as spitting, head turning, and holding food in the mouth, are not unusual among children who have feeding problems. There are feeding questionnaires that address the changing nutritional and developmental needs of young children, along with the social environment of mealtime, such as "About Your Child's Eating" (Davies, Noll, Davies, & Bukowski, 1993). In addition to asking parents about their children's behavior during feeding, clinicians should observe parents and children together during feeding to capture the affective quality of the interaction.

Attention to the parent–child interaction is a critical component of the evaluation of children with feeding problems. In keeping with Bronfenbrenner's (1993) recommendations, parents and children should be observed in multiple contexts. Assuming that observations are conducted during feeding, it is ideal to include an observation during play. The two contexts vary in structure and purpose and, thus, provide a comprehensive view of parent–child interaction.

The Growth and Nutrition Clinic at the University of Maryland Medical Center is a multidisciplinary clinic that is dedicated to providing family-focused evaluation and intervention for children who have growth deficiencies and/or feeding problems (Black, Dubowitz, Hutcheson, Berenson-Howard, & Starr, 1995). The multidisciplinary team includes clinicians who have training in nutrition, pediatrics, social work, and psychology, with specialists available through consultation. The initial evaluation is conducted in the clinic, and a social worker observes a typical meal during a home visit. In addition, caregivers and children are videotaped having lunch. Prior to the evaluation, parents are told that a videotape will be made of them with their child during lunch and the evaluation is scheduled for a time when the parent thinks that the child will be hungry. Parents are advised that they may bring food or eat the food that is available in the clinic (baby food, microwavable meals, applesauce, pudding, crackers, milk, and juice). Feeding occurs in a room that is equipped with a highchair, child's table and chair, and adult chairs. Families are instructed to sit wherever they prefer, to feed their children as they do at home, and to take as long as necessary. The video camera is visible in the room but does not require an operator to be present. The family remains in the room alone until they signal that they have finished.

Feeding may also be observed during a home visit. Observing the child and family in their natural environment enables clinicians to consider the contextual variables that may influence feeding, including the physical environment and the presence of other family members.

Observations should be directed toward both parents and children rather than focused exclusively on parental behaviors. There are several coding systems that have been used during feeding: 1) Nursing Child Assessment Satellite Training Feeding Scale (NCAST, F) (Sumner & Spietz, 1994), 2) Parent Child Early Relational Assessment (PCERA) (Black et al., 1996; Clark, 1985), and 3) A Developmental Classification of Feeding Disorders (Chatoor et al., 1985) (see Appendixes C and D).

INTERVENTION FOR FEEDING PROBLEMS

Feeding occurs within a social context, and, in keeping with ecological theory, feeding problems cannot be treated without considering the influences from the family and the broader culture. Wolke and Skuse (1992) provided a comprehensive list of feeding behavior problems and interventions that can be incorporated into clinical practice. Family-focused intervention may be an optimum strategy to promote healthy growth and development because it is based on ecological theory and recognizes that the development of children's feeding behavior occurs within a multilevel social context (Black, 1995).

Modeling and Videotape

Modeling is an important mechanism that influences children's acceptance of novel or nonpreferred foods. When preschool-age children observed others eating and enjoying the food, they shifted their preferences and joined the social activity of eating the previously novel food (Birch, 1980). Thus, children benefit from eating with others.

Modeling relies on identification with culturally sensitive models to demonstrate optimum behavior (Bandura, 1986). Television and video are effective ways of providing models and occupy a central position within the lives of many families, but their use has been confined almost exclusively to entertainment. By using the techniques of fast-moving dialogues and quick editing in a context that is culturally and developmentally familiar to parents, messages to promote healthy nutrition and to build interactional skills can be presented to parents in an appealing manner that can be shared with peers or with other family members in their own home. Videotapes have been used effectively to encourage breast-feeding (Grossman, Larsen-Alexander, Fitzsimmons, & Cordero, 1991) and to promote favorable mealtime attitudes and behaviors among adolescent mothers (Black & Teti, 1997).

In the Growth and Nutrition Clinic at the University of Maryland, videotapes that are made by families during the evaluation are reviewed by the staff and then used in a therapeutic session with the family. Other clinicians have described the use of videotapes to aid in diagnosing feeding problems and to help families develop alternative interactional strategies (Koniak-Griffin, Verzememnieks, & Cahill, 1992; McDonough, 1993, 1995; Wolke & Skuse, 1992). For example, McDonough (1993, 1995) has demonstrated that videotape can be used successfully in brief psychotherapy as part of interaction guidance to help parents learn to enjoy their children, to understand them better, and to reduce feeding problems. In the Growth and Nutrition Clinic, videotaping becomes familiar to families because it is repeated frequently and incorporated into routine clinical evaluation and intervention procedures. Caregivers learn to look at their personal behavior, at their child's behavior, and, finally, at the feeding partnership.

Caregiver Behavior

One objective of incorporating the videotape into a therapeutic session is to help caregivers recognize how important they are to their child and to enhance the value of the child to them. Caregivers of children who have feeding disorders may feel frustrated and disappointed with their lack of success in feeding their child or with their child's noncompliance and/or rejection. Yet, in every videotape, there are concrete examples of the strength of the caregiver–child relationship, such as the child's looking to the caregiver for guidance, cues, or reactions. This strategy emphasizes the caregiver's importance in the partnership and helps the caregiver develop a sense of efficacy in improving the relationship.

Caregivers often need help in separating their own emotional needs from those of their child. Children of parents who are depressed, hostile, or anxious are less likely to benefit from home intervention than children of caregivers who do not have these symptoms (Hutcheson et al., 1997). In some cases, caregivers may benefit from a therapeutic intervention that addresses their own mental health needs.

Child Behavior

Viewing interaction on videotape helps caregivers see the relationship from the child's perspective. As participants in the interaction, caregivers are often dominated by their own feelings and reactions and cannot consider either the child's perspective or the overall partnership. By watching the videotape, caregivers learn to view the interaction from the child's point of view. They see how the child reacts to a smile or to a criticism. Recognizing the child's perspective is a critical step in intervention because it helps caregivers understand that children are influenced not only by internal regulatory processes but also by the behavior of others. Caregivers who understand that children are influenced by caregiver behavior are more receptive to behavioral interventions.

Partnership

Videotaped interactions can help caregivers recognize the communicative value of children's feeding problems by watching their own reactions. Some children signal satiety by throwing food or turning the bowl upside down. Caregivers who anticipate their children's actions can prevent the disruptive behavior and help children use more socially appropriate methods to signal their desire to terminate the meal. In many cases, caregivers are passive and silent and their interactions are limited to directives to their child to eat. Thus, the child who does not eat is more successful in engaging the caregiver, albeit in negative interactions, than the child who eats the entire meal. This concept often is difficult for caregivers to understand until they observe the interaction on videotape and see for themselves how their child tries to engage them and finally uses problem behaviors to attract their attention.

By watching themselves interacting with their child, caregivers learn to differentiate successful from unsuccessful strategies. Caregivers serve as their own models and are empowered by identifying strategies that work for them and their child. By practicing newly acquired skills through repeated videotaped observations, caregivers learn to analyze interaction patterns and identify aspects of their own behavior that contribute to feeding problems or success in their children. The therapeutic use of videotaped interactions has been effective with caregivers, including those who have cognitive limitations or who experience multiple stressors (McDonough, 1993, 1995; Wolke & Skuse, 1992). The clinician does not instruct or teach the caregiver how to interact with his or her child, but through the use of videotapes the clinician helps the caregiver gain a better understanding of the feeding partnership and how behavior in one partner influences the entire interaction. Caregivers practice alternative methods of interacting with their child with the goal of improving and clarifying their communication so that it is not based on feeding problems.

Reinforcement Controversy

Behavioral principles form the basis of many interventions that are used to eliminate feeding behavior problems (Linscheid, Budd, & Rasnake, 1995). For example, if children refuse to eat, then caregivers can be taught to use reinforcements, such as praise, after children have taken a bite to encourage them to continue to eat. In addition, parents may use other reinforcements, such as access to television (after the meal), to encourage a child once he or she has demonstrated the desired behavior. Negative consequences (e.g., withdrawing social attention or privileges) are used after the child engages in an inappropriate behavior to reduce the likelihood that the negative behavior will continue.

In working with children who do not have feeding behavior problems, Birch, Marlin, and Rotter (1984) reported that reinforcement strategies in which preferred foods were given as rewards for eating nonpreferred foods did not lead to increased consumption of nonpreferred foods. They have suggested an overjustification hypothesis to explain why rewards do not achieve the desired effects with food. Children reason that if a reward is necessary to eat the target food, then it must not be good. Birch and colleagues also argued that feeding should be guided by internal regulatory mechanisms and not by external reinforcement strategies that are imposed by caregivers.

Much of the research on the application of behavioral principles to feeding disorders has been conducted in hospital or institutional settings among children who have severe feeding problems in combination with medical disorders or mental retardation. Children are fed by trained staff with attention directed toward the child's response to each bite that is presented. Children who have severe feeding disorders or disabilities may require external behavioral controls to eat successfully because they are less able to regulate their nutritional needs, to communicate with caregivers, or to acquire feeding skills. There has been little research in which behavioral principles have been integrated into an ecological context or used with children who are living with their families and exhibit mild feeding problems. Therefore, less intrusive strategies, such as modeling, should be considered when encouraging children who do not have severe behavior problems to eat nutritious foods.

APPLICATIONS AND RECOMMENDATIONS

The following recommendations to promote healthy mealtime behavior are based on ecological theory as applied to feeding. They may be incorporated into anticipatory guidance to prevent feeding problems or into intervention programs for young children who are exhibiting feeding problems. They are designed to assist families with enhancing their communication system with their child so that meals are a pleasant social time to meet nutritional requirements rather than an occasion for upsetting or emotion-laden battles for control.

Mealtime Setting

- Infants and young toddlers need to eat more frequently than adults. Encourage caregivers to incorporate healthy snacks into children's daily diets.
- Encourage caregivers to establish a predictable mealtime schedule so that children learn to expect food on a regular basis.
- Discourage caregivers from allowing children to graze or eat freely throughout the day because they will not experience the mild hunger that stimulates appetite.
- Position children during feeding so that their bodies are well supported for eating. Infants should be held so that they feel the security of their caregiver. As children get older, they should be seated so that they can see others, and their arms and hands should be free so that they can self-feed. Highchairs and booster seats enable children to join the family at the table.
- Encourage caregivers to feed children in an area where spills will not be important. Making a mess is part of the process of learning to eat. Dressing children in old clothes or bibs and placing plastic bags or newspapers on the floor can prevent damage that is associated with messes and spills.
- Encourage caregivers to separate mealtime from playtime and not to use toys or television to distract the child during mealtime.
- Emotional family discussions or arguments may distract children from eating and should not happen during mealtime.

- Meals should last no less than about 10 minutes and no more than 20–30 minutes. When possible, children should be encouraged to remain at the table during the entire meal.

Food and Nutrition

- Ensure that caregivers are aware of children's nutritional needs.
- Emphasize the importance of gradually introducing children to novel foods, recognizing that their initial response may be rejection. When the caregiver eats the novel food and signals enjoyment, novel foods become familiar and potentially enjoyable.
- Encourage caregivers to present meals in a manner that is appealing for children and that recognizes children's developing ability to self-feed.
- Encourage caregivers to enable children to have some control over meals by giving them choices of foods or utensils and allowing them to help with preparation.

Mealtime Behavior

- Encourage caregivers to eat with their children so that modeling can occur and mealtimes are viewed as pleasant, social occasions.
- Ensure that caregivers are able to recognize signals from their children regarding hunger and satiety or dislike of specific foods.
- Ensure that caregivers communicate their messages clearly to their children.
- Help caregivers recognize that children tend to balance their intake over the entire day and that there may be substantial variability from meal to meal.
- Encourage caregivers to be on the lookout for any changes in normal eating habits that may signal developmental changes. For example, the child who begins to refuse foods may be looking for ways to exercise control. Caregivers can help children with control by providing choices or mealtime responsibilities (e.g., helping with preparations).
- Encourage caregivers to use nurturing guidance with their children rather than harsh disciplinary practices.
- Encourage caregivers to promote feeding through culturally appropriate strategies without using food as a reward, punishment, or threat.
- Discourage caregivers from fighting with their children or forcing them to eat.
- Encourage caregivers to seek assistance from health care providers if their child is experiencing feeding problems.
- Encourage caregivers to promote self-feeding, first with fingers and then with a spoon.
- Encourage caregivers to respect their children's signals of satiety. When children signal that they are finished (perhaps by throwing food), they should be shown a more socially appropriate way to end the meal and then the food should be removed.
- Encourage caregivers not to focus on the amount of food that the child eats. The quantity of food consumed should be guided by the child's hunger, not by external cues.

All of these recommendations require knowledge of the cultural context, the available food resources, the family's beliefs regarding meals, feeding, and growth, and the feeding partnership between the child and the caregiver. By using a culturally based theory such as ecological theory (Bronfenbrenner, 1993) to examine growth and feeding, clinicians can develop intervention strategies that are culturally, developmentally, and nutritionally appropriate, thereby facilitating acceptance. These targeted intervention strategies should promote healthy feeding behaviors and prevent the growth faltering that is often associated with feeding problems.

REFERENCES

Ainsworth, M., & Bell, S. (1974). Mother–infant interaction and the development of competence. In K. Connolly & J. Bruner (Eds.), *The growth of competence* (pp. 97–118). San Diego: Academic Press.

Bandura, A. (1986). *Social foundations of thought and action: A social cognitive theory.* Upper Saddle River, NJ: Prentice-Hall.

Barnard, K., Hammond, M., Booth, C., Bee, H., Mitchell, S., & Speiker, S. (1989). Measurement and meaning of parent–child interaction. In F.J. Morrison & C.E. Lee (Eds.), *Applied developmental psychology* (Vol. 3, pp. 39–80). San Diego: Academic Press.

Bates, J.E., Freeland, C., & Lounsbury, M.L. (1979). Measurement of infant difficultness. *Child Development, 50,* 794–803.

Bayley, N. (1993). *Bayley Scales of Infant Development* (2nd ed.). San Antonio, TX: The Psychological Corporation.

Beauchamp, G.K., Cowart, B.J., & Moran, M. (1986). Developmental changes in salt acceptability in human infants. *Developmental Psychobiology, 19,* 17–25.

Benoit, D., Zeanah, C.H., & Barton, M.L. (1989). Maternal attachment disturbance in failure to thrive. *Infant Mental Health Journal, 10,* 185–202.

Bentley, M.E., Black, M.M., & Hurtado, E. (1995). Child-feeding and appetite: What can programmes do? *Food and Nutrition Bulletin, 16,* 340–348.

Birch, L.L. (1980). Effects of peer models' food choices and eating behaviors on preschoolers' food preferences. *Child Development, 51,* 489–496.

Birch, L.L. (1992). Children's preferences for high-fat foods. *Nutrition Reviews, 50,* 249–255.

Birch, L.L., & Johnson, S.L. (1994). Appetite control in children. In J.D. Fernstrom & G.D. Miller (Eds.), *Appetite and body weight regulation* (pp. 5–15). Boca Raton, FL: CRC Press.

Birch, L.L., Johnson, S.L., Anderson, G., Peters, J.C., & Schulte, M.C. (1991). The variability of young children's energy intake. *New England Journal of Medicine, 324,* 232–235.

Birch, L.L., Marlin, D.W., & Rotter, J. (1984). Eating as the "means" activity in a contingency: Effects on young children's food preference. *Child Development, 55,* 431–439.

Bithoney, W.G., McJunkin, J., Michalek, J., Snyder, J., Egan, H., & Epstein, D. (1991). The effect of a multidisciplinary team approach on weight gain in nonorganic failure-to-thrive children. *Journal of Developmental and Behavioral Pediatrics, 12,* 254–258.

Black, M.M. (1995). Failure to thrive: Strategies for evaluation and intervention. *School Psychology Review, 24,* 171–185.

Black, M.M., Dubowitz, H., Hutcheson, J., Berenson-Howard, J., & Starr, R.H. (1995). A randomized clinical trial of home intervention for children with failure to thrive. *Pediatrics, 95,* 807–814.

Black, M., Hutcheson, J., Dubowitz, H., Berenson-Howard, J., & Starr, R.H. (1996). The roots of competence: Mother–infant interaction among low-income, African-American families. *Applied Developmental Psychology, 17,* 367–391.

Black, M., & Teti, L. (1997). Videotape: A culturally sensitive strategy to promote communication and healthy nutrition among adolescent mothers and their infants. *Pediatrics, 99,* 432–437.

Brinich, E., Drotar, D., & Brinich, P. (1989). Security of attachment and outcome of preschoolers with histories of nonorganic failure to thrive. *Journal of Clinical Child Psychology, 18,* 142–152.

Bronfenbrenner, U. (1993). Ecological systems theory. In R. Wozniak & K. Fisher (Eds.), *Specific environments: Thinking in contexts* (pp. 3–44). Mahwah, NJ: Lawrence Erlbaum Associates.

Bronner, Y.L. (1996). Nutrition status outcomes for children: Ethnic, cultural, and environmental contexts. *Journal of the American Dietetic Association, 96,* 891–903.

Bzoch, K.R., & League, R. (1971). *Assessing language skills in infancy: A handbook for the multidimensional analysis of emergent language.* Baltimore: University Park Press.

Caldwell, B.M., & Bradley, R.H. (1984). *Home Observation for the Measurement of the Environment.* Little Rock: University of Arkansas, Center for Child Development and Education.

Casey, P.H., Barrett, K., Bradley, R.H., & Spiker, D. (1993). Pediatric clinical assessment of mother–child interaction: Concurrent and predictive validity. *Journal of Developmental and Behavioral Pediatrics, 14,* 313–317.

Caulfield, L., Bentley, M., & Ahmed, S. (1996). Is prolonged breastfeeding associated with malnutrition? Evidence from 19 demographic and health surveys. *International Journal of Epidemiology, 25,* 693–703.

Chatoor, I., Dickson, L., Schaefer, S., & Egan, J. (1985). A developmental classification of feeding disorders associated with failure to thrive: Diagnosis and treatment. In D. Drotar (Ed.), *New direc-

tions in failure to thrive: Implications for research and practice (pp. 235–258). New York: Plenum.

Chatoor, I., Hirch, R., & Persinger, M. (1997). Facilitating internal regulation of eating: A treatment model for infantile anorexia. *Infants and Young Children, 9,* 12–22.

Clark, R. (1985). *The Parent–Child Early Relational Assessment: Instrument and manual.* Madison: University of Wisconsin Medical School, Department of Psychiatry.

Crittenden, P. (1987). Non-organic failure-to-thrive: Deprivation or distortion? *Infant Mental Health, 8,* 51–64.

Davies, C.M., Noll, R.B., Davies, W.H., & Bukowski, W.M. (1993). Mealtime interactions and family relationships of families of children who have cancer in long-term remission and controls. *Journal of the American Dietetic Association, 93,* 773–776.

Davis, C. (1928). Self-selection of diets by newly weaned infants: An experimental study. *American Journal of Diseases of Children, 36,* 651–679.

Davis, C.M. (1934). Studies in the self-selection of diet by young children. *Journal of the American Dental Association, 21,* 636–640.

Dettwyler, K.A. (1987). Infant feeding in Mali: Cultural context and hard data. *Social Science and Medicine, 25,* 553–559.

Dettwyler, K.A. (1989). Styles of infant feeding: Parental/caretaker control of food consumption in young children. *American Anthropologist, 91,* 696–703.

Drotar, D., Eckerle, D., Satola, J., Pallotta, J., & Wyatt, B. (1990). Maternal interactional behavior with nonorganic failure-to-thrive infants: A case comparison study. *Child Abuse and Neglect, 14,* 41–51.

Elmer, E. (1960). Failure to thrive: Role of the mother. *Pediatrics, 25,* 717–725.

Engle, P.L. (1991). Maternal work and child-care strategies in peri-urban Guatemala: Nutritional effects. *Child Development, 62,* 954–965.

Frank, D.A., Silva, M., & Needlman, R. (1993, February). Failure to thrive: Mystery, myth, and method. *Contemporary Pediatrics,* 114–133.

Grossman, L., Larsen-Alexander, J., Fitzsimmons, S., & Cordero, L. (1991). Promotion of breast feeding among inner-city women. *Clinical Pediatrics, 28,* 38–42.

Harkness, S., & Super, C.M. (1996). *Parents' cultural belief systems: Their origin, expressions, and consequences.* New York: Guilford Press.

Heptinstall, F., Puckering, C., Skuse, D., Start, K., Zur-Szpiro, S., & Dowdney, L. (1987). Nutrition and mealtime behavior in families of growth retarded children. *Human Nutrition: Applied Nutrition, 41A,* 390–402.

Hutcheson, J., Black, M., & Starr, R. (1993). Developmental changes in interactional characteristics of mothers and their children with failure to thrive. *Journal of Pediatric Psychology, 18,* 453–466.

Hutcheson, J., Black, M., Talley, M., Dubowitz, H., Berenson-Howard, J., Starr, R.H., & Thompson, B.S. (1997). Risk status and home intervention among children with failure to thrive: Follow-up at age 4. *Journal of Pediatric Psychology, 22,* 651–668.

Illingsworth, R.S., & Lister, J. (1964). The critical or sensitive period with special reference to certain feeding problems in infants and children. *Journal of Pediatrics, 65,* 839–848.

Johnson, S.L., & Birch, L.L. (1992). Children's sensitivity to energy density is related to parents' eating and disciplinary styles. *Journal of Cell Biochemistry, 16B,* 262.

Koniak-Griffin, D., Verzememnieks, I., & Cahill, D. (1992). Using videotape instruction and feedback to improve adolescents' mothering behaviors. *Journal of Adolescent Health, 13,* 570–575.

Linscheid, T.R. (1992). Eating problems in children. In C.E. Walder & M.C. Roberts (Eds.), *Handbook of clinical child psychology* (2nd ed., pp. 451–473). New York: John Wiley & Sons.

Linscheid, T.R., Budd, K.S., & Rasnake, L.K. (1995). Pediatric feeding disorders. In M.C. Roberts (Ed.), *Handbook of pediatric psychology* (2nd ed., pp. 501–515). New York: Guilford Press.

Macht, J. (1990). *Poor eaters: Helping children who refuse to eat.* New York: Plenum.

McDonough, S.C. (1993). Interaction guidance: Understanding and treating early infant–caregiver relationship disturbances. In C.H. Zeanah, Jr. (Ed.), *Handbook of infant mental health* (pp. 414–426). New York: Guilford Press.

McDonough, S.C. (1995). Promoting positive early parent–infant relationships through interaction guidance. *Child and Adolescent Psychiatric Clinics of North America, 4,* 661–672.

Morris, S.E. (1977). Oral-motor development: Normal and abnormal. In J.M. Wilson (Ed.), *Oral-motor function and dysfunction in children* (pp. 114–128). Chapel Hill: University of North Carolina at Chapel Hill.

Orr, S.T., James, S.A., & Charney, E. (1989). A social environment inventory for the pediatric office. *Journal of Developmental and Behavioral Pediatrics, 10,* 287–291.

Polan, H.J., Leon, A., Kaplan, M.D., Kessler, D.B., Stern, D., & Ward, M.J. (1991). Disturbances of affect expression in failure-to-thrive. *Journal of American Academy of Child and Adolescent Psychiatry, 30,* 897–903.

Powell, G.F., Low, J.F., & Speers, M.A. (1987). Behavior as a diagnostic aid in failure to thrive. *Journal of Developmental and Behavioral Pediatrics, 8,* 18–24.

Pugliese, M.T., Weyman-Daum, M., Moses, N., & Lifshitz, F. (1987). Parental health beliefs as a cause of nonorganic failure to thrive. *Pediatrics, 80,* 175–182.

Ross, E.B. (1989). An overview of trends in dietary variation from hunter-gatherer to modern capitalist societies. In M. Harris & E.B. Ross (Eds.), *Food and evolution: Toward a theory of human food habits* (pp. 7–55). Philadelphia: Lippincott-Raven Publishers.

Ross, P., & Zellner, D. (1985). The role of Pavlovian conditioning in the acquisition of food likes and dislikes. In N. Braverman & P. Bronstein (Eds.), *Experimental assessments and clinical applications of conditioned food aversions* (pp. 189–202). New York: New York Academy of Sciences Press.

Rozin, P. (1990). Development in the food domain. *Developmental Psychology, 26,* 555–562.

Rudolph, C.D. (1994). Feeding disorders in infants and children. *The Journal of Pediatrics, 125,* S116–S124.

Rutter, M. (1987). Psychosocial resilience and protective mechanisms. *American Journal of Orthopsychiatry, 57,* 316–331.

Satter, E. (1987). *How to get your kid to eat . . . but not too much.* Palo Alto, CA: Bull Publishing.

Singer, L.T., Song, L., Hill, B.P., & Jaffee, A.C. (1990). Stress and depression in mothers of failure to thrive children. *Journal of Pediatric Psychology, 15,* 711–720.

Skuse, D., & Wolke, D. (1992). The nature and consequences of feeding problems in infants. In P.J. Cooper & A. Stein (Eds.), *Feeding problems and eating disorders in children and adolescents* (pp. 1–26). Philadelphia: Harwood Academic Publishers.

Smith, M.M., & Lifshitz, F. (1994). Excess fruit juice consumption as a contributing factor in nonorganic failure to thrive. *Pediatrics, 93,* 438–443.

Story, M., & Brown, J.E. (1987). Do young children instinctively know what to eat? The studies of Clara Davis revisited. *New England Journal of Medicine, 316,* 103–105.

Sullivan, P.B., & Rosenbloom, L. (1996). An overview of the feeding difficulties experienced by disabled children. In P.B. Sullivan & L. Rosenbloom (Eds.), *Feeding the disabled child* (pp. 1–10). London: MacKeith Press.

Sullivan, S.A., & Birch, L.L. (1990). Pass the sugar, pass the salt: Experience dictates preference. *Developmental Psychology, 26,* 546–551.

Sullivan, S.A., & Birch, L.L. (1994). Infant dietary experience and acceptance of solid foods. *Pediatrics, 93,* 271–277.

Sumner, G., & Spietz, A. (Eds.). (1994). *NCAST caregiver/parent–child interaction feeding manual.* Seattle: University of Washington, School of Nursing, NCAST Publications.

Underwood, B.A. (1985). Weaning practices in deprived economic environments: The weaning dilemma. *Pediatrics, 75,* 194–198.

Wehler, C. (1991). *Community childhood hunger identification project: A survey of childhood hunger in the United States.* Washington, DC: Food Research Action Center.

Wiecha, J., & Palombo, R. (1989). Multiple program participation: Comparison of nutrition and food assistance program benefits with food costs in Boston, Massachusetts. *American Journal of Public Health, 79,* 591–595.

Wolf, L.S., & Glass, R.P. (1996). The therapeutic approach to the child with feeding difficulty: Assessment. In P.B. Sullivan & L. Rosenbloom (Eds.), *Feeding the disabled child* (pp. 47–61). London: MacKeith Press.

Wolke, D., & Skuse, D. (1992). The management of infant feeding problems. In P.J. Cooper & A. Stein (Eds.), *Feeding problems and eating disorders in children and adolescents* (pp. 27–60). Philadelphia: Harwood Academic Publishers.

Wolke, D., Skuse, D., & Mathisen, B. (1990). Behavioral style in failure to thrive infants: A preliminary communication. *Journal of Pediatric Psychology, 15,* 237–243.

Section III

Medical Aspects of Poor Growth

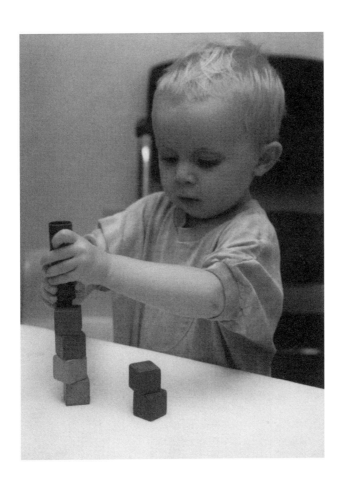

Chapter 9

Medical Assessment and Management and the Organization of Medical Services

Elizabeth A. Rider and William G. Bithoney

Normal childhood growth and development depend on the positive interaction of nutritional, medical, psychosocial, developmental, and environmental factors. When any of these factors are altered, feeding behaviors may be affected and deviations from expected growth and development can result.

There is no universally accepted definition for *failure to thrive* (Wilcox, Nieburg, & Miller, 1989), and a variety of terms are used interchangeably, including *pediatric undernutrition, malnutrition, failure to grow, growth deficiency,* and *growth failure. Growth deficiency* is a clinical syndrome with many etiologies, the common biological issue of which is malnutrition.

Poverty is a major risk factor for growth deficiency. Children who live in poverty and those who have chronic illnesses are at particular risk for malnutrition (Rider, Samuels, Wilson, & Homer, 1996). Meyers et al. (1995) showed a significant association between the nutritional status of children in poor families and the receipt of housing assistance. Ten percent of children from families who are not receiving housing subsidies and 21% of children from families who are on the waiting list for housing subsidies have low growth indicators, compared with 3% of children from families who are receiving housing subsidies. These data suggest that poor urban families may be forced to choose between providing shelter or providing food for their children. In low-income families, nonorganic growth deficiency affects one in seven African American children and one in six Hispanic children who are younger than 1 year (U.S. Department of Health and Human Services, 1991).

Although children who experience growth deficiency more often are from low-income families and poverty is the single greatest risk factor (Frank & Drotar, 1994), growth deficiency occurs in all socioeconomic groups. Hampton (1993) reported that although growth deficiency appears in all social classes in England, the social class of the parent influences whether it is recognized and investigated by health visitors. Professional parents are more likely to be told that their child simply is "small."

The treatment of growth deficiency encompasses medical, developmental, and psychosocial issues. For a given patient and family, appropriate treatment ranges from straightforward management at well-child pediatric visits to consultation with other specialists, referral to a multidisciplinary team, or hospitalization.

This chapter provides a practical outline for the medical assessment of growth deficiency, including history, physical examination, and use of the laboratory. Outpatient management strategies are discussed for the different stages of malnutrition (mild, moderate, and severe). The use of the hospital in the management of growth deficiency is presented, and the multidisciplinary team approach is discussed. Finally, other systems of care are considered.

MEDICAL ASSESSMENT

A thorough history and a physical examination are the crux of the medical assessment of the child who is suspected of experiencing a growth deficiency. The goal is to identify symptoms or conditions that affect the child's growth potential, increase caloric requirements, decrease the use or availability of calories, or affect the parents' ability to meet the child's nutritional needs. Multiple etiologies of growth deficiency exist. Environmental and interactional causes are most prevalent and significantly outnumber organic etiologies. Organic causes most often include gastrointestinal, neurological, pulmonary, cardiovascular, and endocrine disorders (Kessler, 1997).

History

The history starts with the parents' perception of the problem, its onset, and its cause. Historical aspects to consider are presented in Table 1 and are discussed more fully in the following sections.

Prenatal and Perinatal History

Pregnancy and birth history provide important clues to etiology. Frequent miscarriages suggest the need for genetics evaluation. Parental use of tobacco has negative effects on fetal growth, as does maternal use of alcohol or illegal drugs (see Chapter 18). Serious perinatal asphyxia can compromise subsequent growth. Microcephaly or macrocephaly suggests workup for genetic or neurological issues (see Chapter 14). The closely spaced births of several siblings may not allow parents enough time, energy, and personal resources for the child who has been identified as experiencing growth deficiency.

Medical History and Review of Systems

Medical history is important. A detailed **review of systems** elicits information that was omitted inadvertently from the medical history. Recurring respiratory illnesses, **otitis media,** and gastrointestinal illnesses are more common among children who experience growth deficiency (Mitchell, Gorrell, & Greenberg, 1980). Altemeier, O'Connor, Sherrod,

Table 1.   Historical information in the medical assessment of children with growth deficiency

Prenatal History
- Maternal obstetrical history; frequent pregnancies or miscarriages
- Toxic or teratogenic exposures—cigarettes, alcohol, anticonvulsants, other drugs
- Was pregnancy planned?

Perinatal History
- Birth weight, length, head circumference
- Gestational age, prematurity
- Apgars; asphyxia or cerebral palsy
- Small for gestational age or intrauterine growth retardation
- Congenital anomalies, infections
- Length of stay in hospital
- Feeding method (breast or formula)
- Feeding difficulties: failed breast-feeding; poor feeding interactions, bottle propping
- Mother–infant interaction and relationship
- Postpartum depression

Medical History
- Acute illnesses; chronic or recurrent illnesses
- Hospitalizations, surgeries
- Medications, allergies, immunizations

Review of Systems
- Diarrhea; bulky, frequent, or foul-smelling stools; constipation; abdominal distention, cramping
- Vomiting, spitting, gastroesophageal reflux, dysphagia
- Cardiac disease, symptoms of congestive heart failure
- Polyuria, polydipsia, polyphagia
- Respiratory illnesses, chronic rhinitis
- Dysuria, urinary frequency
- Frequent infections (upper respiratory infection, gastroenteritis, otitis media, urinary tract infection, sinusitis); recurrent fevers
- Snoring, mouth breathing, restless sleep, sleep apnea
- Food allergy
- Minor anomalies; dysmorphia

Growth History
- Obtain and plot growth data on growth charts
- Percentage of median value of weight for age, weight for height, height for age
- Growth velocity; crossed percentiles on growth charts
- What occurred at points where growth rate changed (e.g., illness, family stresses)

Nutrition History
- Quantify intake, calories: 3- to 5-day food diary
- Parental beliefs about nutrition, health, food allergies
- If breast-feeding: frequency, comfort, mother's fluid intake and diet, support for nursing
- Formula preparation: frequency, amount; improper preparation, underfeeding
- Delayed introduction of solids; intolerance of new foods
- Appropriateness of food for age
- Food restrictions or promotion: low-fat diets, restrictions for allergy, other diets
- Excessive use of juice, fruit drinks, carbonated beverages

(continued)

Table 1.   (*continued*)

Feeding Behavior
- Feedings or meals per day; "grazing"
- Mealtime environment; who feeds child; parental responses to child's feeding behaviors
- Food refusal, spitting, "picky eater," "food battles," forced feeding
- Pain or discomfort with eating
- Oral-motor function: oral retention; difficulties with sucking, swallowing, or chewing; choking; gagging
- Ability and interest in self-feeding
- Distractions while eating (e.g., TV)

Developmental and Behavior History
- Milestones: gross and fine motor, speech, language
- Sleep, interaction, activity level
- Temperament (e.g., child seen as willful, independent)
- Activity level, distractibility
- Typical day

Family History
- Parental height and weight
- Growth patterns of siblings; physical size of grandparents, aunts, uncles
- Medical problems in family (e.g., growth deficiency, gastrointestinal, neurological, endocrine disorders, diabetes, sickle-cell anemia, cystic fibrosis)
- Psychiatric problems in the family

Psychosocial History
- With whom does child live?
- Age and occupation of parents, caregivers; parents' cognitive capacity
- Living conditions: overcrowding, homelessness, social isolation
- Parents' relationship; parents' own family experience
- Family's strengths, supports, and stresses
- Exposure to tobacco smoke
- Travel history to or from developing countries
- Domestic violence; history of abuse, neglect in nuclear family and parents' families
- Eligibility for additional resources (Special Supplemental Nutrition Program for Women, Infants and Children [WIC], Temporary Assistance for Needy Families [TANF], food stamps, Supplemental Security Income [SSI])

Yeager, and Vietze (1985) found that children who experience nonorganic growth deficiency are smaller at birth and have more illnesses than children who grow normally. Even mild recurrent illnesses (e.g., otitis media) can decrease a child's appetite (see Chapter 12). Acute infections increase metabolic demands and reduce caloric intake via decreased appetite. Recurrent or uncommon infections can signal immunodeficiency such as acquired immunodeficiency syndrome (AIDS) (see Chapter 13). Organic problems that may result in growth deficiency include recurrent vomiting and diarrhea, neurological illness (e.g., cerebral palsy), and chronic upper-airway disease (otitis media and obstruction) (Bithoney & Newberger, 1987; Sills, 1978).

Growth History

An essential part of the history is a review of growth data, plotted on National Center for Health Statistics (NCHS) growth charts, to determine whether a problem is present. The clinical assessment of growth is discussed in Chapter 10.

Nutrition History and Feeding Behavior

Quantitative measurement of caloric intake, obtained from a 24-hour food recall or, more accurately, a 3- to 5-day food diary, is useful (Witschi, 1990). Parental beliefs about nutrition; food and formula preparation; breast-feeding issues; dietary restrictions; and the frequency, amount, and duration of feeds should be explored (see Chapter 6). Inquiry about the existence of pain or discomfort with eating should occur (see Chapter 10). A qualitative assessment of feeding behavior also is important. An assessment of a child's feeding behavior and parental responses can identify contributory interactional problems (see Chapters 7 and 8).

Developmental and Behavior History

Screening assessment of behavior and development is recommended for all children. Children who experience growth deficiency have a higher incidence of developmental delays than the rest of the population; developmental delays are common, with cognitive impairments (decreased IQ score, speech problems, reading delays) most prominent (Berwick, 1980). Gross motor skills and speech often are the most impaired, and cognitive assessment can be affected by depressed mood in the infant or child who experiences growth deficiency (Bithoney & Rathbun, 1983).

Information about temperament and behavioral style should be obtained as well as motor, speech, and language milestones. Children who are viewed as willful may engage in autonomy struggles with food refusal, which may lead to decreased intake. Language delay contributes to impaired interaction (see Chapter 24). Assessment of oral-motor function, including swallowing, lip, and tongue coordination, is important, and children should be referred for further assessments as indicated (see Chapter 23). In-depth language and developmental testing can be useful in evaluating areas of concern (Bithoney, Dubowitz, & Egan, 1992; Bithoney & Rathbun, 1983; Casey, 1992; Schwartz & Abegglen, 1996; see also Chapter 24).

Family History

Growth histories of parents and siblings (see Chapter 10) are helpful. Psychiatric problems as well as a family history of organic medical disease (e.g., cystic fibrosis; diabetes mellitus; other endocrine, metabolic, neurological, or gastrointestinal diseases) that can affect growth should be obtained.

Psychosocial History

A psychosocial history is invaluable in the assessment of growth deficiency. Initial history can be obtained by the primary care provider, and a more detailed social history can be completed by a social worker. Psychosocial and socioeconomic factors, especially those that correlate with the onset of weight loss, provide major etiological information. Mothers of children who experience growth deficiency report more disorganized homes, negative relationships with the child's father (e.g., arguments, separations), social isolation, and less support from families and neighbors (Bithoney & Newberger, 1987; Casey, 1989). Children from low-income families who experience hunger and household food shortages exhibit higher levels of anxiety, irritability, aggression, and oppositional behavior than their low-income peers who do not experience hunger (Kleinman et al., 1998).

The family's stresses as well as their strengths need to be assessed. Parents' age, occupation, cognitive ability, and relationship are important as are their perceptions of their child, their own family experiences, and the father's role. Obtaining information about domestic violence, abuse, and neglect in the present family and parents' families of origin is important. Information about all of the child's caregivers (e.g., child care, relatives) is helpful. Mental health referral is warranted in situations of psychosis, drug abuse, or depression in the child's primary caregiver; marital conflict; disturbances in infant–parent relationships; and other situations that jeopardize the functioning of the child or the family.

Socioeconomic status and eligibility for the Special Supplemental Nutrition Program for Women, Infants and Children (WIC), food stamps, Supplemental Security Income (SSI), medical assistance, and Temporary Assistance for Needy Families (TANF, formerly known as Aid to Families with Dependent Children [AFDC]) should be determined (see Chapters 33 and 36). Such resources are important in planning interventions (see Chapter 35).

Physical Examination

A careful and thorough physical examination should be performed including vital signs and accurate anthropometric measurements (see Chapter 10). Frank and Drotar (1994) identified three goals of the physical examination for children who experience growth deficiency: 1) identification of chronic disease, 2) recognition of potentially growth-retarding syndromes, and 3) documentation of the effects of malnutrition.

Minor dysmorphic features may suggest syndromes that are associated with growth delay, such as fetal alcohol syndrome (see Chapter 18) and Russell-Silver syndrome (see Chapter 14). Short stature may be constitutional, a result of chronic malnutrition or a result of hormone or thyroid deficiencies. Skin findings may be related: scaling in zinc deficiency, rough or hard skin in hypothyroidism, edema in protein deficiency, spoon-shaped nails in iron deficiency (DeGowin & DeGowin, 1976), and **cheilosis** in vitamin deficiencies. Congenital heart disease, renal and endocrine disorders, and malignancy should be ruled out. Oral etiology that could affect eating (e.g., enlarged tongue, dental caries and abscesses, submucous cleft palate, cranial nerve dysfunction resulting in difficulty swallowing) should be evaluated. Large tonsils, with a history of snoring and recurrent otitis media or sinusitis, may indicate tonsillar-adenoidal hypertrophy that can cause growth deficiency via mechanical feeding difficulties (Frank & Drotar, 1994; see also Chapter 12). Abdominal pain can occur as lead levels rise (see Chapter 17). Neurological examination should look for cranial nerve and motor tract dysfunction. Children who experience growth deficiency are described as significantly more rigid or more **flaccid** than control children (Barbero & Shaheen, 1967). Hypertonicity and hyperreflexia can occur from undernutrition as well as cerebral palsy (Bithoney & Rathbun, 1983). Signs of abuse (e.g., unusual skin lesions, severe untreated diaper rash, fractures, burns, retinal hemorrhages) should be considered (Casey, 1992; Frank, Silva, & Needlman, 1993). Table 2 presents physical examination findings in growth deficiency that suggest further evaluation for underlying medical problems.

Parent–Child Interaction

Observation of the interaction between parent and child (see Chapter 7 and Appendixes B, C, D, and E at the end of the book) provides clues to the etiology of growth deficiency. An interactional assessment can be performed by the physician, social worker, primary nurse, clinic or visiting nurse, early intervention team, or others involved in the child's evaluation. Responsiveness to the child's cues, parental warmth and appropriateness with the child, and the child's responsiveness and seeking of interaction and support from the parent elucidate their relationship (Bithoney, Dubowitz, et al., 1992).

Valuable data are gathered by observing a feeding interaction either in the office or, ideally, during a home visit at family mealtime (see Chapter 4). Problems in the child,

Table 2.   Physical examination of infants and children with growth deficiency

	Abnormality	Considerations
Vital signs	Hypotension	Adrenal or thyroid insufficiency
	Hypertension	Renal disease
	Tachypnea/tachycardia	Increased metabolic demands
Skin	Pallor	Anemia
	Poor hygiene	Neglect
	Ecchymoses	Abuse
	Candidiasis	Immunodeficiency
	Eczema	Allergic disease
	Erythema nodosum	Ulcerative colitis; vasculitis
HEENT	Hair loss	Stress
	Chronic otitis media	Immunodeficiency; structural orofacial defect
	Cataracts	Congenital infections; galactosemia
	Papilledema	Increased intracranial pressure
	Uveitis	Vasculitis
	Aphthous stomatitis	Crohn's disease
	Delayed tooth eruption	Delayed bone age
	Milk bottle caries	Neglect
	Thyroid enlargement	Thyroid disease
Chest	Wheezes	Asthma; cystic fibrosis
Cardiovascular	Murmur	Congenital malformations
Abdomen	Distention, hyperactive bowel sounds	Malabsorption
Genitourinary	Hepatosplenomegaly	Liver disease; glycogen storage; tumor
	Anomalies	Associated endocrinopathies
	Diaper rash	Diarrhea; neglect
Rectum	Fistulas	Crohn's disease
	Empty ampulla	Hirschsprung's disease
Extremities	Edema	Hypoalbuminemia
	Loss of muscle mass	Chronic malnutrition
	Clubbing	Chronic lung disease
Nervous system	Abnormal deep tendon reflexes	Cerebral palsy
	Developmental delay	Altered caloric intake or requirements
	Cranial nerve palsy	Dysphagia
Behavior and temperament	Uncooperative	Difficult to feed

From Duggan, C. (1997). Failure to thrive: Malnutrition in the pediatric outpatient setting. In W.A. Walker & J.B. Watkins (Eds.), *Nutrition in pediatrics: Basic science and clinical applications* (p. 712). Hamilton, Ontario, Canada: B.C. Decker; reprinted by permission.

parent, or environment that contribute to poor caloric intake can be identified. Videotaping is a valuable tool for clinical assessment and intervention. It can be used to diagnose specific feeding disorders, such as infant **rumination,** poor suck, forced or inadequate feeding techniques, oppositional feeding patterns, environmental distractions, and distractibility in the child (see Chapter 27). In addition, videotaping can be used to share information with other professionals who are caring for the child, especially team members in a multidisciplinary setting, and with families as a nonjudgmental intervention. Although many centers do not use videotaping routinely, it can be a useful adjunct in the diagnosis and management of growth deficiency (see Chapter 8).

Use of the Laboratory and Other Tests

In many instances, the yield of comprehensive laboratory testing in children who experience growth deficiency is small. The differential diagnosis of growth deficiency is lengthy and can lead to excessive diagnostic testing (Duggan, 1997). Sills (1978), in a study of 185 children who experienced growth deficiency and who had 2,607 laboratory tests, found that only 0.4% of the tests established the diagnosis and that 1% provided useful information. Berwick, Levy, and Kleinerman (1982) found that 0.8% of 4,880 laboratory tests of 122 infants identified the etiology of growth deficiency; however, frugal use of baseline screening tests may be justified, leaving other tests to be used only when indicated by the history or physical examination. Suggested laboratory evaluation is outlined in Table 3. Various investigators (Bithoney & Rathbun, 1983; Cupoli, Hallock, & Barness, 1980; Rathbun & Peterson, 1987) have recommended a minimal initial evaluation consisting of hemoglobin or hematocrit, urinalysis (including specific gravity and pH), and urine culture. Lead and PPD (tuberculosis screening) are recommended in epidemiologically at-risk populations. Cystic fibrosis is the most common genetic disease in the Caucasian population and may be seen more frequently in children who present with malnutrition (W. Bithoney, personal communication, May 1997). A sweat test should be considered in this group, particularly for children who exhibit additional symptoms that are associated with cystic fibrosis (e.g., chronic respiratory or gastrointestinal symptoms).

Iron deficiency and lead toxicity decrease appetite and impair growth (see Chapter 17). Serum ferritin should be considered as hemoglobin and hematocrit are late indicators of depleted iron stores. Sixteen percent of children who experienced growth deficiency in Boston, Massachusetts, had lead levels that were high enough to require chelation therapy, and lead absorption appears to increase in malnourished and calcium-deficient children (Bithoney, 1986). Growth deficiency may result in increased lead absorption; and increased lead levels, malnutrition, and iron deficiency contribute to developmental disabilities that are associated with growth deficiency (Bithoney, 1986). Urinalysis and urine culture detect occult infection or renal tubular acidosis that can cause growth deficiency. Zinc deficiency suppresses growth and affects taste bud function (see Chapter 6). Empirical treatment of zinc deficiency is recommended regardless of whether zinc levels are measured (Frank & Drotar, 1994). If there is a history of blood transfusion or high-risk parental behavior, then human immunodeficiency virus (HIV) testing as well as screening for hepatitis B and C should be considered. If malabsorption is suspected, then stool can be evaluated for fat and reducing substances. Giardia antigen is suggested in immigrant and homeless populations and for children in child care who have diarrhea or abdominal pain; giardiasis is a common cause of growth deficiency in these populations. Other tests, such as bone age to determine the presence of short stature versus constitutional delay and upper GI series or pH probe to evaluate for gastroesophageal reflux, can be conducted when indicated.

Table 3.   Laboratory and other evaluation in growth deficiency

	Test	Diagnostic considerations
General screening	Hematocrit, hemoglobin Consider ferritin[a]	Iron deficiency and lead toxicity impair appetite and growth
	Urinalysis (including specific gravity, pH)	Renal tubular acidosis
	Urine culture	Silent urinary tract infection
Selected populations	PPD with control[b]	TB, anergy[c]
	HIV screen (HBV and HCV)[b] Whole blood lead[b]	Maternal HIV, high-risk behavior or blood transfusion
When specifically indicated	Serum electrolytes BUN, creatinine[c]	Abnormalities seen in vomiting, diarrhea, severe malnutrition, renal pathology
	Stool fat, reducing substances, vitamin A	Malabsorption
	Stool for ova and parasites, Giardia antigen, occult blood	Giardia or other parasites, infection
	Sweat test[b,c,d]	Cystic fibrosis
	Immunoglobulins, serology	Frequent infections caused by immune deficiency
	Alkaline phosphatase, calcium, phosphorus	Alkaline phosphatase is decreased in zinc deficiency, increased in rickets; phosphorus is increased in rickets
	Serum zinc[e]	Zinc deficiency suppresses growth
	Thyroid function tests	Decreased height velocity caused by hypothyroidism
	Blood glucose	Diabetes
	Serum albumin, prealbumin[c]	Severe malnutrition
	Upper GI series, pH probe	Spitting, vomiting seen in gastroesophageal reflux
	Lateral neck X ray	Adenoid hypertrophy

Adapted from Kessler (1997).

[a]Ferritin is an early indicator of depleted iron stores; hemoglobin and hematocrit are relatively late indicators.

[b]Recommended in epidemiologically and environmentally at-risk populations.

[c]May be abnormal secondary to malnutrition.

[d]Transient elevations of sweat electrolytes have been seen with malnutrition and other conditions; genetic testing may be indicated.

[e]May treat empirically without testing.

Laboratory tests (e.g., albumin level, blood urea nitrogen [BUN], creatinine) also may be useful in assessing the degree of nutritional risk in more severe cases of malnutrition (Frank & Zeisel, 1988); however, albumin has a half-life of 20 days and, thus, may not be a useful marker of nutritional status. Prealbumin may be more useful because of its rapid synthesis in the liver; however, it is very sensitive to infection and inflammatory response (Benjamin, 1989; Forse & Shizgal, 1980). In the future, erythrocyte Na+-K+-ATPase

(ENKA) (an enzyme that is involved in basal energy requirements) may prove to be a good marker of subtle malnutrition as its activity correlates with incremental body-weight gain, and diminished energy intake decreases ENKA activity. ENKA is not widely available and is used only on a research basis (Maggioni & Lifshitz, 1995).

Laboratory abnormalities can result from malnutrition itself. Such abnormalities include transient elevations of sweat electrolytes and low levels of thyroid hormone, growth hormone, and somatomedin C. In one study (Bithoney, Epstein, & Kim, 1992), 8% of children who experienced nonorganic growth deficiency had laboratory results that were consistent with renal tubular acidosis (i.e., low serum bicarbonate), which resolved with adequate caloric intake. Anemia also has been shown to correct with nutritional treatment.

In summary, although laboratory testing in growth deficiency generally has a low yield, several screening tests are justified. Additional testing should be guided carefully by the history and physical examination.

MANAGEMENT OF GROWTH DEFICIENCY: THE ORGANIZATION OF CARE

Growth deficiency is a multifactorial, interactive process that involves medical, nutritional, behavioral, developmental, psychosocial, and environmental factors, all of which must be considered in management and long-term follow-up. An interactional–transactional model suggests that both the child and the environment determine a child's developmental outcome, each affecting and being affected by the other (Bithoney, Dubowitz, et al., 1992; Frank & Zeisel, 1988). In the parent–child interaction, the parent may misinterpret the infant's cues of hunger and the infant may begin to interact with irritability and anorexia. This two-way problem eventually results in nurturing and nutritional deficiencies. Given the complexity of growth deficiency, the physician's role extends beyond simply addressing medical issues. The physician or another professional can mobilize and coordinate a team of health professionals who together must ensure that the child and the family receive the interventions that are needed.

All children with clear or suspected growth deficiency warrant a thorough history and physical examination as described previously. The initial evaluation involves gathering comprehensive data and may require several visits (Bithoney, Dubowitz, et al., 1992).

Weight-for-age is the most commonly used index of growth deficiency and, when plotted on numerous occasions, remains the most convenient measure of a child's growth over time (Kessler, 1997); however, using weight-for-height and height-for-age allows the clinician to determine further whether a child is thin or merely short for age (see Chapter 10). Growth parameters can be expressed as a percentage of the median value (i.e., 50th percentile on the NCHS growth chart) for age. Using median values, malnutrition can be categorized as mild, moderate, or severe based on a staging scheme from the work of Gomez et al. (1956) and Waterlow (1972, 1975). Although many use such a staging system, one study demonstrated varying results depending on the indices used (Wright, Ashenburg, & Whitaker, 1994), and others have criticized its use based on statistical reasoning (see Chapter 2). Peterson and Chen (1990) suggested expressing anthropometric measures as z-scores or standard deviation (SD) scores, with the cutoff for undernutrition of -2 SD for weight-for-age, height-for-age, or weight-for-height. Further degrees of undernutrition can be expressed as additional multiples of SD (e.g., -2.5 SD, -3.0 SD, -3.5 SD, -4.0 SD). No uniform agreement exists as to which SD score might correspond to "mild" undernutrition. (For cutoff scores, see Chapter 2; for interpretation of weight-for-age, height-for-age, and weight-for-height, see Chapter 10.) Computer software that provides easy conversion to z-scores is available (see Chapter 2).

Although a question has been raised regarding the validity of the staging scheme of Gomez et al. (1956) and Waterlow (1972, 1975), a staging system for mild, moderate, and severe malnutrition (such as that presented in Table 4) can be used to guide treatment and determine who should be involved in a child's care. The criteria for severity that are used in the table have not yet been converted to SD scores. Management considerations for each stage are presented in Table 5. Specific management is individualized according to the child's and the family's needs and the severity of malnutrition. Bithoney, Dubowitz, et al. (1992) noted that management should address as many contributing factors as are feasible and that even partial solutions may improve a child's growth. For example, nutritional counseling and improving the parent–child interaction may help even when other problems remain unresolved.

Outpatient Management

Using NCHS growth charts routinely, the physician can identify growth faltering as it occurs and intervene early. Any underlying organic disease should be managed aggressively. Growth concerns also may be identified by other providers, such as a WIC dietitian, community health or visiting nurse, or health visitor.

Mild Malnutrition

Office-based interventions begin as soon as slowed weight gain is seen. These consist of addressing problems such as breast-feeding difficulties (Dermer, 1995), incorrect formula preparation, and underfeeding. Suggestions for increasing caloric intake, such as those presented in Table 6, should be provided (see Chapter 6). High-calorie food fortifiers are a mainstay of nutritional therapy as most children cannot sufficiently increase the volume of their intake. Formula can be concentrated gradually to 30 calories per ounce for infants who do not have renal disease. Further formula concentration should be avoided as diarrhea and dehydration can result. A multivitamin that includes iron and zinc is recommended to treat deficiencies that are associated with growth deficiency, to prevent these deficiencies during rapid growth, and to allow parents to focus on calorie rather than vitamin intake (Frank et al., 1993). Unusual dietary beliefs and cultural preferences that may limit caloric intake should be discussed (see Chapter 26).

Parental education regarding effective feeding methods should be provided. Physicians can intervene effectively in many feeding problems that involve behavioral issues, although behavioral consultation should be utilized for complex situations or for those that do not respond to initial interventions (see Chapter 8).

Poverty is a major contributor to malnutrition, and 12%–28% of children in the United States experience repeated food shortages (Wehler, Scott, Anderson, & Parker,

Table 4.   A staging system for classifying the severity of malnutrition

	Underweight Weight-for-age (% of median)	Wasting Weight-for-height (% of median)	Stunting Height-for-age (% of median)
Normal	>90	>90	>95
Mild	75–90	81–90	90–95
Moderate	60–74	70–80	85–89
Severe	<60	<70	<85

Adapted from Gomez et al. (1956) and Waterlow (1972).

Table 5. Management considerations for children with growth deficiency

Mild Malnutrition
- Provide breast-feeding information and support
- Ensure correct formula preparation for formula-fed infants
- Increase caloric intake
- Add multivitamins including iron and zinc
- Address unusual dietary beliefs
- Provide parent education regarding effective feeding methods
- Ask about availability of food
- Use community resources: La Leche League, WIC, TANF, school lunch program, food stamps, visiting nurses
- Consider referral to nutritionist who is experienced with malnutrition in children
- Consider referral to social worker for psychosocial assessment
- Monitor growth frequently

Moderate Malnutrition
- Conduct intensive investigation of medical, nutritional, and social factors
- Evaluate and treat underlying medical problems
- Convey supportive, nonjudgmental concern about child's growth
- Recommend nutritional consultation (nutritionist)
    1. Is caloric intake adequate?
    2. Observe feeding behaviors
- Consider sweat test and stool testing if malabsorption is suspected
- Consider further medical workup if intake adequate and still not growing
- Recommend psychosocial consultation (physician or social worker)
    1. Assess economic circumstances, food availability
    2. Identify family dysfunction
    3. Identify family supports, strengths
    4. Rule out abuse, neglect
- Consider additional interventions
    1. Conduct developmental assessment
        a. Referral for early intervention program or developmental intervention
        b. Behavioral assessment
        c. Cognitive assessment
        d. Speech, physical therapy, occupational therapy assessments as indicated
    2. Provide home supports: social services, visiting nurse, other services
    3. Provide mental health referral when indicated
    4. Monitor growth frequently
- Multidisciplinary team approach (ad hoc or specialized team)

Severe Malnutrition
- Hospitalization criteria
    1. Severe malnutrition
    2. Significant medical problems (e.g., dehydration)
    3. Failure of outpatient treatment
    4. Child abuse or neglect
    5. Significant psychosocial issues (e.g., parental psychosis, drug abuse)
- Referral to multidisciplinary team that specializes in growth deficiency
- Aggressive medical management

Table 6.   High-calorie food fortifiers

Nonfat dry milk—25 kcal/tablespoon
  Stir into potatoes, ground meats, cereals, pudding, and yogurt. Also use to fortify whole milk:
  8 ounces whole milk + 2–3 tablespoons dry milk = 24–26 kcal/ounce. Use only if renal status
  is normal.

Cheese—100 kcal/ounce
  Add melted cheese to a variety of dishes, including vegetables, casseroles, fish.

Sour cream—30 kcal/tablespoon
  Add to beans, squash, potatoes, gravies, casseroles, or salad dressing or use as a dip.

Heavy (whipping) cream—60 kcal/tablespoon
  Mix in gravies, add to casseroles, salad dressings, hot chocolate, cereal, potatoes, and eggs.

Butter, margarine, oil—40 kcal/teaspoon
  Add to gravies, mashed potatoes, cereal, rice, pasta, breads, muffins, and spaghetti sauce.

Peanut butter—100 kcal/tablespoon
  Spread on toast, bread, cookies, apples, bananas.

Instant breakfast preparation—130 kcal/packet

Increased formula concentration
  Example: 13 ounces infant formula concentrate with 10 ounces water = 24 kcal/ounce high-
  calorie formula. Use only if renal status is normal.

From Bithoney, W.G., Dubowitz, H., & Egan, H. (1992). Failure to thrive/growth deficiency. *Pediatrics in Review, 13,* p. 458; reprinted by permission of *Pediatrics in Review.*

1991). Nineteen percent of low-income families with at least one child who is younger than 12 years are hungry 1 month of the year or more (Wehler, Scott, Anderson, Summer, & Parker, 1995); hence, it is essential to ask about the availability of food. Community resources such as WIC, TANF, food stamps, and free school breakfasts and lunches should be facilitated for eligible families (see Chapters 33 and 37). La Leche League and other breast-feeding advocacy organizations can provide valuable support for breast-feeding mothers. The physician also should consider whether a referral to a nutritionist and/or a social worker is indicated.

Moderate Malnutrition

For children with moderate malnutrition and those who do not respond adequately to the management plan that was outlined previously, additional outpatient management strategies should be attempted. A more intensive evaluation of medical, nutritional, and social factors may be needed. Even when growth deficiency primarily is due to organic causes, it is pertinent to address nutritional and psychosocial issues. Frequent visits are recommended, and supportive, nonjudgmental concern about the child's growth should be conveyed.

Complex or difficult cases of moderate malnutrition necessitate the involvement of other health professionals, including a nutritionist and a social worker. The physician or another professional may coordinate this ad hoc team by acting as a liaison between the family and other professionals, integrating information with the medical assessment, and monitoring the child's progress.

Nutritional consultation can determine whether caloric intake actually is low or whether the child consumes adequate calories and does not grow. In the latter situation, malabsorption, decreased utilization of nutrients, or increased metabolic demands should be considered. A sweat test to rule out cystic fibrosis, tests for malabsorption, or gastroenterology consultation may be needed. Metabolic disorders should be considered if these evaluations are negative (Frank et al., 1993).

For children with inadequate caloric intake, 1½–2 times the recommended dietary allowance (RDA) requirements of calories and protein is needed for catch-up growth (Frank & Zeisel, 1988; see also Chapter 6). Nutritional recommendations should be given with close follow-up until normal growth is regained. Medical and psychosocial etiologies must be investigated. Medical etiologies of growth deficiency are numerous. Causes that may be missed include giardia or other parasites, chronic urinary tract infections, sinusitis, adenoid hypertrophy, gastroesophageal reflux, oral-motor dysfunction, lead toxicity, iron or zinc deficiency, celiac disease, malabsorption, and chronic constipation (Frank et al., 1993). In one study (Bithoney et al., 1989), giardiasis was the most common organic cause of growth deficiency.

Psychosocial issues are associated with most instances of inadequate caloric intake, and a thorough psychosocial assessment guides optimum management. Such assessment can occur in extended pediatric visits, depending on the physician's skills and interest, or by a social worker. Psychosocial history reveals relevant information that is related to parent–child interaction, economic circumstances, family stresses, family dysfunction, social supports and isolation, child abuse, parental substance abuse, and domestic violence. Traumatic childhood experiences and unresolved issues—"ghosts in the nursery" (Fraiberg, Adelson, & Shapiro, 1975)—may impair a parent's ability to nurture or to see and respond to a child's needs (see Chapter 30). In addition, children who experience growth deficiency often show temperament and behavior problems including significantly higher reactivity and distractibility to extraneous stimuli, organically determined irritability, temperament disturbances, and altered feeding interactions (Bithoney & Newberger, 1987). Such factors may affect the parent–child interaction and encompass the feeding situation. The small, temperamentally difficult child also can be at high risk for abuse and neglect. These issues indicate the need for behavioral, interactional, and psychosocial interventions. Referral to a mental health professional and a parents' group may be indicated. The use of a behavioral pediatrician, behavioral psychologist, or other interaction expert can be helpful.

Additional consultations and interventions should be considered and may be coordinated by the physician or other professional. Long-term malnutrition in the first 2 years of life affects brain growth and, subsequently, impairs cognition, behavior, and development (see Chapter 3). Hence, developmental assessment (e.g., Bayley Scales of Infant Development [Bayley, 1993], Denver II [Frankenburg, Dodds, Archer, Shapiro, & Bresnick, 1992]), cognitive evaluation, behavioral assessment, speech-language assessment, and occupational and physical therapy evaluations should be obtained as needed. Referral of the child younger than 3 years to early intervention programs and the older child for developmental intervention (sometimes available in preschools and special education programs) should be considered for all children who experience growth deficiency.

The use of home-based interventions by visiting nurses, outreach workers, and home visitors who are trained to deal with stressed families and provide support has been promising. A randomized clinical trial (Black, Dubowitz, Hutcheson, Berenson-Howard, & Starr, 1995) studied 130 children who were younger than 25 months, experienced nonorganic growth deficiency, and received services in a multidisciplinary growth and nutrition clinic. The children who received additional home intervention (e.g., weekly home visits for 1 year by lay home visitors) showed better receptive language over time and more child-oriented home environments (see Chapter 28). Regular services of a homemaker or health visitor provide valuable support for certain families. Klein (1990) noted that home health nurse clinicians not only implement strategies that promote effective parenting but also can locate children with growth deficiency in a manner that is community based and less reliant on the parent for initiation of services.

Severe Malnutrition

Severe malnutrition results in complications such as iron and zinc deficiencies, which can impair growth, and increased lead absorption, which can lead to abdominal pain and anorexia. The immune system is affected (e.g., decreased T-cell function, secretory IgA and complement [components involved in protection against disease]), which may lead to recurrent gastrointestinal or respiratory infections, each of which raises caloric needs and lowers intake. Children who experience severe growth deficiency need intensive medical management including early antibiotic use, annual influenza vaccination, and lactose-free formulas rather than clear liquids for diarrhea (Frank et al., 1993).

Severely malnourished children may be served best by a multidisciplinary team that specializes in growth deficiency. Such teams can also be used for moderately malnourished children. Bithoney et al. (1991) found that multidisciplinary team intervention results in better weight gain than care in a hospital-based primary care clinic. Many university-affiliated and tertiary medical centers have such growth and nutrition teams. These teams usually include a pediatrician, a nutritionist who specializes in treating childhood malnutrition, a social worker, a nurse, a developmental specialist, and sometimes a psychiatrist.

Care in the Hospital

The child who experiences severe malnutrition or mild or moderate malnutrition that does not respond to prolonged treatment may require hospitalization. Indications for hospitalization of the child who experiences growth deficiency include 1) severe malnutrition; 2) significant medical problems (e.g., dehydration); 3) failure of intensive outpatient treatment to achieve catch-up growth over several months; 4) evidence of child abuse or neglect; and 5) other psychosocial circumstances that preclude outpatient treatment, including parental psychosis or drug addiction, extremely problematical parent–child interactions (e.g., hostile or uncaring stance by parent toward child, serious hygiene neglect), or other threat to a child's safety and well-being. Despite health care economic constraints, these children warrant hospital care (see Chapter 20).

In the past, hospital care often was a routine part of the initial management of patients who experienced growth deficiency. Between 1% and 5% of all admissions to pediatric university-affiliated hospitals were for diagnostic workup of growth deficiency (Berwick, 1980; Shaheen, Alexander, Truskowsky, & Barbero, 1968). Although prolonged hospitalizations have been used for intervention (Fryer, 1988; Singer, 1987), a more recent trend has been aggressive outpatient management (Casey, Wortham, & Nelson, 1984; Schmitt & Mauro, 1989). For children who do not meet the criteria for hospitalization, outpatient treatment has the advantages of keeping child and family together as the intervention focus and working with them in their own environment, and it is less costly.

A disadvantage of hospitalization is that hospitalized pediatric patients are themselves at risk for malnutrition (Rider et al., 1996). Hendricks et al. (1995) found that 25% of pediatric inpatients at a tertiary care hospital showed anthropometric or laboratory evidence of acute or chronic malnutrition (down from 50% documented in the same hospital in 1976). Children younger than 2 years of age had the highest rates of malnutrition. Changes in nursing shifts, separating the child from the family, and other distractions can undermine even well-planned feeding schedules. Hospitalization also places malnourished children at risk for hospital-acquired illnesses.

For the child and family who need hospitalization for growth deficiency, however, there are a number of advantages. Fryer (1988), in a meta-analysis of eight studies of children who were hospitalized for growth deficiency, found that hospitalization significantly enhanced the probability of sustained catch-up growth among children who experienced nonorganic growth deficiency. Hospitalization is useful diagnostically and therapeutically. It allows more in-depth observation of parent–child interactions, parenting skills, and the child's feeding ability and style. Refeeding occurs in a controlled and medically safe environment, minimizing cardiovascular or gastrointestinal complications. A nutrition plan can encompass more in-depth knowledge of a child's feeding behaviors, parent–child interaction, and parenting style. Formal referrals or follow-up for medical, nutritional, social work, behavioral, and developmental interventions can be carried out. Careful discharge planning and follow-up are necessary.

Aside from excluding the rare parent whose presence disrupts successful nutritional rehabilitation, parental involvement and presence during hospitalization are important. Most parents feel a sense of failure and will continue to care for the child after discharge. Parental involvement as part of the team promotes better follow-through after discharge and enhances parenting and nurturing skills.

THE MULTIDISCIPLINARY TEAM

The physician or another professional can assemble an effective team, as outlined in Table 7, including the physician, nutritionist, social worker, developmental specialist, behavior specialist, and psychologist or psychiatrist as needed. Visiting nurses, outreach workers, and home visitors who are trained to build relationships with isolated and stressed families can be important members of the team. Close coordination is important as are close monitoring and follow-up, which may last months or years. Long-term treatment of growth deficiency frequently involves ongoing nutritional counseling, developmental and psychosocial interventions, parent–infant therapy, close pediatric monitoring, and coordination of services.

Although physicians or other professionals may form ad hoc teams from available resources, referral to existing multidisciplinary growth deficiency teams also can occur. For children who experience severe malnutrition, a team that specializes in growth deficiency may be best situated to provide the necessary services. Bithoney et al. (1989) studied 86 children who experienced growth deficiency and found that a team intervention—consisting of medical diagnosis and treatment, psychosocial evaluation and referral, and individualized dietary therapy with concentrated calories—resulted in excellent weight gain regardless of etiology.

In a subsequent study, Bithoney et al. (1991) found that children who experienced growth deficiency that was treated by a multidisciplinary team had improved weight gain compared with those who were treated in a hospital-based primary care clinic. Children who attended the primary care clinic often were not seen by a nutritionist, and they received significantly fewer home visits, outreach services, and referrals to federal food assistance programs. Children who were treated by the multidisciplinary team had a service coordinator, who ensured follow-up, and a nutritionist, and most were referred for developmental stimulation. Social workers and a child psychiatrist dealt with issues such as abuse, neglect, and maternal depression as well as housing and federal food program services. Visiting nurse referrals and homemaker services were used as needed. With the intensive services that were provided by the multidisciplinary team, it is not surprising that the weight gain of these children was superior to that of those who were treated in a hospital-based primary care clinic.

The use of a multidisciplinary team in the hospital promotes rapid correction of undernutrition in children who experience growth deficiency. MacPhee, Mori, and Gold-

Table 7. Multidisciplinary management of growth deficiency

Resources[a]	Assessment/management
Child and family	Involvement in assessment and treatment; participatory decision making when appropriate
Physician	Medical diagnosis and management; nutrition history; social assessment; interactional observations; feeding observation and intervention; close pediatric follow-up; may coordinate ad hoc multidisciplinary team; monitor growth
Nutritionist	Nutrition history; dietary assessment; age-appropriate feeding strategies; feeding observations; nutrition counseling
Social worker	Psychosocial assessment and intervention; evaluate parent–child interaction; feeding observations; assess economic circumstances; identify family stresses, strengths, supports, dysfunction; rule out active abuse and neglect; behavioral observation; outreach; locate community and federal resources
Developmental specialists (e.g., pediatrician, psychologist, physical therapist, occupational therapist, speech-language pathologist)	Developmental evaluation including cognitive and behavioral assessments; speech, physical therapy, and occupational therapy evaluations as needed; diagnose and treat developmental and behavior problems; refer to early intervention or infant stimulation programs; developmental intervention
Speech-language pathologist, occupational therapist	Evaluate feeding; rule out oral-motor problems; provide intervention (see Chapter 23)
Nurse practitioner	Medical assessment; feeding and interactional evaluation; nutrition history; social assessment; home visiting; weight checks and follow-up
Child psychiatrist, psychologist, clinical social worker	Treat psychological and behavior problems
Visiting nurses, outreach workers, home visitors	Home-based interventions; family support; parenting skills teaching; case-finding

[a]Team members learn from each other, exchange information and knowledge, and share roles. Who participates in a child's care will depend on the stage of malnutrition and the individual child's and family's situation and needs.

son (1994) described the successful use of an inpatient multidisciplinary team approach and management protocol for the diagnosis and treatment of growth deficiency in a children's hospital. Average length of stay was reduced from 7 days to 4 days. A "team fee" was charged, rather than individual consultation fees, to keep costs down.

Bithoney et al.'s (1991) study points to the need for a "whole child" and "whole family" approach that addresses the various problems that are associated with this complex syndrome. Where a specialized multidisciplinary team is not available and for mildly and moderately malnourished children, the physician or other professional can identify a skilled nutritionist, social worker, and psychologist or psychiatrist in the community to assist in working with these children and their families. The use of visiting nurses and home intervention services also is helpful. In some instances, public health nursing is central to the team. In two local health departments in Colorado, public health nurses work closely with dietitians to provide care to undernourished children and their families. Treatment occurs in the clinic and at home. In one project, home-based services include parent–infant psychotherapy (P. Dawson, personal communication, June 1997).

Frequent communication between caregivers and periodic team meetings increase the effectiveness of treatment (see Chapter 22). There are several models of team work. The multidisciplinary model includes professionals from varied disciplines who function independently, generally at the discretion of the team leader, who usually is a physician in a medical setting or a psychologist or a team coordinator in an educational and early intervention setting (Foley, 1990). In the interdisciplinary model, various professionals make their individual assessments. A more formal structure exists for team communication, and a joint service plan usually is developed (see Chapter 22). Using a transdisciplinary model (Hutchinson, 1978; see also Chapter 1), team members—including the family—may share roles, learn from each other, and exchange information, knowledge, and skills. Crossing traditional disciplinary boundaries may occur, such as early childhood interventionists utilizing a variety of skills.

Finally, it is important to involve the child's parents or other caregivers as a part of the team. Family members should participate in decision making and early intervention. Such involvement decreases their feelings of failure with their child, encourages their involvement and participation, and improves their cooperation with treatment. Continuity of care is important, as are reminders and follow-up for missed appointments. Providing written advice and educational material also is useful.

OTHER SYSTEMS OF CARE

The majority of children who experience growth deficiency have not experienced physical abuse or intentional neglect (Ayoub & Milner, 1985); however, of those children hospitalized for growth deficiency, approximately 10% will experience nonaccidental trauma (Bithoney & Rathbun, 1983; Goldson, Cadol, Fitch, & Umlauf, 1976; Oates & Yu, 1971). If interventions and supports fail and it becomes clear that parents are the major factor in poor growth, then child protective services should be involved (see Chapter 31). If there is no immediate medical, physical, or emotional danger, then placing a child in child care may be preferable to foster care or hospitalization because the parent can retain some responsibility for the child's care and not be excluded from the treatment (Weston et al., 1993).

Professionals working with children who are experiencing growth deficiency can serve in advocacy roles (see Chapter 36). Advocacy includes promoting early identification of these children, prevention by building cooperative relationships with community organizations (e.g., WIC, child care, early intervention programs, child protective services), and political advocacy for food assistance programs and housing subsidies.

CONCLUDING COMMENTS

Growth deficiency in the infant and the child presents a diagnostic and management challenge. It affects many aspects of child development. More often than not without a clear medical etiology, growth deficiency is associated with feeding problems, behavior and interactional difficulties, developmental delay, and cognitive impairments. Complex psychosocial problems often are present, and disturbances in feeding may mirror other family relationship problems.

Given the multidimensional issues in growth deficiency, the physician must consider medical, developmental, and psychosocial issues. Following a comprehensive medical assessment, management can range from intervention during well-child pediatric visits to consultation with other specialists (an ad hoc team), referral to a specialized multidisciplinary team, or hospitalization. Early intervention and close follow-up can make significant differences in developmental and cognitive outcomes; hence, management of this population must be vigorous, comprehensive, and ongoing. Prognosis is hopeful when the medical, psychosocial, and nutritional needs of these children are met.

REFERENCES

Altemeier, W.A., O'Connor, S.M., Sherrod, K.B., & Vietze, P.M. (1985). Prospective study of antecedents for non-organic failure to thrive. *Journal of Pediatrics, 106,* 360–365.

Ayoub, C.C., & Milner, J.S. (1985). Failure to thrive: Parental indicators, types, and outcomes. *Child Abuse and Neglect, 9,* 491–495.

Barbero, G.J., & Shaheen, E. (1967). Environmental failure-to-thrive: A clinical review. *Journal of Pediatrics, 71,* 639.

Bayley, N. (1993). *Bayley Scales of Infant Development* (2nd ed.). San Antonio, TX: The Psychological Corporation.

Benjamin, D.R. (1989). Laboratory tests and nutritional assessment: Protein-energy status. *Pediatric Clinics of North America, 35,* 139–161.

Berwick, D.M. (1980). Nonorganic failure to thrive. *Pediatrics in Review, 1,* 265–270.

Berwick, D.M., Levy, J.C., & Kleinerman, R. (1982). Failure to thrive: Diagnostic yield of hospitalization. *Archives of Diseases of Children, 57,* 347–351.

Bithoney, W.G. (1986). Elevated lead levels in children with nonorganic failure to thrive. *Pediatrics, 78,* 891–895.

Bithoney, W.G., Dubowitz, H., & Egan, H. (1992). Failure to thrive/growth deficiency. *Pediatrics in Review, 13,* 453–459.

Bithoney, W.G., Epstein, D., & Kim, M. (1992). Decreased serum bicarbonate as a manifestation of undernutrition secondary to nonorganic failure-to-thrive. *Journal of Developmental and Behavioral Pediatrics, 13,* 278–280.

Bithoney, W.G., McJunkin, J., Michalek, J., Egan, H., Snyder, J., & Munier, A. (1989). Prospective evaluation of weight gain in both nonorganic and organic failure-to-thrive children: An outpatient trial of a multidisciplinary team intervention strategy. *Journal of Developmental and Behavioral Pediatrics, 10,* 27–31.

Bithoney, W.G., McJunkin, J., Michalek, J., Snyder, J., Egan, H., & Epstein, D. (1991). The effect of a multidisciplinary team approach on weight gain in nonorganic failure-to-thrive children. *Journal of Developmental and Behavioral Pediatrics, 12,* 254–258.

Bithoney, W.G., & Newberger, E.H. (1987). Child and family attributes of failure-to-thrive. *Journal of Developmental and Behavioral Pediatrics, 8,* 32–36.

Bithoney, W.G., & Rathbun, J.M. (1983). Failure to thrive. In M.D. Levine, & A.C. Crocker (Eds.), *Developmental-behavioral pediatrics* (pp. 557–572). Philadelphia: W.B. Saunders.

Black, M.M., Dubowitz, H., Hutcheson, J., Berenson-Howard, J., & Starr, R.H. (1995). A randomized clinical trial of home intervention for children with failure to thrive. *Pediatrics, 95,* 807–814.

Casey, P.H. (1989). The family system and failure to thrive. In C.N. Ramsey (Ed.), *Family systems in medicine* (pp. 348–358). New York: Guilford Press.

Casey, P.H. (1992). Failure to thrive. In M.D. Levine, W.B. Carey, & A.C. Crocker (Eds.), *Developmental-behavioral pediatrics* (2nd ed., pp. 375–383). Philadelphia: W.B. Saunders.

Casey, P.H., Wortham, B., & Nelson, J.Y. (1984). Management of children with failure to thrive in a rural ambulatory setting: Epidemiology and growth outcomes. *Clinical Pediatrics, 23,* 325–330.

Cupoli, J.M., Hallock, J.A., & Barness, L.A. (1980). Failure to thrive. *Current Problems in Pediatrics, 10,* 1–43.

DeGowin, E.L., & DeGowin, R.L. (1976). *Bedside diagnostic examination* (3rd ed.). New York: Macmillan.

Dermer, A. (1995). Overcoming medical and social barriers to breastfeeding. *American Family Physician, 51,* 755–763.

Duggan, C. (1997). Failure to thrive: Malnutrition in the pediatric outpatient setting. In W.A. Walker & J.B. Watkins (Eds.), *Nutrition in pediatrics* (2nd ed., pp. 705–715). Hamilton, Ontario, Canada: B.C. Decker.

Foley, G. (1990). Portrait of the arena evaluation: Assessment in the transdisciplinary approach. In B. Gibbs & D. Teti (Eds.), *Interdisciplinary assessment of infants: A guide for early intervention professionals* (pp. 271–286). Baltimore: Paul H. Brookes Publishing Co.

Forse, R.A., & Shizgal, H.M. (1980). Serum albumin and nutritional status. *Journal of Parenteral Enteral Nutrition, 4,* 450–454.

Fraiberg, S., Adelson, E., & Shapiro, V. (1975). Ghosts in the nursery. *Journal of the American Academy of Child Psychiatry, 14,* 387–422.

Frank, D.A., & Drotar, D. (1994). Failure to thrive. In R.M. Reece (Ed.), *Child abuse: Medical diagnosis and management* (pp. 298–324). Philadelphia: Lea & Febiger.

Frank, D.A., Silva, M., & Needlman, R. (1993). Failure to thrive: Mystery, myth, and method. *Contemporary Pediatrics, 10,* 114–133.

Frank, D., & Zeisel, S. (1988). Failure to thrive. *Pediatric Clinics of North America, 35,* 1187–1206.

Frankenburg, W.K., Dodds, J., Archer, P., Shapiro, H., & Bresnick, B. (1992). The Denver II: A major revision and restandardization of the Denver Developmental Screening Test. *Pediatrics, 89,* 91–97.

Fryer, G.E. (1988). The efficacy of hospitalization of nonorganic failure-to-thrive children: A meta-analysis. *Child Abuse and Neglect, 12,* 375–381.

Goldson, E., Cadol, R.V., Fitch, M.J., & Umlauf, H.J., Jr. (1976). Nonaccidental trauma and failure to thrive. *American Journal of Diseases of Children, 130,* 490–492.

Gomez, F., Galvan, R.R., Frenk, S., Muñoz, J.C., Chavez, R., & Vasquez, J. (1956). Mortality in second and third degree malnutrition. *Journal of Tropical Pediatrics, 2,* 77–83.

Hampton, D. (1993). Tackling feeding problems: A community-based approach. *Health Visitor, 66,* 407–408.

Hendricks, K., Duggan, C., Gallagher, L., Carlin, A., Richardson, D., Collier, S., Simpson, W., & Lo, C. (1995). Malnutrition in hospitalized pediatric patients. *Archives of Pediatric and Adolescent Medicine, 149,* 1118–1122.

Hutchinson, D.J. (1978). The transdisciplinary approach. In J.B. Curry & K.K. Peppe (Eds.), *Mental retardation: Nursing approaches to care* (pp. 65–74). St. Louis: C.V. Mosby.

Kessler, D.B. (1997). Medical evaluation of the poorly growing child. In W.G. Bithoney & J. Wright (Eds.), *Pediatric nutritional challenge: From undernutrition to overnutrition* (pp. 2–13). Columbus, OH: Abbott Laboratories, Ross Products Division.

Klein, M.J.A. (1990). The home health nurse clinician's role in the prevention of nonorganic failure to thrive. *Journal of Pediatric Nursing, 5,* 129–135.

Kleinman, R.E., Murphy, J.M., Little, M., Pagano, M., Wehler, C.A., Regal, K., & Jellinek, M.S. (1998). Hunger in children in the United States: Potential behavioral and emotional correlates [On-line]. *Pediatrics.* Available: http://www.pediatrics.org/cgi/content/full/101/1/e3

MacPhee, M., Mori, C., & Goldson, E. (1994). Change in the hospital setting: Adopting a team approach for nonorganic failure-to-thrive. *Journal of Pediatric Nursing, 9,* 218–225.

Maggioni, A., & Lifshitz, F. (1995). Nutritional management of failure to thrive. *Pediatric Clinics of North America, 42,* 791–810.

Meyers, J., Frank, D., Roos, N., Peterson, K., Casey, P., Cupples, L., & Levinson, S. (1995). Housing subsidies and pediatric undernutrition. *Archives of Pediatric and Adolescent Medicine, 149,* 1070–1084.

Mitchell, W.G., Gorrell, R.W., & Greenberg, R.A. (1980). Failure to thrive: A study in a primary care setting, epidemiology and follow-up. *Pediatrics, 65,* 971–977.

Oates, R.K., & Yu, J.S. (1971). Children with non-organic failure to thrive: A community problem. *Medical Journal of Australia, 2,* 199–203.

Peterson, K.E., & Chen, L.C. (1990). Defining undernutrition for public health purposes in the United States. *Journal of Nutrition, 120,* 933–942.

Rathbun, J.M., & Peterson, K.E. (1987). Nutrition in failure to thrive. In R.J. Grand, J.L. Sutphen, & W.H. Dietz (Eds.), *Pediatric nutrition: Theory and practice* (pp. 627–643). Boston: Butterworth-Heinemann.

Rider, E., Samuels, R., Wilson, K., & Homer, C. (1996). Physical growth, infant nutrition, breast-feeding, and general nutrition. *Current Opinion in Pediatrics, 8,* 293–297.

Schmitt, B.D., & Mauro, R.D. (1989). Nonorganic failure to thrive: An outpatient approach. *Child Abuse and Neglect, 13,* 235–248.

Schwartz, R., & Abegglen, J. (1996). Failure to thrive: An ambulatory approach. *Nurse Practitioner, 21,* 26–32.

Shaheen, E., Alexander, C., Truskowsky, M., & Barbero, G.J. (1968). Failure to thrive: A retrospective profile. *Clinical Pediatrics, 7,* 255–261.

Sills, R.H. (1978). Failure the thrive: The role of clinical and laboratory evaluation. *American Journal of Diseases of Children, 132,* 967–969.

Singer, L. (1987). Long term hospitalization of nonorganic failure to thrive infants: Patient characteristics and hospital course. *Journal of Developmental and Behavioral Pediatrics, 8,* 25–31.

U.S. Department of Health and Human Services. (1991). *Healthy people 2000.* Washington, DC: Author.

Waterlow, J.C. (1972). Classification and definition of protein-calorie malnutrition. *British Medical Journal, 3,* 566–569.

Waterlow, J.C. (1975). Some aspects of childhood malnutrition: Classification, long term effects, experimental analogies. *Australian and New Zealand Journal of Medicine, 5,* 87–96.

Wehler, C.A., Scott, R.I., Anderson, J.J., & Parker, L. (1991). *Community childhood hunger identification project: A survey of childhood hunger in the United States.* Washington, DC: Food Research and Action Center.

Wehler, C.A., Scott, R.I., Anderson, J.J., Summer, L., & Parker, L. (1995). *Community childhood hunger identification project: A survey of childhood hunger in the United States.* Washington, DC: Food Research and Action Center.

Weston, J.A., Colloton, M., Halsey, S., Covington, S., Gilbert, J., Sorrentino-Kelly, L., & Renoud, S.S. (1993). A legacy of violence in nonorganic failure to thrive. *Child Abuse and Neglect, 17,* 709–714.

Wilcox, W.D., Nieburg, P., & Miller, D.S. (1989). Failure to thrive: A continuing problem of definition. *Clinical Pediatrics, 28,* 391–394.

Witschi, J.C. (1990). Short-term dietary recall and recording methods. In W. Willet (Ed.), *Nutritional epidemiology* (pp. 52–68). New York: Oxford University Press.

Wright, J.A., Ashenburg, C.A., & Whitaker, R.C. (1994). Comparison of methods to categorize undernutrition in children. *Journal of Pediatrics, 124,* 944–946.

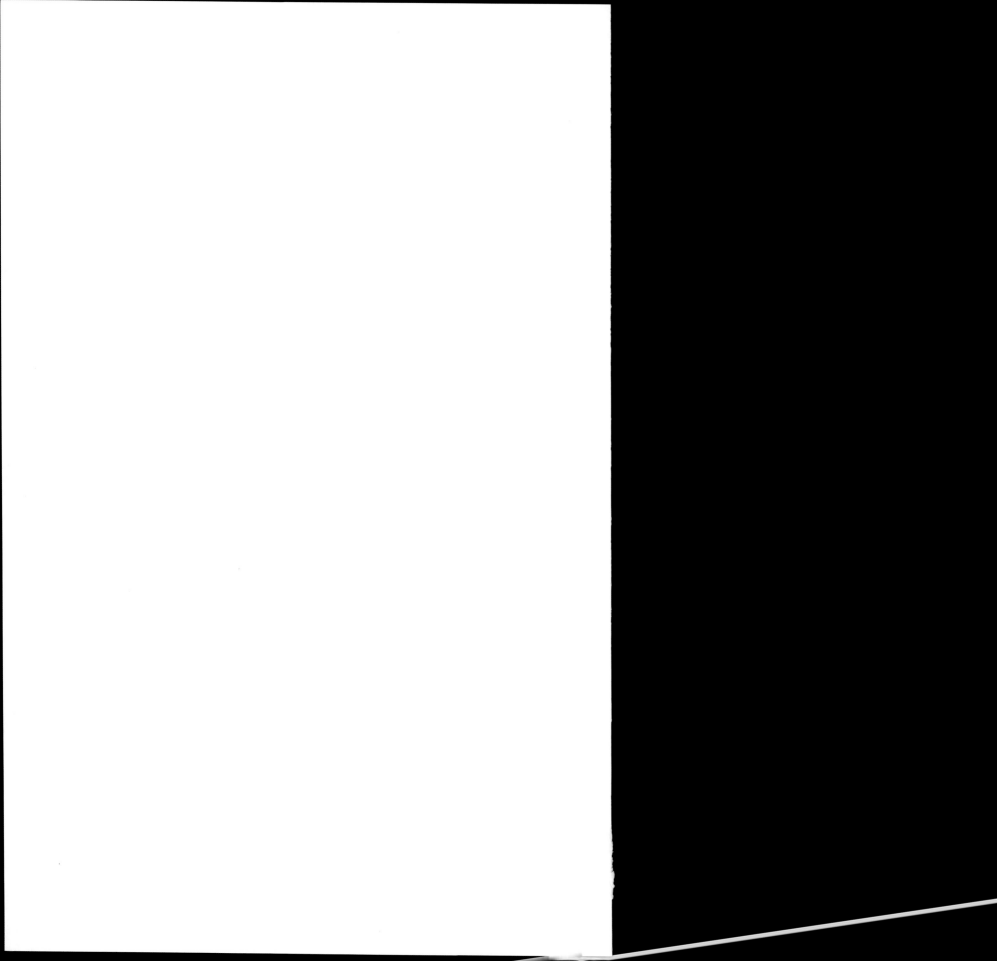

Chapter 10

Clinical Assessment of Growth

Rahel Berhane and William H. Dietz

Serial measurements of children's growth are central to the practice of preventive pediatrics. In most situations, information on attained size and the rate of growth is used as a proxy for nutritional status. Such anthropometric indicators offer an inexpensive and practical tool to identify individuals and populations at nutritional risk; however, proper care should be applied in the interpretation of anthropometric data to avoid making inaccurate conclusions. In this chapter, the various anthropometric indices that are used in the assessment of growth are discussed, with special emphasis on nonpathological conditions that may manifest as growth decelerations on the National Center for Health Statistics (NCHS) growth charts.

MEASUREMENT PROCEDURES

Assessment of growth is based on anthropometric measures; these must be performed accurately. A videotape that demonstrates measurement techniques from the National Health and Examination Survey (NHANES III) (U.S. Department of Health and Human Services, Public Health Service, 1996) is available from the U.S. Government Printing Office. These techniques also are described next.

Weight and Stature

Weight is the easiest anthropometric measure and can be performed with reasonable accuracy on calibrated scales. Infants should be weighed nude and children older than 2 years with light clothing only. For infants younger than 2 years or for older children who are unable to assume an upright posture, recumbent length should be measured. For children between ages 2 and 3 years, record whether the measurement was recumbent length or height. The 0- to 3-year chart should be used to plot measurements of length; the 2- to 19-year charts should be used for height. The measurement of recumbent length is made by placing the infant on a table that has a footboard and exerting gentle pressure at the knees (see Figure 1). The footboard then is brought into firm contact with the child's feet. *Both* feet should be brought against the footboard rather than stretching one leg of a squirming child. A final check on the proper alignment of the head and body should be made before the length measurement is recorded (American Academy of Pediatrics, 1993). Stature should be measured using a stadiometer—a device that is fixed to the wall and that has a ruler and a moveable headboard. The bare feet should be placed so that the heels are together and against the wall. The buttocks, shoulder blades, and back of the head should be in contact with the wall, and the gaze should be horizontal (American Academy of Pediatrics, 1993). Stature measurements often are difficult with children who have cerebral palsy because of the effects of contractures and scoliosis. Anthropometers to measure upper-arm length or lower-leg length as well as charts to interpret levels are available (Snyder, Schneider, Owings, Golomb, & Schork, 1977; Spender, Cronk, Charney, & Stallings, 1989).

Head Circumference

The head circumference is measured by passing a tape from the occipital prominence at the back of the head to the supraorbital ridges in front. Measurements should be taken twice and averaged. Head circumference is mostly affected by prenatal influences such as congenital infections, exposure to teratogens, and genetic factors. It may also be influenced by severe postnatal nutritional deprivation until the age of 36 months. It is widely believed that a fall in head circumference may follow falls in weight and height, although no studies are known to have been conducted.

Skinfold Thickness

Skinfold thickness measurements approximate total body fatness through their association with total subcutaneous fat. They provide an index of body energy stores and are helpful in the evaluation of undernutrition, especially in children with cerebral palsy and other congenital syndromes in which other, nonnutritional factors confound the interpretation of height and weight measurements. Norms are available based on data from the NCHS (Frisancho, 1974). The triceps skinfold is the most commonly used site.

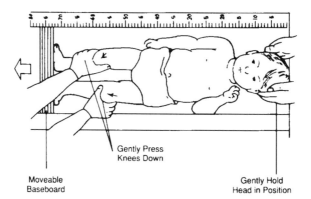

Figure 1.   Measuring an infant's length on a measuring board. (From Pinyerd, B.J. [1992]. Assessment of infant growth. *Journal of Pediatric Health Care, 6,* 305; reprinted by permission.)

Mid–Upper-Arm Circumference

Mid–upper-arm circumference (MUAC) measurement is affected by fat mass, muscle mass, and bone mass. In combination with the triceps skinfold, a calculation can be made to derive the mid-arm muscle circumference. The ease of measurement without need for special equipment made MUAC a popular index in field studies. In the late 1960s, simplified norms that related MUAC to stature were developed for use in crisis situations (Davis, 1971). The QUAC stick, named after the Quaker relief services that introduced it in Nigeria, consists of a measuring rod or board upon which values of arm circumference for specific stature are recorded. In clinical practice in the developed world, serial measurements of MUAC provide an additional index of body composition and can be helpful. Age- and gender-specific nomograms are available (American Academy of Pediatrics, Committee on Nutrition, 1998).

ANTHROPOMETRIC SCALES AND INDICES

Weight, stature, and head circumference are the three most commonly used measures in clinical anthropometry. Several anthropometric indices, such as weight-for-height, weight-for-age, and body mass index (BMI), are derived from these scales by evaluating the relationship of one measurement to another or to age.

Weight and Stature Scales

To assess nutritional status, the growth of a child or a study population is contrasted with anthropometric references. Interpretation of weight and height indices requires knowledge of standard scales for their expression and agreement on acceptable cutoffs. Weight-for-height, height-for-age, and weight-for-age can be described in terms of a percentile score, a standard deviation (SD) unit (z-score), or a percent of median value. In the United States, each scale compares a given measurement with that of a reference population in the NCHS database[1] (see Chapter 2). Percentile curves are used widely by clinicians because of their ease of interpretation; however, they are not helpful if one wishes to describe the extremes of the distributions (e.g., below the 5th percentile).

An easily understood method of describing children with significant degrees of growth delay is to calculate and compare weight-age and height-age (Goldbloom, 1987). The weight-age of a child is the child's age when the present weight is extrapolated horizontally to the 50th percentile on the growth chart. Height-age (and head circumference or head-age) is obtained in the same fashion. It should be remembered that the 50th percentile is not the ideal weight or height for every child. For instance, a healthy 12-year-old girl who is growing along the 5th percentile has a weight-age of 9.5 years but may be normal, especially if her weight has been following the curve, her height matches her weight, and her health and nutrition history is good.

Weight-for-Height Scales and Body Mass Index

Children's weight measurements are affected largely by children's height and do not provide a reliable measure of adiposity. Tall children weigh more for the same level of fatness. Children who are tall for age are classified as overweight, even when appropriately grown; children who are short for age are classified as underweight. To eliminate the height bias,

---

[1]Information about the revised growth charts will become available on the World Wide Web at http://www.cdc.gov/nchswww/

several weight-for-stature indices are available as indicators of body fat. The revised NCHS weight-for-length charts provide such data for children up to age 3 years. Although widely used by clinicians and nutritionists, weight-for-height remains a crude measure and should be used with other nutritional data to identify thin, tall children who are at nutritional risk and who otherwise would be missed if the weight-for-age charts alone were used.

The need for a measure of adiposity that adjusts body weight for individual differences in stature has led to the derivation of several indices of weight-for-height$^{(n)}$ where n is any number between 1 and 3. The most commonly used such index is the BMI, which is weight (kg)/[height (m)]^2. In adults, the BMI has been shown to be a useful measure for the comparison of body fatness when age- and gender-adjusted norms are used (Bray, 1987; Gallehger, 1996). The BMI also correlates significantly with total body fatness in adolescents (Deurenberg, Weststrate, & Seidell, 1991). The revised growth charts from the NCHS have BMI norms for children 2 years and older. BMI changes substantially with age, rising steeply in infancy, falling during the preschool years, and then rising again in adulthood. A study that evaluated the utility of BMI as a measure of body fatness in children and adolescents (Daniels, Khoury, & Morrison, 1997) suggested that maturational stage may be a better correlate of percentage of body fat than age. Thus, sexually mature adolescents have a lower body-fat percentage than do less sexually mature children for the same BMI. Gender, race, and body proportions (waist-to-hip ratio) were also shown to contribute to differences in body fatness for the same BMI. Thus, although the BMI offers a simple anthropometric measure of adiposity that is adjusted for stature, ideally, norms that adjust for maturational age, gender, race, and body proportion would be available to allow accurate comparisons across different groups.

Indices of Undernutrition: Stunting and Wasting

Waterlow (1974, 1994) suggested that the child who is underweight for height be described as *wasted* and that the child who is below normal height-for-age be described as *stunted.* It is widely believed that *wasting,* a deficit of weight relative to height, is a marker for an acute situation, indicating recent weight loss, whereas *stunting* is a marker of long-standing or chronic malnutrition. The association of wasting with an acute insult was supported by studies from developing countries that showed a very high correlation between low weight-for-age and a recent history of intercurrent illnesses (Graitcer, Gentry, Nichaman, & Lane, 1981; Kielmann & McCord, 1978).

The labeling of wasting and stunting as *acute* and *chronic* malnutrition, respectively, suggests that they are different presentations of the same phenomenon, varying only in terms of timing and intensity. If wasting and stunting had the same etiology, however, then one would expect to find a reasonable degree of correlation between the prevalences of the two conditions among children, within populations. Evaluation of a database collected by the World Health Organization (WHO) fails to show a consistent correlation. Countries with a high level of stunting do not necessarily have high levels of wasting (Victora, 1992). For instance, wasting was three times more prevalent in Africa than in Latin America for any given level of stunting. Clinical reports of Peruvian infants in a disadvantaged community showed marked stunting but minimal wasting and, paradoxically, a significant number of children who were overweight (with a high weight-for-height) (Trowbridge et al., 1987). Reports from the Middle East showed that Bedouin infants in the Negev desert, compared with Jewish infants from the same area, showed marked early stunting in the first few months of life with only minimal wasting (Dagan et al., 1983). These findings suggest that different risk factors may be involved in the pathogenesis of stunting and wasting with some possible overlap.

Acute weight loss in relation to intercurrent illnesses and decreased caloric intake is a common risk factor associated with wasting (Graitcer et al., 1981). Accelerated growth rates and remarkable catch-up are documented in response to aggressive nutritional rehabilitation in these children (Ashworth, 1969). The causes of stunting, however, appear to be less straightforward, and response to nutritional intervention programs is not demonstrated consistently (Golden, 1994). The reported lack of response may be related to the timing of the intervention (Huttly, Victora, Barros, Teixeira, & Vaughan, 1991) or to failure to address all of the negative factors that contributed to stunting. A major change in the child's physical environment through adoption and emigration often has been associated with definite catch-up growth, although often not to the NCHS standards (Schumacher, Pawson, & Kretchmer, 1987; Winick, Meyer, & Harris, 1975). Some of the risk factors for stunting identified in studies from developing countries include low socioeconomic status, low birth weight, and a short interval between births (Ricci & Becker, 1996; WHO Working Group, 1986). The mechanisms by which these environmental constraints cause stunting remain to be determined. The complex and multifactorial pathophysiology of stunting argues for a multifaceted intervention program, which, in addition to macro- and micronutrient supplementation, should include family planning and prenatal care to improve birth weight and increase birth intervals as well as efforts to improve the physical environment and decrease frequent infections.

Growth Faltering

In clinical situations in which the growth of individual children is monitored, a single measurement gives very little information on nutritional status. The common practice of defining undernutrition as growth below the 5th percentile is inappropriate and should be discouraged. Malnutrition in the individual patient should not be diagnosed on the basis of anthropometric measurements at a single point in time; rather, the focus should be on the growth pattern over time and the presence of a decrease in growth velocity or growth faltering. A declining growth velocity is a more helpful indicator than attained weight or height. In an extensive review of this subject, Beaton (1989) argued for a distinction between the *process of becoming small* and the *state of being small*. The former is an indicator of a dynamic process potentially amenable to intervention. The latter is a static measure and fails to distinguish the child who started out small and is growing at a normal rate from the child who has experienced growth arrest as a result of disease or adverse environmental conditions. In the clinical evaluation of children, a declining growth velocity can be noted visually as a decrease in the slope of the growth curve. Tabular data for growth increments at fixed intervals also are available (Guo et al., 1991; see Appendix F). The data are based on the Fels cohort that was the basis of the 1977 growth charts. Growth increments could be slightly different in the NHANES sample that is the basis of the revised charts.

In this context, serial monitoring of weight-for-age identifies growth faltering and is the most effective index to follow to identify acute changes. Growth faltering often may be the first and only marker of ill health in children and often triggers further evaluation to identify possible causes. In many cases, however, children may deviate from their earlier percentile positions without pathology. The questions often faced by many clinicians include the following: What is the point beyond which growth deceleration is considered abnormal and further evaluation is required? How does one distinguish physiological fluctuations in growth velocity from pathological growth faltering? In practice, there is no single cutoff point where divergence from a previous percentile becomes pathological. The clinician should exclude potential physiological and artifactual causes in every case by careful history. Diagnosing growth failure without due consideration of these factors provokes anxiety in the parents and tensions in the feeding interaction and may lead to growth failure where none existed previously.

Figure 2 depicts the growth trajectory of a child who is demonstrating a deceleration of growth (weight) at approximately 9 months of age. When an appropriate intervention is applied at 15 months of age, the child's weight gain (catch-up growth) is quickly apparent on the growth curves. The growth faltering and catch-up also are evident by looking at the weight-for-length curve, which shows a drop just below the 5th percentile at 9 months, although the deceleration is noticeable earlier.

Catch-Up Growth

Catch-up growth is a term that was coined by Prader, Tanner, and von Harnach (1963) to refer to the increased growth velocity that occurs during recovery from a growth-impairing influence such as malnutrition or disease. The mechanisms that enable humans and animals to modulate growth velocity in a predetermined channel are not understood fully. In animals, several factors appear to determine the extent of catch-up growth. These

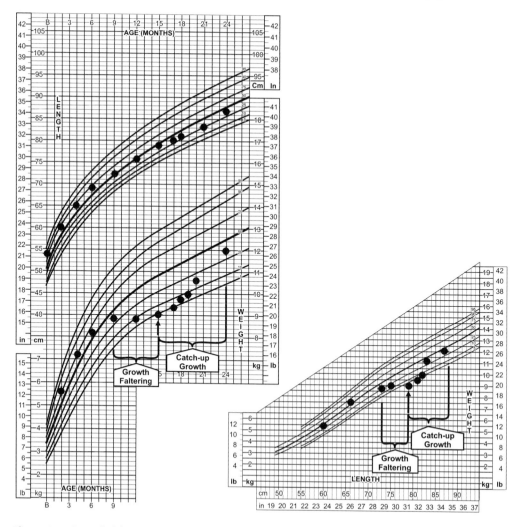

Figure 2.   Growth faltering and catch-up growth.

include the nature of the restricted diet, the severity of undernutrition, the stage of development at the onset of undernutrition, and the duration of undernutrition (Dietz, 1986). In a study of rural Guatemalan children, catch-up growth in undernourished children was most notable in younger children (6–24 months), in those who had more wasting, and in those who were provided nutritional supplementation for a long time (Rivera & Habicht, 1996). Studies of treatment responses of undernourished children have used varying definitions of catch-up growth, which has led to difficulties in comparison between studies. Some investigators defined catch-up growth as the attainment of growth beyond a predetermined threshold, such as weight-for-age above the 3rd percentile (Oates, Peacock, & Forrest, 1985) or weight-for-height greater than 90% of standard (Sturm & Drotar, 1989). Others have used velocity-based measures such as the Growth Quotient (GQ) (Bithoney, McJunkin, Michalek, Snyder, & Munier, 1989; Ellerstein & Ostrov, 1985). *GQ* is defined as observed weight gain in a given period of time divided by expected weight gain in the same period of time. The expected weight gain is the rate of mean weight gain that would result in a patient's paralleling the 5th percentile on the NCHS growth charts. Using a positive change in *z*-score has been suggested as a better velocity measure as it takes into account differing growth rates according to both age and gender (Walravens, 1985).

NONPATHOLOGICAL CONDITIONS THAT MANIFEST AS DECREASING GROWTH VELOCITY ON THE NCHS CHARTS

In clinical practice, a child's growth is serially plotted against the NCHS reference charts over time. Growth faltering warrants evaluation. It may represent undernutrition; however, it also may be due to normal genetic factors or to artifacts that are inherent in the growth charts. Some of the nonpathological causes of growth faltering are discussed next.

Shifting of Percentiles

Several investigators have observed that normal children often shift percentiles for both length and weight in the first 2 years of life (Berkley, Reed, & Valadian, 1983; Smith et al., 1976). Infants with weights at the top of the distribution in the first 3 months of life gradually drop down to percentiles closer to the mean; children at the bottom of the distribution increase. By the age of 1.5–2 years, the growth of most children has settled into a channel and further shifts are very uncommon. The shift in growth percentiles in healthy children in early life is most likely to be a shift toward the 50th percentile rather than away from it (a phenomenon known as *regression toward the mean*). The concept, when first described by Galton (1886), referred to observations in biology whereby tall fathers tended to have tall sons; however, although their sons were taller than average, they tended to be less extreme than their fathers (Galton, 1886; Healy & Goldstein, 1978). Whether regression to the mean is a manifestation of an underlying biological principle or simply a statistical artifact expressing an error function never has been resolved.

Many investigators believe that shifting percentiles in growth reflect a shift from a prenatal, maternally determined growth rate to one that is more genetically controlled (Smith et al., 1976). Regardless of the cause of the phenomenon, the relevant issue in clinical assessment of growth is how to distinguish growth decelerations that are due to a pathological process from normal shift-down of percentiles. Investigators have devised mathematical formulas that adjust for regression to the mean and calculate the predicted percentile or *z*-score for a child, given age, gender, and an earlier percentile position. Any diversion of growth from the predicted percentile thus implies pathological deviation (Berkley et al., 1983; Cameron, 1980; Wright, Mathews, Waterson, & Aynsley-Green,

1994). These mathematical adjustments, although useful for research purposes, are cumbersome and are not clinically helpful. As a general rule, however, in a child between 3 and 12 months who is shifting downward on the percentile curves, other aspects of the medical history including small frame in one of the parents and the absence of other risk factors for growth failure are reassuring and should allow for conservative observation. Similarly, decreasing growth velocity beyond the age at which physiological catch-down is known to occur should call for a more prompt evaluation to identify possible pathology. Low attained growth of an extreme degree (specifically, height more than 3 SD below the mean) also is often associated with pathology and deserves prompt evaluation (Lacey & Parkin, 1974). If a child is shifting downward, then his or her health and nutrition should be evaluated; if no problem is found and if the child is shifting from above the mean toward it, then shifting linear growth may provide reassurance.

Genetic Variation

Several twin and parent–child pair studies have found that the genotype plays a significant role in the determination of several anthropometric dimensions such as length, skeletal breadth, and frame size in the individual. Four common genetic variations are discussed for consideration in the clinical evaluation of children with decreasing growth percentiles.

Familial Short Stature

Children with familial short stature have a family history of short stature and grow at a normal rate. When evaluated in late childhood, these children do not pose diagnostic difficulties because the family history, the normal growth rate, and normal skeletal maturation serve to confirm the diagnosis. In the first 2 years of life as these children decrease their growth velocity and fall to a lower growth channel, parents should be reassured and the child should be monitored conservatively. Parent-specific standards for height that are age- and gender-specific have been developed for the Fels cohort (Himes, Roche, Thissen, & Moore, 1985; see Appendix F). Short parental stature should not be used as an explanation for a child's poor growth if the parents might be short because they experienced undernutrition in childhood—for example, if they grew up poor in a developing country.

Constitutional Leanness

A less-understood genetic factor is the contribution of skeletal breadth to the variation in anthropometric measurements. Although body weight is used universally as a measure of the adequacy of nutritional reserves, weight is a composite measure that is influenced by contributions from bone density, muscularity, and body proportions. Several studies in the anthropological literature have shown that differences in body physique between different tribes are apparent as early as the first few years of life (Eveleth & Tanner, 1976). In fact, differences in body proportions between children of African and European ancestry already are evident at birth (Eveleth, 1978). It is reasonable, therefore, to expect that a child of thin and tall parents will be thin and tall and have a low weight-for-height. Garn and LaVelle (1985), reviewing the family-line origins of lean body mass, suggested that *underweight* does not always mean *underfat*. Low fat mass usually is a direct measure of low energy reserves, whereas low lean body mass reflects several genetic, hormonal, and nutritional influences. In this context, weight-for-frame-size theoretically would provide a better index of nutritional status than weight-for-height.

The Metropolitan Life Insurance Company has published weight-for-frame-size norms for adults, which are used in the evaluation of relative adiposity (Faulkner & Bailey, 1989). Further studies of a large number of children at different ages are required to develop the normative data necessary to evaluate the different measures of frame size through the growth period. In the absence of such norms for children, the evaluation of lean and tall children requires information on parental physique and anthropometric measures, such as the triceps skinfold, to provide information on the adequacy of fat mass. In the absence of such norms, constitutional leanness remains a diagnosis of exclusion. The finding of a normal triceps skinfold, a history of lean physique in the parents, and the absence of any other pathology suggest the diagnosis. (Figure 3 shows the growth chart of a child who was born of lean and tall parents. Note that the child was very thin but that height velocity remained unaffected.)

Constitutional Delay of Maturation (Constitutional Growth Delay)

By 2 years of age, most children have settled into their respective percentiles and are likely to grow parallel to them until puberty. Some children grow substantially below the lower percentiles of growth during childhood, without faltering in weight or height. They may catch up in adolescence, even as late as 17–18 years of age (Lindgern, 1978). Such children may have constitutional delay of maturation or growth. This condition may be suspected if one or both parents experienced a late growth spurt in puberty; however, the distinction of constitutional delay of maturation from chronic undernutrition often is difficult. Evidence that suboptimum nutrition in early infancy may contribute to the course of constitutional delay in some children (Solanes & Lifshitz, 1992) suggests that some cases are due to undernutrition. A thorough evaluation of feeding and nutrition is required before this diagnosis can be made.

Racial Differences in Growth Potential

The WHO has recommended that the 1977 NCHS growth charts be used as an international growth reference. The recommendation is based on the premise that differences in growth in different racial groups largely are a result of environmental inadequacies rather than genetics. One study (Leung & Davies, 1994) compared the growth of a cohort of healthy, full-term Chinese infants in Hong Kong with the 1977 NCHS reference and found that although the calorie and protein intakes of the Chinese infants were well above that recommended by WHO, slightly lower rates of growth were found as early as 2–4 months of age. The Chinese infants continued to grow in the lower channel well into their second birthday. The possibility that these differences are genetic rather than environmental needs to be evaluated by future studies and, if substantiated, argues for specific growth charts for population groups with different growth patterns (Ulijaszek, 1994).

Measurement of Breast-Fed Infants

Several studies indeed have found that breast-fed infants follow a different growth trajectory than what the 1977 NCHS growth charts suggest (Ahn & MacLean, 1980; Dewey et al., 1995; Hitchcock, Gracey, & Owles, 1981; Rider, Samuels, Wilson, & Homer, 1996; Whitehead & Paul, 1984). A WHO working group reviewed the growth of infants who lived under favorable conditions and who were fed according to WHO feeding recommendations (WHO, 1994) (the WHO recommends exclusive breast-feeding from birth to 4–6 months of age, after which the child should continue to be breast-fed while receiving appropriate and adequate complementary foods for up to 2 years and beyond). The working group found significant decreases (0.6 SD) in weight-for-age and smaller decreases (0.3 SD) in length-for-age and weight-for-length in the breast-fed group compared with the NCHS group. WHO has recommended the construction of new standards, based on an international sample that is fed according to recommended rather than existing practices

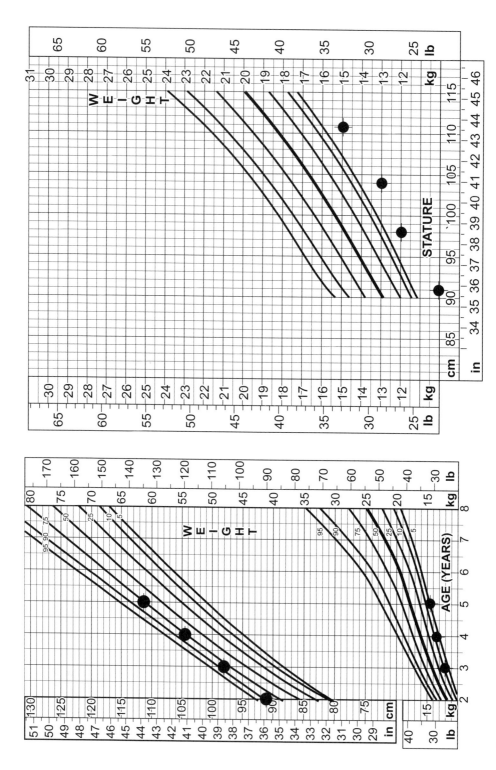

Figure 3. Constitutional leanness.

204

(de Onis, Garza, & Habicht, 1997). WHO has published growth charts for breast-fed infants in the first year of life (WHO Working Group on Infant Growth, 1994).

A comparison of the growth quartiles (25th, 50th, and 75th percentile lines) of infants who where breast-fed for at least 12 months with the 1977 NCHS/WHO reference growth charts (Figure 4) shows that breast-fed infants normally show a slower increase in weight than that indicated in the older reference standard. This is especially prominent in the 1977 weight-for-age curves between 3 and 12 months. The degree of deviation on the length and weight-for-length curves is not as great. For head circumference, the breast-fed group median tracks at about the 75th percentile of the NCHS reference for girls and at or slightly below the 75th percentile for boys (WHO, 1994).

Clinicians should not be alarmed when slight growth deceleration occurs in breast-fed infants beginning around 3–4 months of age if their health and feeding are good. The revised NCHS growth charts have a higher proportion of breast-fed infants than do the 1977 growth charts, which may ameliorate this problem.

Short Interval Between Measurements

The equations that describe the growth curves are statistical approximations. Fluctuations in the growth tempo that are shorter than the measurement intervals are not detected, and longer fluctuations may be lost in the process of curve smoothing. The curves assume that human growth is a continuous process. One report argued that human growth, like many other biological processes, is an intermittent process (Johnson, 1993; Lampl, Veldhuis, & Johnson, 1992). In one study, weekly measurement of normal infants during their first 21 months showed that growth in length occurs by discontinuous, intermittent spurts (Lampl et al., 1992). They found that 90%–95% of normal development during infancy is growth-free and that length accretion is a process of incremental bursts punctuating background stasis sometimes lasting up to 63 days. The findings of this study, if replicated by others, raise intriguing questions about the mechanisms of growth regulation.

Thus, measurement of older children at intervals of 1–2 months may reveal no-growth intervals in height and lead to an erroneous diagnosis of growth faltering. In a study in which 260 well-nourished children between ages 7 and 10 years were measured at intervals of 1 month over a period of 13 months, no measurable growth was observed in normal children for up to 3 months (Marshall, 1971). The study also showed that growth in most children was maximal in the period between March and July and slowest between September and January. The seasonality of growth could bias reference growth charts that are based on cross-sectional surveys if the surveys are performed only at certain times of the year.

The algorithm in Figure 5 is suggested as a guide to the evaluation of slow growth in children.

CLINICAL ASSESSMENT OF GROWTH IN ABNORMAL CHILDREN

The NCHS growth charts are based on measurements of healthy children in the various NHANES surveys. The use of these charts to assess nutritional risk in children who have underlying medical problems poses some difficulty. The nutritional assessment of children who have cerebral palsy or who had low birth weight are two examples of such scenarios and are discussed next.

Growth Assessment of Children with Cerebral Palsy

Children with cerebral palsy are at increased risk for growth problems (see Chapter 14). Reliable measures of weight and height often are impossible to obtain because of fixed

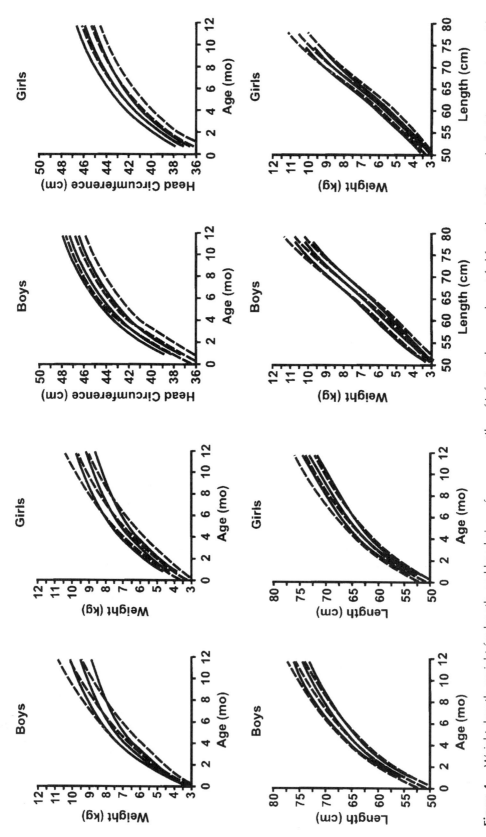

Figure 4. Weight, length, weight-for-length, and head circumference quartiles of infants who were breast-fed for at least 12 months (——) in comparison with the 1977 NCHS growth reference (– – –). (From World Health Organization Working Group on Infant Growth, Nutrition Unit. [1994]. *An evaluation of infant growth* [pp. 52–55]. Geneva, Switzerland: World Health Organization; reprinted by permission of Programme of Nutrition, World Health Organization.)

206

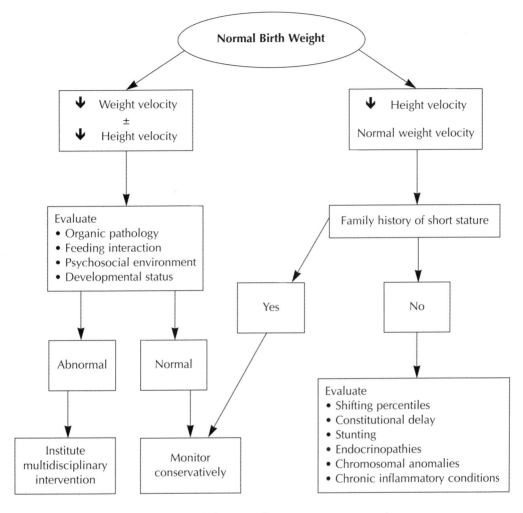

Figure 5.   Guide to the evaluation of slow growth.

joint contractures, scoliosis, involuntary muscle spasms, and poor cooperation in those with cognitive impairments. Anthropometers for segmental measurements such as upper-arm length (UAL) and lower-limb length (LLL) have been introduced (Spender et al., 1989). Age- and gender-specific reference data are available for UAL and LLL (Snyder et al., 1977).

Growth Assessment of Low Birth Weight Infants

The postnatal growth potential of low birth weight (LBW) infants (born at less than 2,500 grams) is a subject of great debate. Earlier studies on term, LBW infants showed that post-natal growth potential depended on body proportionality at birth (Davies, Platts, Pritchard, & Wilkerson, 1979; Holmes, Miller, Hassanien, Lansky, & Goggin, 1977). Infants whose weight was appropriate for length and head circumference (symmetric growth retardation) were believed to be less likely to show accelerated growth than those who were light for their length (asymmetric growth retardation). Extrapolating from animal studies and clinical observations, it was believed that symmetric growth retardation reflected insults that were operating earlier in gestation, thus affecting a critical period of growth during which growth potential is determined (Widdowson & McCance, 1960). Factors such as utero-placental insufficiency, which operates late in gestation, were believed to cause an isolated weight deficit (asymmetric growth retardation). Data from large LBW cohorts, however, do not support the theory that different causal mechanisms account for differences in body proportionality at birth. Instead, they show a continuous spectrum in the distribution of LBW infants. Asymmetric growth retardation was found to be a measure of the severity of growth failure and not necessarily an indicator of a causal mechanism operating at a particular stage of gestation (Kramer, McLean, Olivier, Willis, & Usher, 1989). There also are increasing clinical data from large longitudinal cohorts that suggest that LBW, especially intrauterine growth retardation, carries a limited growth potential irrespective of whether the growth deficit is symmetric or asymmetric (Strauss & Dietz, 1997).

LBW infants are a heterogeneous group that includes premature infants who have attained weights that are appropriate for their gestational age and infants who are small for their gestational age. For premature infants, growth percentile charts that are based on a large longitudinal cohort from the Infant Health and Development Program (IHDP) are available (see Appendix F). The data, collected in the 1980s, reflect the status of premature infants who receive modern neonatal care, and the charts should be used after infants reach term (40 weeks) instead of the Lubchenco charts (Lubchenco, Hansman, & Boyd, 1966), which are based on birth data collected from more than 5,000 Caucasian infants in Denver from 1948 to 1961. (IHDP growth charts for very low birth weight infants [less than 1,500 grams] are available from Ross Products Division, Abbott Laboratories.)

Infants who are born small for gestational age (SGA) frequently are below the 5th percentile, especially when they are born prematurely and are plotted on standard NCHS reference graphs without adjusting for prematurity. Even when the appropriate adjustments are made, they still may plot at or below the 5th percentile; however, if their growth rate is appropriate, then they will grow parallel to but below the standard curves. These children are not undernourished, and their growth should be considered appropriate. It is only when their growth rate decelerates and they demonstrate growth faltering that the possibility of undernutrition should be evaluated further. Figures 6a and 6b show the growth of two infants who were plotted on the IHDP growth curves for premature infants. Figure 6a shows the growth of an infant just below the 5th percentile. There is no growth faltering and no evidence of undernutrition; however, Figure 6b does demonstrate that growth is falling farther from the 5th percentile over time. This is an indication of growth faltering and undernutrition.

Appropriate nutrition of LBW infants is essential to ensure optimum postnatal growth and development; however, in infants with intrauterine growth retardation, failure of compensatory growth may suggest a limited growth potential and is unlikely to be reversed by aggressive nutritional intervention in the postnatal period. Although most causes of intrauterine growth retardation remain to be determined, some, such as chromosomal anomalies and fetal alcohol syndrome (FAS), have been well described (Fitzsimmons, Droste, Shepard, Pascon-Mason, & Fantel, 1990; Jones & Chernoff, 1978). Conditions such as hypothyroidism and celiac disease occur at increased frequency in children with trisomy 21 (Cutler, Benezra-Obeiter, & Brink, 1986; George et al., 1996). Decreasing growth velocity may be the only early manifestation of these conditions and should be evaluated carefully. Similarly, clinical evaluation of growth failure in children with FAS often is difficult because environmental or psychosocial factors also may contribute to growth failure. Serial monitoring of growth velocity and subcutaneous fat reserves with appropriate multi-

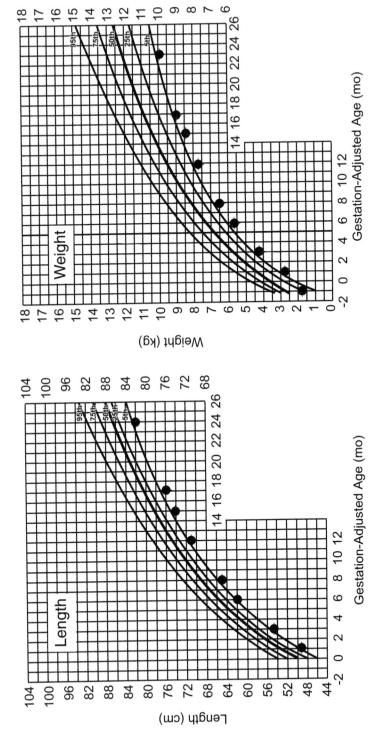

Figure 6a. Small-for-gestational-age infant who is growing along the 5th percentile.

209

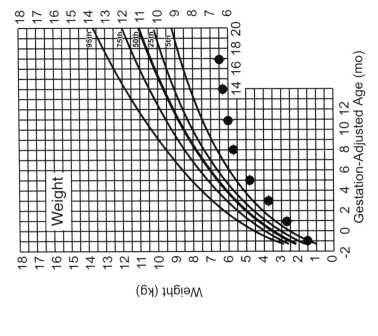

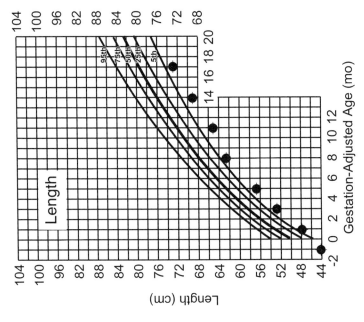

Figure 6b. Small-for-gestational-age infant who is faltering in weight.

disciplinary intervention to optimize the psychosocial environment is required to ensure optimum growth in this population.

SUMMARY

Growth failure in children is the end result of various genetic and environmental influences during both prenatal and postnatal periods. The critical periods during which proper intervention would result in reversal of growth failure are not well known in humans; however, most prenatal insults lead to some permanent curtailment of growth potential that is unresponsive to postnatal nutritional interventions. Decreased growth velocity in the first 2 years of life sometimes may be a result of physiological fluctuations or spurious occurrences that are related to inaccuracies in the reference standards. For a child who presents with low anthropometric measures but otherwise has a normal medical, developmental, and psychosocial history, the possibility of physiological variants of growth should be entertained. The proper distinction of physiological variations from pathological decelerations often requires evaluation over extended periods of time.

REFERENCES

Ahn, C.H., & MacLean, W.C. (1980). Growth of the exclusively breast-fed infant. *American Journal of Clinical Nutrition, 33,* 183–192.

American Academy of Pediatrics. (1993). Assessment of nutritional status. In L.A. Barnes (Ed.), *Pediatric nutrition handbook* (pp. 193–201). Elk Grove Village, IL: Author.

American Academy of Pediatrics, Committee on Nutrition. (1998). *Pediatric nutrition handbook* (4th ed.). Elk Grove Village, IL: Author.

Ashworth, A. (1969). Growth rates in children recovering from protein-calorie malnutrition. *British Journal of Nutrition, 23,* 835–845.

Beaton, G.H. (1989). Small but healthy? Are we asking the right question? *European Journal of Clinical Nutrition, 43,* 863–875.

Berkley, C.S., Reed, R.B., & Valadian, I. (1983). Longitudinal growth standards for preschool children. *Annnals of Human Biology, 10,* 57–67.

Bithoney, W.G., McJunkin, J., Michalek, J., Snyder, J., & Munier, A. (1989). Prospective evaluation of weight gain in both nonorganic and organic failure to thrive children: An outpatient trial of a multidisciplinary team intervention strategy. *Journal of Developmental and Behavioral Sciences, 10,* 27–31.

Bray, G.A. (1987). Overweight is risking fate: Definition, classification, prevention and risks. *Annals of the New York Academy of Sciences, 499,* 14–28.

Cameron, N. (1980). Conditional standards for growth in height of British children from 5.0 to 15.99 years of age. *Annals of Human Biology, 7,* 331–337.

Cutler, A.T., Benezra-Obeiter, R., & Brink, S.J. (1986). Thyroid function in young children with Down's syndrome. *American Journal of Diseases of Children, 140,* 479–483.

Dagan, R., Sofer, S., Klish, W.J., Hundet, G., Saltz, H., & Moses, S.W. (1983). Growth and nutritional status in Bedouin infants in the Negev Desert, Israel: Evidence for marked stunting in the presence of only mild malnutrition. *American Journal of Clinical Nutrition, 38,* 747–756.

Daniels, S.R., Khoury, P.R., & Morrison, J.A. (1997). The utility of body mass index as a measure of body fatness in children and adolescents: Differences by race and gender. *Pediatrics, 99,* 804–807.

Davies, D.P., Platts, P., Pritchard, J.M., & Wilkerson, P.W. (1979). Nutritional status of light-for-date infants at birth and its influence on early postnatal growth. *Archives of Diseases of Children, 54,* 703–706.

Davis, L.E. (1971). Epidemiology of famine in the Nigerian crisis: Rapid evaluation of malnutrition by height and arm circumference in large populations. *American Journal of Clinical Nutrition, 24,* 358–364.

de Onis, M., Garza, C., & Habicht, J.-P. (1997). Time for a new growth reference. *Pediatrics, 100,* e8. Available: http://www.pediatrics.org

Dewey, K.G., Peerson, J.M., Brown, K.H., Krebs, N.F., Michaelson, K.F., Peerson, L.A., Salmen-pera, L., Whitehead, R.G., Young, D.L., & World Health Organization Working Group on Infant Growth. (1995). Growth of breast-fed infants deviation from current reference data: A pooled analysis of US, Canadian and European data sets. *Pediatrics, 96,* 495–503.

Dietz, W.H. (1986). Catch-up growth following undernutrition in children. In S.A. Cohen (Ed.), *The underweight infant, child and adolescent* (pp. 219–231). Norwalk, CT: Appleton-Century-Crofts.

Deurenberg, P., Weststrate, J.A., & Seidell, J.C. (1991). Body mass index as a measure of body fat-ness: Age and sex-specific prediction formulas. *British Journal of Nutrition, 65,* 105–114.

Ellerstein, N.S., & Ostrov, B.E. (1985). Growth patterns in children hospitalized because of caloric-deprivation failure-to-thrive. *American Journal of Diseases of Children, 139,* 164–166.

Eveleth, P.B. (1978). Differences between populations in body shape of children and adolescents. *American Journal of Physical Anthropology, 49,* 373–382.

Eveleth, P.B., & Tanner, J.M. (Eds.). (1976). *Worldwide variation in human growth.* Cambridge, England: Cambridge University Press.

Faulkner, R.A., & Bailey, D.A. (1989). Critical evaluation of frame size determination in the 1983 Metropolitan Life weight-for-height tables. *Canadian Journal of Public Health, 80,* 369–372.

Fitzsimmons, J., Droste, S., Shepard, T.H., Pascon-Mason, J., & Fantel, A. (1990). Growth failure in second-trimester fetuses with trisomy 21. *Teratology, 42,* 337–345.

Frisancho, A.R. (1974). Triceps skinfold and upper arm muscle size norms for assessment of nutri-tional status. *American Journal of Clinical Nutrition, 27,* 1–52.

Gallehger, D. (1996). How useful is body mass index for comparison of body fatness across age, sex and ethnic groups? *American Journal of Epidemiology, 143,* 228–239.

Galton, F. (1886). Regression toward mediocrity in hereditary stature. *Journal of Anthropology Institute, 15,* 246–263.

Garn, S.M., & LaVelle, M. (1985). Family-line origins of low-fat and low-lean child or adolescent. In S.A. Cohen (Ed.), *The underweight infant, child and adolescent* (pp. 15–34). Norwalk, CT: Appleton-Century-Crofts.

George, E.K., Mearin, M.L., Bouquet, J., von Blomberg, B.M., Staple, S.O., van Elburg, R.M., & de Graaf, E.A. (1996). High frequency of celiac disease in Down's syndrome. *Journal of Pediatrics, 128,* 555–557.

Goldbloom, R.B. (1987). Growth failure in infancy. *Pediatrics in Review, 9,* 57–61.

Golden, M.H.N. (1994). Causes and mechanisms of linear growth retardation: Is complete catch-up possible for stunted malnourished children? *European Journal of Clinical Nutrition, 48*(Suppl. 1), S58–S71.

Graitcer, P.L., Gentry, E.M., Nichaman, M.Z., & Lane, J.M. (1981). Anthropometric indicators of nutritional status and morbidity. *Journal of Pediatrics, 27,* 292–298.

Guo, S., Roche, A.F., Fomon, S.J., Nelson, S.E., Chumlea, W.C., Rogers, R.R., Baumgartner, R.N., Ziegler, E.E., & Siervogel, R.M. (1991). Reference data on gains in weight and length during the first two years of life. *Journal of Pediatrics, 119,* 355–362.

Healy, M.J.R., & Goldstein, H. (1978). Regression to the mean. *Annals of Human Biology, 5,* 278–280.

Himes, J.H., Roche, A.F., Thissen, D., & Moore, W.M. (1985). Parent-specific adjustments for eval-uation of recumbent length and stature of children. *Pediatrics, 75,* 304–313.

Hitchcock, N.E., Gracey, M., & Owles, E.N. (1981). Growth in healthy breast-fed infants in the first six months. *The Lancet, 2,* 64–65.

Holmes, G.E., Miller, H.C., Hassaniein, K., Lansky, S.B., & Goggin, J.E. (1977). Post-natal somatic growth in infants with atypical fetal growth patterns. *American Journal of Diseases of Children, 131,* 1078–1083.

Huttly, S.R.A., Victora, C.G., Barros, F.C., Teixeira, A.M.B., & Vaughan, J.P. (1991). The timing of nutritional status determination: Implications for interventions and growth monitoring. *European Journal of Clinical Nutrition, 45,* 85–95.

Johnson, M.L. (1993). Analysis of serial growth data. *American Journal of Human Biology, 5,* 633–640.

Jones, K.L., & Chernoff, G.L. (1978). Drugs and chemicals associated with intrauterine growth defi-ciency. *Journal of Reproductive Medicine, 21,* 365–370.

Kielmann, A.A., & McCord, C. (1978). Weight-for-age as an index of risk of death in children. *The Lancet, 1,* 1247–1250.

Kramer, M.S., McLean, F.H., Olivier, M., Willis, D.M., & Usher, R.H. (1989). Body proportionality and head and length sparing in growth retarded neonates: A critical reappraisal. *Pediatrics, 84,* 717–723.

Lacey, K.A., & Parkin, J.M. (1974). Causes of short stature: A community study of children in Newcastle upon Tyne. *The Lancet, 1,* 42–45.

Lampl, M., Veldhuis, J.D., & Johnson, M.L. (1992). Saltation and stasis: A model for human growth. *Science, 258,* 801–803.

Leung, S., & Davies, D.P. (1994). Infant feeding and growth of Chinese infants: Birth to two years. *Pediatrics and Perinatal Epidemiology, 8,* 301–313.

Lindgern, G. (1978). Growth of school children with early, average and late ages of peak height velocity. *Annals of Human Biology, 5,* 253–267.

Lubchenco, L.O., Hansman, C., & Boyd, E. (1966). Intrauterine growth in length and head circumference as estimated from live births at gestational ages from 26–42 weeks. *Pediatrics, 37,* 403–408.

Marshall, W.A. (1971). Evaluations of growth rate in height over periods of less than one year. *Archives of Diseases of Children, 46,* 414–420.

Oates, R.K., Peacock, A., & Forrest, D. (1985). Long-term effects of nonorganic failure to thrive. *Pediatrics, 75,* 36–40.

Pinyerd, B.J. (1992). Assessment of infant growth. *Journal of Pediatric Health Care, 6,* 302–308.

Prader, A., Tanner, J.M., & von Harnach, G.A. (1963). Catch-up growth following illness or starvation. *Journal of Pediatrics, 62,* 646–659.

Ricci, J.A., & Becker, S. (1996). Risk factors for wasting and stunting among children in Metro Cebu, Philippines. *American Journal of Clinical Nutrition, 63,* 966–975.

Rider, E., Samuels, R., Wilson, K., & Homer, C. (1996). Physical growth, infant nutrition, breast-feeding and general nutrition. *Current Opinion in Pediatrics, 8,* 293–297.

Rivera, J.A., & Habicht, J.P. (1996). The recovery of Guatemalan children with mild to moderate wasting: Factors enhancing the impact of supplementary feeding. *American Journal of Public Health, 89,* 1430–1434.

Schumacher, L.B., Pawson, I.G., & Kretchmer, N. (1987). Growth of immigrant children in the newcomer schools of San Fransisco. *Pediatrics, 80,* 861–868.

Smith, D.W., Truog, W., Rogers, J.E., Greizer, L.J., Skinner, A.L., McCann, J.J., & Harvey, M.A. (1976). Shifting linear growth during infancy: Illustration of genetic factors in growth from fetal life through infancy. *Journal of Pediatrics, 89,* 225–230.

Snyder, R.G., Schneider, L.W., Owings, C.L., Golomb, D.H., & Schork, M.A. (1977). *Anthropometry in infants, children and youths to age eighteen for product safety design.* Bethesda, MD: Consumer Product Safety Commission. (Report No. UM-HSRI-77-17)

Solanes, C.V., & Lifshitz, F. (1992). Body weight progression and nutritional status of patients with familial short stature with and without constitutional delay in growth. *American Journal of Diseases of Children, 146,* 296–302.

Spender, Q.W., Cronk, C.E., Charney, E.B., & Stallings, V.A. (1989). Assessment of linear growth in children with cerebral palsy: Use of alternative measures to height or length. *Devlopmental Medicine & Child Neurology, 31,* 206–214.

Strauss, R., & Dietz, W.H. (1997). Effects of intrauterine growth retardation in premature infants on early childhood growth. *Journal of Pediatrics, 130,* 95–102.

Sturm, L., & Drotar, D. (1989). Prediction of weight for height following intervention in three-year-old children with early histories of non-organic failure to thrive. *Child Abuse & Neglect, 13,* 19–28.

Trowbridge, F.L., Marks, J.S., Lopez de Romana, G., Madrid, S., Boutton, T.W., & Klein, P.D. (1987). Body composition of Peruvian children with short stature and high weight-for-height: Implications for the interpretation of weight-for-height as an indicator of nutritional status. *American Journal of Clinical Nutrition, 46,* 411–418.

Ulijaszek, S.J. (1994). Between-population variation in pre-adolescent growth. *European Journal of Clinical Nutrition, 48,* S1, S5–S14.

U.S. Department of Health and Human Services, Public Health Service. (1996). *NHANES III anthropometric procedures* [Videotape]. Washington, DC: U.S. Government Printing Office. (Stock No. 017-022-01335-5)

Victora, C.G. (1992). The association between wasting and stunting: An international perspective. *Journal of Nutrition, 122,* 1105–1110.

Walravens, P.A. (1985). Growth quotients, z scores and failure to thrive (letter). *American Journal of Diseases of Children, 139,* 862.

Waterlow, J.C. (1974). Some aspects of childhood malnutrition as a public health problem. *British Medical Journal, 4,* 88–90.

Waterlow, J.C. (1994). Causes and mechanisms of linear growth retardation (stunting). *European Journal of Clinical Nutrition, 48*(Suppl. 1), S1–S4.

Whitehead, R.G., & Paul, A.A. (1984). Growth charts and the assessment of infant feeding practices in the Western world and in developing countries. *Early Human Development, 9,* 187–207.

Widdowson, E.M., & McCance, R.A. (1960). The effect of finite periods of undernutrition at different ages on the composition and subsequent development of the rat. *Proceedings of the Royal Society, 158,* 329–342.

Winick, M., Meyer, K.K., & Harris, R.C. (1975). Malnutrition and environmental enrichment by early adoption. *Science, 190,* 1173–1175.

World Health Organization Working Group. (1986). Use and interpretation of anthropometric indicators of nutritional status. *Bulletins of the World Health Organization, 64,* 929–941.

World Health Organization Working Group on Infant Growth Nutrition Unit. (1994). *An evaluation of infant growth.* Geneva, Switzerland: World Health Organization.

Wright, C.M., Mathews, J.N.S., Waterson, A., & Aynsley-Green, A. (1994). What is the normal rate of weight gain in infancy? *Acta Pediatrica, 83,* 351–356.

Chapter 11

Gastrointestinal Problems and Disorders

Nancy F. Krebs

Normal function of the gastrointestinal tract is essential for normal growth. As the clinical subspecialty of pediatric gastroenterology has grown and matured, so has the recognition of the many pathologies of the gastrointestinal tract, many of which can result in impaired growth. This chapter presents a clinical approach to identifying signs or symptoms that may point to the gastrointestinal tract as the possible basis for growth faltering.

Pediatric undernutrition can be viewed as a *net* inadequacy of energy intake and sometimes of specific individual nutrients (macro and micro). The diagnostic approach, thus, can be reduced to two broad headings: inadequate intake and excessive losses. As the clinician approaches evaluation of growth faltering, gastrointestinal dysfunction can most usefully be assessed within this framework.

INADEQUATE INTAKE

Causes of poor intake that are associated with diseases of the gastrointestinal tract may stem from pain or discomfort, dysphagia, or other causes. These are described in more detail next. As with all assessments in pediatrics, the age and the developmental stage of the child have important implications for the likelihood of certain diagnoses.

Pain

Pain that is associated with the eating process may suggest esophageal irritation or **dysmotility.** In the young infant, gastroesophageal reflux (GER) is common and can be accompanied by discomfort and feeding resistance (Hart, 1996; Hillemeier, 1996; Hyman, 1994; Orenstein, 1992).

A history of abdominal pain in an undernourished child is a significant clue that gastrointestinal disease may be present. Pain is often difficult to assess but may be suggested by a history of crying or fussiness in association with eating. In the young infant, such a history suggests GER. A toddler or child may be able to localize pain to the abdomen but not to specific areas that might suggest alternative diagnoses. Other conditions that are associated with a history of crying shortly after feeds include **hiatal hernia,** milk-protein intolerance, overfeeding, and acute gastroenteritis; the last usually is self-limited and accompanied by other symptoms.

Unusual causes of chronic abdominal pain in a toddler or preschool-age child include inflammatory bowel disease, gallstones (cholelithiasis) or other problems with the flow of bile or with the gallbladder itself, infection or irritation of the pancreas (pancreatitis), intermittent volvulus, and intussusception. The last two consist of twisting or sliding of the bowel on itself, which results in compromised blood supply to regions of the intestine. Any of these conditions are potentially quite serious and thus require further diagnostic evaluation when the presentation is suggestive (e.g., lethargy, vomiting, blood in stools, anemia). Lactose intolerance, which may cause gas and distention that may be perceived as pain, should be considered in the older toddler but is quite rare in an infant or young toddler unless there has been preceding diarrhea that may have caused **mucosal** damage in the proximal small bowel. Abdominal pain can also be the result of other systemic illnesses, including pneumonia and diabetes, among others (Roy, Silverman, & Alagille, 1995).

Dysphagia

Dysphagia—difficulty in swallowing—results from problems with the normal neuromuscular integration of sucking, swallowing, and breathing and can reduce a child's ability and willingness to eat. Consideration of oral-motor and pharyngeal functioning is provided in Chapter 23. Esophageal dysphagia can result from numerous anatomic malformations, congenital or acquired, or from primary neuromuscular disorders. Esophageal dysphagia may be suggested by persistent regurgitation or vomiting, choking, coughing, or recurrent episodes of pneumonia or wheezing. Anatomic esophageal abnormalities include communication between the airway and the esophagus (tracheo-esophageal fistula); mass or tumor (within or outside the esophagus itself); or abnormal narrowing, either present at birth or acquired, which causes abnormal movement of the esophagus and thus of material moving through it. Other specific examples are listed in Table 1. Achalasia is a neuromuscular disorder that results in failure of normal relaxation of the lower esophageal **sphincter** and abnormal esophageal **peristalsis.** Although this disorder is typically diagnosed in later childhood, it can present in young children. Furthermore, symptoms often have been present for a number of years prior to diagnosis and are often associated with feeding difficulties and growth impairment. Typical symptoms include dysphagia, retrosternal pain, regurgitation of undigested food, recurrent cough (especially **nocturnal**), and aspiration pneumonia. Mucosal infections and inflammatory disorders of the esophagus are also associated with dysphagia as well as pain with swallowing. In an evaluation of an infant or child with slow growth, the history thus should include questions about perceived difficulties with swallowing. Observation of feeding may also be helpful, but further diagnostic testing usually will be necessary for definitive diagnosis, such as radiological contrast studies (e.g., barium swallow, which highlights the outline of the esophagus); manometry, which provides electrical tracings of changes in pressure within the esophagus, reflecting intensity and coordination of muscle contractions and relaxations; or direct visualization through an endoscope.

Table 1.   Gastrointestinal signs and symptoms that are associated with inadequate intake and excessive losses

Finding	Diagnostic considerations
Inadequate intake	
Pain (esophageal, abdominal)	Gastroesophageal reflux
	Hiatal hernia
	Milk-protein intolerance
	Lactose intolerance
	Overfeeding
	Acute gastroenteritis
	Inflammatory bowel disease
	Inflammation or obstruction of biliary tract
	Pancreatitis
	Intermittent volvulus
	Intussusception
Swallowing difficulties (dysphagia)	Anatomic abnormalities
	• Tracheo-esophageal fistula
	• Mass or tumor
	• Atresia or stenosis
	• Stricture, web, ring
	Neuromuscular dysfunction (achalasia)
	Mucosal infection
	• Viral
	• Fungal
Poor appetite (anorexia) or prolonged satiety	Delayed gastric emptying
	• Excessive gastric acidity
	• Inflammation
	• Dysmotility
	Zinc deficiency
	Ketosis
	• Dehydration
	• Inadequate carbohydrate intake
	• Low total caloric intake
	Acidosis
	• Inborn errors of metabolism
	• Renal tubular acidosis
	• Dehydration
	Constipation
Excessive losses	
Regurgitation/spitting-up	Gastroesophageal reflux
	Esophageal disorders (see above)
Vomiting	
Nonbilious emesis	Gastric outlet obstruction
	• Hypertrophic pyloric stenosis
	• Gastritis
	• Antral ulcer
	Protein hypersensitivity
	Gastroenteritis
	Pancreatitis
	Hepatitis
	Cholecystitis
	Appendicitis
	Inborn errors of metabolism
	Sepsis
	Genitourinary infection
	Pneumonia

(continued)

Table 1. *(continued)*

Finding	Diagnostic considerations
Bilious emesis	CNS pathology Endocrinopathy Intestinal obstruction • Volvulus • Adhesions • Intussusception • Intestinal malformation Sepsis
Diarrhea and malabsorption	Milk-protein hypersensitivity Carbohydrate malabsorption Cystic fibrosis Celiac disease Infection (acute or chronic) Inflammatory bowel disease

Note: This table is not intended to be a complete differential diagnosis for each sign or symptom but rather to provide major diagnoses and diagnostic categories.

Other Causes of Inadequate Intake

Clinical observations link poor dietary intake and chronic constipation, although a specific mechanism is not known. A diet that is low in fiber (and bulk) and inadequate in fluid can cause constipation. Constipation may, in turn, contribute to poor intake. Although clinical experience suggests that appetite and intake often improve when constipation is relieved, controlled investigation of such observations is needed.

Metabolic disorders, such as ketosis or acidosis, often depress the appetite. Ketosis is a metabolic condition in which the body produces large amounts of ketones. It is usually associated with the body's utilization of fat or protein for fuel over carbohydrates. Circumstances that are associated with ketosis include inadequate carbohydrate intake, imbalanced or inadequate caloric intake, dehydration, and insulin insufficiency (diabetes). Acidosis can result from metabolic or respiratory disorders, renal dysfunction, or severe ketosis. **Anorexia** may also be associated with numerous systemic diseases as well as chronic inflammation, acute and chronic infection, malignancy, central nervous system **pathology,** and emotional disturbances (see Chapters 13, 14, and 29).

Even mild zinc deficiency is associated with decreased food intake (see Chapter 6). Whether this is secondary to quantitative or qualitative changes in normal taste perception or to changes in appetite regulation by the brain is unclear. Zinc deficiency may be caused by either inadequate intake or diarrhea and/or malabsorption because the body's zinc balance is regulated primarily through the gastrointestinal tract.

Although psychological and emotional factors are often assumed to be the major influence on food intake, the conditions discussed thus far should be kept in mind as potential contributing factors. Indeed, in many cases, it may be the interaction of such physical conditions with the home and social milieu that predisposes a child to take inadequate energy and nutrients to sustain optimum growth (Rudolph, 1994).

EXCESSIVE LOSSES

Within the category of excessive losses are the obvious gastrointestinal sources of caloric and nutritional losses: vomiting, diarrhea, and malabsorption. This section approaches these symptoms as possible contributing factors to poor growth. Because of the relatively common occurrence of GER, this condition is discussed in somewhat more detail.

Gastroesophageal Reflux

GER is the movement of gastric contents back into the esophagus. GER is very common in young infants; as many as 40%–50% of 1- to 2-month-old infants are found to have episodes of reflux at least twice daily. Discussed next are GER's clinical presentation, evaluation, and treatment.

Clinical Presentation

Refluxed material may be obvious as spit-up or emesis, but reflux can be relatively "silent" as well. Growth impairment may stem from absolute losses, from decreased intake, or from associated problems. Thus, as noted previously, the possibility of reflux should be considered when the history indicates such symptoms as crying or arching (hyperextension) during or after feeds. Infants' crying in response to GER may not be recognized as a response to "heartburn," especially when it is not accompanied by visible regurgitation. Furthermore, because of immaturity of their nervous system, infants may experience sensations from their organs more intensely than do adults. If symptoms persist without treatment, then infants may respond either by refusing to eat or by limiting intake. The setting thus can be in place for difficult infant–caregiver interaction, which can then further perpetuate feeding difficulties.

For most infants (more than 80%), GER resolves between the ages of 6 months and 1 year. Factors that are associated with resolution of GER include maturation of gastrointestinal reflexes, which influence esophageal function and emptying of the stomach; change in anatomic position of lower esophageal sphincter to below the diaphragm; intake of more solid foods; and increased upright posture. Factors that predispose the child to persistence of symptoms include neurological impairments and psychomotor delays, prolonged reliance on a primarily liquid diet, hiatal hernia, pulmonary disease, overfeeding, and obesity.

Evaluation

Because GER is very common and is often benign, it is important to recognize when an evaluation is necessary. Diagnostic studies are indicated either when there are significant associated symptoms, such as dysphagia, growth failure, breathing problems (e.g., choking or not breathing for more than 30 seconds), recurrent pneumonia from **aspiration** of refluxed material, cough, or reactive airway disease (asthma) or when there is evidence of tissue injury. This may manifest as irritation, inflammation, or actual bleeding in the esophagus. Blood loss may be visible in vomitus or may be detectable chemically in stools.

Evaluation for GER often includes an upper gastrointestinal (UGI) X-ray series in which barium is swallowed and can be seen to outline the esophagus, stomach, and the first part of the small intestine. Although reflux can often be seen during the study, failure to document it during this relatively short-term study does *not* indicate its absence at other times. The UGI is most useful to rule out anatomic abnormalities and to evaluate obstruction of stomach emptying.

An esophageal pH probe study consists of an acid-sensitive probe that is swallowed (as part of a small soft tube through the nose) and left in the esophagus for several hours. The probe senses how often and for how long acid from the stomach refluxes into the esophagus. Although such information is rarely necessary to make the diagnosis of GER, it may be helpful to quantify the amount of time that acid reflux is occurring. It also can be done in conjunction with monitoring of breathing and oxygenation, which allows correlation of reflux with other clinical problems.

A gastroesophageal scintiscan, or "milk scan," consists of ingestion of **radionuclide**-labeled formula and allows calculation of the rate of its movement through the stomach. It is most widely used to assess gastric emptying in children who are undergoing surgical **fundoplication** and to assess the indication for a procedure to facilitate emptying. The scintiscan lacks the sensitivity of a UGI for identifying anatomic abnormalities and fails to quantify GER as well as a pH probe does.

Fiber-optic endoscopy allows direct visualization of the mucosa (or lining) of the esophagus, stomach, and duodenum; mucosal biopsies are also used to determine existence and severity of inflammation. It may be helpful in assessing effects of "silent" reflux and in assessing need for and effectiveness of therapy.

Treatment

The mainstays of conservative treatment of GER are instituting small-volume, frequent feeds; positioning after feeds (upright or head elevated, prone); and thickening feeds or more reliance on nonliquid foods. Such approaches are quite benign and should be tried, with or without pharmacological treatment. The rationale for pharmacological therapy is twofold: 1) to reduce gastric acid production and the risk of esophagitis and its associated pain and dysfunction and 2) to enhance gastric emptying to reduce the volume of gastric contents that is available to reflux. The former can be achieved with antacids, which buffer gastric acid, or with H_2 receptor antagonists, such as cimetidine and ranitidine, which reduce acid production. The prokinetic agent cisapride stimulates smooth muscle contraction throughout the gastrointestinal tract and is used to stimulate gastric motility and emptying. Clinical trials suggest therapeutic benefit for children as well as adults with GER (Vandenplas, de Roy, & Sacre, 1991). Agents such as metaclopramide and bethanechol act primarily to increase lower esophageal sphincter tone. Prior to the availability of cisapride, these were used widely but with, at best, mixed results.

Indications for medical therapy include the presence of associated serious symptoms, as described previously. Parents and caregivers alike may need to be reminded of these indications and be reassured that reflux or spitting up is usually not worrisome unless it is associated with other clinical problems. If unacceptable complications of GER cannot be managed with conservative and/or medical interventions or if the child is at risk for persistence of GER symptoms, then a surgical fundoplication should be considered. Although this is an effective procedure, it is not without complications, and the potential benefits must be weighed carefully. If a fundoplication is performed, then the surgeon often will also recommend placing a feeding tube into the stomach (a gastrostomy tube) as a way to relieve pressure if necessary. This is done because the fundoplication usually prevents vomiting.

Vomiting

Vomiting is distinguished from regurgitation or spitting up by its nature: forceful ejection of stomach contents. *Spitting up* refers to stomach contents gently "spilling," not being forcefully ejected, out of the infant's mouth. In essence, this is exaggerated GER. It can occur with jostling, squeezing, or even just laying down the infant. Spitting up is harmless, though often annoying and sometimes frightening to parents, unless it becomes so severe that it interferes with normal growth or causes other problems as described previously. If temperament, intake, and growth are appropriate, then parents should be reassured that spitting up is common, is benign, and has an excellent prognosis. Sometimes it may be helpful to discuss with parents that the only way to stop the infant from spitting up is through fundoplication and that this measure carries some risks as well.

True vomiting carries more serious connotations and, if established and associated with poor weight gain, should be evaluated thoroughly by the clinician. Historical information that is useful in evaluating etiological possibilities includes whether the emesis contains bile, indicated by greenish-yellow coloring; contains blood (the amount and whether it is brownish or bright red); or contains curdled milk or undigested milk or food. Also useful are details of the timing of the vomiting in relation to feeds as well as the quantity and type of feeds and a description of the circumstances that preceded and followed episodes of vomiting.

Persistent vomiting without bile (nonbilious) suggests a gastric outlet obstruction, such as hypertrophic pyloric **stenosis** in a young infant in which the muscular channel that leads from the stomach to the small intestine is thick and too tight for normal stomach emptying; an ulcer or irritation in the stomach near the pylorus, which also results in delayed gastric emptying; a hiatal hernia; or possibly milk-protein allergy, the last especially if associated with other symptoms such as diarrhea, blood in stool, wheezing, or rash (see Chapter 16). Other infectious or inflammatory gastrointestinal diseases also are often associated with vomiting and are listed in Table 1. They are generally accompanied by other signs or symptoms that provide important diagnostic clues.

Bilious emesis always should bring to mind intestinal obstruction or severe illness such as **sepsis.** Because of the potentially severe consequences of intestinal obstruction, bilious emesis should be evaluated promptly, at a minimum with plain X-rays and often with **contrast studies**.

Nongastrointestinal causes of vomiting include inborn errors of metabolism. These should be considered particularly in the infant or child with developmental delays, seizures, or other evidence of neurological abnormality. A large liver on exam or evidence of hepatitis on blood testing would also be suggestive of a metabolic disorder. Significant infections, such as sepsis, pneumonia, or genitourinary infections, can be associated with vomiting, as can central nervous system and endocrine disorders. Generally, acute infections will be relatively obvious in the evaluation of a child who is experiencing growth failure. Central nervous system pathology and endocrine disorders may require more active consideration and pursuit of the underlying cause of unexplained, persistent vomiting.

Diarrhea and Malabsorption

The history or review of systems for an undernourished child should always include questions about stool frequency and character. The clinician is looking for clues about losses of energy and nutrients from the intestines. These may be a result of either abnormal digestion and absorption of nutrients from food or inability to reabsorb nutrients that are secreted into the gastrointestinal tract during digestion, such as proteins, amino acids, minerals, and electrolytes. Because the term *diarrhea* may mean different things to different people, inquiring about its presence or absence may not be enlightening; inquiry should focus on the frequency and the size of stools, water content, color, and presence of blood or mucus. A history of associated symptoms should be sought, such as cramping, abdominal distention or bloating, and flatulence. In addition, the relationship of symptoms to changes in dietary intake should be sought. Although malabsorption often occurs in conjunction with diarrhea, it also can be relatively subtle. For example, constipation as a presenting symptom of celiac disease has been well documented, and constipation is a common clinical problem in children who have cystic fibrosis (see Chapter 12), even in the face of pancreatic insufficiency.

In a young infant, milk-protein hypersensitivity (see Chapter 16) may manifest as watery diarrhea, often accompanied by visible flecks or streaks of blood. Changing to a predigested formula, such as **semi-elemental protein hydrolysate,** or an **elemental for-**

mula with fully digested protein should result in diminished symptoms. Similar symptoms can occur in breast-fed infants who are sensitive to antigens that cross from the mother's diet into the milk. Relief of symptoms in such cases usually is accomplished by the mother's avoidance of the offending substance, such as cow milk, legumes, eggs, or fish.

A history of watery diarrhea, flatulence, and/or cramping may suggest carbohydrate intolerance or malabsorption. Although there are rare conditions with congenital saccharide (simple carbohydrates) malabsorption, carbohydrate malabsorption occurs more commonly after intestinal mucosal damage, such as postinfectious gastroenteritis, celiac disease, cystic fibrosis, and inflammatory bowel disease.

One common cause of flatulence, abdominal distention, and diarrhea in the older infant and toddler is fructose and sorbitol malabsorption. Fructose, the **monosaccharide** that is present in high amounts in fruit and fruit juice, especially apple and pear juices, is absorbed by a process that does not require energy but that does involve a protein carrier. When the child consumes more than what the intestine can absorb, unabsorbed fructose provokes an **osmotic diarrhea** because of the fluid that is drawn into the intestine. Sorbitol, a polyalcohol that is used in dietetic candies and gums and that is present in apple, pear, and prune juices, is absorbed slowly from the gut. At high intakes, especially in conjunction with fructose, it also can cause an osmotic diarrhea. Orange and white grape juices do not have these effects. Such carbohydrate malabsorption that is associated with excessive juice consumption is considered a frequent cause of chronic nonspecific diarrhea, also known as toddler's diarrhea. The distinction should be made, however, that because this malabsorption is not a result of any intestinal pathology, it typically does not cause growth failure (Judd, 1996; Kneepkens & Hoekstra, 1996). Nevertheless, the dietary pattern that is characterized by excessive juice intake, often in the context of a lack of structured mealtime routines, grazing, and other dietary inadequacies (see Chapters 6 and 27), may result in inadequate and/or imbalanced intake of energy and nutrients.

Acute infectious gastroenteritis is generally a self-limited disease and not a primary cause of significant growth failure, except in young infants. In some instances, however, the initial infectious insult can result in intestinal mucosal damage—or, possibly, other conditions that are not understood entirely—that leads to persistent diarrhea, with malabsorption and growth faltering. In the case of dehydration that results from acute diarrhea, recommendations are to rehydrate with standard glucose-electrolyte solution. Feeding should be resumed immediately after the rehydration phase has been accomplished (usually in less than 12 hours). Prolonged use of electrolyte solutions or other clear liquids increases the risk of malnutrition more than any benefit of so-called "gut rest." In fact, early feeding has not been associated with worse symptoms or longer duration of diarrhea and allows earlier nutritional recovery.

Chronic infectious gastroenteritis is commonly caused by the parasites *Giardia lamblia* or *Cryptosporidium,* both of which are transmitted and contracted frequently in child care centers. *Giardiasis* is typically associated with foul-smelling stools, anorexia, and abdominal distention; it also can cause vomiting. Although watery diarrhea may be the initial symptom, fat malabsorption (steatorrhea) generally occurs, along with growth faltering. Symptoms can be variable, intermittent, and prolonged. Diagnosis can be challenging because the organism is shed only intermittently in stool. Newer tests that detect antigen in the stool may facilitate diagnosis. Detection of cysts of the organism in the feces can be made from a variety of stains; but these may not be routine in all laboratories, and they require a specific request to test for the organism. Treatment with appropriate antibiotics is usually effective. Acute infection with *Cryptosporidium* is typically associated with fever, abdominal discomfort, vomiting, and a profuse watery diarrhea. In a child with a normal immune system, the infection is usually cleared within a few days, although symptoms can persist for 2–3 weeks. No antimicrobial therapy has been found to be effective consistently in eradicating the organism, and treatment is supportive, such as providing adequate fluid intake to avoid dehydration and food as tolerated. In a child with a compromised immune system in whom infection may be prolonged, intravenous fluids and nutritional support may be necessary. In either case, significant weight loss can result from the combination of anorexia, feeding intolerance, and increased losses.

Cystic Fibrosis

A high index of suspicion should be maintained for cystic fibrosis in any infant or toddler who is experiencing growth faltering. Stools are characteristically large, foul, oily, foamy, and pale, reflecting fat malabsorption (steatorrhea). In an infant, however, these characteristics may not be apparent, especially to a new parent, and a history of increased frequency may be more prominent. History of chronic cough or frequent lower respiratory infections are important supportive clues but are often not present or immediately obvious. Because of the profound maldigestion as well as malabsorption as a result of both pancreatic insufficiency and abnormal intestinal mucosa, infants and toddlers may present with significant wasting as a result of inadequate energy intake relative to losses and, in older children, increased requirements. Other findings may include edema and low albumin levels in the blood (hypoalbuminemia) as a result of muscle and protein breakdown (catabolism) secondary to negative energy balance and exacerbated by infections and marginal protein intake. Young infants who have cystic fibrosis also may present with a severe rash, which has a distribution and character that are typical of severe zinc and/or protein deficiency. Essential fatty acid and other micronutrient deficiencies may also contribute to the rash. In such cases, the rash is a result of deficiency of these nutrients, which is caused by the malabsorption. Rash as a presenting sign of cystic fibrosis is most common in infants because they have relatively high requirements and can develop frank deficiency quite quickly. Diagnosis of cystic fibrosis is confirmed by obtaining an elevated sweat chloride (greater than 60 mEq/L) by an experienced laboratory. If a child is diagnosed with cystic fibrosis, then he or she should be referred, if possible, to a cystic fibrosis clinical center.

Undernutrition and poor growth often remain problems for infants and children who have cystic fibrosis, despite initiation of appropriate therapies, including pancreatic enzyme replacement. The reasons for this usually are multiple, including some persistent malabsorption, anorexia related to chronic inflammation in the lungs, chronic constipation, and behavioral and psychosocial issues that are related to chronic disease. Because malnutrition is associated with worsening lung disease, gastrostomy tubes often are recommended when a child is persistently at or below 85% of the weight that is appropriate for the child's height. The feeding tube allows supplemental intake of high-calorie and nutritious liquids, which can, for example, be given during the night. This mode of feeding also can be helpful to provide nutritional support during episodes of worsened lung disease when the child may be unable to eat by mouth (Shakib & Adelson, 1996).

Celiac Disease

Diarrhea, abdominal distention, weight loss, anorexia, and irritability are among the most common presenting symptoms for infants and children who have celiac disease, a malabsorptive disease of the proximal small intestine that is associated with permanent intolerance to gluten. Because gluten is one of the proteins found in wheat (and rye), correlation of onset of symptoms with introduction of this grain into the diet provides helpful historical evidence that is suggestive of the diagnosis. Although the basic mechanism of intestinal injury is not entirely clear, the pathology is well described: flat, small intestinal mucosa that results in substantial loss of absorptive surface area. Stools commonly are pale, loose, and very foul smelling; frequency may be variable, from one large, bulky stool per day to two or three per day. As noted previously, presentation with constipation and only intermittent diarrhea also may occur. Growth faltering is the common denominator. The classic patient description is of a miserable toddler with distended abdomen and wasted extremities and buttocks, but this diagnosis should be entertained in any older infant (older than 9 months) or child, especially of northern European ancestry, with evidence of undernutrition and a history of gastrointestinal symptoms. Blood tests that suggest or support the diagnosis include anemia (due to either iron or folate deficiency), low serum albumin, and prolonged coagulation time (hypoprothrombinemia) due to vitamin K deficiency. Microscopic examination of stool for malabsorbed fat also is strongly supportive of the diagnosis of celiac disease, although it is not specific to this disease. Diagnosis is confirmed by clinical response to gluten-free diet, relapse of symptoms following a gluten challenge, finding circulating antigliadin and antiendomysial antibodies, and small intestinal biopsy, with abnormal mucosa (Troncone, Greco, & Auricchio, 1996).

In addition to the conditions that were described in this chapter, chronic diarrhea may be caused by other infections and infestations, inflammatory bowel disease, and a host of other disorders. For the child who presents with growth faltering, the primary clinician's responsibility is to determine the likelihood that pathology that is related to the gastrointestinal tract is contributing to the presenting constellation of findings, via inadequate intake or excessive losses (Lavy & Bauer, 1978; Roy et al., 1995). Once such determination is made, indications for further diagnostic studies or referral to an appropriate subspecialist usually will become clear.

TUBE-FEEDING

In some cases of undernutrition, tube-feeding should be considered. The decision to institute tube-feeding should be based on several factors, including the child's age and diagnosis and the severity of the undernutrition. In all cases, attempts to achieve nutrition orally should be vigorously explored first, and tube-feeding should seldom be the first treatment used.

Tube-feeding is indicated most commonly in cases of medical conditions that are associated with either impaired intake or increased requirements and that are likely to persist. Examples include children with chronic malabsorption, who are dependent on specialized formulas or on slow, continuous delivery of formula; children with cystic fibrosis, who often have some degree of ongoing malabsorption, frequent impairment of appetite due to pulmonary exacerbations, and increased nutritional requirements; and children with neurological and oral-motor impairment. In the last case, it is important to consult a speech-language pathologist or an occupational therapist (see Chapter 23).

The severity of undernutrition and the age of the child help determine the urgency of intervention (see Chapter 9). For example, a severely undernourished infant (less than 70% of median body weight for height) presents a much more fragile situation than a similarly undernourished adolescent. Short-term tube placement for nutritional and fluid resuscitation may be indicated if the child is too lethargic or weak to be fed orally. When the degree of undernutrition is moderate (more than 70%) or mild (more than 80%), the clinician may be able to wait before instituting tube-feeding.

If a child's undernutrition is due to psychological, behavioral, or environmental issues, as with a toddler who refuses to eat, then placement of a feeding tube may make the feeding problem worse. A toddler may pull out the tube, requiring that the parents replace it, an invasive and upsetting experience. A better understanding of the child and the family, although it may take more time and effort, is more likely to lead to effective feeding (see Chapters 7 and 8). Tube-feeding may also simply replace oral intake: The greater the intake provided by tube, the less the intake by mouth is likely to be. Although weight gain and linear growth may be improved by tube-feeding, cessation of tube-feeding often will be associated with recurrence of growth faltering if the fundamental causes have not been addressed.

If tube-feeding is indicated, then nasogastric (NG) tubes are best for short-term needs (from a few weeks to a few months). They can be placed and replaced safely by parents on a weekly basis. Long-term use also is possible, usually with the tube placed at night for overnight feeding and removed in the morning, although this usually is done by older children who can place the tube themselves. The complications of NG tubes include otitis media and sinusitis, vomiting with tube misplacement or dislodgment (e.g., with coughing), and increased GER and possible aspiration because the presence of the tube may impair the child's ability to protect the airway.

When long-term tube-feeding is indicated (more than a few months), a gastrostomy tube should be placed, either surgically or by endoscopy. The placement of a gastrostomy tube also may increase GER and the risk of aspiration, and in some instances a fundoplication may be required. Considerations for the use of feeding tubes, including bolus versus continuous feedings and choice of formulas, have been reviewed (Moore & Greene, 1985).

REFERENCES

Hart, J.J. (1996). Pediatric gastroesophageal reflux. *American Family Physician, 54,* 2463–2472.

Hillemeier, A.C. (1996). Gastroesophageal reflux: Diagnostic and therapeutic approaches. *Pediatric Clinics of North America, 43,* 197–212.

Hyman, P.E. (1994). Gastroesophageal reflux: One reason why baby won't eat. *Journal of Pediatrics, 125,* S103–S109.

Judd, R.H. (1996). Chronic nonspecific diarrhea. *Pediatrics in Review, 17,* 379–384.

Kneepkens, C.M.F., & Hoekstra, J.H. (1996). Chronic nonspecific diarrhea of childhood: Pathophysiology and management. *Pediatric Clinics of North America, 43,* 375–390.

Lavy, U., & Bauer, C.H. (1978). Pathophysiology of failure to thrive in gastrointestinal disorders. *Pediatric Annals, 7,* 743–749.

Moore, M.C., & Greene, H.L. (1985). Tube feeding of infants and children. *Pediatric Clinics of North America, 32,* 401–417.

Orenstein, S.R. (1992). Gastroesophageal reflux. *Pediatrics in Review, 13,* 174–182.

Roy, C.C., Silverman, A., & Alagille, D. (1995). *Pediatric clinical gastroenterology* (4th ed.). St. Louis: Mosby-Year Book.

Rudolph, C.D. (1994). Feeding disorders in infants and children. *Journal of Pediatrics, 125,* S116–S124.

Shakib, L.B., & Adelson, J.W. (1996). Cystic fibrosis: Gastrointestinal complications and gene therapy. *Pediatric Clinics of North America, 43,* 157–196.

Troncone, R., Greco, L., & Auricchio, S. (1996). Gluten-sensitive enteropathy. *Pediatric Clinics of North America, 43,* 355–373.

Vandenplas, Y., de Roy, C., & Sacre, L. (1991). Cisapride decreases prolonged episodes of reflux in infants. *Journal of Pediatric Gastroenterology and Nutrition, 12,* 44–47.

Chapter 12

Cardiopulmonary Problems and Disorders of the Head and Neck

Carol D. Berkowitz

Organic disturbances may affect a child's growth. This chapter discusses cardiac, pulmonary, and head and neck conditions that may impair growth.

CARDIAC CONDITIONS

Growth impairment in children who have congenital heart disease has been recognized for a long time (Mehziri & Drash, 1962). Studies have shown that up to 64% of children who are hospitalized as a result of congenital heart disease have signs of chronic malnutrition (Cameron, Rosenthal, & Olson, 1995), and children with **cyanotic** heart disease have a decreased number of fat cells (Baum & Stern, 1977). Most such children already will have been diagnosed with their cardiac condition, and the question will be whether the cardiac disorder is responsible for the poor growth. In a few cases, poor growth may be the presenting complaint, and it is on the basis of the history and physical examination that a cardiac problem is detected.

Etiology of Growth Impairment that Is Related to Cardiac Conditions

Cardiac lesions are responsible for poor growth in several ways (Pittman & Cohen, 1964): by abnormal function of the heart, causing low oxygen levels in the blood (hypoxia) or poor circulation (cardiac failure or **congestive heart failure** [CHF]) (Cheek, Grastone, & Rowe, 1969); by increasing the demand for energy; or as part of a group of multiple congenital malformations (Cameron et al., 1995; Neill, 1982). Large **ventricular septal de-**

The author thanks Sally Montoya for typing and coordination services in preparing this chapter.

fects (VSDs) and complex **atrial septal defects** (ASDs), which cause large left-to-right **shunts** and **pulmonary hypertension,** also are associated more commonly with impaired growth. Reduced **somatomedin levels** also have been reported in some children with chronic disease (Kappy, 1987).

It is important to remember that many common cardiac conditions do not impair growth. For example, simple ASDs and VSDs usually do not. The most common cardiac finding on physical examination, an innocent heart **murmur,** has no effect on growth. Young infants who experience impaired growth may exhibit the murmur of **peripheral pulmonic stenosis** (PPS), and this murmur may become louder as infants recover from undernutrition because of an increase in the volume of blood flowing through the lungs. In young children, nearly all cardiac conditions are the result of malformations that are present at birth and are referred to as *congenital heart defects* (CHD).

In cyanotic congenital heart disease (**tetralogy of Fallot** or **transposition of the great vessels**), in which the heart and lungs do not provide enough oxygen to the blood, 38% of hospitalized children in one study (Cameron et al., 1995) experienced malnutrition. Although the degree of malnutrition does not correlate exactly with oxygen level (Page, Dervall, Watson, & Scott, 1978), the degree and frequency of growth impairment generally are greater when oxygen levels are lower (Levy, Rosenthal, Fyler, & Nadas, 1978). Another indication that low oxygen has a role in growth impairment is that children frequently gain weight and improve their growth following surgical correction of their defect (Levy et al., 1978; Neill, 1982; Page et al., 1978). Failure to exhibit this catch-up growth postoperatively suggests the presence of an extracardiac reason for the poor growth. In cases of structural abnormalities, anatomic defects impose on the heart extra demands that the heart is unable to meet. In addition, the child may tire easily and not be able to feed adequately. The usual clinical picture of CHF is of an infant who is an eager, rapid feeder, who becomes short of breath and falls asleep exhausted or becomes irritable and inconsolable (Neill, 1982). CHF, which is exacerbated by fluid overload, also may require restriction of fluids and sodium, which may further impair growth.

Medications may have a direct or indirect affect on growth by impairing appetite. **Digitalis** may cause anorexia, especially at high blood levels. **Diuretics**, which are used to reduce fluid overload, also may contribute to anorexia by causing metabolic changes known as **hypochloremic alkalosis** (Gingell & Hornung, 1989).

In some cases, a cardiac lesion, such as tetralogy of Fallot or VSD, may be part of a genetic syndrome. Disorders that are associated with growth problems and CHD include **Turner, Williams, DiGeorge,** and **Noonan syndromes; fetal alcohol** and **rubella syndromes**; and **trisomies 13, 18, and 21** (see Chapter 14).

Evaluating Children Who Have Growth Impairment for Undiagnosed Cardiac Disease

Some children with growth impairment will have heart disease that has not been diagnosed. The medical history and the physical examination will raise suspicion about the correct diagnosis.

History

The history often provides the clue that there is a cardiac condition or that the known cardiac condition is contributing to the growth impairment. There may be a history of easy fatigability. Young infants may manifest this by tiring out during nursing, and older children may manifest this by inability to keep up with age-mates during play. Sweating also may be noted in young infants, especially during a feeding. Feedings may be unusually slow, taking an infant with a cardiac problem 30 minutes to ingest 1–2 ounces. Maternal use of alcohol, certain prescribed medications, and some illicit drugs has been associated with growth impairment as well as structural heart disease. Maternal illness during pregnancy might raise concern about congenital infections such as rubella.

Physical Examination

On exam, **cyanosis** may be present. It is important to distinguish cyanosis, which is noncardiac in origin (often associated with cold or crying), from that which suggests an underlying heart condition. Cyanosis of the extremities (acrocyanosis) or cyanosis around the mouth (circumoral cyanosis) is not uncommon in young infants. Central cyanosis (which is a result of cardiac or pulmonary problems) can be distinguished from noncardiac cyanosis because it involves not just the area around the mouth but also the lips, tongue, and gums. **Clubbing** is a sign of long-standing reduced oxygen levels and suggests underlying cardiac or pulmonary disease.

The physical examination is helpful in detecting the presence of heart disease. The presence or absence of cyanosis should be noted. The cardiac examination should be executed carefully. The size of the heart, the presence of **thrills**, and the presence of murmurs all should be noted. Murmurs suggest structural anomalies, and the murmurs should be graded, localized (both in relation to **systole** and **diastole** and place on the chest wall), and described (e.g., harsh, blowing). The child should be assessed for the presence of dysmorphic features, which would suggest a genetic condition, or exposure to alcohol, drugs, or infection in utero.

Diagnostic Studies

The diagnostic evaluation of the infant with suspected cardiac disease usually includes an **electrocardiogram** (ECG) and a chest X-ray. Most conditions that the noncardiologist can diagnose and manage readily are not associated with poor growth; therefore, if poor growth is suspected to be related to a cardiac problem, then consultation with a pediatric cardiologist is appropriate. The diagnostic workup may include an **echocardiogram,** which would further define the cardiac anatomy.

Genetics consultation is appropriate when a genetic syndrome is suspected. A skeletal survey may reveal a delay in bone age as well as a decrease in the thickness of the cortical bone, a finding sometimes noted with congenital heart disease (White et al., 1971). In assessing all children with growth impairment, a diet history is important to determine the level of nutritional adequacy. If a child is taking medications, then blood tests that include serum drug levels and electrolytes may be useful (see previous discussion).

Management

The management of cardiac disease includes both medical and surgical approaches. CHF should be treated with appropriate agents such as diuretics and digitalis. Surgical correction of structural lesions also may be needed and results in significant improvement (Fyler, Rothman, & Buckley, 1982). The degree of growth improvement varies with the type of lesion. Postoperative growth spurts have been noted with correction of transposition, tetralogy of Fallot, and VSDs with large shunts and associated CHF (Levy et al., 1978; Levy, Rosenthal, Miettinen, & Nadas, 1977). Failure to exhibit catch-up growth postoperatively suggests the presence of an extracardiac reason for impaired growth (Neill, 1982). Nutritional intake should be ensured, taking into account the need for both fluid and sodium restriction.

In all cases, adequate nutritional intake is needed not just to ensure adequate growth but also to help reduce postoperative morbidity (Schwarz, Gewitz, & See, 1990). Formula should be concentrated, and feeders with soft nipples should be used to facilitate nursing. Increasing carbohydrates, specifically in the form of **glucose polymers,** is recommended because carbohydrates are beneficial to stressed heart muscle (Jackson & Poskitt, 1991; Poskitt, 1993; Tripp, 1989). Infant rice cereal (1 tablespoon per 60 cubic centimeters of formula) has been used to increase the caloric density of the formula (Schwarz et al., 1990; see also Chapter 6). The caloric needs of infants who have CHD should be calculated on ideal (median weight for the infant's length) rather than actual body weight (Menon & Poskitt, 1985). **Nasogastric** feedings may be given either as **bolus** or as slow, continuous feedings (Barton, Hindmarsh, Scrimgeour, Rennie, & Preece, 1994). In one study, only continuous 24-hour nasogastric alimentation achieved intake of over 140 kilocalories per kilogram (kcal/kg) per day and improvement in weight and length, when compared with oral feedings with or without 12-hour nasogastric infusions (Schwarz et al., 1990). The use of gastrostomy tube–feeding for infants with cardiac problems has not been evaluated to date.

PULMONARY DISORDERS

Disorders that involve the lungs and respiratory tract can affect growth. The mechanisms by which pulmonary disturbances alter growth are similar to the mechanisms that are involved in cardiac disease. Hypoxia, increased energy needs, and increased energy expenditures are three of the more prominent factors by which growth is impaired in the presence of pulmonary disease. Some of the most common pulmonary conditions are discussed next.

Bronchopulmonary Dysplasia

One of the most common lung conditions that may be associated with poor growth is bronchopulmonary dysplasia (BPD). BPD is a condition of impaired pulmonary function, which develops in about 15%–20% of neonates who are admitted to neonatal intensive care units (NICUs) and who require assisted ventilation (Abman & Groothius, 1994). The condition develops in infants who have been born prematurely and who have experienced respiratory difficulties during the neonatal period.

BPD is characterized by the following three findings when present in an infant who is older than 4 weeks of age: 1) persistent supplemental oxygen requirement to maintain adequate oxygen saturation, 2) a characteristic chest X-ray, and 3) clinical manifestations of respiratory distress (e.g., **tachypnea,** retractions). In addition to tachypnea, affected infants may have abnormal lung findings on physical examination, such as **rhonchi** or **wheezes,** as well as **intercostal retractions** and an increased **anteroposterior** size. Some of these children will require medications to manage their pulmonary disease. The most common medications used include bronchodilators (e.g., theophylline), diuretics (e.g., furosemide), and corticosteroids.

Etiology of Growth Impairment

The etiology of growth impairment of infants with BPD is multifactorial. Premature infants may have low weight and length related to their prematurity. As a rule, age must be corrected when plotting the measurements of a premature infant on a growth curve (see Chapter 10). Catch-up growth should have occurred by 18 months for head circumference, 24 months for weight, and 40 months for length. Conditions other than BPD also may complicate the postnatal course of a premature infant. Neurological problems from **intra-**

ventricular hemorrhage or perinatal hypoxia may lead to the subsequent development of **cerebral palsy** (see Chapter 14).

Pulmonary disease also may affect growth. Infants with BPD expend extra energy in breathing and often require an increased intake to ensure a normal rate of growth. Hypoxia has a profound effect on the growth of the infant with BPD (Groothius & Rosenberg, 1987; Pinney & Cotton, 1978). Medications, such as bronchodilators and diuretics, may alter appetite and lead to decreased intake. **Hypokalemic alkalosis,** a side effect of some diuretics, also serves to suppress the appetite. Other side effects, such as gastrointestinal symptoms (e.g., vomiting, diarrhea, abdominal pain), also may affect food intake. Some infants who have BPD are fluid restricted as a means of minimizing the risk of pulmonary **edema.** Fluid restriction often results in calorie restriction. The work of breathing may interfere with the task of eating. Parents may report that their infants become fatigued during eating and that they therefore have a low intake. Chronic **endotracheal intubation** may be associated with a decreased ability to suck. Some infants who have BPD also may experience GER, which impairs their growth (see Chapter 11).

Management

The challenge for the health care provider is to diagnose any underlying associated conditions that are related to prematurity, to treat the BPD appropriately, and to maximize the nutrition of the infant. It also is important to keep in mind the psychosocial factors that may play a role. Premature infants, particularly those who have spent extended periods of time in a NICU, separated from their parents, are at increased risk for child abuse and neglect (see Chapter 31).

The nutritional management of the infant who has BPD necessitates the delivery of calorie-dense feedings. These can be accomplished through the use of specially prepared formulas, including those that have a lower sodium load. Alternatively, regular infant formula can be prepared to be more concentrated (usually to 24 calories per ounce [cal/oz]) simply by using more formula and less water (three scoops of powdered formula to 5 oz of water, or 13 oz of liquid formula to $8\frac{1}{2}$ oz of water). The addition of glucose polymers or infant rice cereal also may increase the caloric density of the formula. Nasogastric feedings have not been recommended routinely for the management of impaired growth that is associated with BPD. Vitamins, zinc, and iron therapy should be included in the dietary management.

Other Pulmonary Conditions

In addition to BPD, other pulmonary conditions may be associated with growth impairments. Three of these conditions are asthma, cystic fibrosis, and deformities of the chest wall. Children who have asthma and chest wall deformities, like those who have BPD, may already have been diagnosed, and the question will be which factors are contributing to their poor growth. It is important to note that not all children who have these conditions will experience impaired growth. Children who have cystic fibrosis, however, may present with growth impairment and a chronic cough, and the challenge will be for the physician to make the correct diagnosis and institute appropriate management.

Asthma

Children who have asthma exhibit symptoms of a variable degree. Some children are relatively asymptomatic, experiencing one to two episodes of wheezing per year. Other children are symptomatic most of the time. Most children who have asthma do not exhibit growth impairment, although delay in puberty and growth is considered a feature of asthma

(Ferguson, Murray, & Tze, 1982; Hauspie, Susanne, & Alexander, 1967; Murray, Fraser, Hardwick, & Pirie, 1976; Spock, 1965). Children who develop asthma before age 3 years are more likely to exhibit growth impairment (Murray et al., 1976). Some children who have asthma also may have food allergies (see Chapter 16).

The medications that are used to treat asthma seldom reduce appetite. Prednisone, in fact, may increase appetite but may lead to stunted late prepubertal growth (Balfour-Lynn, 1986; Crowley, Hindmarsh, Matthews, & Brook, 1995; Ninan & Russell, 1992).

Cystic Fibrosis

Cystic fibrosis is an **autosomal recessive inherited disorder** that occurs with variable frequencies in different ethnic populations. The major defect in cystic fibrosis is the impaired ability to move sodium and chloride across the cell membrane. The clinical features of cystic fibrosis are multiple and include respiratory problems, **sinusitis, nasal polyps,** gastrointestinal disturbances including **meconium ileus** and rectal prolapse, **pancreatic insufficiency** with **malabsorption** and malnutrition, diabetes (reported in 8%–12% of individuals who reach 16–20 years of age), and **cirrhosis** of the liver (Colin & Wohl, 1994). Cystic fibrosis is suspected in the child with chronic cough and recurrent respiratory infections, especially when growth is poor. The child who is suspected of having cystic fibrosis usually is evaluated with a sweat test, a procedure in which sweat is collected and analyzed for sodium chloride level.

Etiology of Growth Impairment

Growth impairment in children who have cystic fibrosis is reported to be the most common feature of the disease in infancy and in childhood. Pancreatic insufficiency occurs in about 85% of patients who have cystic fibrosis and is a major contributing factor to poor growth. Low oxygen levels from chronic lung impairment also impair growth and affect both weight gain and stature. Studies of infants who had presymptomatic cystic fibrosis have shown that these infants have normal energy expenditure (Bronstein, Davies, Hambridge, & Accurso, 1995).

Management of Growth Impairment

The management of cystic fibrosis involves a three-pronged approach: promoting normal growth and good nutrition, minimizing the development of lung disease, and preventing and managing other complications such as **esophageal varices** (Colin & Wohl, 1994).

Pancreatic enzyme replacement is essential to help normalize nutrition because the child does not have normal digestive abilities. Fat-soluble vitamins should be taken throughout the individual's life. The aim should be to maintain the body mass index (see Chapter 10) at close to the 50th percentile. To do this, caloric intake of 120%–150% of that recommended for a normal child has been suggested (Hubbard & Mangrum, 1982). Newer recommendations suggest that the daily energy requirement for the child who has cystic fibrosis is the same as for a healthy, normal child if growth is normal and there is minimal loss of fat in the stools (Ramsey, Farrell, & Pencharz, 1992). The logical approach to growth and nutrition for the child who has cystic fibrosis is to monitor growth and adjust caloric intake accordingly. Other treatment modalities are aimed at reducing the risk of lung disease (Knowles et al., 1990; Ramsey et al., 1993).

Chest Wall Deformities

Chest wall deformities may develop on their own or because of another condition, such as **diaphragmatic hernia.** Although some chest wall deformities are believed not to be of clinical significance, others may impair pulmonary or cardiac function. The evaluation of affected children includes an ECG, chest X-ray, and, when appropriate, an echocardiogram. Pulmonary function studies also should be obtained (see Chapter 14).

Some children have a more global genetic syndrome, and the chest wall deformity represents just one component of the disorder. The presence of one major congenital **anomaly** suggests the possibility of other major or minor anomalies, and a careful physical examination should be conducted to determine whether any syndrome is present (see Chapter 14).

The management for children who experience poor growth and chest wall deformities is to ensure adequate pulmonary functioning. Sometimes, surgical intervention is needed to accomplish this. Optimum nutritional intake should be maintained.

Undiagnosed Pulmonary Conditions

Some children who experience poor growth have not been diagnosed with any predisposing pulmonary condition. A thorough history might raise the possibility of an underlying pulmonary complaint. Suspicion of an underlying pulmonary disorder would be raised by a history of chronic cough, wheezing or recurrent pulmonary infections, or other symptoms. For instance, children who have cystic fibrosis may have large, foul-smelling stools, rectal prolapse, or jaundice. Persistent cough, as is seen in young infants who have **pertussis,** may be associated with poor weight gain. Cough, as well as post-tussive emesis (vomiting after coughing), may persist for several months following pertussis infection. Chronic cough may be secondary to GER and intermittent aspiration (see Chapter 11). Cough in association with growth impairment also may be seen in children who are infected with the human immunodeficiency virus (HIV) (see Chapter 13).

The physical assessment of children who experience impaired growth should include a determination of the respiratory rate (which may be elevated in the presence of lung disease), an examination of the lungs for the presence of abnormal breath sounds (such as wheezes or **rales**), and an assessment of the anteroposterior diameter of the chest and chest configuration. The examiner also should look for clubbing. The presence of dysmorphic features might suggest a genetic syndrome, with lung disease as one component. The presence of jaundice is suggestive of some conditions including alpha-1-antitrypsin deficiency or cystic fibrosis. Alpha-1-antitrypsin deficiency is an inherited disorder in which the protein that prevents certain enzymes from working is deficient. Individuals develop pulmonary disease as well as cirrhosis of the liver.

Diagnostic studies to be considered include a chest X-ray, sweat chloride, and pulmonary function studies. Pulse oximetry is a noninvasive procedure to determine whether the patient is **hypoxemic.** Cultures may be indicated if the patient appears to have a chronic infection. Levels of alpha-1-antitrypsin are indicated in the child with jaundice as a component of his or her clinical picture.

DISORDERS OF THE HEAD AND NECK

Growth impairment may occur secondary to disturbances in the head and neck region. Such disturbances may be congenital or acquired.

Cleft Lip and Palate

Multiple factors impair the growth of children with **clefts of the lip and palate** (Bowers et al., 1988; Duncan, Shapiro, Soley, & Turet, 1983; Kaufman, 1991). Foremost are problems related to feeding and inadequate food intake. These difficulties are especially common during the first few weeks of life. The birth of a child with an obvious facial anomaly is particularly stressful and may challenge parents' ability to cope (Kaufman, 1991). Children with clefts are particularly prone to otitis media, and this also may impair their growth. In addition, the cleft may be just one component of a genetic syndrome that includes growth impairment (Suslak & Desposito, 1988). Increased incidence of growth hormone deficiency has been reported in children with clefts (Rudman et al., 1978).

Specialty care is best provided by a team that includes a pediatrician, plastic surgeon, audiologist, dentist, speech-language pathologist or occupational therapist, and ear, nose, and throat (ENT) physician. Management is directed at correcting the cleft through surgical repair. Repair of palatal clefts usually is carried out at about 12–18 months of age. Until that time, management consists of facilitating feeding through the use of special nipples and plastic bottles that are especially designed for feeding infants with clefts (Clarren, Anderson, & Wolf, 1987). Otitis media should be managed with antibiotics. Pressure equalization tubes (PETs) are indicated when ear infections have been recurrent. Concentrated formula (24 cal/oz) also should be used. The addition of cereal, **MCT oil,** or glucose polymers also may be helpful (see Chapter 6).

Recurrent Infections of the Head and Neck

Chronic or recurrent infections of the head and neck may impair growth by interfering with the child's ability to eat. Otitis media is one of the most common problems of childhood and is reported to have a prevalence of 15%–20%. The peak age of occurrence is 6–36 months of age, with a second peak occurring between the ages of 4 and 6 years (Sifuentes, 1996). Acute bouts of otitis may have a transient impact on growth, particularly weight gain. Recurrent infections, especially when associated with fever and ear pain, may affect long-term weight gain and result in wasting. It is important to keep in mind that recurrent otitis may be related to some underlying condition, such as a craniofacial anomaly including subtle ones such as a **submucous palatal cleft** (Berera, 1993), immunodeficiency syndromes, and disorders related to **ciliary motility.** In the last two cases infections also may be present in other areas, such as the respiratory tract. Infections of the throat also may recur on a chronic basis and impair a child's ability to eat.

Although decreased intake is the major reason for growth impairment in association with infections of the throat or ears, other factors also may contribute to the growth problem. Fever may lead to a **hypermetabolic state** so that even when intake seemingly is adequate, it might not meet the heightened caloric requirements. In addition, there may be increased nutritional losses through vomitus or stool (Granot, Matoth, & Feinmesser, 1990; Sifuentes, 1996). It is not uncommon for infants with otitis media to experience the symptoms of secondary gastroenteritis in conjunction with a bout of otitis media.

The medical management of otitis media includes obtaining a careful medical history to determine whether there are factors that may be contributing to the infant's predisposition to recurrent ear infections. In any infant with failure to thrive and recurrent infections, concern about an immunodeficiency condition, including infection with HIV, is not unreasonable (see Chapter 13). Other environmental conditions also may predispose the infant to ear infections. Although breast-feeding is noted to be protective, parental smoking, child care attendance, and bottle propping are associated with a higher incidence of otitis media (Bluestone & Klein, 1988).

The physical examination would provide the answer to whether otitis media is present. Examination may reveal **erythema,** pus behind the eardrum, distorted landmarks, and decreased mobility. Documentation of tympanic membrane dysfunction can be obtained through the use of a **tympanogram.** Other diagnostic studies usually are not indicated unless the child has failed antibiotic therapy and there is concern about the presence of an unusual **pathogen** in the middle ear. In such cases, a diagnostic **tympanocentesis** can be performed. Similarly, children with recurrent sore throats should be evaluated with throat cultures.

The mainstay of medical management is the use of appropriate antibiotics. In general, appetite improves and vomiting and diarrhea cease once the infection is under control. Weight gain then resumes along the expected curve. Unfortunately, some infants develop new infections before they have fully recovered their weight. There are two approaches to the long-term management of recurrent otitis media (Teele, 1991). One involves the use of prophylactic antibiotics, whereby children are maintained on a protracted course of medication in an effort to suppress any smoldering infection. The other approach to recurrent otitis media is surgical and involves the placement of PETs. Such tubes are particularly useful in patients with craniofacial anomalies in which there is documentable **Eustachian tube dysfunction.**

In addition to these intervention strategies, nutritional intake should be ensured. Infants with otitis media frequently are reluctant to feed from a bottle because increased pressure is experienced in the middle ear during sucking. In fact, refusal to suck may be the first sign of an ear infection. Some infants respond to being fed from a spoon or a syringe during their acute illness. In general, the prognosis for normal growth and stature is excellent once the children have their otitis managed or are no longer at an age when they are predisposed to such types of infections.

Tonsillar Hypertrophy and Upper-Airway Obstruction

Most children who are experiencing problems related to tonsillar and adenoid hypertrophy and upper-airway obstruction present with complaints related to snoring, sleep **apnea,** or daytime drowsiness (Deutsch & Isaacson, 1995). Some of these children will be obese. There is, however, a subset of children with tonsillar hypertrophy who present with growth impairment, particularly with wasting (Everett, Koch, & Saulsbury, 1987; Rains, 1995; Singer & Saenger, 1990). In some children, the mechanism of growth impairment has been related to mechanical difficulties with eating and swallowing. Sometimes there is the complaint of choking or of vomiting food that has been only partially chewed. Intermittent reduction of oxygen and elevation of carbon dioxide have been reported in some affected children (Schiffman, Faber, & Eidelman, 1985; Southall et al., 1989). Reduced levels of oxygen impair growth (Page et al., 1978).

Mouth breathing and noisy respiration usually are noted. On physical examination, tonsillar hypertrophy (marked enlargement) may be readily apparent. Often, the tonsils are described as "kissing," meeting in the midline. The child may have an open bite and be a mouth breather, a sign that adenoid hypertrophy also is present. Occasionally, **serous otitis media** may be an associated finding.

Although suggested management would be removal of the tonsils and adenoids, documentation of their negative effect on the child's health may be required. Studies to assess this effect would include an ECG to determine whether there are signs of right heart strain from the airway obstruction, as well as overnight studies in a sleep laboratory to determine whether sleep apnea is present. Children with documented recurrent infections of the ears or tonsils, sleep apnea, or signs of right heart strain should be referred to an ENT specialist. **Tonsillectomy,** often in association with **adenoidectomy,** frequently results in dramatic improvement in these children. Improved appetite, food intake, and weight gain rapidly follow after surgical removal of the hypertrophied tissues.

Airway obstruction also may be associated with laryngomalacia. This condition occurs when the tissues above the opening to the windpipe, in the area around the vocal cords, are floppy or redundant. As a result, the infant manifests noisy respirations that are referred to as *stridor*. Although many such affected infants experience no problems with their growth and their symptoms resolve without medical intervention, a number of infants with laryngomalacia have feeding difficulties and poor weight gain (Kavanagh & Babin, 1987). There also is an association between laryngomalacia and gastroesophageal reflux, which can predispose to growth impairment (Belmont & Grundfast, 1984). Infants with symptomatic laryngomalacia may respond dramatically to surgical correction and demonstrate accelerated growth after an operative repair of the larynx.

CONCLUSION

Conditions that involve the heart and lungs and the head and neck areas may interfere with normal growth. Certain conditions are congenital, whereas others are acquired. Occult conditions require a careful history and physical examination to detect their presence and institute an appropriate treatment plan.

REFERENCES

Abman, S.H., & Groothius, J.R. (1994). Pathophysiology and treatment of bronchopulmonary dysplasia. *Pediatric Clinics of North America, 41,* 277–315.

Balfour-Lynn, L. (1986). Growth and childhood asthma. *Archives of Disease in Childhood, 61,* 1049–1055.

Barton, J.S., Hindmarsh, P.C., Scrimgeour, C.M., Rennie, M.J., & Preece, M.A. (1994). Energy expenditure in congenital heart disease. *Archives of Disease in Childhood, 70,* 5–9.

Baum, D., & Stern, M.P. (1977). Adipose hypocellularity in cyanotic congenital heart disease. *Circulation, 55,* 916–920.

Belmont, J.R., & Grundfast, K. (1984). Congenital laryngeal stridor (laryngomalacia): Etiologic factors and associated disorders. *Annals of Otology, Rhinology and Laryngology, 93,* 430–437.

Berera, G. (1993). Index of suspicion: Submucous cleft palate. *Pediatric Review, 14,* 191–192.

Bluestone, C.D., & Klein, J.O. (1988). *Otitis media in infants and children.* Philadelphia: W.B. Saunders.

Bowers, E., Mayro, R., Whitaker, L., Pasquariello, P.S., Larossa, D., & Randall, P. (1988). General body growth in children with cleft palate and related disorders: Age differences. *American Journal of Physiological Anthropology, 75,* 503–515.

Bronstein, M.N., Davies, P.S.W., Hambridge, K.M., & Accurso, F.J. (1995). Normal energy expenditure in the infant with presymptomatic cystic fibrosis. *Journal of Pediatrics, 126,* 28–33.

Cameron, J.W., Rosenthal, A., & Olson, A.D. (1995). Malnutrition in hospitalized children with congenital heart disease. *Archives of Pediatric and Adolescent Medicine, 149,* 1098–1102.

Cheek, D.B., Grastone, J.E., & Rowe, R.D. (1969). Hypoxia and malnutrition in newborn rats: Effects of RNA, DNA and protein in tissues. *American Journal of Physiology, 217,* 64–65.

Clarren, S., Anderson, B., & Wolf, L. (1987). Feeding infants with cleft lip, cleft palate, or cleft lip and palate. *Cleft Palate Journal, 24,* 244–249.

Colin, A.A., & Wohl, M.E.B. (1994). Cystic fibrosis. *Pediatric Review, 15,* 193–200.

Crowley, S., Hindmarsh, P.C., Matthews, D.R., & Brook, C.G.D. (1995). Growth and the growth hormone axis in prepubertal children with asthma. *Journal of Pediatrics, 126,* 297–303.

Deutsch, E.S., & Isaacson, G.C. (1995). Tonsils and adenoids: An update. *Pediatric Review, 16,* 17–21.

Duncan, P., Shapiro, L., Soley, R., & Turet, S.E. (1983). Linear growth patterns in patients with cleft lip or palate or both. *American Journal of Diseases of Children, 137,* 159–163.

Everett, A.D., Koch, W.C., & Saulsbury, F.T. (1987). Failure to thrive due to obstructive sleep apnea. *Clinical Pediatrics, 26,* 90–92.

Ferguson, A.C., Murray, A.B., & Tze, W.J. (1982). Short stature and delayed skeletal maturation in children with allergic disease. *Journal of Allergy and Clinical Immunology, 69,* 461–466.

Fyler, C.D., Rothman, K.J., & Buckley, L.P. (1982). Long term prognosis of the surgical treatment of congenital heart disease. *Transactions of Association of Life Insurance of Medical Directors of America, 65,* 101–118.

Gingell, R.L., & Hornung, M.G. (1989). Growth problems associated with congenital heart disease in infancy. In E. Lebenthal (Ed.), *Testbook of gastroenterology and nutrition in infancy* (pp. 639–649). New York: Raven Press.

Granot, E., Matoth, I., & Feinmesser, R. (1990). Chronic middle ear effusion—A possible cause of protracted vomiting and failure to thrive in infancy. *Clinical Pediatrics, 29,* 722–724.

Groothius, J.R., & Rosenberg, A.A. (1987). Home oxygen promotes weight gain in infants with BPD. *AJDC, 141,* 992–995.

Hauspie, R., Susanne, C., & Alexander, F. (1967). Maturational delay and temporal retardation in asthmatic boys. *Journal of Allergy and Clinical Immunology, 59,* 200–206.

Hubbard, V.S., & Mangrum, P.J. (1982). Energy intake and nutrition counseling in cystic fibrosis. *Journal of the American Dietetic Association, 80,* 127–131.

Jackson, M., & Poskitt, E.M. (1991). The effects of high-energy feeding on energy balance and growth in infants with congenital disease and failure to thrive. *British Journal of Nutrition, 65,* 131–143.

Kappy, M. (1987). Regulation of growth in children with chronic illness: Therapeutic implication for the year 2000. *AJDC, 141,* 489–493.

Kaufman, F.L. (1991). Managing the cleft lip and palate patient. *Pediatric Clinics of North America, 38,* 1127–1147.

Kavanagh, K.T., & Babin, R.W. (1987). Endoscopic surgical management for laryngomalacia: Case report and review of the literature. *Annals of Otology, Rhinology and Laryngology, 96,* 650–653.

Knowles, M.R., Church, N.L., Waltner, W.E., Yankaskas, J.R., Gilligan, P., King, M., Edwards, L.J., Helms, R.W., & Boucher, R.C. (1990). A pilot study of aerosolized amiloride for the treatment of lung disease in cystic fibrosis. *New England Journal of Medicine, 322,* 1189–1194.

Levy, R.J., Rosenthal, A., Fyler, D.C., & Nadas, A.S. (1978). Birthweight of infants with congenital heart disease. *American Journal of Diseases of Children, 132,* 249–254.

Levy, R.J., Rosenthal, A., Miettinen, O.S., & Nadas, S. (1977). Determinants of growth in patients with ventricular septal defect. *Circulation, 57,* 793–797.

Mehziri, A., & Drash, A. (1962). Growth disturbance in congenital heart disease. *Journal of Pediatrics, 61,* 418–429.

Menon, G., & Poskitt, E.M. (1985). Why does congenital heart disease cause failure to thrive? *Archives of Disease in Childhood, 60,* 1134–1139.

Murray, A.B., Fraser, B.M., Hardwick, D.F., & Pirie, G.E. (1976). Chronic asthma and growth failure in children. *The Lancet, 2,* 197–198.

Neill, C.A. (1982). Congenital heart disease: Hemodynamic growth retardation. In P.J. Accardo (Ed.), *Failure to thrive in infancy and early childhood* (pp. 169–178). Baltimore: University Park Press.

Ninan, T., & Russell, G. (1992). Asthma, inhaled corticosteroid treatment, and growth. *Archives of Disease in Childhood, 67,* 703–705.

Page, R.E., Dervall, P.B., Watson, D.A., & Scott, O. (1978). Height and weight gain after total correction of Fallot's tetralogy. *British Heart Journal, 40,* 416–420.

Pinney, M.A., & Cotton, E.K. (1978). Home management of BPD. *Pediatrics, 61,* 856–859.

Pittman, J.G., & Cohen, P. (1964). The pathogenesis of cardiac cachexia. *New England Journal of Medicine, 271,* 403–409.

Poskitt, E.M. (1993). Failure to thrive in congenital heart disease. *Archives of Disease in Childhood, 68,* 158–160.

Rains, J.C. (1995). Treatment of obstructive sleep apnea in pediatric patients. *Clinical Pediatrics, 34,* 535–541.

Ramsey, B.W., Astley, S.J., Aitken, M.L., Burke, W., Colin, A.A., Dorkin, H.L., Eisenberg, J.D., Gibson, R.L., Harwood, I.R., & Schidlow, D.V. (1993). Efficacy and safety of short term administration of aerosolized recombinant human deoxyribonuclease in patients with cystic fibrosis (CF). *American Review of Respiratory Disease, 148,* 145–151.

Ramsey, B.W., Farrell, P.M., & Pencharz, P. (1992). Nutritional assessment and management in cystic fibrosis: A consensus report. *American Journal of Clinical Nutrition, 55,* 108–116.

Rudman, D., Davis, T., Priest, J., Patterson, S.H., Kutner, M.H., Heymsfield, S.B., & Bethel, R.A. (1978). Prevalence of growth hormone deficiency in children with cleft lip or palate. *Journal of Pediatrics, 93,* 378–382.

Schiffmann, R., Faber, J., & Eidelman, A.I. (1985). Obstructive hypertrophic adenoids and tonsils as a cause of infantile failure to thrive: Reversed by tonsillectomy and adenoidectomy. *International Journal of Pediatric Otorhinolaryngology, 9,* 183–187.

Schwarz, S.M., Gewitz, M.H., & See, C.C. (1990). Enteral nutrition in infants with congenital heart disease and growth failure. *Pediatrics, 3,* 368–373.

Sifuentes, M. (1996). Otitis media. In C.D. Berkowitz (Ed.), *Pediatrics: A primary care approach* (pp. 176–181). Philadelphia: W.B. Saunders.

Singer, L.P., & Saenger, P. (1990). Complications of pediatric obstructive sleep apnea. *Otolaryngologic Clinics of North America, 23,* 665–676.

Southall, D.P., Croft, C.B., Stebbens, V.A., Ibrahim, H., Gurney, A., Buchdahl, R., & Warner, J.O. (1989). Detection of sleep-associated dysfunctional pharyngeal obstruction in infants. *European Journal of Pediatrics, 148,* 353–359.

Spock, A. (1965). Growth patterns in 200 children with bronchial asthma. *Annals of Allergy, 23,* 608–615.

Suslak, L., & Desposito, F. (1988). Infants with cleft lip/cleft palate. *Pediatric Review, 9,* 331–334.

Teele, D.W. (1991). Strategies to control recurrent otitis media in infants and children. *Pediatric Annals, 20,* 609–616.

Tripp, M.E. (1989). Developmental cardiac metabolism in health and disease. *Pediatric Cardiology, 10,* 150–158.

White, R.I., Jr., Jordan, C.E., Fischer, K.C., Dorst, J.P., Nagy, J.M., Garn, S.M., & Neill, C.A. (1971). Delayed skeletal growth and maturation in adolescent congenital heart disease. *Investigative Radiology, 6,* 326–332.

Chapter 13

Infectious Disease and Nutrition

Harland S. Winter and James Oleske

The interaction between humans and microbes is a complex relationship that begins before birth and continues for a lifetime. Most bacteria that reside in and on the human body contribute to health. Bacteria that inhabit the gastrointestinal tract break down foods and provide additional nutrition. In the newborn, the breakdown of **lactose** by bacteria in the colon is an important source of energy. Health is maintained by a complex interaction between bacteria and the immune system. Changes in **immune function** or microbial virulence can alter this balance. Because host and infectious agents depend on the same source of nutrition for survival, a symbiotic relationship has evolved between host and normal flora. Excesses or deficiencies of almost every known macronutrient or micronutrient can impair the body's ability to control infection. Conversely, infection alters nutritional status, which causes deficiencies that may enhance the survival of the microbe. This interrelationship among microbes, nutrition, and immune function usually is in balance; but when perturbed by infectious disease, undernutrition, or **immunodeficiency,** the entire cycle is affected and altered growth or illness results.

IMMUNE FUNCTION AND UNDERNUTRITION

Undernutrition impairs the ability of the immune system to respond to **pathogens.** The earlier that undernutrition occurs in life, the greater the impact on the developing immune system. Among low birth weight infants, weight for gestational age may reflect prenatal nutrition. Undernutrition in the infant who is small for gestational age can result in decreased numbers of lymphocytes and impaired immune function that can persist for many months after birth. In contrast, the infant who is appropriate for gestational age frequently recovers immune function by 3 months of age. These observations support the hypothesis that nutrition rather than gestational age is an important element of immune development (Chandra, 1981).

At every age, protein-energy malnutrition (PEM) contributes to one's susceptibility to infections by depressing immune function. For many reasons, adults, as well as children, who are undernourished acquire more frequent infections and have a longer course of illness. Although antibody production is relatively preserved in adults, malnourished children may not make antibodies after immunizations and may not react appropriately to skin tests such as that for tuberculosis; thus, the ability to prevent an infection or to respond to a pathogen is impaired. In chronically undernourished children, studies are ongoing to determine whether specific replacement with vitamin A may enhance immune function in individuals with vitamin A deficiency (Semba et al., 1993) and correct other immunological abnormalities (Lie, Ying, Wang, Brun, & Geissler, 1993).

In addition to PEM, specific nutrient deficiencies, such as zinc, may affect a child's response to vaccinations. Other micronutrient deficiencies, such as vitamin C, vitamin E, B-complex vitamins, iron, selenium, copper, magnesium, and beta-carotene, can reduce the ability of white blood cells to fight infection; however, care should be taken with nutritional replacement therapy. For example, excessive zinc, provided in infant formula, can compete with copper absorption and induce copper deficiency. Because children rarely have a single defined nutrient deficiency, supplementation with single nutrients may be ineffective and possibly hazardous to immune function. Maintaining balanced diets that are appropriate for calories, protein, fat, carbohydrates, micronutrients, and vitamins will prevent and reverse most nutritionally induced immunological dysfunction.

ACUTE INFECTION AND UNDERNUTRITION

The reasons for undernutrition in a child with an acute illness may be difficult to identify. Most children with an acute infectious disease will decrease their caloric intake because of anorexia. For the child with normal nutrition, a sudden, short-term decrease in caloric intake is compensated by the use of stored **glycogen** and fat. After depleting **hepatic glycogen** and fat stores, muscle mass will be utilized for energy. Some acute infections, such as recurrent otitis media, may not affect nutritional status unless they are associated with an underlying immune deficiency. Recurrent pneumonia, chronic sinusitis, or chronic diarrhea most commonly are thought to be associated with immunodeficiency. These conditions or a persistent decrease in weight-for-height, especially in an infant or young child, should be a tip-off for a possible deficiency in immune function. Most children with frequent ear infections grow normally, but some will be undernourished only because they do not consume enough calories. Some viral infections, such as **herpetic stomatitis,** cause oral lesions that make swallowing painful and result in decreased caloric intake. Altered mental status in a child also can result in decreased caloric intake; however, the most common reason for a child with an acute illness to lose weight is a combination of decreased caloric intake and fever. The metabolic impact of fever not only increases **resting energy requirements** but also causes levels of micronutrients such as iron and zinc to decrease in the serum and be sequestered in the liver, bone marrow, and **reticuloendothelial system.** This creates a functional deficiency. Replacing these nutrients may not be beneficial in the acute setting. For example, although iron-containing compounds may impair growth of some bacteria, iron supplementation may increase the growth of other bacteria (Bullen, Rogers, & Leigh, 1972).

Increased losses of nutrients most commonly occur in diarrheal states, which may be prolonged in the child who has a chronic illness. Infectious agents that cause bacterial

dysentery, viral gastroenteritis, and parasitic diseases frequently result in intestinal injury and **malabsorption.** The intestine loses its ability to absorb nutrients, which makes malnutrition worse. Vomiting also may occur but usually resolves within 24 hours of the onset of illness. For immigrant families, diarrheal illnesses may cause anxiety and concern for the child's well-being. In many developing countries, diarrheal illness is associated with death. Many first-generation immigrant families will know of family members or friends who have had children die from diarrheal disease. In the United States, an adequately nourished infant who lives in an environment with clean water and good sanitation will have an excellent chance of total recovery. Clinicians who care for children of immigrants should be sensitive and anticipate the concerns of the family. Acknowledging their apprehensions while reassuring them that the differences in nutritional status will help with recovery will alleviate anxiety. Respecting cultural diversity and how immigrant parents may interpret nutritional intervention for acute diarrheal illnesses is an important aspect of care.

CHRONIC INFECTION AND UNDERNUTRITION

Chronic illnesses such as **cystic fibrosis** (CF) (see Chapter 12) and acquired immunodeficiency syndrome (AIDS) are associated with chronic and recurrent infections. In CF, recurrent acute pulmonary infections evolve into chronic illnesses. Children who are infected with the human immunodeficiency virus (HIV) develop **sino-pulmonary** and gastrointestinal disease, either of which ultimately may impair nutritional status. Treatment of nutritional problems in the child with chronic infections requires a multidisciplinary approach that is best illustrated by using AIDS as the example.

As of December 1997, the Centers for Disease Control and Prevention have received 8,086 reports from the United States of AIDS in children younger than 13 years (Centers for Disease Control and Prevention, 1997). During this same time period, the **pandemic** has reached even greater magnitude throughout the world. Estimates are that 8.8 million women and 800,000 children have AIDS and that 1.3 million children already have died (Joint United Nations Programme on HIV/AIDS, 1996). Although transmission from mother to infant can be reduced with perinatal **antiretroviral** treatment, many HIV-exposed infants become infected (Connor et al., 1994). In regions of the world where prenatal care and medication are not available easily, transmission rates are not affected.

Failure to thrive is an ill-defined term that is used in different contexts to describe a child who is not growing. Usually, clinicians mean that a child is not gaining weight at the expected rate and that the weight for height is lower than the 10th percentile. Prolonged undernutrition that results in decreased weight-for-height eventually will cause stunting of linear growth. In contrast, children with short stature from genetic or endocrine causes will, in general, have increased weight-for-height. Thus, undernutrition that is associated with chronic infections such as HIV or CF will be characterized by a decline in weight percentiles followed by fall off in linear growth. Declines in linear growth that are not preceded by a decreased ratio of weight for height may be related to other factors.

With AIDS, failure to gain weight is a widely recognized problem in the young child, whereas short stature is a common observation in long-term survivors. **Candida** infections can cause undernutrition because painful swallowing limits intake, but other disorders characterized by **hepatosplenomegaly,** pneumonia, and diarrhea may cause undernutrition because of increased metabolic demands or losses of nutrients. In children who are not infected with HIV and whose weight-for-height is normal, mortality is 0.5%, whereas in children whose weight-for-height is decreased, mortality increases to more than 18% (Scrimshaw, Taylor, & Gordon, 1968). For these and many other reasons, appropriate nutrition is a fundamental and necessary part of a child's medical therapy. Preliminary observations suggest that wasting and gastrointestinal disorders contribute significantly to mortality in children who are infected with HIV.

Because of these multiple effects, nutritional support should be an integral part of the transdisciplinary approach to management of children and parents who are infected with HIV. The nutritional status of the nurturing parent may play a role in the health of the child and cannot be neglected when creating a family care plan. Social workers, nurses, mental health workers, nutritionists, and physicians bring a special expertise to the care of families with children who are infected with HIV. Socioeconomic conditions, such as availability of food and child care resources, also are factors in determining the success of nutritional intervention.

Recognition by health care providers of the important role that nutrition plays in the treatment of children with chronic disease should result in early nutritional intervention and anticipation of both clinical situations that impair nutrient availability, absorption, or utilization and psychosocial issues that affect nutritional assessment and intervention in underserved populations.

GUIDELINES FOR EVALUATING NUTRITIONAL STATUS

The evaluation of nutritional status depends on accurate measurements of growth, energy requirements, and caloric intake.

Longitudinal Assessment of Growth

The simplest measures for assessing a child's nutritional status are growth in weight, height, and head circumference. Parental stature as well as intrauterine growth, reflected by birth weight and length, play an important role in assessment. In the child with chronic infection, growth measurements should be standardized and made by the same individual at each visit. Height should be measured three times to ensure reliable measurements.

Estimating Energy Requirements

Adults with asymptomatic HIV infection have increased resting energy expenditure and total energy expenditure (Grunfeld et al., 1992; Hommes, Romijn, Endert, & Sauerwein, 1991), but extensive data are not available for children. Clinical experience suggests that energy requirements are normal during times of well-being but that the child who has HIV infection may not compensate for periods of stress (e.g., infection) when energy requirements are increased. Fever and inflammation may increase energy requirements further and potentiate undernutrition in an already compromised child.

The recommended dietary allowance (RDA) is the most easily obtainable measure of caloric needs. Alternatively, resting energy expenditure plus activity or stress factors (e.g., febrile illness) should be used to estimate energy needs. During times of stress, caloric requirements may increase to 150% of the RDA; therefore, energy needs of a child with recurrent infections that are associated with an immune deficiency, CF, or recurrent sinusitis will require increased calories to maintain normal growth. If this child also has impaired absorption or decreased oral intake, then the problem of undernutrition is amplified.

Evaluating Body Composition

Anthropometric measurements of arm circumference and skinfold thickness provide more reliable measures of body composition but may not be readily available. Precise measures of body composition using dual energy X-ray absorptiometry (**DEXA**) scans are most reliable but generally are not available except at research centers.

In most clinical situations, one can obtain an estimation of lean body mass from anthropometric measurements. Having a nutritionist as part of a multidisciplinary team will provide this expertise. Most normal children will lose fat mass in response to chronic undernutrition. Once fat reserves are depleted, loss of lean body mass occurs. Measuring arm circumference and triceps skinfold thickness enables the nutritionist to calculate lean body mass.

Estimating Caloric Intake

Use of either a 72-hour diet diary or a 24-hour diet recall is the best, albeit imperfect, tool available for estimating caloric intake. Estimation of caloric intake along with assessment of available food resources is an essential part of a complete evaluation (see Chapter 6). Determining caloric intake enables the team to assess whether the child is receiving sufficient caloric support to grow. Undernourished children who seem to eat sufficient calories to grow should be evaluated for malabsorption. If caloric intake is decreased, then access to food sources, pain with chewing or swallowing, and anorexia need to be considered. A diet history is beneficial for assessing the cause of undernutrition.

PREVENTION

For the child with chronic disease, preventing infection is the best strategy for enhancing nutritional status. In environments in which economic factors are the leading cause of undernutrition, economists, community leaders, and politicians can provide resources and access to food. When immunodeficiency contributes to recurrent infection, nutrients and medications that enhance immune function are the most beneficial. For families who have members who are infected with HIV, health care providers must provide information about the value of "safe" foods, such as well-cooked meat and eggs. This means that families should be educated about adequate refrigeration and appropriate food preparation (see Chapter 28). Although therapeutic interventions such as appetite stimulants and tube-feeding have resulted in increased weight for children who are infected with HIV, most of the gain has been in fat mass with little improvement in lean body mass and linear growth. In addition to the care of the undernourished child, the health and nutritional status of the nurturing parent may benefit the health of the child more directly.

Although AIDS is used as a model for undernutrition, any child with chronic infections or recurrent illness and who has parents who are unavailable is at risk for more severe undernutrition. The nurturing that is provided by a parent or other caregiver is essential for successful intervention.

TREATMENT

The goals of nutritional management for the child with chronic infection and undernutrition include treating underlying gastrointestinal or infectious diseases, such as **Mycobacterium avium intracellulare** or **cryptosporidiosis;** maintaining normal growth and development; providing sufficient nutrition for catch-up growth; preventing immunocompromise; and maintaining a sense of well-being to permit age-appropriate activities. Successfully integrating these goals into a comprehensive treatment plan requires the participation of an experienced pediatric nutritionist. **Enteral** supplements should be provided to increase nutrient intake by increasing the frequency of feedings, concentrating formulas, and using cream or whole milk (if the child is not lactose intolerant). Calorically dense foods such as fats, peanut butter, or cheese also increase calories. Close monitoring of growth will permit nutritional intervention to begin at a time when nutritional therapy may be beneficial in preventing sequelae of undernutrition. For children with chronic infections that cannot be eradicated, appetite stimulants result in weight gain by increasing fat mass, but lean body mass is not altered (Von Roenn et al., 1994). Similarly, tube-feeding may be beneficial in increasing weight but does not help lean body mass (Henderson et al., 1994). If prolonged tube-feeding is anticipated, then it can be provided by gastrostomy, which will not restrict normal activities (see Chapter 11). **Parenteral** feedings should be restricted to children who are unable to tolerate enteral feedings.

CONCLUSION

In North America, the relationship among undernutrition, immunity, and infection is most relevant for children with chronic disease. Strategies in addition to calorie- or nutrient-enhancing formulas may be needed to improve growth in children with chronic illness. The importance of a transdisciplinary approach to nutritional intervention and early detection of nutritional deficiencies may prevent long-term complications of undernutrition.

REFERENCES

Bullen, J.J., Rogers, H.J., & Leigh, L. (1972). Iron-binding proteins in milk and resistance to Escherichia coli infection in infants. *British Medical Journal, 1,* 69–75.

Centers for Disease Control and Prevention. (1997). HIV/AIDS Surveillance Report, 1997. *Morbidity and Mortality Weekly Report, 45*(46), 1005–1010.

Chandra, R.K. (1981). Serum thymic hormone activity and cell-mediated immunity in healthy neonatal, preterm infants and small-for-gestational age infants. *Pediatrics, 67,* 407.

Connor, E.M., Sperling, R.S., Gelber, R., Kiselev, P., Scott, G., et al. (1994). Reduction of maternal–infant transmission of human immunodeficiency virus type 1 with zidovudine treatment. *New England Journal of Medicine, 331,* 1173–1180.

Grunfeld, C., Pang, M., Shimizu, L., Shigenaga, J.K., Jensen, P., & Feingold, K.R. (1992). Resting energy expenditure, caloric intake, and short-term weight gain in human immunodeficiency virus infection and the acquired immunodeficiency syndrome. *American Journal of Clinical Nutrition, 55,* 455–460.

Henderson, R.A., Saavedra, J.M., Perman, J.A., Hutton, N., Livingston, R.A., & Yolken, R.H. (1994). Effect of enteral tube feeding on growth on children with symptomatic human immunodeficiency virus infection. *Journal of Pediatric Gastroenterology and Nutrition, 18,* 429–434.

Hommes, M.J.T., Romijn, J.A., Endert, E., & Sauerwein, H.P. (1991). Resting energy expenditure and substrate oxidation in human immunodeficiency virus (HIV)-infected asymptomatic men: HIV affects host metabolism in the early asymptomatic stage. *American Journal of Clinical Nutrition, 54,* 311–315.

Joint United Nations Programme on HIV/AIDS. (1996). *The HIV/AIDS situation in mid 1996: Global and regional highlights. Fact-sheet.* Geneva, Switzerland: World Health Organization.

Lie, C., Ying, C., Wang, E.L., Brun, T., & Geissler, C. (1993). Impact of large-dose vitamin A supplementation on childhood diarrhoea, respiratory disease and growth. *European Journal of Clinical Nutrition, 47,* 88–96.

Scrimshaw, N.S., Taylor, C.E., & Gordon, J.E. (1968). Interactions of nutrition and infection. *World Health Organization Monograph Series, 57.*

Semba, R.D., Ward, B.J., Griffin, D.E., Scott, A.L., Natadisastra, G., West, K.P., Jr., & Sommer, A. (1993). Abnormal T-cell subset proportions in vitamin deficient children. *The Lancet, 341,* 5–8.

Von Roenn, J.H., Armstrong, D., Kotler, D.P., Cohn, D.L., Klimas, N.G., Tchekmedyian, N.S., Cone, L., Brennan, P.J., & Weitzman, S.A. (1994). Megesterol acetate in patients with AIDS-related cachexia. *Annals of Internal Medicine, 121,* 393–399.

Chapter 14

Neurological and Genetic Disorders

Edward Goldson

Poor growth has been of concern to child care providers for generations. The etiology and differential diagnosis of poor growth is enormous, encompassing disorders of every organ system and including a wide variety of psychosocial factors. This chapter addresses neurological and genetic disorders that are associated with poor weight gain, primarily in the young child.

NEUROLOGICAL DISORDERS

Among the neurological disorders that are associated with poor growth are **microcephaly,** cerebral palsy (CP), tumors of the central nervous system (CNS), and myopathy.

Microcephaly

Microcephaly is a physical finding that is associated with many chromosomal disorders, a wide variety of other syndromes, pre- and perinatal difficulties that result in brain damage, and many neurodegenerative disorders. Microcephaly has also been encountered among children who have sustained profound nutritional deprivation without having had any of the previously noted conditions. The data concerning the cognitive, behavioral, and physical outcomes of undernutrition are drawn primarily from developing countries; thus, generalizing those data to the American experience should be done with caution. Nevertheless, the information is instructive. Galler (1984), in an extensive review of the literature, noted that microcephaly has been reported to be associated with early protein-energy malnutrition occurring in the first 2 years of life. She divided the studies into three groups: those that described the concurrent effects of malnutrition, the intermediate effects, and the long-term effects.

Among the concurrent effects of malnutrition, researchers identified microcephaly. Moreover, the results of autopsy studies on these children revealed a decrease in the number of nerve cells and a decrease in the connections between the various parts of the brain. These changes, aside from the observed microcephaly, are also associated with cognitive and behavioral impairments (see Chapter 3). The changes in the brain are noted most prominently when malnutrition occurs in the first year of life, at a time when there is much brain development and when the brain is particularly vulnerable to a wide variety of insults.

The intermediate effects of malnutrition are also significant. It appears that children who experienced severe malnutrition in the first 12 months of life were the least likely to attain a normal head circumference in measurements up to 50 months, even though their malnutrition was corrected (Graham, 1966). They also demonstrated more impaired cognition. This was not the case for children who experienced malnutrition after the first year of life.

Finally, early, severe malnutrition had long-term effects. Galler (1984) reviewed a number of studies and found that children who experienced severe malnutrition continued to have reduced head circumference as well as significant cognitive impairments. These impairments are probably the result of the early insult when the brain was developing rapidly, suggesting that there is a critical period for growth, which, if perturbed, will result in an adverse outcome.

When the clinician encounters a child with microcephaly, he or she must not conclude prematurely that it is secondary to malnutrition but should begin a neurological evaluation for etiology (Fenichel, 1997). Primary microcephaly indicates that the brain never formed properly as the result of a genetic or chromosomal abnormality. In secondary microcephaly, the brain started to form normally until a disease process interfered with further growth (Fenichel, 1997). Microcephaly at birth establishes the antepartum time of brain injury but does not distinguish primary from secondary causes. When presented with a child who has microcephaly, the clinician must determine whether there is a family history of small head size and whether associated features such as seizures or mental retardation are present in the child or in affected family members.

Cerebral Palsy

CP is one of the most common neurological disorders encountered among children. More than 100,000 Americans younger than 18 years have some neurological disability attributed to this disorder, which affects 1 child in 1,000 (Kuban & Leviton, 1994). CP is an "umbrella term covering a group of non-progressive, but often changing, motor impairments secondary to lesions or anomalies of the brain arising in the early stages of its development" (Mutch, Alberman, Hagberg, Kodama, & Perat, 1992, p. 549).

CP is divided into several categories that are related not only to nutritional needs and growth but also to functional outcome (Aicardi & Bax, 1992). The first is hemiplegia, or hemiparesis, which is defined as a unilateral (one-sided) motor disability, mostly spastic (increased muscle tone) in type. The second group of disorders is the diplegias. They are characterized by involvement of both sides of the body with the lower limbs being more affected than the upper limbs. Diplegia is one of the most common forms of CP. Included among the diplegias is spastic diplegia, which has a high incidence among preterm infants. A rarer form of diplegia is spastic-ataxic diplegia, which is usually congenital in origin and usually not related to perinatal disturbances. The third form is tetraplegia, or quadriplegia (bilateral hemiplegia), which is the most severe form of the disorder. It is characterized by spasticity of all extremities and involvement of the bulbar muscles (muscles that control facial movements and swallowing). Tetraplegia is usually accompanied by microcephaly and mental retardation requiring extensive supports. The final form of CP is dyskinetic CP (extrapyramidal or athetoid CP). This is characterized by abnormal movements or postures that are related to defective coordination of movements or regulation of muscle tone or both (Aicardi, 1992).

Growth in children with CP is impaired by nutritional and other, unknown factors. Nutritional factors appear to have their greatest influence on weight gain (Rempel, Colwell, & Nelson, 1988; Shapiro, Green, Krick, Allen, & Capute, 1986), whereas nonnutritional factors may limit linear growth (Stevenson, Roberts, & Vogtle, 1995). Factors that influence nutritional intake, particularly in the more severely involved children, include oral-motor dysfunction (Reilly & Skuse, 1992; see also Chapter 23), food refusal (Goldson, Milla, & Bentovim, 1985), gastroesophageal reflux (GER) (Reyes, Cash, Green, & Booth, 1993), and hypoxemia (Rogers, Arvedson, Msall, & Demerath, 1993). All of these conditions are associated with a risk of **aspiration** and the development of chronic lung disease; thus, children with CP who have growth delays, particularly those with quadriplegic CP, need to have complete physical evaluations and nutritional assessments. This is best accomplished by a team and should include a full medical and dietary history that focuses on intake, vomiting, gagging with feeds, and food refusal and includes an oral-motor assessment, a swallowing study to determine whether aspiration is occurring, and a radiographic and/or pH study to determine whether GER is occurring (see Chapter 11). Treatment will depend on the nature of the condition and its effect on the child's well-being.

A second group of children with CP are those with very low birth weight and other complications of prematurity, such as chronic lung disease. These children under the best of circumstances remain smaller and lighter than their peers (Goldson, 1996). When chronic lung disease is an additional factor, nutritional status can be compromised significantly.

Tumors of the Central Nervous System

Tumors of the CNS are rare in children, although they occasionally may present with growth impairment without neurological symptoms. They more commonly present with expanding head size (in very young children), ataxia, vomiting, and chronic irritability from headache. Tumors of the CNS, particularly gliomas, which are located in the region of the hypothalamus or diencephalon and the third ventricle, may present with poor growth. The symptom complex of these rare tumors has been called the *diencephalic syndrome* (DS) (Russell, 1951). DS is characterized by a hyperalert state, motor hyperactivity, euphoria, **tremor**, vomiting, lid retraction (Collier's sign), irritability, optic atrophy, multidirectional nystagmus (the presenting feature in 43% of individuals), emaciation without gastrointestinal disturbances, and pallor without anemia and without signs of increased intracranial pressure (Addy & Hudson, 1972; Burr, Slovis, Danish, Gadoth, & Butler, 1976; Russell, 1951; Solomon, Frank, & Gold, 1969). Other findings associated with these tumors include **ataxia,** tremor, **hyperreflexia, hemiparesis,** and **strabismus** (Starrett, 1982).

Poor growth begins in the first 6 months of life despite what appears to be a normal appetite. Some of these children eat abnormally large amounts of food, whereas others eat very little. A number of these children, however, do have feeding difficulties, the most common being recurrent vomiting, which tends to occur more frequently in children with posterior fossa tumors.

Other tumors, such as brain stem gliomas, can present with prolonged growth failure without the constellation of the DS. These children can have **cachexia** and vomiting without the typical symptoms of ataxia, **diplopia,** and headache. Wagner and Granditsch (1986) reported three children who had brain tumors and who presented for a considerable period of time with only poor growth but without any abnormal neurological findings.

Intracranial tumors should be included in the differential diagnosis of children who experience poor weight gain and growth impairment, particularly if there are CNS signs.

The diagnosis of these tumors is most easily made with the use of computed tomography (CT) or magnetic resonance imaging (MRI). The outcome for these children is usually poor, although some children do survive for a number of years when treated with irradiation (Namba, Nishimoto, & Yagyu, 1985).

Myopathy

Myopathy is a disorder in which the primary abnormality resides in the muscle as opposed to the CNS, although there can be a CNS component to the disease. Myopathies result in muscle weakness and muscle wasting, which is usually proximal in distribution. Although there often may be nutritional compromise in the final stages of a myopathy, it is rare that the presenting complaint is undernutrition. This is true of myotonic dystrophy and some of the other muscular dystrophies; however, the one reported exception to this clinical experience is Duchenne's dystrophy.

Duchenne's dystrophy is the most common lethal X-linked disease, with an incidence of approximately 1 in 3,500 male births (Rapisarda, Muntoni, Gobbi, & Dubowitz, 1995). It has its onset in early childhood and is slowly progressive. The initial symptoms in the birth to 3-year range usually involve difficulty climbing stairs, problems rising from the floor, or symptoms of pelvic weakness. With time, a waddling gait and some degree of muscle atrophy develop. Other symptoms include progressive muscle weakness, scoliosis, and a decrease in deep tendon reflexes. Respiratory failure occurs, and there also is cardiac involvement, which is initially seen only on the electrocardiogram, although it may progress to cardiac decompensation (Aicardi, 1992). MRI scans and other studies reveal no abnormalities of the CNS.

Although it occurs rarely, the appearance of Duchenne's dystrophy in the first year of life can be associated with poor weight gain. This is not well appreciated, but the diagnosis of Duchenne's dystrophy should be considered in an infant who presents with poor weight gain, associated delays in motor development, and muscle weakness. The evaluation for this constellation of findings should include a serum creatinine kinase level. If this enzyme level is elevated, then the diagnosis of Duchenne's dystrophy needs to be considered. An electromyogram and muscle biopsy can help diagnose this disorder.

GENETIC DISORDERS

Genetic disorders are usually characterized by developmental delays and dysmorphic features. Such observations made by the parent, physician, or other care provider usually lead to referral and diagnosis. The more atypical the infant or child, the earlier the initiation of the investigation and, frequently, the earlier the diagnosis; however, several conditions that are associated with poor growth may not be obvious. Conversely, there are syndromes in which the child is undernourished in the presence of what appears to be adequate caloric intake.

Fragile X Syndrome

Fragile X syndrome, also an X-linked condition, is not associated frequently with growth problems but more with abnormal behavior, prominent ears, mental retardation, and macroorchidism (enlarged testes). The syndrome is the most common human chromosomal anomaly that is associated with heritable mental retardation and the second most frequent cause of mental retardation after Down syndrome (Jacky, 1991). Young boys with fragile X syndrome have been found to have puffiness around the eyes, strabismus, narrow and broad palpebral fissures, a large head relative to body size, and prominent ears, which often are long, wide, cupped, or protruding. **Epicanthal folds, ptosis,** and low-set ears have been noted but appear in less than 25% of the affected children; however, these findings may not be very striking in the young infant.

Although hypotonia is a common finding in young males with fragile X syndrome, focal, abnormal neurological signs do not occur frequently in these individuals. Poor weight gain has been reported in some young males with fragile X syndrome. This has been associated with hypotonia and with GER. Although these problems seem to improve with time, in infancy they can result in feeding and weight gain problems that can be quite intractable (Goldson & Hagerman, 1992).

Fragile X syndrome should be considered in any male infant or very young boy who presents with a history of early undernutrition, vomiting, food refusal, and hypotonia. An important clue is a family history of mental retardation, particularly when it is sex linked. The diagnosis of fragile X syndrome can be pursued by a referral to a geneticist or by chromosomal and DNA analysis.

Down Syndrome

Down syndrome (trisomy 21) is the most common chromosomal anomaly that is identified with mental retardation and has an incidence in 1 in 600 live births. Children with Down syndrome have physical characteristics that include midface hypoplasia with a depressed nasal bridge, upward slant to the palpebral fissure, epicanthal folds, short neck, and single palmar creases (Pueschel, 1992). Children with Down syndrome have short stature and low birth weight and continue to be small (Cronk & Annerén, 1992); however, there are some children who fail to gain weight over and above their short stature and genetic potential. This weight problem is associated with cardiac, respiratory, and gastrointestinal disorders as well as feeding problems and inadequate nutrition, particularly in early childhood (Pipes, 1992).

The young infant with Down syndrome who fails to maintain adequate weight gain should be evaluated. Often, the etiology is quite evident, such as when congenital heart disease or abnormalities of the bowel are present; however, there can be difficulties associated with upper-airway obstruction, oral-motor dysfunction, food refusal, and chronic infection, which warrant investigation. Usually, with treatment, the problem of poor nutrition resolves and adequate weight gain is established. This can be monitored readily as there are growth charts for children with Down syndrome (Cronk et al., 1988).

Trisomies 13 and 18

Although trisomy 21 is the most common form of trisomy, at least two other trisomies are associated with poor growth. Trisomy 13 (D1 trisomy syndrome) is characterized by defects of the eye, nose, lip, and forebrain, polydactyly, skin defects of the posterior scalp, cardiac defects, renal anomalies, and intestinal problems. The prognosis for these children is grim: 82% succumb within the first month (Jones, 1997). Those who do survive often have seizures and fail to gain weight and to grow.

Trisomy 18 syndrome is characterized by clenched hands, a short sternum, and abnormal dermal ridge patterns on the fingertips; however, there are more than 130 different abnormalities noted in this syndrome involving all organ systems. These children usually are feeble, and mortality is high, with 50% of the infants dying within the first week of life (Jones, 1997). A poor suck is characteristic of these infants and often necessitates the use of nasogastric feeding to sustain life. Almost all of these infants and children demonstrate a failure to grow and a failure to gain weight. The diagnosis of both trisomy 13 and trisomy 18 can often be made on a clinical basis; however, the definitive diagnosis can be made only by obtaining chromosomes.

Prader-Willi Syndrome

Prader-Willi syndrome (PWS) (Prader, Labhart, & Willi, 1956) has two very different stages (hypotonia of infancy and obesity of childhood) that, if not recognized, may lead to delay in diagnosis.

The clinical features that are experienced during infancy and early childhood include poor weight gain; delays in achieving motor and language milestones, and typical facies characterized by **dolicocephaly**, narrow bifrontal diameter, almond-shaped lips, thin upper lip, and down-turned corners of the mouth (Butler, 1990; Donaldson et al., 1994; Holm et al., 1993). Approximately 70% of affected individuals have a deletion of the long arm of chromosome 15 at q11q13 (Jones, 1997), which is detected by high-resolution chromosome analysis or fluorescent in situ hybridization (FISH).

Clinical diagnostic criteria for PWS have been established (Holm et al., 1993). Major criteria include the presence of hypotonia and poor suck, feeding problems in infancy with failure to thrive, the characteristic facial features that were described previously, **hypogonadism,** global developmental delays, and cytogenetic markers of PWS. Minor criteria include decreased fetal movements, weak cry, hypopigmentation, and thick, viscous saliva. Early recognition of the clinical picture is essential if one is to be able to care for these children effectively and successfully. The clinician should include PWS in the differential diagnosis of the very hypotonic infant who exhibits an abnormal cry and feeding difficulties.

XO Syndrome

A syndrome that is strongly associated with short stature and, more recently, with poor weight gain is XO syndrome, or Turner syndrome (Turner, 1938). It consists of a constellation of findings including infantilism, congenital webbed neck, and **cubitus valgus.** These physical findings have been found to be associated with the deletion of one X chromosome. One in 2,000 live-born girls is affected by the disorder. There also is a spectrum of the disease that is associated with **mosaics** such as XX/XO, XY/XO and situations in which only a part of the X chromosome is missing. Children are frequently identified by their short stature, congenital lymphedema and associated puffiness over the dorsum of the hand, webbing of the neck and a low posterior hairline, broad chest and widely spaced hypoplastic nipples, a narrow palate and relatively small mandible, cardiac defects, and a horseshoe kidney. Some of these children also have small palates and mandibles.

Mathisen, Reilly, and Skuse (1992) reported on the presence of oral-motor dysfunction and feeding disorders in children who have Turner syndrome. Mothers in that study reported that their children had significant feeding difficulties that were characterized by gagging and vomiting and poor weight gain in the first year of life.

The diagnosis of Turner syndrome is frequently made at birth. If not, then in the presence of suspicious physical features and poor weight gain associated with feeding difficulties, the clinician should consider Turner syndrome and obtain chromosomes.

Russell-Silver Syndrome

Russell-Silver syndrome (RSS) is associated not only with short stature but also with poor weight gain. What is most striking in this syndrome are the skeletal asymmetry, short stature, and small, triangular face with a normal head circumference. Because of the small face and normal head circumference, a false impression of hydrocephalus is sometimes conveyed. Many of these children have difficulty with hypoglycemia during the first 2–3 years of life, and some have been noted to have growth hormone deficiency as evidenced by poor linear growth that requires endocrine evaluation (Jones, 1997). Finally, some of these children have feeding disorders, which can result in poor weight gain. In infancy, these children may demonstrate delays in achieving developmental milestones despite having normal intelligence. The etiology of this disorder remains unknown. RSS should be considered in a child with short stature, often of prenatal onset, triangular face, and asymmetry of the limbs. Close monitoring for hypoglycemia should be a part of the counseling that is provided to parents.

Other Syndromes that Are Associated with Poor Growth

Other syndromes are associated with undernutrition and poor growth. When considering an infant with these characteristics, the clinician must decide when to embark on a genetic evaluation. Jones stated that

> Any infant with three or more minor anomalies should be evaluated for a major malformation, many of which are occult. . . . These minor anomalies are most common in areas of complex and variable features such as the face, auricles, hands, and feet. Before ascribing significance to a given anomaly in a patient, it is important to note whether it is found in other family members. (1997, p. 727)

Following are several relatively rare and newly identified syndromes in which there are minor as well as major anomalies in children who experience growth delays. These conditions are worthy of consideration when a clinician is confronted with a child who has the described characteristics.

Smith-Lemli-Opitz Syndrome: Described in 1964, this syndrome is characterized by unusual facial characteristics including partially closed eyelids and skinfolds in the corners of the eyes, curved second and third toes, and undescended testes. Other associated anomalies include cataracts, cleft palate, and small chin.

Deletion 13q Syndrome: First described by Lele, Penrose, and Stallarf in 1963, it is characterized by a deletion of the long arm of chromosome 13 localized to band q14. Children who have this syndrome have a high nasal bridge, eye defects that include tumors, and underdeveloped thumbs.

Familial White Matter Hypoplasia, Agenesis of the Corpus Callosum, Mental Retardation, and Growth Deficiency: Described by Curatolo et al. in 1993, children who have this very rare syndrome have mid-line facial abnormalities, long eyebrows, widely spaced eyes, and a small chin.

Familial Olivopontocerebellar Atrophy: This was described by Harding, Dunger, and Grant in 1988. Two siblings who were reported to have had this rare condition had low muscle tone, limited joint movement, and visual impairment.

MEDICAL EVALUATION

Diagnosis of the conditions that are described in this chapter starts with a complete history and physical examination. For children who have dysmorphic features and who are strongly suspected of having a genetic disorder, particular emphasis should be placed on the family history. A three-generation family history is strongly recommended, particularly when one is concerned with a sex-linked disorder such as fragile X syndrome. If the child who is being evaluated is suspected of having CP, then the examiner should gather history concerning the prenatal and perinatal periods, although brain damage at birth is no longer considered to be the primary cause of this disorder (Nelson, 1988).

The history and physical examination will very often provide the clinician with a diagnosis. When this is not the case, the laboratory can be employed. When syndromes are considered, high-resolution chromosomes, DNA testing, and FISH can be of help in making the diagnosis. Often, the aid of a dysmorphologist or a geneticist is required. When myopathies are considered, a muscle biopsy and an EMG can be of help along with the expertise of a neurologist. When tumors are considered, cranial imaging is warranted along with the involvement of an oncologist and a neurosurgeon if a tumor is identified.

CONCLUSION

Poor growth is the common pathway for a wide variety of diseases that involve different organ systems. This chapter has focused on neurological and genetic disorders. The disorders discussed in this chapter rarely present initially as growth problems. Some of them, such as Down syndrome, are quite common, whereas others, such as familial white matter hypoplasia, are very rare. No matter what their frequency in the population, a knowledge of their association with pediatric undernutrition can be very helpful in the early diagnosis and management of children who have these problems.

REFERENCES

Addy, D.P., & Hudson, F.P. (1972). Diencephalic syndrome of infant emaciation. *Archives of Disease in Childhood, 47,* 338–343.

Aicardi, J. (1992). Primary muscle disease. In J. Aicardi (Ed.), *Diseases of the nervous system in childhood* (pp. 1172–1237). London: MacKeith Press.

Aicardi, J., & Bax, M.C.O. (1992). Cerebral palsy. In J. Aicardi (Ed.), *Diseases of the nervous system in childhood* (pp. 330–374). London: MacKeith Press.

Burr, I.M., Slovis, A.E., Danish, R.K., Gadoth, N., & Butler, I.J. (1976). Diencephalic syndrome revisited. *Journal of Pediatrics, 88,* 439–444.

Butler, M.G. (1990). Prader-Willi syndrome: Current understanding of cause and diagnosis. *American Journal of Medical Genetics, 35,* 319–332.

Cronk, C.E., & Annerén, G. (1992). Growth. In G.M. Pueschel & J.K. Pueschel (Eds.), *Biomedical concerns in persons with Down syndrome* (pp. 19–37). Baltimore: Paul H. Brookes Publishing Co.

Cronk, C., Crocker, A.C., Pueschel, S.M., Shea, A.M., Zackai, E., Pickens, G., & Reed, R.B. (1988). Growth charts for children with Down syndrome: 1 month to 18 years of age. *Pediatrics, 81,* 102–110.

Curatolo, P., Cilio, M.R., Del Giudice, E., Romano, A., Gaggero, R., & Pessagno, A. (1993). Familial white matter hypoplasia, agenesis of the corpus callosum, mental retardation and growth deficiency: A new distinctive syndrome. *Neuropediatrics, 24,* 77–82.

Donaldson, M.D.C., Chu, C.E., Cooke, A., Wilson, A., Greene, S.A., & Stephenson, J.B.P. (1994). The Prader-Willi syndrome. *Archives of Diseases in Children, 70,* 58–63.

Fenichel, G.M. (1997). *Clinical pediatric neurology: A signs and symptoms approach* (3rd ed.). Philadelphia: W.B. Saunders.

Galler, J.R. (1984). The behavioral consequences of malnutrition in early life. In J.R. Galler (Ed.), *Nutrition and behavior* (pp. 63–117). New York: Plenum.

Goldson, E. (1996). The micropremie: Infants with birth weights < 800 grams. *Infants and Young Children, 8,* 1–10.

Goldson, E., & Hagerman, R.J. (1992). Fragile X syndrome and failure to thrive. *American Journal of Diseases of Children, 147,* 605–607.

Goldson, E., Milla, F.J., & Bentovim, A. (1985). Failure to thrive: A transactional issue. *Family Systems Medicine, 3,* 205–213.

Graham, G. (1966). Growth during recovery from infantile malnutrition. *Journal of the American Medical Women's Association, 21,* 737–742.

Harding, B.N., Dunger, D.B., & Grant, D.B. (1988). Familial olivopontocerebellar atrophy with neonatal onset: A recessively inherited syndrome with systemic and biochemical abnormalities. *Journal of Neurology, Neurosurgery, and Psychiatry, 51,* 385–390.

Holm, J.A., Cassidy, S.B., Butler, M.G., Hanchett, J.M., Greenswag, L.R., Whitman, B.Y., & Greenberg, F. (1993). Prader-Willi syndrome consensus diagnostic criteria. *Pediatrics, 91,* 398–402.

Jacky, P. (1991). Cytogenetics. In R.J. Hagerman & A.C. Silverman (Eds.), *Fragile X syndrome: Diagnosis, treatment and research* (pp. 98–145). Baltimore: The Johns Hopkins University Press.

Jones, K.L. (1997). *Smith's recognizable patterns of human malformation* (5th ed.). Philadelphia: W.B. Saunders.

Kuban, K.C.K., & Leviton, A. (1994). Cerebral palsy. *New England Journal of Medicine, 330,* 188–195.

Lele, K.P., Penrose, L.S., & Stallarf, H.B. (1963). Chromosome deletion in a case of retinoblastoma. *Annals of Human Genetics, 27,* 171–174.

Mathisen, B., Reilly, S., & Skuse, D. (1992). Oral-motor dysfunction and feeding disorders of infants with Turner syndrome. *Developmental Medicine and Child Neurology, 34,* 141–149.

Mutch, L., Alberman, E., Hagberg, B., Kodama, K., & Perat, M.V. (1992). Cerebral palsy epidemiology: Where are we now and where are we going? *Developmental Medicine and Child Neurology, 34,* 547–551.

Namba, S., Nishimoto, A., & Yagyu, Y. (1985). Diencephalic syndrome of emaciation (Russell's syndrome). *Surgical Neurology, 23,* 581–588.

Nelson, K.B. (1988). What proportion of cerebral palsy is related to birth asphyxia? *Journal of Pediatrics, 112,* 572–574.

Pipes, P.L. (1992). Nutritional aspects. In S.M. Pueschel & J.K. Pueschel (Eds.), *Biomedical concerns in persons with Down syndrome* (pp. 39–46). Baltimore: Paul H. Brookes Publishing Co.

Prader, A., Labhart, A., & Willi, H. (1956). Ein syndrom von adipositas, kleinwuchs, kryptorchismus und oligophrenie zustand im neugeborenalter. *Schweizerischer Medizin Wochenschrift, 86,* 1260–1261.

Pueschel, S.M. (1992). Phenotypic characteristics. In S.M. Pueschel & J.K. Pueschel (Eds.), *Biomedical concerns in persons with Down syndrome* (pp. 1–12). Baltimore: Paul H. Brookes Publishing Co.

Rapisarda, R., Muntoni, F., Gobbi, P., & Dubowitz, V. (1995). Duchenne muscular dystrophy presenting with failure to thrive. *Archives of Disease in Childhood, 72,* 437–438.

Reilly, S., & Skuse, D. (1992). Characteristics and management of feeding problems of young children with cerebral palsy. *Developmental Medicine and Child Neurology, 34,* 379–388.

Rempel, G.R., Colwell, S.O., & Nelson, R.P. (1988). Growth in children with cerebral palsy fed via gastrostomy. *Pediatrics, 82,* 857–862.

Reyes, A.L., Cash, A.J., Green, S.H., & Booth, I.W. (1993). Gastroesophageal reflux in children with cerebral palsy. *Child: Care, Health, and Development, 19,* 109–118.

Rogers, B.T., Arvedson, J., Msall, M., & Demerath, R.R. (1993). Hypoxemia during oral feeding of children with severe cerebral palsy. *Developmental Medicine and Child Neurology, 35,* 3–10.

Russell, A.A. (1951). Diencephalic syndrome in infancy and children. *Archives of Disease in Childhood, 26,* 274.

Shapiro, B.K., Green, P., Krick, J., Allen, D., & Capute, A.J. (1986). Growth of severely impaired children: Neurological versus nutritional factors. *Developmental Medicine and Child Neurology, 28,* 729–733.

Smith, D.W., Lemli, L., & Opitz, J.M. (1964). A newly recognized syndrome of multiple congenital anomalies. *Journal of Pediatrics, 64,* 210–217.

Solomon, G.E., Frank, D.J., & Gold, A.P. (1969). "Failure to thrive" of cerebral etiology. *New England Journal of Medicine, 280,* 769–770.

Starrett, A.L. (1982). Neurological and developmental disorders causing growth failure in infancy. In P.J. Accardo (Ed.), *Failure to thrive in infancy and early childhood* (pp. 135–151). Baltimore: University Park Press.

Stevenson, R.D., Roberts, C.D., & Vogtle, L. (1995). The effects of non-nutritional factors on growth in cerebral palsy. *Developmental Medicine and Child Neurology, 37,* 124–130.

Turner, H.H. (1938). A syndrome of infantilism, congenital webbed neck, and cubitus valgus. *Endocrinology, 23,* 566.

Wagner, U., & Granditsch, G. (1986). Gedeihstörung al hauptsymptom intrakranieller tumor im frühen kindesalter. *Pädiatrie un Pädiologie, 21,* 147–153.

Chapter 15

Endocrine Disorders

Andrea Maggioni and Fima Lifshitz

Pediatricians often are consulted by parents who are worried about poor growth in their children, and they often seek consultation with a pediatric endocrinologist to help in the diagnosis and management of children with growth disturbances. Few children younger than 3 years who are seen for growth concerns will have endocrine disorders, but it is important to identify the ones who might. Generally, those with endocrine disorders will have short stature; however, even in a pediatric endocrine referral center, a large proportion of children with short stature are healthy. This is because either poor and inaccurate measurements are taken or the patient and the family need to be reassured by a pediatric endocrinologist that the child is growing normally but in the low-normal range.

This chapter reviews two common variations of growth that, although worrisome, are considered to be normal. It will assist the clinician in addressing other endocrine disorders that are not very frequent but that should not be missed. Finally, the chapter briefly discusses psychosocial dwarfism. (See Chapter 10 for other aspects of growth evaluation.)

ASSESSMENT OF GROWTH

Disease-related growth charts have been developed for some specific conditions that are associated with growth retardation, such as Turner syndrome (Lyon, Preece, & Grant, 1988), Down syndrome (Cronk et al., 1988), Noonan syndrome (Witt, Keena, Hall, & Allanson, 1986), and achondroplasia (Horton, Rptter, & Rimoin, 1978). Because growth is an active process, growth velocity charts are more accurate than cross-sectional growth charts in determining growth pattern; thus, growth velocity should be evaluated over a period of at least 6–12 months (Brook, Hindmarsh, & Healy, 1986). Children with abnor-

The authors thank Dr. Diego Botero for reviewing this chapter.

mal growth velocity should be evaluated for possible pathological conditions. It is important to take into account that there also is a significant seasonal variation in growth (Tiwary, 1993). Peak growth rates have been observed to occur in the summer and the spring with a low point in the winter and the fall.

A more sensitive method for assessing body weight and length progression is to compare the reference data developed by Guo et al. (1991) on the expected incremental gains in weight and length for clinically meaningful age intervals during the first 2 years of life (see Chapter 10 and Appendix F).

The X ray of the wrist for bone age determination is another helpful tool in differentiating the type of short stature. The ossification centers of the skeleton appear and mature in a predictable way, which has allowed the development of normal age-related standards. The two most commonly used methods for assessing the skeletal age are the Greulich and Pyle (1950) and the Tanner-Whitehouse (Tanner et al., 1983) methods. Usually, a significant delay in the maturation of the bone age is seen in pathological short stature such as in malnutrition, hypothyroidism, growth hormone deficiency, or chronic diseases.

VARIATIONS OF NORMAL GROWTH

Because the size of an infant at birth is more related to maternal size and intrauterine influences than to genetic factors, an adjustment in growth velocity occurring in the first 2–3 years of life is to be expected in many children. There may be a decrease in growth velocity across two major percentiles as the child's growth reaches a channel that is normal for his or her genetic potential; therefore, specific growth patterns in the first years of life may represent normal variations in growth velocity (Maggioni & Lifshitz, 1995). These patterns include patients with familial short stature (FSS) and constitutional growth delay (CGD).

Familial Short Stature

FSS has also been defined as genetic short stature. Some children who are larger at birth than what their parents might have predicted will readjust their growth percentile downward sometime between 6 and 18 months of age according to their genetic potential. After this deceleration phase, they will grow along their new growth channel, which is more appropriate to their genetic potential for height, without further deceleration to a lower percentile. These patients are short throughout life as are their parents. In contrast with patients with CGD, children with FSS do not exhibit a weight deficit for height, and their bone age is within 2 standard deviations (SD) of the mean for their chronological age (Maggioni & Lifshitz, 1995).

The diagnosis of FSS is made when the child's height is appropriate to the parents' heights and the predicted adult height falls within the parents' target height. These children keep growing at a normal rate along the lower percentiles of the growth chart. One cannot use short parental stature to explain a child's small size if the parents were themselves malnourished.

Constitutional Growth Delay

Patients with CGD are called "slow growers" and "late bloomers." Studies have shown that the major deceleration of growth occurs during the first 2 years of life. Thereafter and throughout the prepubertal years, they grow parallel to but below the 3rd percentile showing a catch-up growth at a time later than the pubertal growth spurt (Horner, Thorsson, & Hintz, 1978). These children usually have a 2- to 3-year delay in the bone age. In 60%–90% of the cases, there is a positive family history of delay in growth and pubertal development (Bierich, 1987). When adolescence begins and the growth spurt occurs, the bone age increases proportionally to the height.

CGD is seen more often in boys and only occasionally in girls. The diagnosis of CGD in girls should be made only after eliminating other possibilities for pathological growth patterns. An easy way to differentiate this group of patients from infants with FSS is based on the deficit in their weight-to-length ratio and weight-to-height ratio profiles from 4 months to 12 years of age (Solans & Lifshitz, 1992). In children who have CGD, body weight gain slows (see Figure 1), whereas in FSS it does not. Thus, infants who have CGD appear to fail to thrive with body weight deficits for length, whereas infants who have FSS maintain a normal or even an excess body weight for length. During puberty, the body weight-to-height increases, and the patient will grow and develop appropriately. Differences have also been reported in some nutritional parameters, such as mean creatinine-height index, retinol binding protein, and serum iron values, that were lower among children with CGD (Solans & Lifshitz, 1992).

Similar findings of slow weight and length progression were reported in a long-term study of children who experienced a moderate to severe protein-energy malnutrition during their first year of life (Galler, Ramsey, & Solimano, 1985). Their pattern of growth strikingly resembled the pattern in CGD. On this basis, it can be postulated that inadequate food intake for age may be the cause of poor weight gain in infancy of children with CGD. Children with CGD should have a nutritional evaluation for adequate intake.

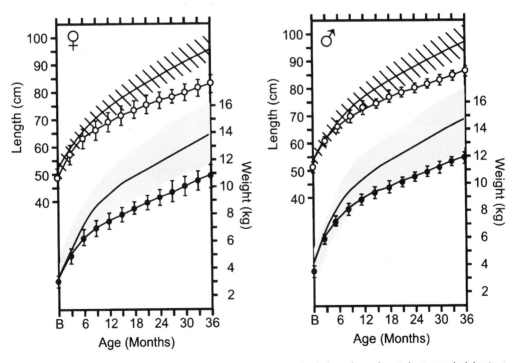

Figure 1. In constitutional growth delay, deceleration in both length and weight (growth faltering) occurs in the first 3 years of life. (From Horner, J.M., Thorsson, A.V., & Hintz, R.L. [1978]. Growth deceleration patterns in children with constitutional short stature: An aid to diagnosis. *Pediatrics, 62,* 531–532; reprinted by permission.)

PATHOLOGICAL SHORT STATURE

Short stature has been defined as height that is below the 3rd percentile; therefore, by definition, 3% of normal children would be classified as being short. *Dwarfism,* the severe form of short stature, is defined as height that is more than 3 SD below the mean. Pathological growth should be considered in children who do not grow well regardless of their height.

Any child who falls behind in growth, crossing 2 major percentiles on the growth chart, should undergo a complete evaluation even if the height still is above the 3rd percentile. Included in this group are children with CGD who are seen during the deceleration phase of their growth in the first 2–3 years.

Because there are multiple causes of short stature and growth retardation, laboratory investigation should be based on the information obtained from the history and the physical examination. History of chronic illnesses, drug intake (see Chapter 18), mid-parental and target height, birth size, growth pattern, nutritional state, body segment proportions, and bone age are the most important points to take into consideration. The following simple laboratory screening tests should be performed initially: complete blood count, sedimentation rate, venous blood gases, thyroid function tests, liver and kidney function tests, and urinalysis (Lifshitz & Cervantes, 1996).

Hypothyroidism

Since the implementation of newborn screening programs that have provided for the prompt diagnosis of congenital hypothyroidism, the presence of this condition as a cause of growth failure is very rare. Acquired cases of hypothyroidism in children must always be considered in the presence of a deceleration in growth and a relative obesity (Rivkees, Bode, & Crawford, 1988). Other symptoms are less common, and slow growth rate is usually the only presenting symptom. The mechanism of slow growth in hypothyroidism is related to the thyroid hormone's being an important regulator of growth hormone (GH) secretion. Children with a family history of autoimmune disease as well as children with Down syndrome, Turner syndrome, Klinefelter syndrome, or diabetes mellitus are at increased risk of developing thyroid autoimmune disease such as **Hashimoto's thyroiditis**. The laboratory evaluation will show a high level of thyroid stimulating hormone (TSH) and a low or normal thyroxine (T4) level. Positive thyroid antibodies are usually present. The bone age is delayed markedly. Replacement therapy with thyroid hormone (T4) leads to a rapid normalization of GH secretion and catch-up growth.

Skeletal Dysplasias

Children who demonstrate skeletal abnormalities on X rays or upon physical examination deserve evaluation for metabolic bone diseases (e.g., achondroplasia, hypochondroplasia, rickets, osteosclerosis). Most of the skeletal dysplasias are associated with short stature. Other findings that suggest a skeletal dysplasia are strong family history, extreme short stature, and abnormal body proportions.

Hypophosphatemic rickets is a metabolic bone disease that may present with short stature and signs of rickets (Verge, Cowell, Howard, Donaghue, & Silink, 1993). The latter includes **frontal bossing, rachitic rosary,** bowing of the legs, and widening of the wrists. Therapy with phosphate and vitamin D will improve the condition and the prognosis for final adult stature.

Growth Hormone Deficiency

GH deficiency may be congenital or acquired. The congenital form is usually associated with mid-line defects (e.g., cleft lip and palate, optic nerve hypoplasia or dysplasia) or may be inherited. Rarely, functional GH deficiency may occur because of an abnormal GH molecule. Usually, infants have a normal size at birth and manifest poor linear growth by 3 years of age. The acquired form may be associated with birth trauma, mid-line tumors, and head trauma. Both forms (congenital and acquired) may be associated with isolated GH deficiency or with multiple pituitary hormone deficiencies (panhypopituitarism) (Schaff-Blass, Burstein, & Rosenfield, 1984).

The diagnosis of GH deficiency is based on findings of short stature, slow growth rate for age, delayed bone age, and subnormal GH levels in response to stimulation tests with two different pharmacological stimuli. GH levels measured randomly (unstimulated) are of limited value in the diagnosis of GH deficiency. Therapy with GH is highly effective in children with classic GH deficiency. Treatment is needed until epiphyses have fused. There still is a lot of controversy in regard to whether some children with mild or subtle forms of GH deficiency are missed by the classic laboratory criteria.

Glucocorticoid Excess

Glucocorticoid excess, whether endogenous or exogenous, has a profound effect on growth. The attenuation in growth is predominantly a direct effect of glucocorticoid on the growth plate; thus, a child who presents with a decrease in growth rate and a marked increase in weight should be suspected of having Cushing syndrome, although it is rare in childhood. Children who take pharmacological doses of glucocorticoids for chronic conditions are at high risk for growth failure (Allen, 1996). Alternate-day dosing regimens do allow for normal growth to some extent. Catch-up growth does occur upon removal of the steroids or a decrease in the therapeutic dosage.

Turner Syndrome

The diagnosis of Turner syndrome should be considered in any girl who presents with short stature and low growth velocity. It is important to have a high index of suspicion because, in many girls, the physical features are not obvious; therefore, a chromosomal assessment and measurement of luteinizing hormone (LH) and follicle stimulating hormone (FSH) levels are imperative in every girl with short stature even in the absence of the stigmata of Turner syndrome (Rosenfield, 1996).

PSYCHOSOCIAL DWARFISM

Several syndromes are characterized by growth failure in association with emotional deprivation, and they can occur from infancy through adolescence. They are named syndromes of *psychosocial short stature, emotional deprivation dwarfism, functional hypopituitarism,* or *psychosocial growth failure.* An extensive review of the psychodynamics of these syndromes has been published elsewhere (Blizzard & Bulatovic, 1996).

At least three different subtypes of psychosocial dwarfism have been recognized. Type 1 occurs usually in infants younger than 2 years of age. There is no evidence that these children have a GH deficiency, and they usually recover when adequate nutrition is provided. Type 2 is characteristic of children older than 3 years. GH deficiency is a common finding in this group; however, they respond poorly to growth hormone therapy, and a major psychological component is always present. Type 3 is more characteristic of older children. They do not have a GH deficiency when tested, but they will respond with a significant increase in growth when given GH. Endocrine dysfunction and growth inhibition are usually reversible when these patients are removed from the adverse environment. It is evident that psychological causes of poor growth can present in patients from early infancy through adolescence and that their occurrence spans all socioeconomic groups.

REFERENCES

Allen, D.B. (1996). Growth suppression by glucocorticoid therapy. *Endocrine and Metabolic Clinics of North America, 25,* 699–717.

Bierich, J.R. (1987). Constitutional delay of growth and development. *Growth, Genetics and Hormones, 3,* 9.

Blizzard, R.M., & Bulatovic, A. (1996). Syndromes of psychosocial short stature. In F. Lifshitz (Ed.), *Pediatric endocrinology* (3rd ed., pp. 83–93). New York: Marcel-Dekker.

Brook, G.G.D., Hindmarsh, P.C., & Healy, M.H.R. (1986). A better way to detect growth failure. *British Medical Journal, 293,* 1186.

Cronk, C., Crocker, A.C., Pueschel, S.M., Shea, A.M., Zackai, E., Pickens, G., & Reed, R.B. (1988). Growth charts for children with Down's syndrome: 1 month to 18 years of age. *Pediatrics, 81,* 102–110.

Galler, J.R., Ramsey, F., & Solimano, G. (1985). A follow-up study of the effects of early malnutrition on subsequent development: I. Physical growth and sexual maturation during adolescence. *Pediatric Research, 19,* 518.

Greulich, W.W., & Pyle, S.I. (1950). *Radiographic atlas of skeletal development of the hand and wrist.* Stanford, CA: Stanford University Press.

Guo, S., Roche, A.F., Fomon, S.J., Nelson, S.E., Chumlea, W.C., Rogers, R.R., Baumgartner, R.N., Ziegler, E.E., & Siervogel, R.M. (1991). Reference data on gains in weight and length during the first two years of life. *Journal of Pediatrics, 119,* 355–362.

Horner, J.M., Thorsson, A.V., & Hintz, R.L. (1978). Growth deceleration patterns in children with constitutional short stature: An aid to diagnosis. *Pediatrics, 62,* 529–534.

Horton, W.A., Rptter, J.I., & Rimoin, D.L. (1978). Standard growth curve for achondroplasia. *Journal of Pediatrics, 93,* 435–438.

Lifshitz, F., & Cervantes, C.D. (1996). Short stature. In F. Lifshitz (Ed.), *Pediatric endocrinology* (3rd ed., pp. 1–18). New York: Marcel-Dekker.

Lyon, A.J., Preece, M.A., & Grant, D.B. (1988). Growth curves for girls with Turner's syndrome. *Archives of Diseases of Childhood, 60,* 932–935.

Maggioni, A., & Lifshitz, F. (1995). Nutritional management of failure to thrive. *Pediatric Clinics of North America, 42,* 791–810.

Rivkees, S.A., Bode, H.H., & Crawford, J.D. (1988). Long-term growth in juvenile acquired hypothyroidism. *New England Journal of Medicine, 318,* 599–602.

Rosenfield, R.L. (1996). Essentials of growth diagnosis. *Endocrine and Metabolic Clinics of North America, 25,* 743–758.

Schaff-Blass, E., Burstein, S., & Rosenfield, R. (1984). Advances in diagnosis and treatment of short stature, with special reference to the role of growth hormone. *Journal of Pediatrics, 104,* 801.

Solans, C.V., & Lifshitz, F. (1992). Body weight progression and nutritional status of patients with familial short stature with and without constitutional delay in growth. *American Journal of Diseases of Children, 146,* 296–302.

Tanner, J.M., Whitehouse, R.H., Cameron, N., Marshall, W.A., Healy, M.J.R., & Goldstein, H. (1983). *Assessment of Skeletal Maturity and Prediction of Adult Height (TW2 Method).* London: Academic Press.

Tiwary, C. (1993, June). Seasonal and latitudinal effects on growth in patients on Protropin growth hormone in the U.S. and Canada. *Genentech National Cooperative Growth Study Summary Report, 15.*

Verge, C.F., Cowell, C.T., Howard, N.J., Donaghue, K.C., & Silink, M. (1993). Growth in children with X-linked hypophosphatemic rickets. *Acta Paediatrica Scandinavica, 388*(Suppl.), 70–75.

Witt, D.R., Keena, B.A., Hall, J.G., & Allanson, J.E. (1986). Growth curves for height in Noonan syndrome. *Clinical Genetics, 30,* 150–153.

Chapter 16

Adverse Reactions to Foods

John M. James and A. Wesley Burks

Adverse symptoms following the ingestion of food may be observed in young children and can be a challenge for families and health professionals. This chapter provides a practical approach to identifying these reactions. Particular emphasis is placed on reactions that may impair weight gain in the first 3 years of life. Accepted treatment measures are discussed with an emphasis on the unnecessary restriction of the diet, which, in some cases, may lead to nutritional deficiencies and even growth problems characterized historically as "failure to thrive."

DEFINITIONS

An *adverse food reaction* is any abnormal clinical response following the ingestion of a food or a food additive (Sampson, 1989). These reactions are divided into two major categories:

1. *Food allergy:* an immunologically mediated food reaction that is unrelated to any physiological effect of the food (e.g., a reaction that is mediated by specific **IgE** antibodies to a food, such as cow-milk allergy)
2. *Food intolerance:* any abnormal physiological response to food that is not mediated by the immune system (e.g., lactose intolerance)

PREVALENCE

Although surveys have reported that as many as 15%–30% of households in the United States had at least one member who believed that he or she was allergic to some food ingredient (Altman & Chiaramonte, 1996; Sloan & Powers, 1986), this belief was not confirmed when patient histories were tested with food challenges (Bock, 1987; Kajosaari,

1982; Niestijl Jansen et al., 1994). Overall, the actual prevalence of food allergy in children who are younger than 3 years is less than 8% (Bock, 1987; Kajosaari, 1982); in adults, food allergy is estimated to be less than 2% (Niestijl Jansen et al., 1994; Young, Stoneham, Petrudhevitch, Barton, & Rona, 1994). This is much less than what is perceived by the general public.

NATURAL HISTORY

Most adverse food reactions, 80% in one study (Bock, 1987), occur in the first year of life; the majority of children return to a normal diet by age 3. Key factors in the development of tolerance include the food allergen involved and the ability to completely restrict it in the diet (Bock & Atkins, 1989, 1990; Sampson & Scanlon, 1989). Unfortunately, allergies to peanuts, tree nuts (e.g., cashews, pecans, walnuts), fish, and shellfish are rarely "outgrown" (Bock & Atkins, 1989; Daul, Morgan, & Lehrer, 1990). Overall, approximately one third of children younger than 3 years with food allergy can tolerate the food after 1–2 years of avoidance (Pastorello et al., 1989; Sampson & Scanlon, 1989).

CLINICAL MANIFESTATIONS

Adverse food reactions including food allergy typically present with symptoms involving the skin, gastrointestinal tract, and respiratory system. These symptoms may occur alone or in combination and, in some cases, may result in severe generalized reactions (e.g., anaphylaxis). It is rare for an infant or young child to be allergic to more than one or two foods. Eight foods together cause most cases of food allergy: egg, peanuts, milk, soy, wheat, fish, tree nuts, and shellfish. These points may help one to assess the likelihood that a reaction is due to food allergy.

Food Allergy: IgE-Mediated Reactions

Food allergy can impair weight gain in infants and young children by causing gastrointestinal symptoms. These symptoms include nausea, vomiting, abdominal pain, cramping, and, less frequently, diarrhea. They typically occur within 1 hour of the food ingestion. Infants with the food-induced IgE-mediated form of allergic eosinophilic gastroenteritis can present with weight loss or poor growth. This disease is characterized by an allergic history, elevated blood levels of IgE antibody and **eosinophils**, and positive skin tests to a variety of foods and inhalants (Kettlehut & Metcalfe, 1988).

Unwarranted concern about food allergy can lead some parents to restrict their children's diet, which may result in poor weight gain. Investigators evaluated 11 toddlers with histories of multiple food allergies despite little or no supporting evidence (Roesler, Barry, & Bock, 1994). The children presented with significant, long-standing failure to thrive secondary to diminished calorie intake. Only two of the children had their food allergy histories confirmed following well-controlled food challenges. Other than feeding difficulties and caloric restriction, no specific organic cause was found for the failure to thrive in the remaining nine children. This illustrates that invalid beliefs about food allergies can result in improper dietary restriction, which, in turn, may result in poor weight gain and serious long-term consequences for children.

Other manifestations of food allergy affect the skin, such as a red, itchy rash (e.g., hives) or worsening eczema. In fact, skin symptoms are the most common finding in IgE-mediated food allergy. Although hives and swelling usually present acutely (i.e., in less than 24 hours) (James & Sampson, 1992), chronic daily hives (i.e., greater than 6 weeks in duration) are rarely the result of food allergy (Champion, Roberts, Carpenter, & Roger, 1969). Finally, food allergy may be a significant triggering factor in approximately 30% of children with eczema who present in an outpatient clinic setting (Burks, Mallory, Williams, & Shirrell, 1988).

Respiratory reactions also have been reported during food challenges. Nasal congestion, sneezing, and runny nose frequently have been observed (James, Bernhisel-Broadbent, & Sampson, 1994). Moreover, wheezing has been documented in a subset of individuals with asthma who experienced adverse food reactions during food challenges. Isolated respiratory symptoms as the sole clinical finding of food allergy, however, are rare (Bock, 1992; James et al., 1994).

Severe allergic reactions (e.g., anaphylaxis) and even fatalities can occur following the ingestion of foods (James & Burks, 1995; Sampson, Mendelson, & Rosen, 1992). Peanuts, milk, eggs, and tree nuts have been implicated in the majority of these reactions. Children may experience these reactions after the ingestion of even very small amounts of these foods. Common clinical features include the presence of asthma, previous episodes of anaphylaxis with the incriminated food, a failure to recognize early symptoms of anaphylaxis, and a delay or lack of immediate use of emergency medications (e.g., epinephrine, antihistamines).

Food Allergy: Non–IgE-Mediated Reactions

Some immunologically mediated food reactions do not appear to be caused by IgE antibodies. For example, food-induced enterocolitis syndrome, which is most often triggered by cow milk or soy protein, commonly presents in infants who are younger than 3 months (Powell, 1978). This syndrome presents with delayed vomiting and diarrhea (usually 2–6 hours after the food ingestion) with secondary dehydration, and children with this disease may present with poor weight gain. Food-induced enterocolitis syndrome is an uncommon systemic reaction to food ingestion, for which the precise mechanism remains unknown. Diagnostic tests to determine specific IgE antibodies to the offending foods are usually negative. The diagnosis can be confirmed with a food challenge. Tolerance to the offending protein usually is achieved by the child's second or third birthday.

Food Intolerance

As mentioned previously, food intolerance represents any abnormal physiological response to food that is not triggered by the immune system (James & Sampson, 1992; Sampson, 1989). In lactose intolerance, the small intestine is unable to digest lactose, the main sugar in cow milk. This condition most often follows viral diarrhea. The hereditary form of lactose intolerance is common in families of African and Mediterranean origin and rarely presents in children younger than 3 years. The main symptoms of this condition include diarrhea, stomach cramping, and excess gas. Other examples of food intolerance include bacterial food poisoning and physiological side effects of food additives (e.g., diarrhea from sorbitol in some fruit juices; headache, chest tightness, nausea, and sweating following the ingestion of monosodium glutamate).

DIAGNOSIS

The medical history is very useful in differentiating adverse reactions to food (James & Sampson, 1992; Sampson, 1986). A detailed description of each symptom (e.g., skin, gastrointestinal, respiratory) should be obtained. Important historical points include the timing of the reaction in relation to food ingestion, the minimum quantity of food required to cause symptoms, the reproducibility of the symptoms, and the length of time elapsed since the last reaction. Documentation of the treatment received and of the response to treatment is also very useful. It is usually easier to tell which food is causative when the reaction occurs infrequently (e.g., first episode of hives) than when it is chronic (e.g., eczema). Diet diaries are occasionally helpful in identifying which food is the cause of an adverse reaction. Finally, a family history that is positive for allergy can be useful in identifying those who are at increased risk for food allergy.

The physical examination is useful in assessing overall nutritional status, growth, and signs of allergy, such as eczema. Moreover, this examination will help rule out other conditions, such as food intolerances, that may mimic food allergy (Sampson, 1986).

The possibility of food allergy can best be evaluated by an allergist. Skin tests may be done using the prick or puncture technique to screen for IgE-mediated food allergies (Atkins, Steinberg, & Metcalfe, 1985; Sampson, 1983). These can be performed on infants as early as the first few months after birth. When high-quality extracts are used in conjunction with standard criteria of interpretation, these tests give useful, reproducible clinical information in a short period of time (15–20 minutes). Skin testing is a reliable method of excluding IgE-mediated food allergies; a negative test is more than 95% accurate. A positive test, however, only is suggestive of food allergy with an accuracy of less than 50%. This emphasizes the need to confirm the clinical history and positive skin test with a food challenge, unless the history is convincing for anaphylaxis. Finally, the laboratory assessment of food allergy may include the measurement of food-specific IgE antibodies in the blood (i.e., **radioallergosorbent testing**), which provides information similar to skin testing.

Elimination diets, usually done for 7–14 days, are difficult to use by themselves for the diagnosis of food allergy. In fact, they are rarely diagnostic of food allergy. Their success depends on identifying the correct allergen and completely eliminating it in all forms from the diet. Elimination diets may, in some cases, impair the child's nutrition, especially when more than one food is suspected as an allergen. Allergy to multiple foods is a rare occurrence (Bock, 1987; James & Sampson, 1992; Roesler, Bock, & Leung, 1995). Strict elimination of the responsible food is the only proven therapy for food allergy and other adverse food reactions, and a properly managed elimination diet can lead to resolution of food reactions. Before recommending ongoing dietary restrictions (i.e., elimination diets lasting longer than 1 month), one should make every attempt to confirm the clinical and laboratory evidence of a food reaction with a food challenge.

Food challenges are the best way to confirm the diagnosis of food allergy and other adverse food reactions (Atkins et al., 1985; Burks et al., 1988; Pastorello et al., 1989; Sampson, 1983). These challenges, which include the double-blind, placebo-controlled food challenge, should be conducted in a clinic or hospital, especially when true food allergy is suspected. Trained personnel and equipment for severe reactions (e.g., anaphylaxis) must be present (Executive Committee of the Academy of Allergy and Immunology, 1986). A published guide reviewed the combined clinical experience of six centers doing blind food challenges (Bock et al., 1988).

In summary, if no specific foods are implicated in the history and if skin tests to foods are negative, then further workup for IgE-mediated allergy is not indicated. With positive skin tests and/or symptoms associated with specific foods, an elimination diet may be instituted for 7–14 days. If symptoms persist, then food is not likely to be the problem, except in some cases of chronic eczema or asthma. Symptoms that recur after a regular diet is resumed should be evaluated with a food challenge.

TREATMENT

Strict elimination of the causative food is the only proven therapy for food allergy and other adverse food reactions (Bock & Atkins, 1990; Pastorello et al., 1989; Sampson, 1989; Sampson & McCaskill, 1985). A properly managed elimination diet can lead to resolution of food reactions and will avoid malnutrition (David, Waddington, & Stanton, 1984; Lloyd-Still, 1979). Restriction diets should exclude only those foods that have been proved to provoke food allergy (Bock & Atkins, 1990; Sampson & McCaskill, 1985).

Occasionally, individuals who are on elimination diets may experience adverse food reactions following accidental ingestion of the eliminated food allergen (David, 1984). Educating families about how to read food labels and identify common words for the allergen of concern (e.g., casein and whey are cow-milk proteins) is crucial to avoiding the ingestion of hidden ingredients (Barnes-Koerner & Sampson, 1991). Diet sheets or pocket-size cards also are useful references for individuals who have food allergies. The Food Allergy Network[1] is an organization that has been developed to serve as a resource to individuals with food allergies and their families, physicians, and other caregivers.

Appropriate nutritional counseling is important to ensure that an elimination diet is well balanced and avoids any anticipated nutritional deficiencies. For example, calcium deficiency can result from an improperly implemented milk-restriction diet (Davidovits, Levy, Avramovitz, & Eisenstein, 1993; McGowan & Gibney, 1993). Finally, several cow-milk protein hydrolysate formulas are available commercially and have provided safe substitutes for individuals with allergies to cow- and soy-milk proteins.

CONCLUSION

Adverse reactions to foods are an unusual cause of poor nutrition and inadequate weight gain in children younger than 3 years. In some instances, however, they may be important reactions to consider. This chapter has provided the practitioner with guidelines as to when to suspect these reactions, as well as their evaluation and treatment.

REFERENCES

Altman, D.R., & Chiaramonte, L.T. (1996). Public perception of food allergy. *Journal of Allergy and Clinical Immunology, 97,* 1247–1251.

Atkins, F.M., Steinberg, S.S., & Metcalfe, D.D. (1985). Evaluation of immediate adverse reactions to foods in adult patients: I. Correlation on demographic, laboratory, and prick skin test data with response to controlled oral food challenge. *Journal of Allergy and Clinical Immunology, 75,* 348–355.

Barnes-Koerner, C., & Sampson, H.A. (1991). Diets and nutrition in food allergy. In D.D. Metcalfe, H.A. Sampson, & R.A. Simon (Eds.), *Food allergy: Adverse reactions to foods and food additives* (pp. 332–354). Boston: Blackwell Scientific Publications.

Bock, S.A. (1987). Prospective appraisal of complaints of adverse reactions to foods in children during the first 3 years of life. *Pediatrics, 79,* 683–688.

Bock, S.A. (1992). Respiratory reactions induced by food challenges in children with pulmonary disease. *Pediatric Allergy and Immunology, 3,* 188–194.

---

[1]Food Allergy Network: 10400 Eaton Place, Suite 107, Fairfax, VA 22030-2208; telephone: (703) 691-3179; FAX: (703) 691-2713; World Wide Web site: http://www.foodallergy.org; e-mail address: fan@worldweb.net

Bock, S.A., & Atkins, F.M. (1989). The natural history of peanut allergy. *Journal of Allergy and Clinical Immunology, 83,* 900–904.

Bock, S.A., & Atkins, F.M. (1990). Patterns of food hypersensitivity during sixteen years of double-blind placebo-controlled oral food challenges. *Journal of Pediatrics, 117,* 561–567.

Bock, S.A., Sampson, H.A., Atkins, F.M., Zeiger, R.S., Lehrer, S., Sachs, M., Bush, R.K., & Metcalfe, D.D. (1988). Double-blind placebo-controlled food challenge as an office procedure: A manual. *Journal of Allergy and Clinical Immunology, 82,* 986–997.

Burks, A.W., Mallory, S.B., Williams, L.W., & Shirrell, M.A. (1988). Atopic dermatitis: Clinical relevance of food hypersensitivity reactions. *Journal of Pediatrics, 113,* 447–451.

Champion, R.H., Roberts, S.O., Carpenter, R.G., & Roger, J.H. (1969). Urticaria and angioedema: A review of 554 patients. *British Journal of Dermatology, 81,* 588–597.

Daul, C.B., Morgan, J.E., & Lehrer, S.B. (1990). The natural history of shrimp hypersensitivity. *Journal of Allergy and Clinical Immunology, 86,* 88–93.

David, T.J. (1984). Anaphylactic shock during elimination diets for severe atopic eczema. *Archives of Disease in Childhood, 59,* 983–986.

David, T.J., Waddington, E., & Stanton, R.H.J. (1984). Nutritional hazards of elimination diets in children with atopic dermatitis. *Archives of Disease in Childhood, 59,* 323–325.

Davidovits, M., Levy, Y., Avramovitz, T., & Eisenstein, B. (1983). Calcium-deficiency rickets in a four-year-old boy with milk allergy. *Journal of Pediatrics, 122,* 249–251.

Executive Committee of the Academy of Allergy and Immunology. (1986). Personnel and equipment to treat systemic reactions caused by immunotherapy with allergic extracts. *Journal of Allergy and Clinical Immunology, 77,* 271–273.

James, J.M., Bernhisel-Broadbent, J., & Sampson, H.A. (1994). Respiratory reactions provoked by double-blind food challenges in children. *American Journal of Respiratory and Critical Care Medicine, 149,* 59–64.

James, J.M., & Burks, A.W. (1995). Food-induced anaphylaxis. *Immunology Clinics of North America, 15,* 477–488.

James, J.M., & Sampson, H.A. (1992). An overview of food hypersensitivity. *Pediatric Allergy and Immunology, 3,* 67–78.

Kajosaari, M. (1982). Food allergy in Finnish children aged 1 to 6 years. *Acta Paediatrica Scandinavica, 71,* 815–819.

Kettlehut, B.V., & Metcalfe, D.D. (1988). Adverse reactions to foods. In E. Middleton, C.E. Reed, E.F. Ellis, N.F. Adkinson, & J.W. Yunginger (Eds.), *Allergy: Principles and practice* (pp. 1481–1502). St Louis: C.V. Mosby.

Lloyd-Still, J.D. (1979). Chronic diarrhea of childhood and the misuse of elimination diets. *Journal of Pediatrics, 95,* 10–13.

McGowan, M., & Gibney, M.J. (1993). Calcium intakes in individuals on diets for the management of cows' milk allergy: A case control study. *European Journal of Clinical Nutrition, 47,* 609–616.

Niestijl Jansen, J.J., Kardinaal, A.F.M., Huijbers, G., Vlieg-Boerstra, B.J., Martens, B.P.M., & Ockhuizen, T. (1994). Prevalence of food allergy and intolerance in the adult Dutch population. *Journal of Allergy and Clinical Immunology, 93,* 446–456.

Pastorello, E.A., Stocchi, L., Pravetonni, V., Bigi, A., Schilke, M.L., Incorvaia, C., & Zanussi, C. (1989). Role of the elimination diet in adults with food allergy. *Journal of Allergy and Clinical Immunology, 84,* 475–483.

Powell, G.K. (1978). Milk and soy induced enterocolitis of infancy: Clinical features and standardization of challenge. *Journal of Pediatrics, 93,* 553–560.

Roesler, T.A., Barry, P.C., & Bock, S.A. (1994). Factitious food allergy and failure to thrive. *Archives of Pediatric and Adolescent Medicine, 148,* 1150–1155.

Roesler, T.A., Bock, S.A., & Leung, D.Y.M. (1995). Management of the child presenting with allergy to multiple foods. *Clinical Pediatrics, 34,* 608–612.

Sampson, H.A. (1983). Role of immediate food hypersensitivity in the pathogenesis of atopic dermatitis. *Journal of Allergy and Clinical Immunology, 71,* 473–480.

Sampson, H.A. (1986). Differential diagnosis in adverse reactions to foods. *Journal of Allergy and Clinical Immunology, 78,* 212–219.

Sampson, H.A. (1989). Food allergy. *Journal of Allergy and Clinical Immunology, 84,* 1062–1067.

Sampson, H.A., & McCaskill, C.M. (1985). Food hypersensitivity and atopic dermatitis: Evaluation of 113 patients. *Journal of Pediatrics, 107,* 669–675.

Sampson, H.A., Mendelson, L., & Rosen, J.P. (1992). Fatal and near-fatal food anaphylaxis reactions in children. *New England Journal of Medicine, 327,* 380–384.

Sampson, H.A., & Scanlon, S.M. (1989). Natural history of food hypersensitivity in children with atopic dermatitis. *Journal of Pediatrics, 115,* 23–27.

Sloan, A.E., & Powers, M.E. (1986). A perspective on popular perceptions of adverse reactions to foods. *Journal of Allergy and Clinical Immunology, 78,* 127–133.

Young, E., Stoneham, M.D., Petrudhevitch, A., Barton, J., & Rona, R. (1994). A population study of food intolerance. *The Lancet, 343,* 1127–1129.

Chapter 17

Anemia, Lead Exposure, Renal Disease, and Dental Caries

Diana Becker Cutts and Joni Geppert

What is an appropriately aggressive evaluation of the seemingly healthy but undernourished child who is completely asymptomatic and whose examination reveals no abnormalities other than depressed growth measurements? This chapter reviews several important, common, and often asymptomatic conditions that may be significant to childhood growth delays: iron deficiency anemia, lead exposure, renal disease, and dental caries.

IRON DEFICIENCY ANEMIA

The United States reports an overall 3% national prevalence of iron deficiency anemia for children 1–2 years of age and less than 1% for children 3–5 years of age (Looker, Dallman, Carroll, Gunter, & Johnson, 1997). These numbers indicate a significant declining trend (Looker et al., 1997; Yip, Binkin, Fleshood, & Trowbridge, 1987) and commonly are attributed to the increased use of iron-fortified foods and infant formulas (Yip et al., 1987) and the increased bioavailability of iron in fortified foods (Rees, Monsen, & Merrill, 1985). Young children who live in low-income families are at substantially higher risk for anemia, however, with 20% of children younger than 2 years and 17% of children 3–4 years having a hemoglobin or hematocrit below the 5th percentile (Centers for Disease Control and Prevention, 1995). Low-income African American children younger than 5 years are affected disproportionately, with an anemia prevalence of 27% (Centers for Disease Control and Prevention, 1995). Although it is known that African children have slightly lower hemoglobin levels than Caucasian children even when iron status is comparable (Perry, Byers, Yip, & Margen, 1992), this high rate of anemia cannot be explained by racial differences alone. In most cases, anemia in young children can be attributed to poor iron nutrition (Boutry & Needlman, 1996; Dallman, Yip, & Johnson, 1984).

The child who experiences growth delay is at even higher risk for inadequate iron nutrition (Bithoney, Van Sciver, Foster, Corso, & Tentindo, 1995). When food intake is inadequate to meet nutrient needs, iron stores may be depleted at a time when iron requirements may be increased. The consumption of large amounts of iron-poor milk, which may replace iron-containing foods such as fortified grains, also is concerning. Children whose use of bottles is prolonged inappropriately or is extensive or children who have difficult transitions to solids are, therefore, vulnerable to developing iron deficiency anemia. Children who are not being breast-fed should receive iron-fortified formula for the first year of life and begin iron-fortified cereals between 4 and 6 months. Introduction of cow milk before age 1 year also is associated with an increased risk of iron deficiency.

The link to long-lasting developmental disadvantage for children with iron deficiency anemia has been demonstrated in multiple investigations (Lozoff, Brittenham, Jimenez, & Wolf, 1991; Walter, Andraca, Chadud, & Perales, 1989; see also Chapter 3). There also is evidence that iron deficiency in the absence of anemia affects cognitive abilities in preschoolers (Pollitt, Leibel, & Greenfield, 1983), suggesting that by the time anemia develops, a significant adverse impact on health already may have occurred.

Iron deficiency has been associated with an impairment in the immune response (Dallman, 1986). This association is complicated further because infection may decrease iron absorption and anemia may increase the risk for infection (Beresford, Neale, & Brooks, 1971; Dallman, 1986). Furthermore, iron deficiency is not infrequently accompanied by deficiencies of zinc (Hallberg, 1989), which itself has been shown to be an important cofactor for somatic growth and for changes in brain functioning (Fredrickson, 1989). Alterations of the intestinal mucosa also occur in the presence of iron deficiency, resulting in an increased absorption of toxic substances—notably, lead—from the diet (Mahaffey, 1981). These interactive effects of iron deficiency create multiple jeopardies for the affected child.

Children between the ages of 6 months and 5 years generally should be treated for iron deficiency anemia if their hemoglobin is less than 11 g/dl or their hematocrit is less than 34. The distribution of hemoglobin and hematocrit differs slightly by race and altitude. For African American children, the hemoglobin cutoff may be lowered to 10.6 and the hematocrit to less than 33 (Centers for Disease Control and Prevention, 1998). Oral iron therapy is usually given in a dosage of 3–6 mg/kg/day of elemental iron in two or three divided doses. If hemoglobin levels improve by 1 gram per deciliter (g/dl) or normalize after 28 days, then iron supplementation should be continued for an additional 2 months. If no improvement is evident, then further evaluation regarding patient compliance or other causes of the anemia should be conducted (Institute of Medicine, Food and Nutrition Board, National Academy of Sciences, 1993).

Dietary education on strategies to improve iron intake and referral, when appropriate, for enrollment in the Special Supplemental Nutrition Program for Women, Infants and Children (WIC)—a program that serves only 80% of those who are eligible nationally (U.S. Department of Agriculture, 1998)—is an important adjunct to medical treatment of iron deficiency.

LEAD EXPOSURE

Elevated blood-lead concentrations have been associated with symptoms of abdominal pain, anorexia, vomiting, constipation, irritability, lethargy, developmental regression, seizures, and ataxia. Most children, however, are clinically asymptomatic. The silent and long-term damage caused by increased lead levels includes altered neuropsychological functioning and cognitive impairments as well as deleterious effects on child development

(Baghurst et al., 1992; Bellinger, Stiles, & Needleman, 1992; Dietrich, Berger, Succop, Hammond, & Bornschein, 1993).

Impaired growth also has been correlated with increased lead levels. An analysis of the second National Health and Nutrition Examination Survey data showed a significant negative correlation of height, weight, and chest circumference with childhood blood-lead level (Schwartz, Angle, & Pitcher, 1986). Direct neuroendocrine effects of lead, resulting in diminished secretion of growth hormone and insulin-like growth factor, are seen in children with increased lead levels (Huseman, Varma, & Angle, 1992). The profile of the child at greatest risk includes factors of low-income status, residence in housing that was built prior to 1950 or residence in recently remodeled housing that was built prior to 1978, and non-Caucasian race (Mahaffey, Annest, Roberts, & Murphy, 1982). The Centers for Disease Control and Prevention estimates that there are 1.7 million children in the United States who have elevated blood-lead levels (Satcher, 1997), and children with growth delays are a particularly noteworthy group of higher prevalence (Bithoney, 1986; Schwartz et al., 1986). Increased absorption of lead apparently occurs when the stomach is empty. Several investigators have questioned whether lead levels that previously were thought to be of little consequence are, in fact, clinically toxic (Baghurst et al., 1992; Bellinger et al., 1992; Schwartz, 1994). The evolution of current screening policies has reflected these concerns (Satcher, 1997), noting that there may be no threshold level of exposure that is completely benign. Current screening policies also have noted that although national data clearly point to specific risk factors for lead exposure, there are significant local differences that need to be taken into account by community public health agencies in designing screening protocols (Satcher, 1997).

Managing elevated lead levels includes educating the family about lead exposure reduction practices, including dietary manipulations to increase calcium and iron intake, decrease fat intake, and ensure regular meals. Close monitoring and follow-up is indicated, and chelation therapy is advised for children with persisting significant elevation of blood-lead levels. Coordination of developmental and educational services and involvement of housing assistance programs, public health departments, and environmental inspection agencies are important to the successful amelioration of adverse health effects that are the result of this environmental toxin.

RENAL DISEASE

Growth impairment is associated with a lengthy list of congenital and acquired renal diseases, usually on the basis of renal failure, although the exact mechanism of action is unclear (Chesny, 1987). Isolated tubular defects also can cause growth impairment (Donckerwolcke, Yang, & Chan, 1989; Santos & Chan, 1986) as can the chronic or recurrent urinary tract infections such as are seen in the presence of obstruction, vesicoureteral reflux, or structural renal anomalies (Freidman & Lewy, 1978). The lack of specific symptoms to suggest renal disease may mislead the clinician, although there may be intermittent fevers, nausea or vomiting, poor feeding, preference for liquids over solid foods, polyuria, decreased activity, or irritability (Freidman & Lewey, 1978). Bony changes that result from decreased vitamin D and calcium absorption also may occur in children with chronic renal disease (Chesney, 1984). Chronic renal failure, which accounts for the majority of growth failure associated with renal disease, is discovered easily with screening laboratory tests, which include a BUN and creatinine blood level. Because serum creatinine concentration reflects muscle mass, the young child normally has a low creatinine, and levels greater than 0.4 milligram (mg)/dl may indicate significant alteration of normal kidney function (Atiyeh, Dabbagh, & Gruskin, 1996).

The body depends on the kidneys to regulate acid-base homeostasis, thus maintaining blood pH in a relatively narrow range. Renal acidosis results from tubular dysfunction that prevents the normal acidification of urine and consequent acid excretion. The diagnosis of Classic, or Type I, distal renal tubular acidosis (RTA) can be suspected on the basis of a persistent serum carbon dioxide less than 17.5 mEq/dl and a urine pH of more than 6 (Strive, Clardy, Varade, Prada, & Waldo, 1993). Serum chloride concentrations typically are elevated, whereas potassium levels can be elevated or depressed. Distal RTA is the result of a deficiency of hydrogen ion secretion by the distal renal tubule and collecting duct, leading to a complete loss of the distal bicarbonate recovery mechanism. Alkali treatment protects against the development of kidney stones. Most children with distal RTA have a permanent defect and require lifelong treatment (Donckerwolcke et al., 1989; Santos & Chan, 1986), although some have demonstrated disappearance of the acidification defect over time (Leuman & Steinmann, 1975).

Proximal, or Type II, RTA is the result of the proximal renal tubule's losing its capacity to reabsorb bicarbonate, which causes a large amount of bicarbonate to be delivered to the distal tubule. As there is a limited capacity to reabsorb bicarbonate in the distal tubule, a large amount is wasted in the urine. Because the distal tubule maintains function, the urine of children with proximal RTA can be acidified to a pH of less than 6. Although treatment typically necessitates larger dosages of alkali, this condition is more commonly transient, lasting only 1–2 years (Petersen-Smith, 1995). Proximal RTA also occurs as part of Fanconi's syndrome, a condition of proximal tubule dysfunction resulting in **glycosuria, aminoaciduria,** and **phosphaturia** (Kurtzman, 1985). Children whose screening laboratory tests reveal abnormally low serum bicarbonate and high serum chloride deserve further evaluation and may warrant consultation with a nephrologist.

Diagnosis of RTA is confounded, however, by the finding of serum bicarbonate levels between 16 and 20 mEq/dl in approximately 10% of children with growth impairment who were seen at a referral center clinic for failure to thrive (Bithoney, Epstein, & Kim, 1992). These children were without any evidence of renal disease, and their laboratory abnormalities and growth delays subsequently corrected with institution of adequate caloric intake. None of these children were treated with alkali therapy. Undernutrition itself may interfere with tubular renal function (Bithoney et al., 1992), and clinicians must be alert to differentiate between primary and secondary processes.

DENTAL CARIES

The dietary practices associated with baby-bottle tooth decay include excessive and prolonged use of bottles with carbohydrate-rich fluids accompanied by a "grazing" pattern of intake. Baby-bottle tooth decay typically occurs when an infant or child is put to bed with a bottle that contains carbohydrate-rich liquids, such as milk, formula, juice, and sweetened soft drinks. The same syndrome also can occur when an infant is allowed to breastfeed for extended periods of time or is provided with a pacifier that is dipped in a sweetened substance such as jam. These practices frequently are associated with poor growth and malnutrition through inadequate iron intake, increased or decreased caloric intake, and development of poor eating habits. Because baby-bottle tooth decay affects the primary teeth that are used for chewing solid foods, children may prefer liquids and very soft foods and may decrease intake intentionally to minimize pain.

Prevalence estimates among low-income Head Start participants in the United States range from 11% in Ohio to well over 50% in Native American populations (Bruerd & Jones, 1996; Milnes, 1996). Because several studies have directly linked extensive dental caries and baby-bottle or nursing tooth decay in young children with impaired growth

(Acs, Lodolini, Kaminsky, & Cisneros, 1992; Ayhan, Suskan, & Yildirim, 1996), the contribution of the accompanying poor dentition, chronic oral infections, and mouth pain in children with inadequate growth cannot be ignored.

A dental examination, particularly of the child with a history of concerning dietary habits, is an important part of the evaluation of any child with nutritional problems. Prompt referral to dentists who are skilled in the care of young children should be made when any signs of decay are present in the primary teeth. Families should be encouraged to introduce babies to cup use at 6 months and weaning from the bottle by 1 year of age. Limiting juice consumption to less than 6 ounces per day is reasonable for the young child. Educational efforts to decrease the prevalence of baby-bottle tooth decay should be directed to all parents and child care workers.

CONCLUSION

The medical practitioner who cares for children who exhibit the symptom of poor growth must consider all potential contributing and, perhaps, exacerbating factors. Anemia, lead exposure, renal disease, and dental caries are important comorbidities in young, malnourished children.

REFERENCES

Acs, G., Lodolini, G., Kaminsky, S., & Cisneros, G.J. (1992). Effect of nursing caries on body weight in a pediatric population. *Pediatric Dentistry, 14,* 302–305.

Atiyeh, B.A., Dabbagh, S.S., & Gruskin, A.B. (1996). Evaluation of renal function during childhood. *Pediatrics in Review, 17,* 175–180.

Ayhan, H., Suskan, E., & Yildirim, S. (1996). The effect of nursing or rampant caries on height, body weight and head circumference. *The Journal of Clinical Pediatric Dentistry, 20,* 209–212.

Baghurst, P.A., McMichael, A.J., Wigg, N.R., Vimpani, G.V., Robertson, E.F., Roberts, R.J., & Tong, S. (1992). Environmental exposure to lead and children's intelligence at the age of seven years: The Port Pirie cohort study. *New England Journal of Medicine, 327,* 1279–1284.

Bellinger, D.C., Stiles, K.M., & Needleman, H.L. (1992). Low-level lead exposure, intelligence and academic achievement: A long-term follow-up study. *Pediatrics, 90,* 855–861.

Beresford, C.H., Neale, R.J., & Brooks, O.G. (1971). Absorption and pyrexia. *The Lancet, 1,* 568–572.

Bithoney, W.G. (1986). Elevated lead levels in children with nonorganic failure to thrive. *Pediatrics, 78,* 891–895.

Bithoney, W.G., Epstein, D., & Kim, M. (1992). Decreased serum bicarbonate as a manifestation of undernutrition secondary to nonorganic failure-to-thrive. *Journal of Behavioral Pediatrics, 13,* 278–280.

Bithoney, W.G., Van Sciver, M.M., Foster, S., Corso, S., & Tentindo, C. (1995). Parental stress and growth outcome in growth-deficient children. *Pediatrics, 96,* 707–711.

Boutry, M., & Needlman, R. (1996). Use of diet history in the screening of iron deficiency. *Pediatrics, 98,* 1138–1142.

Bruerd, B., & Jones, C. (1996). Preventing baby bottle tooth decay: Eight-year results. *Public Health Reports, 111,* 63–65.

Centers for Disease Control and Prevention. (1995). *Pediatric Nutrition Surveillance System annual summary.* Atlanta: National Center for Chronic Disease Prevention and Health Promotion, Division of Nutrition and Physical Activity.

Centers for Disease Control and Prevention. (1998). Recommendations to prevent and control iron deficiency in the United States. *Morbidity and Mortality Weekly Report, 47*(No. RR-3), 1–28.

Chesney, R.W. (1984). Metabolic bone disease. *Pediatrics in Review, 5,* 227–237.

Chesney, R.W. (1987). Growth retardation in childhood renal disease: A hormonal or nutritional problem? *American Journal of Nephrology, 7,* 253–256.

Dallman, P.R. (1986). Biochemical basis for the manifestations of iron deficiency. *Annual Review of Nutrition, 6,* 13–40.

Dallman, P.R., Yip, R., & Johnson, C. (1984). Prevalence and causes of anemia in the United States, 1976 to 1980. *American Journal of Clinical Nutrition, 39,* 437–445.

Dietrich, K.N., Berger, O.G., Succop, P.A., Hammond, P.B., & Bornschein, R.L. (1993). The developmental consequences of low to moderate prenatal and postnatal lead exposure: Intellectual attainment in the Cincinnati Lead Study Cohort following school entry. *Neurotoxicology and Teratology, 15,* 37–44.

Donckerwolcke, R., Yang, W., & Chan, J.C.M. (1989). Growth failure in children with renal tubular acidosis. *Seminars in Nephrology, 9,* 72–74.

Fredrickson, C.J. (1989). Neurobiology of zinc and zinc-containing neurons. *International Review of Neurobiology, 31,* 146–238.

Friedman, J., & Lewy, J.E. (1978). Failure to thrive associated with renal disease. *Pediatric Annals, 7,* 73–82.

Hallberg, L. (1989). Search for nutritional confounding factors in the relationship between iron deficiency and brain function. *American Journal of Clinical Nutrition, 50,* 598–606.

Huseman, C.A., Varma, M.M., & Angle, C.R. (1992). Neuroendocrine effects of toxic and low blood lead levels in children. *Pediatrics, 90,* 186–189.

Institute of Medicine, Food and Nutrition Board, National Academy of Sciences. (1993). Recommended guidelines for prevention, detection, and management of iron deficiency anemia. In R. Earl & C.E. Woteki (Eds.), *Iron deficiency anemia: Recommended guidelines for the prevention, detection, and management among U.S. children and women of childbearing age* (pp. 14–18). Washington, DC: National Academy Press.

Kurtzman, N.A. (1985). Renal tubular acidosis: A constellation of symptoms. *Hospital Practice, 22,* 173–188.

Leuman, E.P., & Steinman, B. (1975). Persistent and transient distal renal tubular acidosis with bicarbonate wasting. *Pediatric Research, 9,* 767–773.

Looker, A.C., Dallman, P.R., Carroll, M.D., Gunter, E.W., & Johnson, C.L. (1997). Prevalence of iron deficiency in the United States. *Journal of the American Medical Association, 277,* 973–976.

Lozoff, B., Brittenham, G.M., Jimenez, E., & Wolf, A.W. (1991). Long-term developmental outcome of infants with iron deficiency. *New England Journal of Medicine, 325,* 687–694.

Mahaffey, K.R. (1981). Nutritional factors in lead poisoning. *Nutrition Reviews, 39,* 353–362.

Mahaffey, K.R., Annest, J.L., Roberts, J., & Murphy, R.S. (1982). National estimates of blood lead levels: United States, 1976–1980. Association with selected demographic and socioeconomic factors. *New England Journal of Medicine, 307,* 573–579.

Milnes, A.R. (1996). Description and epidemiology of nursing caries. *Journal of Public Health Dentistry, 56,* 38–50.

Perry, G.S., Byers, T., Yip, R., & Margen, S. (1992). Iron nutrition does not account for the hemoglobin differences between blacks and whites. *Journal of Nutrition, 122,* 1417–1429.

Petersen-Smith, A.M. (1995). Renal tubular acidosis: When kids won't grow. *Journal of Pediatric Health Care, 9,* 131–133.

Pollitt, E., Leibel, R.L., & Greenfield, D.B. (1983). Iron deficiency and cognitive test performance in preschool children. *Nutrition and Behavior, 1,* 137–146.

Rees, J.M., Monsen, E.R., & Merrill, J.E. (1985). Iron fortification of infant foods: A decade of change. *Clinical Pediatrics, 24,* 707–710.

Santos, F., & Chan, J.C.M. (1986). Renal tubular acidosis in children: Diagnosis, treatment and prognosis. *American Journal of Nephrology, 6,* 289–295.

Satcher, D. (1997). *Screening young children for lead poisoning: Guidance for state and local public health officials.* Atlanta: Centers for Disease Control and Prevention.

Schwartz, J. (1994). Low-level lead exposure and children's IQ: A meta-analysis and search for a threshold. *Environmental Research, 65,* 42–55.

Schwartz, J., Angle, C., & Pitcher, H. (1986). Relationship between childhood blood lead levels and stature. *Pediatrics, 77,* 281–288.

Strive, C., Clardy, C., Varade, W., Prada, A., & Waldo, F. (1993). Urine to blood carbon dioxide tension gradient and maximal depression of pH to distinguish rate-dependent from classic distal tubular acidosis in children. *Journal of Pediatrics, 122,* 60–65.

U.S. Department of Agriculture. (1998). *Special Supplemental Nutrition Program for Women, Infants and Children (WIC): Eligibility and coverage estimates 1998 update—U.S. and outlying areas.* Washington, DC: Author.

Walter, T., Andraca, I., Chadud, P., & Perales, C.G. (1989). Iron deficiency anemia: Adverse effects on infant psychomotor development. *Pediatrics, 84,* 7–17.

Yip, R., Binkin, N.J., Fleshood, L., & Trowbridge, F.L. (1987). Declining prevalence of anemia among low-income children in the United States. *Journal of the American Medical Association, 258,* 1619–1623.

Chapter 18

Effects of Prenatal Exposures to Alcohol, Tobacco, and Other Drugs

Deborah A. Frank and Frieda Wong

The clinician evaluating the child who has been referred for failure to thrive must determine to what extent the child's growth deficits reflect prenatal factors that limit the potential efficacy of postnatal interventions. Such an evaluation becomes particularly complex when the child has a history of prenatal exposure to psychoactive substances, whether legal (e.g., cigarettes, alcohol) or illegal (e.g., marijuana, cocaine, opiates). It is critical that the clinician who is evaluating any child who is experiencing failure to thrive tactfully ascertain in detail the child's prenatal history of exposure to psychoactive substances. This history should include not only which substances the mother used but also, ideally, some estimate of frequency, quantity, and timing of use (e.g., packs of cigarettes per day, average number of drinks per day, maximum number of drinks on a single occasion, number of milligrams of methadone, number of days per week of cocaine use). Mothers often will respond most readily to the question, "How much did you use before you found out that you were pregnant?" The interviewer can then go on to inquire about the second and third trimesters.

Prenatal exposures may influence the risk of later growth failure not only by depressing the child's size at birth (from decreased gestational age or intrauterine growth retardation) but also by transient or persistent alterations in the child's neurological and gastrointestinal functioning, which can be linked to feeding difficulties. Prematurity and intrauterine growth retardation of whatever cause are intricately related to postnatal growth patterns (see Chapter 10). The discussion in this chapter is restricted to growth impairments that are linked specifically to prenatal exposures to psychoactive substances.

Commonly used psychoactive substances not only may exert toxic effects prenatally but also may influence the postnatal caregiving milieu to the detriment of the child's growth. It is important to identify caregivers' ongoing psychoactive substance use because, unlike prenatal history, this can be modified by clinical intervention. A parent who is intoxicated chronically with alcohol or illegal drugs and whose material resources and psychic energies are focused primarily on satisfying an addiction often fails to provide the nutrition and care that is necessary for children to realize their growth potential.

The fetus rarely is exposed to only one psychoactive substance in pregnancy (multiple exposures are common) (Frank & Zeisel, 1988); however, for simplicity of presentation, the effects on postnatal growth of each commonly used substance are discussed one by one. It is important to note that most studies report between-group differences in aggregate but do not define clearly the percentage of children, with and without a psychoactive substance exposure, who would have attained growth or growth rate so decreased as to come to clinical attention as "failure to thrive."

ALCOHOL

When addressing prenatal alcohol effects on later growth, clinicians must distinguish between children who fit the diagnosis of fetal alcohol syndrome (FAS)—a pattern of growth deficiency that includes microcephaly, distinctive craniofacial dysmorphology (including shortened palpebral fissures, smooth philtrum, and thin upper lip), and central nervous system dysfunction found in offspring of chronically alcoholic women—and children with a history of exposure to alcohol prenatally but who do not fit a syndrome diagnosis. Spohr and Steinhausen (1987), in a sample of 54 German children with FAS, found that the number of children with weight, length, and head circumference above the 3rd percentile increased with maturation from preschool to school age. One long-term follow-up study in the United States (Streissguth et al., 1991) suggested that children with diagnosed FAS tend to have short stature and microcephaly that persist into adolescence and adulthood, with less pronounced deficits in weight. In a subsample of 31 subjects in that study, the weight-for-height distribution approximated that of the National Center for Health Statistics (NCHS) norms.

The growth effects of prenatal alcohol exposure without FAS are less clearly delineated and appear to be related to demographic factors, the age of the mother, the stability of the home environment, and the amount and the timing of in utero exposure. Infants who are exposed to alcohol in utero, particularly in the second and third trimesters (Coles et al., 1990; Day, Richardson, & Robles, 1994), as a group show decreased weights and lengths and, usually, head circumference at birth regardless of ethnicity or socioeconomic status (Day et al., 1994; Day et al., 1990; Fried & O'Connell, 1987; Greene et al., 1991; Jacobson, Jacobson, & Sokol, 1994; Sampson, Bookstein, Barr, & Streissguth, 1994). The threshold for negative prenatal alcohol effects on size at birth is not clearly defined, ranging from one drink per day during the second and third trimesters (0.5 ounces absolute alcohol) (Day et al., 1990) to four drinks per day (2 ounces absolute alcohol) (Jacobson et al., 1994), when confounding factors are controlled statistically.

The literature diverges as to what extent in utero exposure to alcohol affects postpartum growth in the absence of recognized FAS. In predominantly Caucasian, middle-class samples, negative prenatal alcohol effects on child size are transient and no longer found after 8–12 months of age (Fried & O'Connell, 1987; Sampson et al., 1994). In contrast, some studies have found that in utero alcohol exposure exerts long-lasting effects on growth in economically deprived, ethnically mixed, or predominantly African American populations. Greene et al. (1991) concluded that the effect of prenatal alcohol exposure on weight and stature through 4 years, 10 months of age was small and not statistically significant. In repeated measurements of low-income children at 8 and 18 months and 3 and 6 years of age, Day and colleagues (Day, Goldschmidt, et al., 1991; Day et al., 1994; Day et al., 1990; Day, Robles, et al., 1991) showed that children who were exposed in utero to one or more drinks per day throughout pregnancy showed consistently smaller height, weight, and head circumference at each measurement interval. Effects at later ages were mediated by growth parameters at 8 months, suggesting little relative catch-up growth (Day et al., 1994). Russell, Czarnecki, Cowan, McPherson, and Mudar (1991) found significant decrements in height and head circumference but not in weight in 6-year-old children whose mothers admitted to two or more drinks per day before the recognition of pregnancy. Coles et al. (1990) also identified significant decrements in head circumference but not in weight or length between the ages of 5 and 8 years among children whose mothers continued to drink throughout pregnancy. Jacobson et al. (1994) found slower rates of gain in weight and length from birth to 6.5 months and increased likelihood of weight and length below the 10th percentile among offspring of women whose average intake was 2 ounces of absolute alcohol per day. At 13 months, deficits in length but not in weight were associated with prenatal alcohol exposure but only among children of mothers who were older than 30.

The mediating mechanisms of prenatal alcohol effects on postnatal growth are not well understood. In FAS, a number of clinically obvious factors, including oral malformations, inefficient sucking, and delayed oral-motor development, have been noted by clinicians, but no pathognomonic pattern of oral-motor dysfunction has been identified (Van Dyke, Mackay, & Ziaylek, 1982). In children with prenatal alcohol exposure without FAS, both impaired appetite regulation and neuroendocrine effects on the growth hormone axis have been postulated but not confirmed (Day et al., 1994; Middaugh & Boggan, 1995). Whether the extent of decreased skeletal growth in children with prenatal alcohol exposure predicts the severity of cognitive impairments is a matter of controversy (Janzen, Nanson, & Block, 1995).

COCAINE

Cocaine exposure in utero is associated independently with decrements in gestational age (Chasnoff, Griffith, Freier, & Murray, 1992; Jacobson et al., 1994; Weathers, Crane, Sauvain, & Blackhurst, 1993) and consistently with lower birth weight (Handler, Kistin, Davis, & Ferre, 1991) and usually lower length and head circumference for gestational age (Chasnoff et al., 1992; Harsham, Keller, & Disbrow, 1994; Tronick, Frank, Cabral, Mirochnik, & Zuckerman, 1996; Weathers et al., 1993; Zuckerman et al., 1989). A single small study of infant feeding behavior at 7–16 weeks of age (Neuspiel, Hamel, Hochberg, Greene, & Campbell, 1991) found no difference between newborns who were exposed to cocaine and those who were not exposed. Postnatal catch-up in weight has been described in several follow-up studies; weights of infants who were and were not exposed became indistinguishable between 3 (Chasnoff et al., 1992) and 6 months of age (Harsham et al., 1994; Jacobson et al., 1994), reflecting faster-than-average rates of gain (Jacobson et al., 1994). Catch-up in length (Chasnoff et al., 1992; Jacobson et al., 1994; Weathers et al., 1993) has been reported by some (Harsham et al., 1994) but not others, who found relative increased weight for length at 1 year among infants who were exposed, because weight caught up before length. One study described persistent decrement in head circumference to age 2 years (Chasnoff et al., 1992), but two others (Jacobson et al., 1994; Weathers et al., 1993) found no such decrement by 12–13 months of age. In long-term follow-up to 6 years of age, 28 children with light to moderate cocaine exposure did not differ in adjusted weight, height, or head circumference from comparison children (Richardson, Conroy, & Day, 1996).

NICOTINE AND MARIJUANA

Smoking either tobacco or marijuana by women during pregnancy has been associated with decreased weight and length and, sometimes, head circumference in the newborn (Fried & O'Connell, 1987), probably associated with increased maternal carbon monoxide levels and decreased fetal oxygenation (Frank et al., 1990; Zuckerman et al., 1989). Prenatal marijuana exposure has not been associated with depressed postnatal growth in any follow-up study (Day et al., 1994; Fried & Watkinson, 1988; Jacobson et al., 1994). Passive exposure to cigarettes postnatally has been associated with increased risk of recurring otitis, sinusitis, and lower respiratory illness (DiFranza & Lew, 1996), a cumulative burden of infections that can impede growth. Although some investigators (Fried & Watkinson, 1988) have noted in the first 2 years of life a trend for small decrements in length, weight, and head circumference associated with prenatal tobacco exposure, two studies found no such effects once prenatal alcohol exposure was controlled statistically (Day et al., 1994; Jacobson et al., 1994).

OPIATES

Heroin use during pregnancy (Wilson, Desmond, & Wait, 1981) has been linked with decreased weight, length, and head circumference at birth as has methadone. Methadone exerts fewer negative effects on in utero growth than heroin, probably because of better maternal compliance with prenatal care (Doberczak, Thornton, Bernstein, & Kandall, 1987). Neonatal narcotic abstinence syndrome is characterized by disturbances in sucking as well as vomiting and diarrhea, which may be severe enough to impede early weight gain and even hydration if not managed carefully (Finnegan, 1985). As Hans (1992) summarized, long-term growth outcomes following prenatal opiate exposure vary from sample to sample: Some show no differences by the preschool years from children who were not exposed, whereas others manifest increased rates of depressed head circumference and linear growth. No studies have shown later weight-for-age deficits following early opiate exposure (Hans, 1992).

CONCLUSIONS

Although most commonly used psychoactive substances, including cocaine, marijuana, tobacco, and opiates, are associated with lower birth weight, length, or head circumference, catch-up postnatal somatic growth occurs when adequate nutrition and environment are provided. In terms of clinical expectations for later growth, catch-up somatic growth following all of these exposures tends to occur in the first year of life, so growth faltering in the early months should be addressed promptly. Microcephaly may persist following prenatal opiate exposure.

Growth outcomes following in utero alcohol exposure in the second and third trimesters, even at levels sufficient to cause FAS, are quite variable with potential for at least partial recovery beyond infancy. Alcohol effects are more likely to be seen in stature and head circumference than in weight. Depressed weight-for-height cannot be attributed to prenatal alcohol exposure.

Clinicians should not accept any of the psychoactive substances discussed in this chapter as sufficient explanation for a child who is underweight for height or who is faltering from a previously established growth trajectory. Like other children who "fail to thrive," children with histories of prenatal exposure to psychoactive substances merit intensive multidisciplinary intervention.

REFERENCES

Chasnoff, I.J., Griffith, D.R., Freier, C., & Murray, J. (1992). Cocaine/polydrug use in pregnancy: Two-year follow-up. *Pediatrics, 89,* 284–289.

Coles, C.D., Brown, R.T., Smith, I.E., Platzman, K.A., Erickson, S., & Falek, A. (1990). Effects of prenatal alcohol exposure at school age: I. Physical and cognitive development. *Neurotoxicology and Teratology, 13,* 357–367.

Day, N.L., Goldschmidt, L., Robles, N., Richardson, G., Cornelius, M., Taylor, P., Geva, D., & Stoffer, D. (1991). Prenatal alcohol exposure and offspring growth at 18 months of age: The predictive validity of two measures of drinking. *Alcoholism: Clinical and Experimental Research, 15,* 914–918.

Day, N.L., Richardson, G.A., & Robles, N. (1994). Alcohol, marijuana, and tobacco: Effects of prenatal exposure on offspring growth and morphology at age six. *Alcoholism: Clinical and Experimental Research, 18,* 786–794.

Day, N.L., Richardson, G., Robles, N., Sambamoorthi, U., Taylor, P., Scher, M., Stoffer, D., Jasperse, D., & Cornelius, M. (1990). Effect of prenatal alcohol exposure on growth and morphology of offspring at 8 months of age. *Pediatrics, 85,* 748–752.

Day, N.L., Robles, N., Richardson, G., Geva, D., Taylor, P., Scher, M., Stoffer, D., Cornelius, M., & Goldschmidt, L. (1991). The effects of prenatal alcohol use on the growth of children at three years of age. *Alcoholism: Clinical and Experimental Research, 15,* 67–71.

DiFranza, J.R., & Lew, R.A. (1996). Morbidity and mortality in children associated with the use of tobacco products by other people. *Pediatrics, 97,* 560–568.

Doberczak, T.M., Thornton, J.C., Bernstein, J., & Kandall, S.R. (1987). Impact of maternal drug dependency on birth weight and head circumference of offspring. *American Journal of Diseases of Children, 141,* 1163–1167.

Finnegan, L.P. (1985). Effects of maternal opiate abuse on the newborn. *Federation Proceedings, 44,* 2314–2317.

Frank, D.A., Bauchner, H., Parker, S., Huber, A.M., Kyei-Aboagye, K., Cabral, H., & Zuckerman, B. (1990). Neonatal body proportionality and body composition after in utero exposure to cocaine and marijuana. *Journal of Pediatrics, 117,* 622–626.

Frank, D.A., & Zeisel, S.H. (1988). Failure to thrive. *Pediatric Clinics of North America, 35,* 1187–1206.

Fried, P.A., & O'Connell, C.M. (1987). A comparison of the effects of prenatal exposure to tobacco, alcohol, cannabis and caffeine on birth size and subsequent growth. *Neurotoxicology and Teratology, 9,* 79–85.

Fried, P.A., & Watkinson, B. (1988). 12- and 24-month neurobehavioural follow-up of children prenatally exposed to marihuana, cigarettes and alcohol. *Neurotoxicology and Teratology, 10,* 305–313.

Greene, T.A., Ernhart, C.B., Sokol, R.J., Martier, S., Marler, M.R., Boyd, T.A., & Ager, J. (1991). Prenatal alcohol exposure and preschool physical growth: A longitudinal analysis. *Alcoholism: Clinical and Experimental Research, 15,* 905–913.

Handler, A., Kistin, N., Davis, F., & Ferre, C. (1991). Cocaine use during pregnancy: Perinatal outcomes. *American Journal of Epidemiology, 133,* 818–825.

Hans, S.L. (1992). Maternal opioid drug use and child development. In I.S. Zagan & T.A. Slotkin (Eds.), *Maternal substance abuse and the developing nervous system* (pp. 177–214). San Diego: Academic Press.

Harsham, J., Keller, J.H., & Disbrow, D. (1994). Growth patterns of infants exposed to cocaine and other drugs in utero. *Journal of the American Dietetic Association, 94,* 999–1007.

Jacobson, J.L., Jacobson, S.W., & Sokol, R.J. (1994). Effects of prenatal exposure to alcohol, smoking, and illicit drugs on postpartum somatic growth. *Alcoholism: Clinical and Experimental Research, 18,* 317–323.

Janzen, L.A., Nanson, J.L., & Block, G.W. (1995). Neuropsychological evaluation of preschoolers with fetal alcohol syndrome. *Neurotoxicology and Teratology, 17,* 273–279.

Middaugh, L.D., & Boggan, W.O. (1995). Perinatal maternal ethanol effects on pregnant mice and on offspring viability and growth: Influences of exposure time and weaning diet. *Alcoholism: Clinical and Experimental Research, 19,* 1351–1358.

Neuspiel, D.R., Hamel, C., Hochberg, E., Greene, J., & Campbell, D. (1991). Maternal cocaine use and infant behavior. *Neurotoxicology and Teratology, 13,* 229–233.

Richardson, G.A., Conroy, M.L., & Day, N.L. (1996). Prenatal cocaine exposure: Effects on the development of school-age children. *Neurotoxicology and Teratology, 18,* 627–634.

Russell, M., Czarnecki, D.M., Cowan, R., McPherson, E., & Mudar, P.J. (1991). Measures of maternal alcohol use as predictors of development in early childhood. *Alcoholism: Clinical and Experimental Research, 15,* 991–1000.

Sampson, P.D., Bookstein, F.L., Barr, H.M., & Streissguth, A.P. (1994). Prenatal alcohol exposure, birthweight, and measures of child size from birth to age 14 years. *American Journal of Public Health, 84,* 1421–1428.

Spohr, H.L., & Steinhausen, H.C. (1987). Follow-up studies of children with fetal alcohol syndrome. *Neuropediatrics, 18,* 13–17.

Streissguth, A.P., Aase, J.M., Clarren, S.K., Randels, S.P., LaDue, R.A., & Smith, D.F. (1991). Fetal alcohol syndrome in adolescents and adults. *Journal of the American Medical Association, 265,* 1961–1967.

Tronick, E.Z., Frank, D.A., Cabral, H., Mirochnick, M., & Zuckerman, B. (1996). Late dose-response effects of prenatal cocaine exposure on newborn neurobehavioral performance. *Pediatrics, 98,* 76–83.

Van Dyke, D.C., Mackay, L., & Ziaylek, E.N. (1982). Management of severe feeding dysfunction in children with fetal alcohol syndrome. *Clinical Pediatrics, 21,* 336–339.

Weathers, W.T., Crane, M.M., Sauvain, K.J., & Blackhurst, D.W. (1993). Cocaine use in women from a defined population: Prevalence at delivery and effects on growth in infants. *Pediatrics, 91,* 350–354.

Wilson, G.S., Desmond, M.M., & Wait, R.B. (1981). Follow-up of methadone-treated and untreated narcotic-dependent women and their infants: Health, developmental, and social implications. *Journal of Pediatrics, 98,* 716–722.

Zuckerman, B., Frank, D.A., Hingson, R., Amaro, H., Levenson, S., Kayne, H., Parker, S., Vinci, R., Aboagye, K., Fried, L.E., Cabral, H., Timperi, R., & Bauchner, H. (1989). Effects of maternal marijuana and cocaine use on fetal growth. *New England Journal of Medicine, 320,* 762–768.

Chapter 19

Diagnostic Coding of
Children with Failure to Thrive

Patrick H. Casey

Diagnostic coding of children with failure to thrive (FTT) long has been fraught with problems. FTT has been called a descriptive condition, a sign, or a symptom rather than a diagnosis, with no uniform understanding of etiology, course, treatment, and prognosis (see Chapter 1). Even within pediatrics, the clinical field that developed and uses the term *FTT*, there is no uniformity in perception of terminology or classification; in fact, there is considerable and growing concern regarding the ongoing use of the term *FTT*. Despite this concern, the term *FTT* is used in this chapter per convention and because this chapter describes how various classification schemes deal with FTT.

Related clinical disciplines involved in the management of children with FTT have developed different terminology and classifications. This chapter provides a brief overview of various terminology and classifications. The coding and classification approach of the major diagnostic classification schemes, the *Diagnostic and Statistical Manual of Mental Disorders, Fourth Edition* (DSM-IV) (American Psychiatric Association, 1994) and the *International Classification of Diseases, Ninth Revision* (ICD-9) (1994), is presented. Two new diagnostic classification schemes, the *Classification of Child and Adolescent Mental Diagnoses in Primary Care: Diagnostic and Statistical Manual for Primary Care* (DSM-PC) *Child and Adolescent Version* (American Academy of Pediatrics, 1996) and the *Diagnostic Classification of Mental Health and Developmental Disorders of Infancy and Early Childhood* (ZERO TO THREE: National Center for Infants, Toddlers and Families, 1994), are described, and the ways in which they deal with FTT are presented.

CLASSIFICATION AND CLINICAL CATEGORIZATIONS

As noted by Rutter (1978), clinical classifications allow the ordering of information and grouping of clinical phenomena and provide for the grouping of clinical types in an operational fashion based on facts, not concepts. Classifications allow communication among researchers and clinicians, which ultimately provide understanding in treatment and prognosis. From a practical perspective, classifications allow coding of clinical conditions for administrative purposes such as billing and compiling statistics. The following clinical categories of FTT have been developed. Unfortunately, there is inadequate empirical data to support uniformly any one classification system. This problem is reflected in coding issues described next.

Medical Classification

The historical categories that are most consistently utilized in the pediatric literature are organic and nonorganic FTT (Berwick, 1980; Bithoney, Dubowitz, & Egan, 1992). *Organic FTT* is used when the clinician believes that the FTT results from a specific medical condition, such as cystic fibrosis or congenital heart disease. *Nonorganic FTT* is used to describe a situation in which extreme problems in the child's environment are judged to be the cause of the FTT. This dichotomy has proved to be unacceptable, except in the minority of children with FTT. Many clinicians and theorists are moving to a transactional model of categorizing FTT (transactional FTT) (Casey, 1992; Skuse, 1985). Multiple and, often, subtle aspects of the child (e.g., temperament, feeding difficulties, mild health conditions) that may be seen in a child who has no specific medical diagnosis or in children who have historical characteristics, such as low birth weight or intrauterine growth retardation, interact with features of the parents (e.g., lack of experience, temperamental or emotional variability) and the environment (e.g., unstable or inadequate living environment, social isolation, inadequate finances). No one characteristic is so extreme as to be considered the specific cause of growth difficulties.

Nutritional Classification

Most medical experts believe that pediatric undernutrition (malnutrition) is central to the etiology of FTT (Black & Dubowitz, 1991; Frank & Zeisel, 1988). Most research work with malnutrition has been done with children who live in developing countries, and these researchers have developed classifications of mild, moderate, or severe malnutrition based on weight-for-age, height-for-age, or weight-for-height (Frank, Silva, & Needlman, 1993; see Chapter 9). A review applied these classifications to a large sample of children with FTT in the United States; although there were some discrepancies regarding classification, the majority had mild to moderate malnutrition (Wright, Ashenburg, & Whitaker, 1994).

Developmental Classification

A compelling classification of children with FTT is based on developmental age of onset in the context of problems in parent–child interactions that occur at that stage (Chatoor, Schaefer, Dickson, & Egan, 1984; Lieberman & Birch, 1985). FTT in this classification is conceptualized as a feeding disturbance resulting from breakdowns in the successful achievement of developmental issues and a failure in the mutually satisfactory regulation of relationship between infant and caregiver.

- *Disorder of homeostasis:* Disorder of homeostasis occurs in the first 2–3 months of life, with major contribution from the infant relating to variability in normal physiological functions such as sleep, breathing, elimination, and feeding organization and stabilization. Any biological event, such as prematurity, central nervous system injury, or mechanical feeding problems, increases the likelihood of this condition, depending on the ability of the parent to negotiate the transition to organization in these functions.

- *Disorder of attachment:* The attachment relationship, resulting in and from a synchronized reciprocal interaction between parent and infant, evolves from 2 to 6 months of age. Failure in development of attachment may result in FTT (see Chapters 29 and 30). Infants who have problems with homeostasis and challenging temperaments may contribute to the development of this attachment problem.

- *Disorders of separation and individuation:* The infant begins to function with increasing emotional and physical independence between 6 and 36 months of age. As the child grapples increasingly with the need for autonomy while dependent, mealtime may become a focus of struggle for control over what, when, and how the meal transpires. This struggle may result in food refusal or other negative mealtime behaviors, ultimately resulting in FTT because of inadequate nutritional intake.

Psychiatric Diagnoses

Mental health providers typically have used the following diagnoses when treating children with FTT:

- *Feeding disorder of infancy or early childhood:* The most specific diagnosis for classification of FTT in the DSM-IV is the so-called Feeding Disorder of Infancy. This is discussed in more detail in the section "Formal Coding Schemes."

- *Depression:* Some experts have argued that the criteria used to diagnose major depressive disorder in the *Diagnostic and Statistical Manual of Mental Disorders, Third Edition, Revised* (DSM-III-R) (American Psychiatric Association, 1987) and the DSM-IV can be applied usefully to infants with FTT (Powell & Bettes, 1992). This would suggest that some infants with FTT are, in fact, depressed.

- *Reactive attachment disorder:* Reactive attachment disorder results in disturbed and developmentally inappropriate social relatedness and has its onset during the preschool years (Richters & Volkmar, 1994). This disorder results from grossly pathological caregiving that fails to meet the child's emotional or physical needs. This diagnosis may be causatively associated with FTT.

Feeding Disorder: Physiological

A different perspective from the psychiatric model of feeding has been provided by speech and occupational therapists, gastroenterologists, and others. This approach conceptualizes feeding in a more physiological fashion (Rudolph, 1994). Although no specific diagnostic categories have been recommended in this area, the following clinical categories have been described.

- *Oral-motor feeding problem:* Feeding requires chewing, sucking, ingesting, and swallowing. These various aspects of feeding are dependent on coordination of sensory and motor skills and split-second timing of tongue, pharynx, larynx, and cessation of breathing. Problems in this area often are subtle but may result in difficulties that are sufficient to cause inadequate caloric intake, resulting in nutritional problems and FTT (Mathisen, Skuse, & Wolke, 1989; Ramsay, Gisel, & Boutry, 1993; see Chapter 23).

- *Food aversion:* Some children actively avoid eating because of aversive experiences during eating at earlier ages. This may result from discomfort that is associated with gastroesophageal reflux, gagging, or aspiration. The food aversion may persist beyond the ongoing presence of the underlying medical condition. Other children may miss the opportunity to develop age-appropriate feeding skills during various developmental phases because of dependence on tube-feeding.

FORMAL CODING SCHEMES

The coding and classification approach to FTT of the major and newer diagnostic classification schemes is described in this section.

International Classification of Diseases

Most health organizations utilize the code entitled "Lack of Expected Normal Physiologic Development" (783.4) of the ICD-9 for coding children with FTT. Failure to thrive specifically is mentioned under this code, along with delayed milestones, failure to gain weight, lack of growth, physical retardation, and short stature. Unfortunately, this nonspecific terminology overlaps with several distinct and separate clinical circumstances seen in primary care settings. This code, thus, is very problematic from both clinical and research perspectives because of its lack of specificity.

Related codes in the ICD-9 that may be considered include abnormal weight gain (783.1), feeding difficulties and mismanagement (783.3), and other and unspecified disorders of eating (307.5) including psychogenic rumination (307.53) and "other" infantile feeding disturbance or loss of appetite of nonorganic origin (307.59). Related nutritional codes include malnutrition of mild (263.1) or moderate (263.0) degree; arrested development following protein-calorie malnutrition (263.2) or child maltreatment syndrome; and emotional and/or nutritional maltreatment of child (995.5).

Diagnostic and Statistical Manual of Mental Disorders

Feeding Disorder of Infancy or Early Childhood (307.59) is the diagnostic category in the DSM-IV that is most specific for use for children with FTT. Criteria include 1) feeding disturbance manifested by persistent failure to eat adequately with significant failure to gain weight or significant weight loss over at least 1 month; 2) not due to associated gastrointestinal or other medical condition; 3) not better accounted for by another mental disorder or lack of food; and 4) onset before 6 years of age. Problems with this category include lack of specific anthropometric criteria to determine "significant failure to gain weight" and emphasis on "failure to eat" to the neglect of failure to feed, for whatever mechanical or environmental cause. As noted previously, Reactive Attachment Disorder of Infancy or Early Childhood (313.89) or Major Depressive Disorder (e.g., 296.20) may be considered for some children with FTT.

Diagnostic Classification of Mental Health and Developmental Disorders of Infancy and Early Childhood

ZERO TO THREE: National Center for Infants, Toddlers and Families published a diagnostic classification in 1994. The *Diagnostic Classification of Mental Health and Developmental Disorders of Infancy and Early Childhood* purports to address the need for a systematic, developmentally based approach to classifying mental health and developmental disorders in the first 4 years of life. This is a multi-axial system of classification, similar to the DSM-IV, but no attempt was made to use the same codes as exist in the DSM-IV. In fact, many new categories were created in this system.

Eating Behavior Disorder (600) is the diagnostic code in this system that is most specific for children with FTT. This code should be considered "when an infant or young child shows difficulties in establishing regular feeding patterns or appropriate food intake (e.g., nonorganic failure to thrive)" (p. 39).

This classification scheme includes Regulatory Disorder (400) and subtypes, similar to the homeostatic disorder described previously in the section "Developmental Classification." The Eating Behavior Disorder should not be used if Regulatory Disorder is present, which is characterized by difficulties with regulating behavior and physiological, sensory, attentional, motor, or affective processes and with organizing a calm, alert, or affectively positive state.

Diagnoses related to DSM-IV diagnoses with different codes and modified terminology include Reactive Attachment Deprivation/Maltreatment Disorder of Infancy (206) and Depression of Infancy and Early Childhood (203). A second volume of case descriptions is available (Lieberman, Wieder, & Fenichel, 1997) to assist with the use of these classification categories.

The Classification of Child and Adolescent Mental Diagnoses in Primary Care: Diagnostic and Statistical Manual for Primary Care—Child and Adolescent Version

The American Academy of Pediatrics (1996) in cooperation with the American Psychiatric Association, which oversees the development of the DSM, has published a coding system, the DSM-PC. The product of many years' work, the DSM-PC attempts to provide a classification scheme and coding system that is usable for primary care providers. This system uses codes and classifications of the ICD-9 and the DSM-IV, but it has several unique characteristics. This system assumes that behavioral manifestations reflect a spectrum from normal to disorder; thus, each symptom cluster has three categories: developmental variation, problem, and disorder. In addition, these categories are presented from a developmental perspective in four distinct age categories: infancy (birth–2 years), early childhood (3–5 years), middle childhood (6–12 years), and adolescence (13 years and older). Differential diagnoses of medical and mental health problems are included as both alternative causes and comorbid conditions.

FTT is depicted as a presenting complaint in the irregular feeding behavior cluster, along with poor appetite, finicky eating, and poor weight gain. This system uses Inadequate Nutrition Variation (V65.49) for children with weight and height less than the 30th percentile but greater than the 3rd percentile and less-than-average intake for age and Inadequate Nutrition Intake Problem (V40.3) for children who fail to grow in a normal fashion (weight and height less than the 3rd percentile and failure to maintain growth velocity greater than 6 months). Feeding Disorder of Infancy or Early Childhood (307.59), as discussed in the DSM-IV, is the final disorder in this spectrum. Reactive Attachment Disorder (313.89) and Major Depressive Disorder (296.20) are listed as common comorbid conditions in this scheme.

CONCLUSION

No optimum classification and coding scheme exists for use with children with FTT. Lack of uniform terminology and different perspectives of etiology and clinical subtypes among various clinical specialists have led to different coding schemes. This is compounded by the fact that pediatricians and other primary care providers typically do not use the DSM coding system because of lack of experience and training, and, in many cases, they cannot be reimbursed when using those clinical codes. Clearly, further research is required to better categorize children with FTT. Perhaps the DSM-PC coding scheme developed for use in primary care will cross some of the clinical gaps and enhance the use of more uniform coding schemes across disciplines.

REFERENCES

American Academy of Pediatrics. (1996). *The classification of child and adolescent mental diagnoses in primary care: Diagnostic and statistical manual for primary care (DSM-PC) child and adolescent version.* Elk Grove Village, IL: Author.

American Psychiatric Association. (1987). *Diagnostic and statistical manual of mental disorders* (3rd ed., rev.). Washington, DC: Author.

American Psychiatric Association. (1994). *Diagnostic and statistical manual of mental disorders* (4th ed.). Washington, DC: Author.

Berwick, D.M. (1980). Non-organic failure-to-thrive. *Pediatrics in Review, 1,* 265–270.

Bithoney, W.G., Dubowitz, H., & Egan, H. (1992). Failure to thrive/growth deficiency. *Pediatrics in Review, 13,* 453–460.

Black, M., & Dubowitz, H. (1991). Failure-to-thrive: Lessons from animal models and developing countries. *Developmental and Behavioral Pediatrics, 12,* 259–267.

Casey, P.H. (1992). Failure to thrive. In M.B. Levine, W.B. Carey, & A.C. Crocker (Eds.), *Developmental-behavioral pediatrics* (2nd ed., pp. 275–383). Philadelphia: W.B. Saunders.

Chatoor, I., Schaefer, S., Dickson, L., & Egan, J. (1984). Non-organic failure to thrive: A developmental perspective. *Pediatric Annals, 13,* 829–843.

Frank, D.A., Silva, M., & Needlman, R. (1993). Failure to thrive: Mystery, myth, and method. *Contemporary Pediatrics, 10,* 117–133.

Frank, D.A., & Zeisel, S.H. (1988). Failure to thrive. *Pediatric Clinics of North America, 35,* 1183–1206.

Lieberman, A.F., & Birch, M. (1985). The etiology of failure to thrive: An interactional developmental approach. In D. Drotar (Ed.), *New directions in failure to thrive: Implications for research and practice* (pp. 240–252). New York: Dlenan Press.

Lieberman, A.F., Wieder, S., & Fenichel, E. (1997). *The DC: 0–3 casebook: A guide to the use of ZERO TO THREE's* Diagnostic Classification of Mental Health and Developmental Disorders of Infancy and Early Childhood *in assessment and treatment planning.* Washington, DC: ZERO TO THREE: National Center for Infants, Toddlers and Families.

Mathisen, B., Skuse, D., & Wolke, D. (1989). Oral-motor dysfunction and failure to thrive among inner-city infants. *Developmental Medicine and Child Neurology, 31,* 293–297.

Powell, G.F., & Bettes, B.A. (1992). Infantile depression, non-organic failure to thrive, and DSM-III-R: A different perspective. *Child Psychiatry and Human Development, 22,* 185–198.

Ramsay, M., Gisel, E.G., & Boutry, M. (1993). Non-organic failure to thrive: Growth failure secondary to feeding skills disorder. *Developmental Medicine and Child Neurology, 35,* 295–297.

Richters, M.M., & Volkmar, F.R. (1994). Reactive attachment disorder of infancy or early childhood. *Journal of the American Academy of Child & Adolescent Psychiatry, 33,* 328–332.

Rudolph, C.D. (1994). Feeding disorders in infants and children. *Journal of Pediatrics, 125,* S116–S124.

Rutter, M. (1978). Diagnostic validity in child psychiatry. *Advances in Biological Psychiatry, 2,* 2–22.

Skuse, D.H. (1985). Non-organic failure to thrive: A re-appraisal. *Archives of Disease in Childhood, 60,* 173–178.

Wright, J.A., Ashenburg, D.A., & Whitaker, R.D. (1994). Comparison of methods to categorize undernutrition in children. *Journal of Pediatrics, 124,* 944–946.

World Health Organization. (1994). *International classification of diseases (9th rev.) code book.* Reston, VA: St. Anthony Publishing.

ZERO TO THREE: National Center for Infants, Toddlers and Families. (1994). *Diagnostic classification of mental health and developmental disorders of infancy and early childhood.* Arlington, VA: Author.

Chapter 20

Managed Care as Part of Family-Centered Service Systems

Catherine A. Hess

The rapid growth of managed care has significant implications for access to care, quality of care, and health outcomes for all Americans. This is especially true for children who have special health care needs, such as intervention for pediatric undernutrition. Children's health services and the broader array of child and family services such as education, child welfare, and social services must be aimed at and must work together to promote both health *and* development. Success in achieving these outcomes relies heavily on working effectively with children's families. Tenets of *family-centered* and *integrated* or *coordinated* services have been promoted widely by public- and private-sector leaders in policy and program development for children (Carnegie Task Force on Meeting the Needs of Young Children, 1994; National Commission on Children, 1991; Schorr, 1988; U.S. Department of Health and Human Services, Maternal and Child Health Bureau, Division of Services for Children with Special Needs, 1996).

The special needs of undernourished children exemplify the issues and challenges in ensuring that managed care is an effective component of community service systems that foster healthy growth and development of children. With both biological and psychosocial determinants and consequences for health, growth, development, and learning, pediatric undernutrition often requires a multidisciplinary clinical approach that provides primary and specialty medical care, nutrition, and mental health services. Child and family support

The author gratefully acknowledges the contributions of current and former Association of Maternal and Child Health Programs staff in writing the Principles on which this chapter is based: Barbara Aliza, former Director of Policy; Treeby Brown, Senior Policy Analyst; Amy Fine, Senior Policy Analyst; and Lisa Gallin Lynch, former Policy Analyst.

services such as home visiting, transportation, and child care often are critical, as is access to other community programs, especially the Special Supplemental Nutrition Program for Women, Infants and Children (WIC) and other food and nutrition resources and early intervention services for infants and toddlers. Purchasing specifications and payment rates under managed care arrangements may not cover adequately the provision or referral and coordination of these services. Furthermore, managed care organizations, which historically have not served large numbers of individuals who are enrolled in Medicaid or other populations that are at high risk or have special needs, often lack knowledge and experience with children's special health care needs and with other community resources and programs for these children and their families.

Managed care has grown rapidly in both the public and the private sectors. Growth in managed care enrollment in Medicaid, which insured one in every four children in 1995, has been dramatic, increasing from 800,000 in 1983 to more than 12 million in 1996 (Rosenbaum et al., 1997). This managed care transformation, particularly in Medicaid, may determine the future course of nascent policy and program initiatives to ensure family-centered, comprehensive, coordinated service systems for children, especially those who have special health care needs. The poorest children who have the most severe disabilities and medical needs are enrolled in Medicaid, and state and federal initiatives are expanding further the numbers of children who are enrolled in Medicaid and other state health insurance plans for children.

The passage of federal legislation for state Child Health Insurance Programs (CHIP, or Title XXI of the Social Security Act) as part of the 1997 Balanced Budget Act will help the states insure an estimated 5 million additional children through Medicaid or separate state plans. Whichever financing mechanism is used, it is expected that states will continue to increase the use of managed-care arrangements to deliver services.

Medicaid comprehensively covers all health and related services that children need to prevent, treat, or ameliorate health conditions and has become a major source of revenue for many components of child and family service systems, including early intervention, special education–prescribed therapies, nutrition, mental health, and case management or care coordination services. With the public sector's increasing clout as a major purchaser of managed care, how Medicaid and other public programs address—or fail to address—the scope of services and the coordination of services that are needed by children will shape how managed care responds to these needs for all children. The addition of federally supported CHIP and the flexibility that states were given under this program make these issues of benefits and service coordination even more salient than before.

This chapter suggests principles that can guide public- and private-sector purchasers, policy makers, service providers, professionals, and consumers in further developing and shaping managed care to fit and work with existing and evolving child and family service systems and achieve better health and developmental outcomes.

PRINCIPLES FOR ADDRESSING
PEDIATRIC UNDERNUTRITION IN MANAGED CARE

Public health professionals who are responsible for administering programs for children, including children who have special health care needs, have identified a set of basic principles to guide design of managed care arrangements (Association of Maternal and Child Health Programs, 1996). These principles are applicable and highly relevant to care for undernourished children. The first is that *managed care arrangements should contribute to a seamless system of care.* For the undernourished child, this means that managed care should have effective working agreements with other community programs and services, such as WIC, early intervention, child care, child welfare, and public health, that can offer expertise and resources to meet the child's and family's needs. Coordination or integration of all of these resources also can promote continuity of care for children and families whose financial and insurance status may change over time.

Second, *families and professionals should participate in designing, implementing, and monitoring managed care.* Consumers and providers who are knowledgeable about pediatric undernutrition should work with policy makers, public and private purchasers, and managed care organizations and providers to share and help apply their expertise to systems design and monitoring. *Community-based, coordinated, family-centered health and support services should be at the core of these designs.* System design should recognize and respect each family's unique needs and strengths. *Care should be comprehensive and responsive to the unique developmental and changing needs of children and families.* This principle is particularly important for children who have pediatric undernutrition, given that undernutrition has multiple determinants and consequences for health and development.

Third, *managed care should work collaboratively with state and local public health agencies to support and contribute to community-wide strategies to improve the health of populations. The expertise and resources of both the public and the private sectors should be recognized and shared to build comprehensive service systems that improve health.* In relation to pediatric undernutrition, for example, public and private sectors can collaborate in such areas as surveillance and training. Managed care organizations can join forces with other community leaders and stakeholders to address food and hunger issues, working together to build and link community resources such as food pantries with public and private food and nutrition programs. Such collaborative community efforts can help managed care organizations address their bottom-line concerns by fostering good public relations and maximizing community resources that can help prevent the costly consequences of severe undernutrition.

PUTTING THE PRINCIPLES INTO PRACTICE

Means to achieve these principles can be broken down into a number of key functions that are necessary to building effective family-centered systems.

Providing Outreach, Enrollment, and Information

Particularly with the new kinds of service delivery and financing systems that are represented in managed care, outreach, information and education to consumers, professionals, providers, and other community resources are critical to the effective functioning and appropriate use of the system. Families need good information about plans prior to their enrollment in order to make informed choices about which plans will best meet their needs. The family of an undernourished child, for example, would want to know whether the plan's provider panel includes the multiple disciplines, with pediatric specialists, that are needed to address this special need. Communication methods and content should be designed to reach and inform the diversity of families who are enrolling in managed care, including those with low literacy skills and those whose primary language is not English. Informing and educating community agencies about managed care plans not only can help those agencies develop appropriate linkages but also can enable them to reach and assist families with choosing plans that will best meet their needs.

Partnerships between managed care plans and community agencies in outreach, information, and education remain important after families are enrolled. Helping families understand their rights and responsibilities and how to use the system appropriately can help ensure that they get the services that they need when they need them. Particularly important for Medicaid recipients are information and education on services that may remain available to them outside the managed care plan. Many states have "carved out" some special services or groups of individuals, such as those who receive Supplemental Security Income (SSI), from reimbursement through managed care arrangements; however, families and providers may not be aware of these options. Parents of an undernourished child need to understand the policies and procedures for obtaining multidisciplinary care within the plan and also know whether Medicaid still reimburses services that are offered in early intervention, public health or mental health, or school settings. For example, knowing that they still are entitled to transportation services and how those services are being arranged in the context of managed care can be critical to many parents' abilities to ensure that their children get care.

Ensuring Sound Financial Structures

Fundamental to the capacity to provide quality care are resources that are adequate to ensure solvency, recruit and retain good providers, and provide comprehensive services. Particularly important to the families of children at high risk or with special needs, such as those who are undernourished, are payment rates that are sufficient to cover the specialty and ancillary services that these children require. Where capitated payments are utilized, risk adjustment methodologies need to be developed, applied, evaluated, and readjusted as necessary. Given that these methods still are in their infancy, consideration should be given to "carving out" these children or some of the special or supplemental services that they need or developing and piloting special models for delivering and financing their care. All of these approaches are being tried in states and communities throughout the United States.

Sound financing policies for managed care also should ensure that any cost sharing for families encourages and does not inhibit appropriate utilization of preventive, primary, and specialty care. Families of children who have special health care needs can face extraordinary out-of-pocket costs, making it even more critical for them that cost-sharing requirements not impose barriers to obtaining necessary services, including specialty care.

Developing Standards and Guidelines

The foundation for quality assurance and improvement standards is a key tool for accountability to consumers and purchasers. As with other components of family-centered systems, standards should be developed in active collaboration with knowledgeable parents, professionals, providers, and other community representatives. Standards for content of care should be based on nationally recognized standards that have been developed by professional organizations such as the American Academy of Pediatrics and by public agencies such as the U.S. Public Health Service (Green, 1994). Particularly critical for children who have special health care needs, such as those who are undernourished, is that the standards for care and the covered benefits be based on a definition of *medical necessity* that is specific to children. Such a definition includes services to promote development and prevent adverse outcomes rather than restricts services to those that ameliorate a condition or restore a function, limitations that are found commonly in definitions of *medical necessity* that are intended for adults. Medicaid's Early Periodic Screening, Diagnosis and Treatment (EPSDT) program is based on a pediatric-specific definition, allowing children to receive critical preventive and developmental services.

States, working in partnership with communities, should develop minimum standards that address not only content of care but also temporal and geographical access to care, cultural competence, provider credentialing and panel or network composition, and referrals and care coordination. Clear guidelines in these last two areas especially are important to children who have special health care needs in ensuring access to appropriately qualified providers within and outside the managed care plan and in coordinating the services of multiple health care specialists and other community services such as education and food and nutrition programs. Managed care compliance with established standards should be encouraged with assistance, incentives, and remedies that include penalties when necessary.

Ensuring Quality Services Through Contracting

Concomitant with the new approaches to health care financing and delivery that are represented in managed care is the need for new legal frameworks to govern the relationships among purchasers, plans, providers, and consumers. Contracts are an essential and evolving component of the legal framework for managed care, which also includes laws and regulations. Managed care contracts between purchasers (such as Medicaid and employers) and plans, as well as between plans and providers, must delineate clearly and precisely expectations of the plans and providers if they are to be held accountable.

A baseline study of 1995 contracts between state Medicaid agencies and managed care plans (Rosenbaum et al., 1997) found great variability among the states on a number of dimensions, including many that are critical to children who have special health care needs. Examples of these elements include the degree of discretion that is given to plans in structuring delivery systems, including network composition and access features; the degree of guidance on medical necessity criteria; and the extent to which the contracts identify Medicaid services that the state will retain responsibility for providing outside the plan. The study found that few contracts addressed referrals or coordination of care with providers or community agencies outside the plan. Relevant to pediatric undernutrition is the finding that only 8 of the 37 states' contracts that were studied included any provisions regarding the WIC nutrition program, and only 9 had any provisions regarding individualized family service plans that are required under federal law for children from birth to age 3 who are served under the Individuals with Disabilities Education Act (IDEA) of 1990 (PL 101-476) and its Amendments of 1997 (PL 105-17). Even among those states that addressed these linkages, there was great variability in the clarity and specificity of the language. Clear and specific requirements in these and other areas that are essential to access to quality, family-centered care are necessary for Medicaid agencies and other purchasers to hold plans accountable.

Collecting, Analyzing, and Reporting Data

Data are essential for assessing and addressing needs, planning and evaluating system design and performance, and monitoring and improving quality. Collecting, analyzing, and reporting data from managed care plans are critical not only to efforts to improve plan performance but also to efforts to improve the health status of all residents of a community. Uniform, comparable data are necessary to compare plan performance and to allow aggregation within communities, states, regions, and the United States to support systems planning and policy development. The *Health Plan Employer Data and Information Set* (HEDIS) (National Committee for Quality Assurance, 1997), developed voluntarily by the managed care industry in consultation with the public sector and other key stakeholders, represents an important effort toward these ends. Further work is needed to refine and build on this data set, particularly in developing appropriate measures of plan performance in serving children who have special health care needs.

Collaboration and partnerships among purchasers, managed care plans, and public health agencies regarding data collection, analysis, and reporting are essential to maintaining and improving population-based surveillance of health status, including nutritional status. Many public health surveillance systems have relied heavily on reporting from public clinics, which have heretofore served large proportions of Medicaid recipients. The movement into private systems of these populations that are at high risk and that have special needs makes it essential for managed care plans to work with public agencies to maintain these surveillance systems and identify other means, such as special studies, to analyze and address trends, new and emerging diseases and conditions, contributing factors, effective interventions, and groups and areas at highest risk. Such collaboration will serve the public's health and, in so doing, aid managed care plans in preventing or reducing adverse health outcomes.

Monitoring and Evaluating

Informed by the data discussed in the previous section, monitoring and evaluating the processes, structures, and outcomes of managed care are essential to quality improvement (Grason & Guyer, 1995). From a broadly conceived public health perspective, quality encompasses the health of the community; therefore, monitoring and evaluating managed care should include attention to the contributions of managed care and its impact on family and community health. A community process that involves families and community agencies should be utilized for the ongoing cycle of problem identification and corrective plan development, implementation, and review.

Ensuring Appropriate Provider Networks and Settings

All children have service needs that are different from those of adults, requiring providers who are trained and experienced specifically in pediatric and family services. Children who have special health care needs require care from providers who have more specific expertise. In the case of undernourished children, these providers may include primary and specialist physicians and nurses, nutritionists, social workers, and mental health clinicians who have experience in pediatric undernutrition. Managed care plans should ensure that such multidisciplinary, experienced providers are available and readily accessible within the plan or through arrangements with out-of-plan providers, including public- and community-based agencies, and that these providers work together as a team. An adequate number and mix of providers relative to the populations to be served and the incidence of special conditions such as pediatric undernutrition should be ensured, with consideration given to supporting or developing regional arrangements when appropriate.

As much as possible, services for children who have special needs should be readily available and accessible at locations within the communities in which they live, including child care sites and the home. Where highly specialized care cannot reasonably be available in all communities, arrangements should be made for transporting families to care or, alternatively, transporting the care to the families.

Ensuring Access to Needed Services
Through Service Planning and Care Coordination

Developing individual or family service plans and coordinating the services that are contained in the plans are particularly important for children who are at high risk for developing special needs or who have special needs that require multiple services; many undernourished children are among those who need these services. As developed through such programs as maternal and child health, early intervention, family preservation and support, developmental disability, and mental health, individual service plans outline the services that the child and the family need and assign agency responsibility for their payment and provision. It is critical that managed care plan providers join teams of agency personnel and parents in developing and implementing these plans to promote a comprehensive, coordinated, and family-centered approach. A single, comprehensive care plan and designation of one individual to work with the family and health, social services, education, and other service providers can reduce fragmentation and duplication in services. Such care coordination extends beyond the more traditional medical model of case management to ensure and coordinate community services such as child care and transportation.

Providing Technical Assistance and Training

The rapid growth of managed care has spawned new organizations and arrangements with varying capacities and expertise in integrating financing and delivery of care. These new plans, as well as many of those that are well established, are entering the Medicaid managed care market. The women and children who are enrolled in Medicaid generally have levels of risk and need that greatly exceed those of the commercially enrolled groups that managed care plans are accustomed to serving. Significant proportions of children who have special health care needs also are enrolled in Medicaid. Public agencies at national, state, and local levels, as well as public and private providers who traditionally have served Medicaid recipients, can work with purchasers and plans to provide technical assistance and training that can increase plans' capacities and competencies in serving these populations. Training and technical assistance should cover areas such as individual, family, and community needs assessment; standards and protocols for care, especially for groups that are at high risk for developing special needs and that have special needs; service planning and coordination of care with other community agencies; methods for outreach and education; cultural competence; and family-centered approaches to care.

Linking Resources

There are many federal, state, and local public- and private-sector programs and resources that offer services and benefits to children and their families. Given the extent to which children rely on their parents and community resources and the extent to which their health and well-being are linked to environmental, social, and biological determinants, fostering their healthy growth and development requires coordinating, integrating, and maximizing the resources that are available. Again, managed care organizations may be unfamiliar with these resources and the benefits that they can provide in preventing or ameliorating health problems. Purchasers, particularly Medicaid, should ensure that managed care plans have agreements and arrangements in place to link children and families to these community resources. For undernourished children, linkages with WIC, early intervention, and the programs that are provided for by Title V of the Social Security Act of 1935 (PL 74-271) for maternal and child health and children with special health care needs (see Chapters 25 and 33) are particularly important. Linkage mechanisms should include clear protocols for referral, follow-up, and care coordination and be formalized in memorandums of agreement or contractual relationships. These agreements can address many of the other components of family-centered systems that are outlined in this chapter (see also Chapter 35).

Ensuring Access to a Dispute Resolution Process

Particularly in the time period when managed care arrangements are still new and evolving in many parts of the United States, it is essential to have formal processes for receiving and resolving disputes and complaints about these plans. These processes are particularly important for children who have special needs such as with pediatric undernutrition, given their needs for care that are above and beyond those of the majority of children. Differences in expectations and in understandings can arise around benefits coverage, access to specific providers, quality, or continuity of care. Formal processes are needed to ensure resolution of differences and can be important components of quality assurance systems. These processes should facilitate prompt resolution of issues, limiting interruptions in care. Care that is in dispute but that is essential to the child's health and development should continue to be provided during the period in which the dispute is being resolved. Families should receive clear information on grievance procedures and their rights and responsibilities as well as assistance from an enrollee representative, advocate, or ombudsman. Reports on the number and types of grievances and their resolution should be available publicly and should form part of the plan's report card on its performance.

CONCLUSION

Managed care offers the promise and potential to ensure many of the elements of a system of care that are critical to promoting the health and development of children. Managed care's emphases on prevention, quality, and coordination of services represent important foundations for building responsive service systems. To best meet the needs of children, particularly children who have special needs such as with pediatric undernutrition, managed care plans must work in partnership with families, other providers, and professionals to build on this foundation and make it an integral part of family-centered, community-based, culturally competent, and coordinated systems of care.

REFERENCES

Association of Maternal and Child Health Programs. (1996). *Partnerships for healthier families: Principles for assuring the health of women, infants, children, and youth under managed care arrangements.* Washington, DC: Author.

Carnegie Task Force on Meeting the Needs of Young Children. (1994). *Starting points: Meeting the needs of our youngest children.* New York: Carnegie Corporation of New York.

Grason, H., & Guyer, B. (1995). *MCH policy research brief: Quality, quality assessment, and quality assurance considerations for maternal and child health populations and practitioners.* Baltimore: The Johns Hopkins University, Child and Adolescent Health Policy Center.

Green, M. (Ed.). (1994). *Bright futures: Guidelines for health supervision of infants, children, and adolescents.* Arlington, VA: National Center for Education in Maternal and Child Health.

Individuals with Disabilities Education Act (IDEA) of 1990, PL 101-476, 20 U.S.C. §§ 1400 *et seq.*

Individuals with Disabilities Education Act Amendments of 1997, PL 105-17, 20 U.S.C. §§ 1400 *et seq.*

National Commission on Children. (1991). *Beyond rhetoric: A new American agenda for children and families.* Washington, DC: U.S. Government Printing Office.

National Committee for Quality Assurance. (1997). *Health plan employer data and information set (HEDIS) 3.0.* Washington, DC: Author.

Rosenbaum, S., Shin, P., Smith, B.M., Wehr, E., Borzi, P.C., Zakheim, M.H., Shaw, K., & Silver, K. (1997). *Negotiating the new health system: A nationwide study of Medicaid managed care contracts.* Washington, DC: George Washington University, Center for Health Policy Research.

Schorr, L.B. (1988). *Within our reach: Breaking the cycle of disadvantage.* New York: Anchor Press.

Social Security Act of 1935, PL 74-271, 42 U.S.C §§ 301 *et seq.*

United States Department of Health and Human Services, Maternal and Child Health Bureau, Division of Services for Children with Special Needs. (1996). *Children with special health care needs in managed care organizations: Summaries of Expert Work Group Meetings.* Rockville, MD: Author.

Chapter 21

Pediatric Undernutrition and Managed Health Care

Madeleine U. Shalowitz and Joel I. Shalowitz

Studies show that children who are undernourished are at increased risk for illness and adverse developmental outcomes (see Chapter 3). Although management of this condition requires little technological support, the more complex cases are expensive to manage because of the multiple professionals who must be involved in the care of the child. Early, intensive management of these children, however, can circumvent both the undernutrition and its consequences. A healthier child ultimately will require fewer medical services. Indirect benefits also may accrue if the child requires fewer special education services and has increased lifelong productivity.

The management of pediatric undernutrition mirrors the philosophy of managed care at its best: coordinated care by a multidisciplinary team of professionals across a continuum of sites and services. At its worst, financial constraints can disrupt long-standing professional relationships or postpone, deny, or otherwise limit necessary services. The unique developmental aspects of childhood coupled with the low incidence of individual chronic illnesses in the general pediatric population challenge managed care organizations (MCOs) to define and fund services for children's special needs. *Pediatric undernutrition* is a diagnosis that identifies a child as being at risk for developing—but not yet having—a disability or a chronic illness and often is viewed as a social disorder, so the case for referral for subspecialty team management is even more difficult. Professionals who care for such children, therefore, must build a cogent and compelling justification for services within the MCOs. To develop successful strategies for such services, pediatric health care providers

The Continuing Education Program for Managed Care Providers was generously funded by a grant from the Genentech Foundation for Growth and Development.

must move beyond a reactive, uninformed, and negative stance to a real understanding of the theory and organization of managed care. To that end, the next section offers a summary of managed care's key elements.

ORGANIZATION OF MANAGED CARE

Rising health care costs provided the impetus for rapid expansion of MCOs. MCOs have begun to address concerns about quality and accountability for care. Several types of MCOs have developed: 1) health maintenance organizations (HMOs), 2) preferred provider organizations (PPOs), and 3) point of service (POS) plans.

Cost Management

In both the fee-for-service and the PPO systems (in which the MCO pays health care providers a discount on their fee-for-service charges), the physician experiences identical financial incentives: More services generate more revenue. An alternative payment mechanism, called *capitation,* is a fixed monthly payment that the HMO pays the practitioners for each assigned patient or family unit. Unlike fee-for-service and PPO systems, this method of physician compensation creates a monthly budget for the care of a patient and covers the cost of primary care as well as other services, described next. The financial incentives with capitation also reflect budget management.

In capitated HMOs, primary care providers (PCPs) provide a specified set of services for a defined population during a given time period in exchange for a fixed per-person payment per month. HMO premiums typically are calculated based on the cost of care for an "average" patient. This amount frequently is adjusted by age and gender of the individual but not for *individual* health risk. Because of wide variations in patient health characteristics, health care providers who receive capitation must care for sufficient numbers of patients to diversify the financial risks attendant in their care. If providers can furnish services for less than the capitation rates that they receive, then they make a profit. If expenses exceed capitations, then they incur losses.

Capitated payments to PCPs in HMOs usually are of three types. First, plans may pay them for their primary care services only. The HMO pays for referral services such as laboratory, X ray, and specialist fees. This method is called *primary care–only capitation.* In a second method, called *full risk capitation,* PCPs may accept a larger capitation but assume financial responsibility for referral services. A third type pays the PCPs a primary care capitation but returns to them at the end of a year any surplus in a fund created to pay for referrals. Unlike fee-for-service practice and PPO payments, a capitated system does not reward physicians for increasing utilization of their services or ordering more tests. In fact, the opposite economics apply.

Another important feature of physician payment under HMO contracts involves profit sharing with the plan. HMOs achieve their cost savings and make their profits by reducing inpatient utilization rates (Miller & Luft, 1993). Plans pay for hospitalizations along with other costs from a fund that the plan sets aside once it collects premiums. If money remains in this fund at the end of a year, then HMOs may pay PCPs part of this surplus. If the fund has a deficit, then the HMO usually absorbs it. For general pediatrics, where inpatient utilization typically is low, surpluses can be substantial.

The combination of risk-based capitation and potential for payments from the aforementioned fund creates an incentive system in which physicians eliminate unnecessary discretionary services or substitute less-costly alternatives to care such as outpatient surgery and home health care (Miller & Luft, 1993). Utilization of nondiscretionary services is similar in MCOs and the fee-for-service system. For example, one study showed no difference in the utilization of intensive care services for a Medicare population (Angus et al., 1996).

Quality and Accountability

Businesses, government agencies, and individual patients have begun to demand measurable quality standards for health care services. The media have focused their attention on problems that have occurred when MCOs have failed to provide timely access to care.

Sophisticated HMOs have discovered that they can improve health outcomes and decrease costs by coordinating care across a continuum of services ranging from prevention to acute care to services for chronic illnesses. The patient's PCP coordinates all services, either alone or, ideally, with the help of the HMO. This coordination is easy when the patient requires only uncomplicated outpatient care. Difficulties can arise, however, when patients develop chronic and, particularly, debilitating illnesses.

Different payment methods cause significant systematic changes in physician behavior. Although concerns abound on the negative aspects of these behavior changes, capitation forces physicians to question not only the cost-effectiveness of some services but also whether the services are necessary at all. Patients should not have to endure unnecessary procedures as the financial benefit for performing them no longer exists. Research studies show that HMOs provide more preventive services than do fee-for-service providers and that the quality of care in HMOs is equal or superior to that in the fee-for-service sector (Miller & Luft, 1993). These studies primarily were limited to the care of adults in systems in which physicians were employees of the plans. Although more research needs to be conducted on quality of care in other types of physician organizations, Berwick noted, "If anything, the data suggests hazards and ethical problems in the overuse of services in fee-for-service settings, rather than its underuse in capitated care" (1996, p. 1228).

CHILDREN WHO HAVE SPECIAL
HEALTH CARE NEEDS UNDER MANAGED CARE

A detailed discussion of children who have special health care needs under managed care is beyond the scope of this chapter. Much of the available literature on the impact of managed health care for populations who have special health care needs focuses on older adults and has limited applicability to pediatric populations (Forrest, Simpson, & Clancy, 1997). The value placed by MCOs on coordinated care, home-based interventions, and preventive management offers potential advantages to children who have special health care needs; however, either the employer (in commercial managed care plans) or the state government (in Medicaid managed care plans) must fund the plan adequately so that needed services and specialty providers are, in fact, covered benefits (Fox, Wicks, & Newacheck, 1993; Hughes, Newacheck, Stoddard, & Halfon, 1995). Every effort should be made to ensure continuity of primary and subspecialty care. Continuity of care can be enhanced when the PCP, subspecialist, and health plan work together to coordinate the child's care.

In an effort to contain costs, states are converting Medicaid from fee-for-service reimbursement to case management and budgetary control under Medicaid managed care. In 1994, Medicaid managed care programs were in various stages of development or implementation in more than 40 states (Freund & Hurley, 1995). Those who are enrolled in these programs most rapidly are children and adults in poor families who receive public assistance (Iglehart, 1995). In response to additional federal funding available beginning in 1997, states may offer health insurance to previously uninsured children. Although implementation of this program will vary by state, these children may be added to the states'

Medicaid enrollment. Therefore, such children will compose an additional potential cohort of enrollees in Medicaid managed care (Children's Defense Fund, 1997).

Based on site visits to several states whose Medicaid managed care programs have been in place for several years, Gold, Sparer, and Chu concluded that "managed care is not a magic bullet for solving all access and cost concerns and that no amount of managed care can substitute for adequately financed programs" (1996, p. 162). They recommended that the health care providers and plans show that they can handle the risk for medical delivery that is associated with caring for low-income populations. Special attention must be paid to policies, systems, and reimbursement for the care of individuals who have chronic illnesses.

The fate of children who have chronic illnesses under Medicaid managed care is of particular concern. Many studies have documented the impact of poverty on the acute and chronic health care needs of children. Fowler and Anderson (1996) suggested that demographic variables alone are not sufficient to predict future health care resource use for children. Multiple predictors will be necessary to ensure that children who have chronic illnesses will fare equally under managed health care. Unfortunately, the baseline data on health services and outcomes for the poor have been so inadequate that appropriate comparisons between fee-for-service and managed care systems cannot be made (Gold et al., 1996).

As Medicaid managed care programs are implemented, the existing individual community-based PCPs often become organized into a loosely aligned network of PCPs. Despite the need to attract highly qualified physicians to care for populations with greater potential morbidity, some evidence exists that practicing physicians will fall short of typical MCO professional standards for board certification. In a New York survey of 33 physicians who were practicing pediatrics under Medicaid, fewer than half were board certified (Fairbrother, DuMont, & Friedman, 1995). Questions, therefore, must be raised about whether the goal of enhanced quality can be realized with the available pool of community-based PCPs.

AREAS OF CONCERN FOR TREATING PEDIATRIC UNDERNUTRITION IN MANAGED CARE SETTINGS

In primary care settings, early identification and intervention offer the key to managing pediatric undernutrition. Early identification finds children whose growth has slowed but whose weight may not yet be abnormal. Family dysfunction is of shorter duration, and the behaviors are more amenable to treatment. Family education that is provided in the context of primary care may resolve the child's undernutrition. Cases that do not respond quickly to straightforward nutritional guidance should be referred promptly for multidisciplinary team management.

Although pediatric undernutrition may occur across socioeconomic strata, the vast majority of patients are poor and receive Medicaid. In the past, under fee-for-service health care, unrestricted access for referral to multidisciplinary programs offered a partial safety net for the care of undernourished children, compensating in part for any lack of sophistication of the PCPs. Under managed care, as under fee-for-service, an unsophisticated PCP may not recognize pediatric undernutrition until the problem is long standing. Even when pediatric undernutrition is identified, the physician may be unable to assemble the appropriate professional support. Under managed care, the PCP also may fail to refer when necessary for subspecialty team management because of the short-sighted view of the cost of the referral. The potential long-term consequences for the patient and the cost to the plan are enormous.

The management of pediatric undernutrition under managed care, therefore, relies on the PCP's ability to 1) identify undernourished children and intervene early, 2) advocate for referral to and payment for appropriate specialists and services, and 3) coordinate care. The following case illustrates these points.

During her first trimester of pregnancy, Sam's mother had a ruptured cerebral arteriovenous malformation and had general anesthesia and neurosurgery. Sam was born 6 weeks prematurely and required mechanical ventilation initially but was discharged at 4 weeks of age. He was fed standard infant formula and showed poor weight gain.

Sam's mother was a member of a commercial MCO. Sam's grandmother was an employee of a local children's hospital. Because of the grandmother's relationship to the hospital, the hospital's multidisciplinary team evaluated Sam at 11 months of age even though the PCP of the MCO would not make the referral (so no payment to the team was ever made). Sam was significantly underweight and had moderate gross motor and language delays. The team recommended nutritional supplementation, physical therapy, and cognitive intervention, all implemented without authorization for payment by the PCP.

When Sam returned to the hospital at 19 months, his undernutrition had worsened, he was not talking, and he had clinical signs of upper-airway obstruction (snoring and frequent ear infections) and possible obstructive sleep apnea (OSA), all of which the team believed contributed to his poor weight gain (see Chapter 12). The team implemented an intensive intervention program to improve his nutritional status, including weekly home visits. On the written request of the hospital program director, the PCP authorized a hearing test and an ears, nose, and throat (ENT) evaluation. Sam, unfortunately, was sent to an adult ENT specialist, who thought that a hearing test on this child could be done only with sedation and therefore did not try to perform the test.

Sam's weight fell further from the 5th percentile. The program director asked the PCP to authorize admitting Sam into the hospital to institute nasogastric (NG) feedings, and Sam began to gain weight. A hearing test that was conducted during the inpatient stay showed a moderate hearing loss.

It took 8 months for Sam's doctor to authorize a pediatric ENT evaluation at the children's hospital. The ENT physician requested a sleep study to rule out OSA; the PCP arranged to have the test conducted at a community hospital. An inadequate study was conducted and read as normal. The program director and the ENT specialist intervened, arranging for an overnight study (again absorbing the cost). The study (conducted without the NG tube in place) showed such severe OSA that NG feeds had to be discontinued (the tube would increase the obstruction). A tonsillectomy and an adenoidectomy with **tympanostomy tube** *placement were performed. After surgery, Sam's weight improved rapidly on oral supplements alone without further feeding intervention. His hearing and his sleep study now are normal, but he has cognitive delays and attends a special education program.*

This case illustrates how the concern for minimizing outside referrals can compromise the care of a child. Fortunately for Sam, because of his grandmother's relationship to the children's hospital, the team provided a partial safety net to advocate for appropriate services. Other children would not have had the same access to subspecialty support. Many parents might not recognize the need to seek other resources or even know where to look if they did identify a problem. Sam's case highlights problems with delayed identification and intervention, the use of specialists who are unfamiliar with the care of children with special needs, and inadequate advocacy for and coordination of services. All of these factors contributed in an unquantifiable way to the prolonged course of Sam's problems. All resulted in substantial extra cost for the insurer. The manner in which Sam's case was handled is not the fault of managed care as a construct; however, the incentives that are in place under managed care demand the expertise of a sophisticated practitioner who can distinguish serious from routine care and can advocate effectively to justify necessary services.

RECOMMENDATIONS

Confronting the challenges of managed care for children who have special health care needs will demand basic research on health outcomes for children (Forrest et al., 1997; Newacheck et al., 1996). This section outlines how a multidisciplinary team can construct a proposal to an MCO for services for pediatric undernutrition and suggests three ways to create a partnership with the MCO: education, demonstration, and creative packaging of multidisciplinary services.

Education

The role of continuing education for PCPs, utilization review coordinators, and case managers is critical. To raise the level of understanding, the ability to diagnose pediatric undernutrition, and the team's visibility as a resource to the PCP, the program should proactively seek multiple forums to provide continuing education. The first author of this chapter developed and received grant funding for a continuing education module for PCPs in managed care settings and presented the program at two HMOs. Both HMOs were very supportive, paying for mailings and providing meeting space and refreshments; the PCPs participated enthusiastically.

Demonstration

The incidence of and the morbidity that is associated with undernutrition in populations that are at risk must be demonstrated to the MCO to justify the need for a special policy regarding their management. Proposals to MCOs will have to justify the expense of providing multidisciplinary services by making a case for 1) the savings in inpatient hospitalization, 2) improved health outcome, and 3) efficient and effective models of care. In addition, because some of the services may lie beyond traditional medical care (e.g., social services, transportation, feeding intervention), the MCO may require documentation of the medical need to provide such services and of the lack of alternative funding mechanisms to pay for them. To demonstrate the value of early intervention and referral for pediatric undernutrition, programs must show that referral to an outpatient multidisciplinary program has a superior outcome for the patient than does routine primary care and costs less overall (Bithoney et al., 1989; Bithoney et al., 1991). In the long run, clinicians who are caring for undernourished children must demonstrate superior clinical outcomes through well-designed health outcomes research. Financial analysis must be part of these evaluations.

In the short run, a quick analysis can show that the cost of referral for outpatient multidisciplinary team management is less than the cost of hospitalization. This comparison is called a *cost tradeoff.* By using a typical hospital per diem rate for inpatient stay, the program can calculate a typical hospital bill for managing an undernourished child. For example, at $1,000 per day, a 7-day stay for a single child would cost the plan $7,000. If outpatient assessment and treatment by the team avoid a hospital stay and cost $2,000, then outpatient multidisciplinary services for children who do not respond to primary care management are a cost-effective alternative to hospitalization.

Creative Packaging

The services of the multidisciplinary team can be packaged in creative ways. Sometimes the management of pediatric undernutrition requires more observation or supervision than can be provided in a typical outpatient program; however, unless the child has an acute illness, many admissions for acute nutritional management are either prospectively or retrospectively reviewed, and payment is denied because of the use of an acute care setting. This denial of payment has some merit in that the services that are used to manage pediatric undernutrition require time and cognitive professional expertise but limited technology. To justify a longer stay, the package of inpatient services might use an alternative site, such as a subacute facility or the equivalent of a halfway house, at a lower rate to the plan. The program may choose to reconfigure its services including, for example, a day treatment program with transportation, an intensive home-visiting program, or homemaker services. Any such options should have a systematic evaluation of process and outcome.

An outpatient multidisciplinary program can propose several possible relationships among itself, the PCP, and the MCO. The multidisciplinary team offers the PCP and the MCO something that they might not be able to assemble otherwise: a group of professionals who have special knowledge and experience and who will provide coordinated care for the child and the family. In the language of managed care, the team has added value as a ready resource to the practitioner that he or she cannot or may not want to duplicate on his or her own. The team must be prepared to provide a spectrum of services from technical assistance only to a temporary transfer of primary and specialty care to the team for intensive intervention. If only technical assistance is authorized, then the team can provide a framework for evaluating the child. The practitioner then would have to assemble and coordinate all of the pieces to develop a treatment plan that makes sense for the patient and the family; however, because a high frequency of visits is integral to the management of pediatric undernutrition, a preferable approach would authorize the program to assume the total care of the patient for a defined and monitored period of time. This approach would reduce the total burden of care for both the PCP and the family. The program would negotiate a different cost for each option.

At the health care system level, if data show that the incidence of and the morbidity and costs that are associated with pediatric undernutrition are high, then the plan may consider separating the cost of this care from capitation and the institutional fund. This situation, called a *carve-out,* commonly is used by MCOs for such services as transplantations and open-heart procedures. In this case, when a child is undernourished, the MCO would cover directly the cost that is associated with this diagnosis, thus removing the PCP's financial disincentive for referral. The multidisciplinary team then would assume the case management of the child across the continuum of inpatient and outpatient services, interfacing both with the PCP and directly with the MCO. A health plan case manager would coordinate care with the team. In seeking a carve-out, the definition of *pediatric undernutrition* must be very specific, the affected children must be defined clearly, and the covered services must be precise.

CONCLUSION

The management of pediatric undernutrition presents a challenge under managed care, but not because of a philosophical incompatibility. In fact, continuity of care and case management are the cornerstones of success for each. If the PCPs are experienced and well trained, then they may have the expertise to make the diagnosis of pediatric undernutrition, differentiate the simple from the more complex cases, and refer appropriate patients for multidisciplinary management. Through a better understanding of the language and the mechanics of managed care and a systematic analysis of the epidemiology of pediatric undernutrition and its treatment, creative approaches to packaging services for undernourished children will become easier to design and market to the MCOs.

REFERENCES

Angus, D.C., Linde-Zwirble, W.T., Sirio, C.A., Rotondi, A.J., Chelluri, L., Newbold, R.C., Lave, J.R., & Pinsky, M.R. (1996). The effect of managed care on ICU length of stay: Implications for Medicare. *Journal of the American Medical Association, 276,* 1075–1082.

Berwick, D.M. (1996). Quality of health care: Part 5. Payment by capitation and the quality of care. *New England Journal of Medicine, 335*(16), 1227–1231.

Bithoney, W.G., McJunkin, J., Michalek, J., Egan, H., Snyder, J., & Munier, A. (1989). Prospective evaluation of weight gain in both nonorganic and organic failure-to-thrive children: An outpatient trial of a multidisciplinary team intervention strategy. *Journal of Developmental and Behavioral Pediatrics, 10,* 27–31.

Bithoney, W.G., McJunkin, J., Michalek, J., Snyder, J., Egan, H., & Epstein, D. (1991). The effect of a multidisciplinary team approach on weight gain in non-organic failure-to-thrive children. *Journal of Developmental and Behavioral Pediatrics, 12,* 254–258.

Children's Defense Fund. (1997, August 8). *Summary of child health provisions in the 1997 Budget Reconciliation Act* [On-line]. Washington, DC: Author. (Available: http://www.childrensdefense. org/health_newsum.html)

Fairbrother, G., DuMont, K.A., & Friedman, S. (1995). New York City physicians serving high volumes of Medicaid children: Who are they and how do they practice? *Inquiry, 32*(3), 345–352.

Forrest, C.B., Simpson, L., & Clancy, C. (1997). Child Health Services research: Challenges and opportunities. *Journal of the American Medical Association, 277*(22), 1787–1793.

Fowler, E., & Anderson, G. (1996). Capitation adjustment for pediatric populations. *Pediatrics, 98*(1), 10–17.

Fox, H.B., Wicks, L.B., & Newacheck, P.W. (1993). Health maintenance organizations and children with special needs. *American Journal of Diseases in Childhood, 147,* 546–552.

Freund, D.A., & Hurley, R.E. (1995). Medicaid managed care: Contributions to issues of health reform. *Annual Review of Public Health, 16,* 473–495.

Gold, M., Sparer, M., & Chu, K. (1996). Medicaid managed care: Lessons from five states. *Health Affairs, 15*(3), 153–166.

Hughes, D.C., Newacheck, P.W., Stoddard, J.J., & Halfon, N. (1995). Medicaid managed care: Can it work for children? *Pediatrics, 95*(4), 591–594.

Iglehart, J. (1995). Health policy report: Medicaid and managed care. *New England Journal of Medicine, 332*(25), 1727–1731.

Miller, R.H., & Luft, H.S. (1993). Managed care: Past evidence and potential trends. *Frontiers of Health Services Management, 9,* 3–37.

Newacheck, P., Stein, R., Walker, D., Gortmaker, A., Kuhlthau, K., & Perrin, J. (1996). Monitoring and evaluating managed care for children with chronic illnesses and disabilities. *Pediatrics, 98*(5), 952–958.

Chapter 22

Interdisciplinary Teamwork

Patience Sampson

Within a poor population in a major city, many, if not most, families live in extremely difficult situations. These situations may have affected the parents' ability to nurture the particular child who carries the diagnosis of pediatric undernutrition, also called *failure to thrive* (FTT) (Cupoli, Hallock, & Barnes, 1980). Working with families to alleviate or resolve these situations is a demanding, draining process.

Singling out one circumstance to focus on and treat is not particularly useful or diagnostically accurate when developing a treatment plan. Historically, the parent–child dyad has been evaluated for the cause of FTT (Alderette & deGraffenried, 1986). Certainly there may be some dynamic between the mother and the child—a difficult pregnancy or birth or the child's temperament—that affects their attachment; however, many factors may be important. The etiology also may be organic. Some other event within or outside the family may be overwhelming the family's ability to nurture. The nurturer may be isolated, depressed, anxious, or unsupported (Cupoli et al., 1980).

For the children who are treated by the Growth and Development Clinic at Boston Medical Center, exposure to urban and domestic violence is common. Poverty and isolation from basic resources—food, shelter, and clothing—are routine. Many families experience at least some of these difficulties; some experience many of these difficulties simultaneously. The diagnosis of FTT, however, is not exclusive to poor, inner-city populations. Regardless of the setting, an effective treatment plan must address the rehabilitation of the caregiving environment as well as the nutritional, medical, and developmental rehabilitation of the child (Rathbun & Peterson, 1987).

A team intervention is particularly effective in this difficult field. Not only does the intervention require the specific expertise of the different professionals, but the support that team members give and receive from one another is essential for the provision of good treatment.

WHAT IT TAKES TO KEEP A TEAM RUNNING WELL

It is the team leader's responsibility to provide an environment in which one can be comfortable asking for help and support. Demonstrating mutual respect for the individual team members' professional and personal expertise supports the members' sense of competence and relevance in the team process. Continuous communication is essential not only for support but also to ensure a coordinated treatment plan. It is important to have regular meetings to review activity and treatment plans on each case. In the specialty clinic at Boston Medical Center, each case is reviewed before and after each week's clinic session. Team members discuss interim progress (or lack of it) and assign parts of an action plan to take place before the next clinic visit.

Interdisciplinary issues such as differences of opinion are worked out in these meetings with respect and joint participation. Differences of opinion not only may be based on differences in professional perspectives but also may reflect the feelings that a particular team member has as an individual working with a particular family. Input from all team members is supported, and clinical decisions are made within the team process. If a major difference continues to exist, then it is presented to the family openly as a difference. Open and direct communication with families supports their participation in the treatment plan. In addition, the ability of the providers to express their different opinions to the family, while still working together, provides a healthy model for handling conflict. If a difficult decision is made—for example, whether to report a family to the Department of Social Services—then conditions for reporting the family will have been agreed on by team members in previous discussions. Families also have been informed of the level of concern, and team interventions have focused on bringing in resources to rectify potentially reportable situations. Of course, not all situations can be handled that ideally. In situations in which an immediate decision must be made, team members identify objective information and support the members who are upset by the referral.

Working together as a team to treat a family is nurturing for the team members. A team provides support to acknowledge personal and program limitations. One person does not have the ability or responsibility for a total treatment plan but is accountable to the other members for his or her individual part. Accessibility of the team leader and the team members to each other in both formal and informal ways supports mutual nurturing.

WHEN THERE IS NO TEAM

Simultaneous assessment of nutritional, medical, and psychosocial risk factors is the ideal (Bithoney, 1984; Peterson, Washington, & Rathbun, 1984); however, not all of the disciplines that are required to conduct these assessments may be located in the same facility. Even when the professional who has found the undernourished child is an isolated worker for the Special Supplemental Nutrition Program for Women, Infants and Children (WIC), it is possible to locate others to work with and share responsibility for treatment. A physician, nutritionist, and social worker or other mental health professional may be located at another facility, such as a home health agency, family service agency, or neighborhood health center, and a collaboration begun. (See Bithoney, 1984, and Peterson et al., 1984, for excellent references to consult when identifying resources to meet patient needs.)

Interdisciplinary staff members on a large, hospital-based team often develop a certain familiarity with each other's material knowledge base over time. A new team may need time to research the ways in which their individual expertise is applied to the treatment of undernutrition and to share that information with the other treatment providers.

Each team member remains responsible for his or her own assessment and action plan, but communication ensures well-developed and coordinated treatment interventions. The more knowledge that each team member has of each other's potential contribution, the more comprehensive the treatment plan can be and the more supportive team members can be to each other in the treatment's application.

SUMMARY

Treating the child with FTT is difficult and draining. The members of the interdisciplinary team that is treating the child with FTT need nurturing from their peers and team leader in much the same way that the child needs nurturing from his or her caregiver.

The implications of treating all of the risk factors that contribute to the condition of FTT are overwhelming. Interdisciplinary team treatment provides both the professional capabilities and the resources for nurturing and support that are necessary to sustain the team. Interdisciplinary issues are best resolved in a democratic process; the resolution invests team members in the outcome.

REFERENCES

Alderette, P., & deGraffenried, O. (1986, May–June). Non-organic failure-to-thrive syndrome and the family system. *Social Work, 31,* 207–213.

Bithoney, W.G. (1984). The child with failure to thrive. In R. Howard & H. Winter (Eds.), *Nutrition and feeding of infants and toddlers* (pp. 285–296). Boston: Little, Brown.

Cupoli, J., Hallock, J., & Barnes, L. (1980). Failure to thrive. In L. Gluck (Ed.), *Current problems in pediatrics* (pp. 1–42). Chicago: Yearbook Medical Publishers.

Peterson, K., Washington, J., & Rathbun, J. (1984). Team management of failure to thrive. *Journal of the American Dietetic Association, 84,* 810–815.

Rathbun, J., & Peterson, K. (1987). Nutrition in failure to thrive. In R.J. Grand, J.L. Sutphen, & W.H. Dietz (Eds.), *Pediatric nutrition: Theory and practice* (pp. 627–643). Boston: Butterworth-Heinemann.

Section IV

Child Development

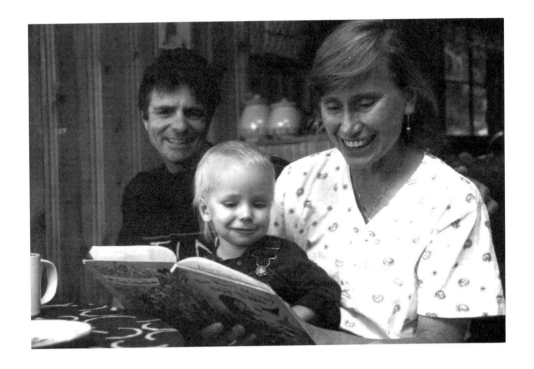

Chapter 23

Oral-Motor Skills and Swallowing

Nancy Creskoff and Angela Haas

Throughout the life span, the mouth plays a critical role in the areas of comfort, nutrition, and communication. Although it is compact in relation to the rest of the body, the mouth's impact is profound on growth, development, and well-being. A child's ability to eat safely and successfully is dependent on normal anatomy, well-coordinated muscle activity, sensory processing, and a supportive feeding environment (Stevenson & Allaire, 1991).

When there is concern about the eating process, including poor intake or poor weight gain, a referral to a feeding specialist may be warranted. A feeding specialist may be any professional who has specific training in anatomy, physiology, normal development, psychology, and neurology as they relate to eating. Occupational therapists and speech-language pathologists generally function as feeding specialists. Optimally, the feeding specialist is one member of an interdisciplinary team that also includes the family for optimum treatment planning and outcome. A framework for assessing a child's eating abilities and implications for treating oral-motor difficulties are presented in this chapter.

NORMAL STRUCTURE AND FUNCTION

Normal oral function during eating is supported by intact structures of the mouth and the pharynx. In general, the structures should be symmetric, free of clefts, and well aligned. Normal muscle tone and sensation should be present. The quality of oral-motor skills depends on normal sensory channels not only to receive sensory information but also to process and interpret it appropriately. Normal sensory capacity is a result of the ability to accurately gate or control sensory input and adaptively perceive and interpret that information (Wolf & Glass, 1992). As a result of normal structure, function, and sensation, the lips, cheeks, jaw, palate, teeth, and tongue are able to perform the individual tasks that are necessary for efficient eating. For example, the lips move to allow for mouth opening and lip closure; they form a seal against a nipple, a cup, or a spoon; and they keep food and liquid in the mouth. The cheeks form boundaries to hold food and liquid in the mouth as well, and they aid in establishing negative pressure for sucking. The jaw provides a stable base for controlled or graded mouth movement, as needed for chewing, and functions in pressure changes for sucking. The contour and vault of the hard and soft palate are well shaped, and the soft palate elevates during speech and swallowing. The teeth and gums are pain-free, and the tissue is healthy in appearance. The tongue has full range of motion and is able to assume a variety of shapes and positions, including forming a seal with the lips and palate. Taste sensation is intact. Given the normal anatomy and functional abilities just described, a child's feeding skills develop sequentially. (See Table 1, which details the developmental acquisition of feeding skills.)

ORAL-MOTOR DYSFUNCTION

Oral-motor dysfunction, which is characterized by alterations or defects in structure, movement, sensation, or muscle tone, can contribute to poor nutritional intake as a result of difficulties in sucking, chewing, and swallowing. Although the etiology is not always clear, oral-motor dysfunction is often seen when there is central nervous system involvement (Wolf & Glass 1992), such as prematurity, cerebral palsy, brain injury, seizure disorder, and **sensory processing disorders.** Dysfunction can be measured along a continuum from mild to severe. For example, a child may demonstrate a mildly dysfunctional pattern of tongue protrusion or thrusting when spoon feeding, resulting in loss of food from the mouth and increased time needed to complete a meal. In comparison, a child with severe oral dysfunction may not be able to close his or her mouth, move the food back with his or her tongue, or eat without choking. As a result of these issues, children with oral-motor dysfunction can be difficult to feed. Feedings may require increased vigilance and patience to ensure that these children receive adequate nutrition. (See Table 2 for guidelines for referring a child for an oral-motor assessment.)

Following an oral-motor assessment, treatment with a feeding specialist may be indicated. The child who is having difficulty chewing, for example, can gain strength and coordinated movement of the lips, cheeks, and tongue in therapy. Specific exercises and techniques may be employed to help the child master chewing and improve eating abilities to safely advance his or her diet. Refusal of age-appropriate tastes or textures may be an indication of motor or sensory dysfunction, which warrants further investigation (Palmer & Heyman, 1993).

ORAL TONE AND SENSATION

Oral tone is an important consideration, as it directly influences oral posture and movement. Simply defined, muscle tone is the degree of tension present in a muscle. High tone means that a muscle is stiff, whereas low tone means that it is floppy. A child with high tone may have retracted lips, jaw, and tongue, demonstrating labored oral movements with decreased range of motion (Morris & Klein, 1987). A child who presents with low muscle tone may demonstrate an **open oral rest posture**; have a flat, inactive tongue; show poor lip seal; and have floppy cheeks (Morris & Klein, 1987). A child may present with altered oral sensation, which can be described as **hypersensitivity** or **hyposensitivity** as illustrated in the case examples on pages 313–314.

Table 1. Developmental acquisition of feeding skills

Age	Food types	Positioning	Oral patterns	Self-feeding
1 month	Liquid from bottle or breast	Semi-reclined or sidelying with neck slightly flexed	Sucking pattern, loses some liquid; sequences two or more sucks before pausing to breathe or swallow.	Brings hands to mouth
4–6 months	Liquids, baby cereals, puréed foods	Supported semi-sitting or sitting position	Sucking pattern. No longer loses liquid during sucking, although may lose some when initiating or terminating the suck or as the nipple is removed. By 4 months, sequences 20 or more sucks from breast or bottle. Uses a sucking pattern with puréed foods with tongue protrusion past the lips. Some food is pushed out of the mouth. At 6 months, jaw quiets and remains in a stable, open position until the spoon enters the mouth. The tongue quiets to accept the spoon.	At 4 months, infant pats bottle and holds both hands on the bottle. Infant holds bottle independently with one or both hands at 6 months. Cup may be introduced at 6 months.
9 months	Liquids, puréed foods, ground or junior foods, mashed table foods, teething cookies, soft cookies and crackers	Sitting, usually in a highchair with a tray table for spoon feeding and finger feeding	No longer loses any liquid during sucking initiation or when the nipple is removed from the mouth. Child may use wide jaw excursions with cup drinking, and loss of liquid is common. Upper lip is active in food removal from the spoon. Uses vertical jaw movements when chewing solids. Begins to transfer food from the center of the mouth to the side. Child uses vertical and diagonal rotary jaw movements for chewing.	Capable of independent finger feeding. Holds and bangs spoon. Drinks from cup held by caregiver.
12 months	Liquids and coarsely chopped table foods including easily chewed meats	Sitting unsupported in a highchair or a similar seat (e.g., clip-on chair, booster chair)	Sucking pattern. Takes liquid primarily from a cup. Tongue may protrude slightly for stability. Uses a controlled, sustained bite on a soft cookie. Minimal loss of food from mouth with spoon feeding. Lips are active to clear utensil of food and contain food while chewing.	Child holds cup and drinks with some spilling. Brings a filled spoon to mouth with spilling.

(continued)

Table 1. (continued)

Age	Food types	Positioning	Oral patterns	Self-feeding
18 months	Liquids and coarsely chopped table foods including most meats and some raw vegetables	Sitting unsupported at the family table or at a small child's chair and table	Jaw stabilization is obtained by biting down on the edge of the cup. Upper lip is closed on the edge of the cup, providing a good seal for drinking. Child uses a controlled, sustained bite on a hard cookie. Can chew with the lips closed and does so intermittently. Diagonal rotary jaw movements are smooth and well coordinated.	Child scoops food onto spoon and brings it to the mouth.
24 months	Liquids, wide variety of table foods except for some raw fruits, vegetables, and nuts	Sitting at table	Jaw stabilization is emerging. Jaw movement in chewing is variable and includes diagonal rotary and circular rotary movements. Tongue is used in a free, sweeping motion to clean food from the upper and lower lips. Child swallows solid foods including those with a combination of textures with easy lip closure as needed.	Child brings spoon or fork to mouth with the hand palm-up, uses well. Typically, child is fully weaned from the bottle or breast (may occur earlier) and drinks entirely from the cup.

Table 2.   Referral criteria for oral-motor assessment

- Frequent or excessive drooling not associated with teething; drooling normally may be present in infants or toddlers from 5 to 24 months of age (Stevenson & Allaire, 1991); teething typically is completed between the ages of 12 and 16 months (Morris & Klein, 1987; Sullivan & Rosenbloom, 1996)
- Excessive loss of food or formula from mouth
- Inability to move food from one side of the mouth to the other; most children are proficient with this skill by 24 months of age (Morris & Klein, 1987)
- Swallowing food whole or difficulty breaking down solids prior to swallowing
- Chewing for an extended period of time, pocketing food in cheeks, or spitting out food
- Refusing advanced textures of solid food, such as raw fruits and vegetables, hard crunchy snacks, and meats
- Abnormal oral-motor patterns or reflexes (e.g., tongue protrusion or thrusting beyond the lips, open oral rest posture, tonic bite reflex)
- Easy fatigue while eating
- Extensive time required to complete a meal (over 30 minutes)
- Known movement disturbance (e.g., cerebral palsy, muscular dystrophy, seizure disorder, head injury) that requires specialized positioning, equipment, or techniques

Annie is a 22-month-old girl who is currently taking liquids and purées. Her mother reports that she is a messy eater, losing purées from her mouth. She is unsuccessful with drinking from an open cup and must drink from a cup that has a spouted lid. Her mother also reports that Annie still has food in her mouth when presented with the next bite. Annie prefers to have all of her food warmed and prefers foods that have a strong taste: spicy, salty, distinct flavors. She is having difficulty moving on to solids that require chewing. Upon evaluation, Annie is observed to have low muscle tone, which results in her mouth being open most of the time and frequent drooling. She is not aware of food or drool on her lips and chin. She demonstrates weak, ineffective chewing attempts with soft solids, which result in swallowing foods whole. She tends to pocket hard solids between her teeth and cheek.

Annie demonstrates oral hyposensitivity as evidenced by decreased awareness of saliva and food on the outside of her mouth. She has difficulty keeping puréed foods in her mouth as they provide less sensory information than hard, crunchy solids. She is unaware of food in her mouth that needs to be swallowed, both purées and solids, and does not perceive the need for further breakdown of soft solids before swallowing. Annie prefers strong flavors and warm temperatures because they provide increased sensory information as does the spouted cup lid.

Therapeutic intervention would be beneficial for Annie with an emphasis on increasing facial and oral tone as a necessary foundation for movement, increasing sensory awareness, and improving coordinated oral movement and strength. In therapy, a variety of tools and techniques may be used, such as resistive exercises, whistles and blow toys, and foods with strong flavors and distinct textures.

Christopher is a 15-month-old boy who presents with a narrow range of foods in his diet. He refuses foods that are unfamiliar or different from his preferred foods, which are smooth, bland purées. Christopher's parents report that he is intolerant of foods that are lumpy or bumpy or that have crumbs or pieces. He will gag and occasionally vomit with these textures. Christopher prefers foods and liquids at room temperature. He resists face washing and toothbrushing. During feeding observation, Christopher becomes distressed if his hands or face are messy and cannot resume eating until they are wiped. He will not allow food to touch his lips but rather will use his teeth to clear food from the spoon.

Christopher demonstrates oral hypersensitivity as evidenced by the limited number of foods in his repertoire, all of which are similar with respect to taste, temperature, and texture. His frequent gagging and vomiting are due to an inability to tolerate textured foods. Aversion to touch in or around the mouth and an overreaction to the feel of food on his lips and face while eating are additional signs of hypersensitivity.

A therapy program for Christopher would focus on improving his ability to accept touch, reducing episodes of gagging and vomiting, and expanding the variety of tastes, textures, and temperatures in his diet. Treatment must include techniques to normalize overall sensory integration in order to proceed with feeding therapy. The advancement of taste, temperature, and texture may then be addressed in a sequential fashion.

POSITIONING

Adequate support and stability are necessary for successful eating performance (Morris & Klein, 1987). Alignment of the head, neck, and trunk along with a solid, seated base are recommended for a child to execute the fine motor movements of eating and swallowing. Proximal stability permits distal mobility, which is needed for self-feeding, efficient intake of nourishment, and safe swallowing (Stevenson & Allaire, 1991). In other words, when a child's body is well supported, he or she is better able to use his or her hands and mouth for eating.

An infant should be fed in a semi-reclined, fully supported position. The head and neck should be flexed slightly to allow for comfortable breathing and swallowing. As the child develops and graduates to an independent sitting position, a highchair can provide secure seating. The highchair tray lends support for the arms as self-feeding skills are practiced. When a child is able to join his or her family at the table, he or she needs a chair that allows for stable sitting and close contact with the table.

When movement or tone are altered, as with cerebral palsy, special arrangements may be needed to achieve the best positioning. In some cases, alternative positioning techniques enable children to eat successfully (Morris & Klein, 1987). Optimum alignment for these children may not be standard but may promote optimum function.

SWALLOWING

Typical swallow function includes two voluntary phases—the oral preparatory phase and the oral phase—and two automatic phases—the pharyngeal phase and the esophageal phase (Logemann, 1983). During the oral preparatory phase, which may involve chewing, food and liquid are formed into a cohesive **bolus**, or mouthful. The tongue moves in a posterior wave to move the bolus toward the back of the mouth during the oral phase. The swallow reflex is initiated in the pharyngeal phase: The larynx elevates, the soft palate closes off the nasal passages, the epiglottis and the vocal cords close to protect the airway, and the cricopharyngeus muscle relaxes to allow the bolus to move into the esophagus. In the esophageal phase, the bolus moves through the esophagus and into the stomach.

Table 3 lists clinical signs of swallowing difficulties. It is important to understand that these observations alone do not constitute a full assessment, nor do they allow for accurate

Table 3.   Referral criteria for swallowing assessment

- Coughing, choking, or gagging during or after feeding
- Nasopharyngeal regurgitation (loss of food or liquid through nose)
- Food refusal behaviors such as turning head away, pursing lips together, pushing away food, spitting out foods or liquids
- Vomiting during or after feeding
- Coughing or choking on secretions; inability to manage saliva; excessive drooling
- Voice or cry sounding wet or gurgly after eating or drinking
- Frequent respiratory infections such as pneumonia or bronchiolitis
- Unusual head or body movements or discomfort during feedings
- Overreaction to food or liquids in or around mouth as evidenced by gagging, crying, or strong refusal behaviors
- No reaction to food or liquids in or around the mouth as evidenced by no awareness of food on the lips, no mouth movement, and no attempt to swallow

diagnosis of swallow dysfunction without radiographic testing. (Please note that all of the clinical signs listed in Table 3 also may be indicators of gastroesophageal reflux [GER] [DiPalma & Colon, 1991]. See Chapter 11 for additional information on GER.)

Evaluation

Recommended components of a swallowing evaluation include a parent interview, observation of oral-motor and sensory processes during feeding, nutritional assessment including height, weight, and 3-day diet history, and a videofluoroscopic swallow study. A videofluoroscopic swallow study is the most accurate method of diagnosing a swallowing disorder (Wolf & Glass, 1992) and is indicated when a child displays one or more of the clinical signs that are described in Table 3. With this radiographic procedure, all phases of the swallow may be observed with a variety of tastes and textures in a simulated feeding experience. Positioning and compensatory strategies may be incorporated into the exam for optimum treatment planning. A comprehensive team approach is beneficial (Arvedson & Brodsky, 1993; Jones, 1989; Kramer & Eicher, 1993); a basic team consists of a feeding specialist, a dietitian, and a radiologist. Alternative methods are cited in the literature for evaluating swallow function when the videofluoroscopic swallow study is unavailable or inappropriate (Langmore, Schatz, & Olsen, 1988; Logemann, 1983; Wolf & Glass, 1992).

The videofluoroscopic swallow evaluation may reveal that a child is aspirating or is at risk for aspirating. Risk factors include a delay in initiating the swallow reflex, residue in the pharynx after the swallow, and movement of the X-ray contrast material into the airway or nasal passages. Aspiration increases a child's risk for lung infections and ultimately may weaken a child's ability to fight off and recover from respiratory illness. Compromised respiratory status may then result in reduced energy for physical and mental development.

Intervention

After the comprehensive swallow evaluation, a discussion must take place between the family and the child's primary care team regarding the optimum feeding regimen. This regimen must provide adequate nutrition and maintain oral skills in a safe and reasonable manner. It is important to understand that treatment cannot affect children's reflexive phases of swallowing. Compensatory strategies that are successful with adults, such as using a chin tuck with every swallow, are not possible with infants and small children. The need for language comprehension and self-monitoring prohibits the use of these strategies. Treatment can help, however, by modifying the child's diet, positioning, and oral-sensory and oral-motor skills as described previously. In addition, certain techniques may be employed to address specific issues, such as pacing the meal and limiting the size of each bite or spoonful.

Alternative methods for intake may be necessary (Young, 1993). In some cases, a specific texture, such as thin liquid, may have to be eliminated from the child's diet because of swallow dysfunction. Some children benefit from temporary supplemental tube-feedings that are provided via a **nasogastric tube** (Bazyk, 1990). When long-term supplemental feedings are anticipated, a **gastrostomy tube** may be indicated. In more severe cases, all nutrition and hydration must be provided with gastrostomy or nasogastric tube-feedings. (See Chapter 11.)

In all children fed by tube, it is critical to preserve oral-motor and oral-sensory function as much as possible in order to promote oral feeding interest and ability. A feeding program may range from partial oral intake to a taste stimulation program based on the severity of the swallow dysfunction (Morris & Klein, 1987). Generally, children who are tube-fed receive a prescribed, static volume of formula according to an artificial feeding schedule that may or may not closely resemble usual mealtimes. It is often difficult for children to make the transition from tube-feeding to oral feeding. Some of the challenges in working toward eating by mouth include establishing a typical hunger drive, drawing a conceptual association between the mouth and satiety, and overcoming oral aversion due to lack of experience with eating. Individual therapy or group therapy is recommended to support and guide the child and family through this process.

SUMMARY

Oral-motor, oral-sensory, and swallow dysfunction—separate or together—may reduce a child's ability to safely consume adequate nutrition for growth and development. Volume and variety of oral intake can be affected significantly by an impairment in any of these areas. Children who are having difficulty advancing their diets to age-appropriate tastes and textures may require further assessment of motor and sensory systems. If a child is diagnosed with a structural or functional impairment that limits oral intake, then every effort should be made to maintain and promote oral feeding skills within safe boundaries for that child. Early referral to a feeding therapist is recommended for evaluation and possible treatment.

REFERENCES

Arvedson, J.C., & Brodsky, L. (1993). *Pediatric swallowing and feeding: Assessment and management.* Thousand Oaks, CA: Singular Publishing.

Bazyk, S. (1990). Factors associated with the transition to tube feeding in infants fed by nasogastric tubes. *American Journal of Occupational Therapy, 44,* 1070–1078.

DiPalma, J., & Colon, A.R. (1991). Gastroesophageal reflux in infants. *American Family Physician, 43*(3), 857–864.

Jones, P.M. (1989). Feeding disorders in children with multiple handicaps. *Developmental Medicine and Child Neurology, 31,* 404–406.

Kramer, S.S., & Eicher, P.M. (1993). The evaluation of pediatric feeding abnormalities. *Dysphagia, 8,* 215–224.

Langmore, S.E., Schatz, K., & Olsen, N. (1988). Fiberoptic endoscopic examination of swallowing safety: A new procedure. *Dysphagia, 2,* 216–219.

Logemann, J. (1983). *Evaluation and treatment of swallow disorders.* Boston: College Press Publications.

Morris, S.E., & Klein, M.D. (1987). *Pre-feeding skills.* Tucson, AZ: Therapy Skill Builders.

Palmer, M.M., & Heyman, M.B. (1993). Assessment and treatment of sensory- versus motor-based feeding problems in very young children. *Infants and Young Children, 6*(2), 67–73.

Stevenson, D., & Allaire, J.H. (1991). The development of normal feeding and swallowing. *Pediatric Clinics of North America, 38*(6), 1439–1453.

Sullivan, P.B., & Rosenbloom, L. (1996). Introduction: An overview of the feeding difficulties experienced by disabled children. In P.B. Sullivan & L. Rosenbloom (Eds.), *Feeding the disabled child* (pp. 11–21). London: MacKeith Press.

Wolf, L.F., & Glass, R.P. (1992). *Feeding and swallowing disorders in infancy.* Tucson, AZ: Therapy Skill Builders.

Young, C. (1993). Nutrition. In J.C. Arvedson & L. Brodsky (Eds.), *Pediatric swallowing and feeding: Assessment and management* (pp. 157–208). Thousand Oaks, CA: Singular Publishing.

Chapter 24

Detecting Communication Difficulties in Infants and Toddlers Who Have Feeding Difficulties

Elizabeth R. Crais

Jesse's parents had had some concerns about Jesse's development but were not sure as first-time parents whether they were just being too watchful. In the beginning, Jesse had some feeding problems, but those seemed to be working themselves out with the help of Jesse's pediatrician and a nutritionist. As Jesse began to gain weight and get stronger, his parents began to worry about his lack of interest in them and that he was not making many sounds. They had seen at the doctor's office other infants who were always using a lot of sounds. His parents decided at their next visit with the pediatrician to ask whether they should be worried about Jesse's limited interaction and lack of sound making. They also wondered whether it was normal for a child his age not to be very interested in looking at his parents or in trying to get their attention.

For the professionals who provide services to Jesse and his parents, the questions raised in the scenario are not simple ones, nor are they answered easily by one or two bits of information. To answer questions about Jesse, the professionals and the parents must collaborate to uncover Jesse's current abilities, strengths, and needs and must look across multiple sources of information to confirm the initial concerns. This chapter provides information for professionals and parents who need to make the decision of whether to refer a child for evaluation to an interdisciplinary team and/or a speech-language pathologist.

INTRODUCTION

Communication is a central part of everyday functioning. Through it, people exchange ideas, information, and feelings, get their needs met, share experiences, and plan for the future. Communication is the link to the development of relationships with others and serves as both a means of interaction and a reason for interactions. For some young children, communication is not an easy or natural process, and delays or disorders may be evident at an early age or may become evident only as the child moves out into the world to interact with others in his or her environment.

Communication delays or disorders may be of several different types and may affect different components of language and communication. For example, communication can be nonverbal (e.g., gestures, facial expressions, body posture) or verbal (e.g., speaking, writing, using sign language), and deficits may appear in either or both areas. Communication can also be defined broadly such that any act that influences another can be called communicative. In this sense, communication can occur between and among species, and both newborns and animals can communicate. Two parts of communication that are typically thought to be specific to humans are language and speech. *Language* is a complex system of symbols that are understood mutually and used in a conventional way, and deficits in language typically are referred to as *expressive* and/or *receptive delays* or *disorders.* Speech (producing vocal sounds and sound sequences) is the most common means by which to communicate; disorders in speaking may range from mild (e.g., the child who says wabbit for rabbit) to severe (e.g., the child who is unable to produce any sounds vocally).

Communication delays or disorders may occur alone or may be part of a larger developmental disability such as mental retardation, autism, or cerebral palsy. Delays or disorders in communication may affect a child's social, emotional, cognitive, language, and later academic development. Indeed, Aram and Hall (1989) reported that 60% of children who exhibited language disorders as preschoolers received special education services during the school years. In addition, 5%–10% of children younger than 3 years have delayed communication development (Rossetti, 1996), and 10%–12% of all school-age children have some type of disability. Of those preschool children identified with disabilities, 70% have speech, language, or communication impairments (U.S. Department of Education, 1987); thus identifying young children who have or who are at risk for communication difficulties is an important aspect of service delivery for all children and for all service providers.

To help guide professionals in the referral process, this chapter focuses on the identification of all children who have or who are at risk for communication difficulties, with special emphasis on children who are also undernourished. The chapter first addresses the linkages between the development of feeding and communication skills and disorders, then provides an overview of what to look for in children who are at risk for communication difficulties, and finally previews basic intervention principles for working with children who have communication and feeding difficulties.

LINKS BETWEEN FEEDING AND COMMUNICATION

Feeding and communication are linked in a variety of ways throughout infancy and early childhood. The following sections highlight some of the connections between feeding and communication development and possible points in the process where difficulties may arise.

Risk Factors that Are Important to Feeding and Communication

Many of the same biological and environmental factors that put children at risk for feeding disorders also place them at risk for communication disorders. Biological factors that affect both feeding and communication include prematurity and low birth weight, chronic illness, genetic disorders (e.g., Down syndrome, cystic fibrosis), and neuromuscular disorders (e.g., cerebral palsy, Rett syndrome). Environmental factors such as maternal education, poverty, unemployment, parental abuse or neglect, parental mental or emotional problems, drug use, and level and type of parental support all may play a role in the development of feeding and communication. Furthermore, the cumulative effect of risk factors may be substantial for both feeding and communication processes (Sameroff & Fiese, 1990).

Transactional Nature of Communication and Feeding Development

Communication, like feeding (see description in Satter, 1992, and Chapter 7), is a reciprocal process that depends on the characteristics and abilities of the child as well as those of the interactive partner. The interactionist, or transactional, perspective that is held by many professionals (MacDonald & Gillette, 1989; Sameroff & Fiese, 1990) focuses on the reciprocal nature of communication and the importance of caregivers in establishing basic communication skills. Both communication and feeding have important child and partner variables that may contribute to successful development. Child variables that are important to both communication and feeding include temperament, behavioral characteristics, readability of cues, level of functioning, prematurity, and overall health and stamina (Dunst, Lowe, & Bartholomew, 1990; Satter, 1990). For example, infants who have ongoing illnesses or who were born prematurely may send subtle and inconsistent communication signals, thus making it difficult for caregivers to figure out what they need (Field, 1987; Wyley, 1995). In addition, behavioral characteristics that often accompany malnutrition include irritability, lethargy, and decreased social responsiveness (Sturm & Drotar, 1992); undernourished children also seem to show more negative affect in feeding and nonfeeding situations (Polan et al., 1991). Thus, caregivers may themselves become less responsive, stimulating, or positive to a child who demonstrates these characteristics, and both the development of adequate feeding and communication may be at risk. Important partner variables include the parental risk factors just noted as well as the overall style of the caregiver (e.g., responsive versus directive) and the ability of the caregiver to recognize and respond consistently and appropriately to the child's cues and developmental level (Dunst et al., 1990).

In addition to the transactional nature of the development of both processes between child and caregiver, communication and feeding skills have a transactional relationship with each other. For example, undernourished children have been reported to make little eye contact, rarely vocalize, dislike cuddling, and engage in self-stimulatory acts (Berkowitz & Senter, 1987)—all behaviors that may inhibit the development of good communication skills. As indicated by Satter (1992), high-quality feeding interactions in the first years of life are linked positively to a child's later cognitive and linguistic competence and security of attachment (Barnard et al., 1989). Alternatively, a child's limited ability to communicate may make successful recognition of the infant's cues for feeding less likely and may exacerbate parental overmanaging in feeding (Satter, 1990). Finally, undernutrition generally occurs in the first 2 years of life (see Chapter 2), a critical period for the development of communication and language skills.

Role of Contingency and Responsiveness

In both communication and feeding development, contingency and responsiveness play major parts in helping the infant gain control over the environment. Responsiveness is important, but the ability of the parent to respond contingently or to recognize and respond to what the child wants or needs plays an even greater role. The infant's early signals may indicate a physical or emotional state, such as a need to change position, hunger, or the need for attention or comfort. When an infant's caregivers learn to identify the infant's signals, interpret them appropriately, and respond as quickly and as consistently as possible, they enable the infant to learn that he or she can have an effect on the world (Dunst et al., 1990); this encourages the infant to communicate more frequently and to build trust. Some infants' early communication signals, however, are difficult to interpret, and the infants' caregivers may have trouble learning how to read their children's communication cues (Field, 1987; Wetherby & Prizant, 1993). For example, some children, because of cognitive or physical impairments, have difficulty expressing themselves either verbally or nonverbally (Beukelman & Mirenda, 1998); even those who use verbal means may be limited in their ability to be understood.

For some caregivers and their undernourished children, the failure to develop contingent and responsive relationships presents problems for both feeding and communication. When compared with mothers of typically developing children, mothers of children who have been diagnosed with pediatric undernutrition appear less sensitive and the infants appear more negative and engage in fewer vocal interactions (Berkowitz & Senter, 1987; Polan et al., 1991). These mothers have been reported to make fewer positive vocalizations (e.g., praise, approval, laughter), make more negative vocalizations (e.g., criticism, threats), respond less to their infant's signals, and take part in less mutual gazing and mutual interaction (Berkowitz & Senter, 1987). In addition, they may reject bids from the infant or respond in confusing or unpredictable ways (Benoit, Zeanah, & Barton, 1989). All of these behaviors indicate less-than-favorable results for the development of responsive and contingent relationships and most certainly will have an effect on not only the caregiver–child feeding relationship but also the infant's communicative competence.

Oral-Motor Factors

Although oral-motor skills are critical to infants' and toddlers' eating and oral communication, they are covered in detail elsewhere (see Chapter 23). In summary, it is clear that for some undernourished children, communication difficulties are likely, and the possibility of current or future communication disorders should be investigated.

IDENTIFYING WHAT IS TYPICAL AND WHAT IS NOT

Two methods are used to help professionals identify children who are undernourished and who also may have or may be at risk for communication difficulties. The first is the traditional method of providing key milestones within a chronological age sequence for both comprehension and production (see Table 1). The second method provides a more detailed examination of domains within communication development and offers a chance to identify developmental trends within domains. The following sections provide ideas for what to look for in children who are suspected of having difficulties communicating. Referrals for consultation or evaluation can be made to interdisciplinary early intervention teams or to a speech-language pathologist directly.

Table 1. Children's milestones of communication development

Age	Hearing/understanding	Expressing
Birth to 3 months	• Can be quieted by a familiar, friendly voice • Startles, cries, or wakes when there is a loud sound	• Produces small, throaty noises
3 to 6 months	• Enjoys rattles and other sound-making toys • Responds to pleasant tones by cooing • Stops playing and appears to listen to sounds or speech	• Laughs out loud • Cries differently for pain, hunger, and discomfort • Coos—produces an assortment of oohs, ahs, and other vowel sounds
6 to 9 months	• Responds to soft levels of speech and other sounds • Temporarily stops action in response to "no" • Turns head directly toward voices and interesting sounds • Begins to understand routine words when used with a hand gesture (e.g., bye-bye, up)	• Babbles—repeats consonant–vowel combinations such as ba-ba-ba • Makes raspberry sound • Makes sounds with rising and falling pitches
9 to 12 months	• Follows simple directions presented with gestures (e.g., give it to me, come here) • Responds to his or her own name even when spoken quietly • Will turn and find sound in any direction	• Vocalizes to get attention • Imitates sounds • Produces a variety of speech sounds (e.g., m, b, d) in several pitches
12 to 18 months	• Knows the names of familiar objects, persons, and pets • Follows routine directions presented without gestural or visual cues (e.g., come here, clap hands) • Identifies sounds coming from another room or outside • Enjoys music and may try to dance	• Uses two to three words spontaneously • Imitates simple words • Uses jargon speech (babbling that sounds like real speech) to communicate • Points to request or draw attention to objects, people, and events
18 to 24 months	• Points to two or more body parts • Identifies five or more pictures of common objects when named	• Uses vocabulary of 20+ words • Uses jargon speech with intelligible words • Says "no" or "no-no" in response to questions or commands
24 to 30 months	• Responds to two-part command (e.g., get the shoe and bring it to me) • Listens to simple stories • Understands possessive terms (my, mine, yours)	• Puts together two or more words to make simple sentences • Uses vocabulary of 50+ words • 50% of speech can be understood by unfamiliar listeners

(continued)

Table 1. (*continued*)

Age	Hearing/understanding	Expressing
30 to 36 months	• Answers to "what" and "who" questions • Identifies objects and pictures by use (e.g., show me what you sit on) • Easily follows simple conversation • Understands basic concepts (e.g., big, little, in, on)	• Consistently uses two- to three-word sentences • Asks "what" and "where" questions • Uses some plural (e.g., cars) and verb markers (e.g., running) • 50%–75% of speech can be understood by unfamiliar listeners

From *Your Child's Milestones of Communication Development* [Poster]. (1993). Nashville, TN: Bill Wilkerson Center Press; reprinted by permission.

Milestones

A major difficulty in identifying young children with communication difficulties has been the reliance on particular milestones, specifically, the production of first words and word combinations. Unfortunately, the range of first word use is large, typically ranging from 12 to 20 months of age (Bates, O'Connell, & Shore, 1987); word combinations occur sometime between 18 and 24 months. Referral for a "language delay," therefore, often is not made until the child is at least 24 months and, many times, later because of parent and professional tendencies to take a "wait and see" approach. Research indicates that by profiling a child's abilities across a variety of domains *within* communication it is possible to identify children who are at risk for communication disorders at earlier ages (Wetherby & Prizant, 1996).

Two popular screening tools that were developed within a milestone framework and that are used by health care professionals to identify children with communication and other developmental delays are the Denver II (Frankenburg et al., 1990) and the Early Language Milestone Scales (Coplan, 1987). They both have proved useful for identifying global delays in young children and, when supplemented with discussion with caregivers and observation of the child, can be a starting point for referral. In addition, given the high correlation between parents' concerns about their children's developmental status and the outcome of developmental screening measures (Bricker & Squires, 1989; Glascoe, MacLean, & Stone, 1991), professionals should recognize the positive nature of validating one source of information with the other.

Domains of Communication Development

As with the milestone method, no one single behavior or absence of a behavior typically warrants a referral; however, by looking across domains, the professional may be able to identify multiple domains that indicate at-risk behavior.

Readiness for Social Interaction

An infant's or toddler's readiness for interaction depends on both physiological and environmental factors and the interplay of those factors. In the early stages, infants indicate a readiness to interact by staying calm and alert when presented with stimuli (e.g., visual and/or auditory). For older infants and toddlers, interactive readiness may be indicated by making eye contact, tolerating shared physical space or touch, giving or showing or receiving objects, and/or directing vocalizations or verbalizations toward the family member or the professional.

It is common for young children to show hesitance or even avoidance of interaction with strangers (especially vocal or verbal); thus, the presence of people who are familiar to the child and the use of an observational setting that is as natural as possible are critical. In addition, family members can often provide helpful tips for professionals in facilitating interaction with the child and in teasing apart which "non-readiness" behaviors are related to the environment (e.g., elicited by strangers, medical setting) and which behaviors are typical of the child in all or most settings. Asking the caregiver to describe what the infant or young child does when talked to, shown objects, or smiled at can be helpful.

After the first 2–3 months of life, most typically developing infants should be showing clear signs of interest in and attention to social interactions by caregivers (Barnard, Morisset, & Spieker, 1993); by 3 months, smiling should be an easily won prize for attentive caregivers. Infants who are 4–8 months old should be attentive to social games (e.g., peekaboo, pat-a-cake) and should begin to share two-way communication with caregivers (e.g., caregiver vocalizes and infant vocalizes to caregiver) by the end of this period (Greenspan, 1992). As young children's comprehension grows, they should be able to respond to their own names by looking (at 12 months) and should be able to follow simple commands (e.g., "Come here") given with gestures (by 18 months). Inattentiveness to people, lack of eye contact, or lack of shared mutual gaze with familiar adults all should be signals of a child's risk for communication difficulties.

Intentionality

Initially, an infant's communication is unintentional. Infants send communication signals and, in turn, receive caregivers' responses by using their eyes, ears, and touch. Infants look at faces and make eye contact from birth. Sometimes they communicate feelings of displeasure by crying or turning away from something displeasing. Other times, they communicate these same feelings through hiccuping, yawning, stretching their arms, finger splaying, placing a hand over their eyes, grimacing, or even falling asleep (Fogel, 1991). Over time, through the consistent response of the caregiver to these communicative behaviors, infants learn to associate their action with a certain reaction from the caregiver. Sometime between 8 and 12 months of age, children typically progress from using unintentional communicative behaviors to using intentional behaviors that function to directly affect another's behavior (Dunst et al., 1990). Children in this stage communicate primarily to 1) control someone else's behavior by making a request or protesting; 2) achieve and maintain social interaction by using greetings, playing social games such as peekaboo or pat-a-cake, gesturing, and showing off; and 3) draw joint attention to an object, event, or action that is shared by both the child and the listener (Wetherby & Prizant, 1993). These intentions predominate through the first 2 years of a child's life. Later developing intentions include requesting permission, acknowledging, clarifying, and requesting information and may not emerge until the one-word (12–20 months) or multiword (24+ months) stage (Wetherby & Prizant, 1993).

To help in the referral process, the focus should be on whether the child uses intentional communication. Because it may be difficult at times to determine whether a child has communicated intentionally, Wetherby and Prizant's (1993) criteria for judging intentionality may be helpful: Does the child

1. Alternate eye gaze between the listener and the goal?
2. Persist in signaling or change the signal until a goal is accomplished?

3. Use a conventional signal (e.g., wave "bye") or a ritualized form (e.g., lie down on floor to request diaper changing)?
4. Pause for a response from a listener?
5. Terminate a signal and/or display satisfaction when a goal is met?
6. Display dissatisfaction when a goal is not met?

Feeding and Oral-Motor Skills

The guiding principle in working with caregivers around feeding is to help caregivers find ways that will allow them to be successful with their child (see Chapter 7); therefore, assessment needs to focus dynamically on the feeding relationship and on identifying collaboratively with families the strategies and techniques that may gain success. Feeding skills, if they were of concern to caregivers, and their relationship to caregiver–child interaction and overall communication efforts would be addressed as part of the profiling to identify children who are at risk for communication difficulties. In addition, oral-motor skills would be part of any comprehensive assessment (see Chapter 23).

Play Skills

For many children, there is substantial evidence that language and play skills are highly correlated during some stages of development and that both reflect common underlying cognitive processes (Kennedy, Sheridan, Radlinski, & Beeghly, 1991); thus, using the child's play skills as an indicator of the child's cognitive and communicative potential can be a helpful strategy in making decisions about referral. Two particular types of play that can be observed or inquired about from caregivers are play with objects and pretend play.

Early object play from birth to 4 months is typified by looking at, holding, and mouthing objects. In the 4- to 8-month range, as fine motor skills increase, play includes mouthing, banging, shaking, and manipulating objects. Later, between 8 and 12 months, infants begin to manipulate objects more easily, throwing and dropping them and giving and showing them to adults, and begin to be participants in social games (e.g., pat-a-cake). In the 12- to 18-month range, toddlers typically push, pull, turn on, put in, and take out objects. They begin to stack objects and figure out the relationships between play objects. Most toddlers in this age range use pointing as a way to gain objects or draw attention to objects. Between 18 and 24 months, toddlers play easily with a variety of toys (e.g., blocks, cars, dolls, sandbox toys, toy animals) and should be showing clearly their knowledge of how to use these toys in appropriate ways. In the 24- to 36-month range, more elaborate actions on objects should be evidenced, especially in a pretend, or symbolic, way, discussed next.

In the area of pretend play, single pretend schemes (e.g., child drinks from empty cup) often emerge at approximately 12–20 months along with first words (Kennedy et al., 1991). If children who are 20–24 months old are not exhibiting any pretend play behaviors, then professional suspicions should be raised. Likewise, as children begin to combine words (20–24 months), single pretend schemes are joined (e.g., child stirs and then feeds self); if a child is combining play behaviors but not combining words, then red flags should be raised. By 28 months, children produce longer utterances, produce ordered play sequences, and play-act familiar scenarios (Kennedy et al., 1991; McCune-Nicholich & Bruskin, 1982).

Once professionals and family members have identified a child's approximate play level and have examined the child's other skills (described later), inferences can be made about the child's overall ability to use representational thinking. If children do not exhibit play behaviors that are typical of their chronological age or only exhibit behaviors from much earlier stages, then questions should be raised about their other developmental domains.

Sound Production

To make decisions regarding a child's overall communication level, a look at the child's capabilities for sound making and sound imitation are useful. The work of Rescorla and Ratner (1996) has indicated that children with specific expressive language impairment vocalize less than their typically developing peers, in addition to having proportionately smaller sound inventories and using less mature syllable shapes.

In identifying delays in a child's phonological development, it is useful first to identify critical milestones that serve as comparisons. Infants typically begin by producing reflexive sounds for the first few months, move on to comfort or cooing sounds between 2 and 4 months, begin to produce longer series of syllables and prolonged vowels and consonants with much vocal play between 4 and 6 months, produce reduplicated babbling (e.g., bababa) between 7 and 9 months, and use more varied and complex babbling (e.g., badaba) and their first words sometime after 10 months (Smith, Goffman, & Stark, 1995).

It is important to identify both the child's level of phonological development (e.g., vocalizations, word approximations, words) and the child's breadth of sound-making capabilities at any one level. For example, a child may be producing words but with a very limited repertoire of syllable shapes or consonants and vowels (e.g., ba/ball, baba/bottle, bye-bye). This child's prognosis would be quite different from that of a child who may not yet be producing words but who already uses a large range of consonants and vowels as well as varied syllable shapes. The number of consonant sounds in the child's sound inventory progresses from an average of 3.4 consonant sounds produced by 50% of children at 15 months to 6.3 consonants at 18 months, 6.7 at 21 months, and 9.5 at 24 months (Stoel-Gammon, 1985); thus, both the overall number of vocalizations and the number of consonants that are used by a child can indicate typical or atypical development.

For young children who do not use word approximations or recognizable words, caregiver report and observation of the child's sound production inventory can be compared with what might be expected at the child's age. For young children who are beginning to produce words or word approximations, professionals can ask parents to list the child's words or word approximations to gain an idea of the child's overall number of different consonants used. If the child's inventory is quite limited at a particular age and there are other reasons for concern, then a referral should be made. In addition, when caregivers report that their child who is age 18 months or older avoids imitation of nonspeech (e.g., animal sounds, train sound) or speech sounds, particularly if the child becomes upset by caregiver attempts to elicit imitation, the professional should ask about the child's other production and comprehension skills. If limitations are noted in these other areas, then a referral should be made.

Words and Word Combinations

The acquisition of vocabulary has been argued to be the basis of learning in general and an indication of the child's ability to abstract from the environment the words and concepts that are important in the dominant culture (Sternberg & Powell, 1983). Vocabulary development is a window into the child's experiences, the input language, and the sociocultural influences that surround the child. Middle-class parents report that their children produce an average of 3.6 words or word-like sounds at 10 months, 11.9 at 12 months, 43.4 at 15 months, 79 at 16 months, 178.9 at 20 months, and 317 by 24 months (Fenson et al., 1990).

For identifying emerging words and word approximations, parental report and obser-vation can provide the data around which referral decisions are made. As children acquire a larger set of words, parent report tools such as the MacArthur Communicative Devel-opment Inventories (Fenson et al., 1990) can be used to document production vocabular-ies from 9 to 30 months of age. In addition, the MacArthur form for 9- to 16-month-olds (Words and Gestures) allows a look at both production and comprehension vocabularies. The form for 16- to 30-month-olds (Words and Sentences) also documents some aspects of morphological and syntactic development. Normative data then can help determine which children are in need of referral, specifically those who fall below the 10th percentile.

Word combinations typically emerge between 18 and 24 months, but some typically developing children do not produce word combinations until after 24 months (Fenson et al., 1990). Most children begin to combine words when their vocabularies reach between 50 and 100 words (Fenson et al., 1990). An early red flag for a 24-month-old child is the failure to have a production vocabulary of 50 words and/or no two-word combinations (Paul, 1991; Rescorla, 1989); however, as indicated by the work of Paul, Looney, and Dahm (1991), half of these "late talkers" by age 3 will perform at age level on standard-ized measures. Thus, the distinction between who will and who will not "outgrow" these early "delays" can be difficult (Paul, 1991). Although vocabulary size is important, factors such as phonological, social, cognitive, and imitative skills can also help sort out the "late talkers" from children who have expressive language disorders.

In examining a child's word combinations, the length of the child's utterances can be predictive of the child's overall language development (Miller, 1981). The term used most often, *mean length of utterance* (MLU), refers to counting both the words and the "mor-phemes" (e.g., -ing, -ed, plural "s") that are used by the child and averaging across utter-ances. The typical MLU is 1.0–1.6 at 18 months, 1.1–2.1 at 21 months, 1.5–2.2 at 24 months, 2.0–3.1 at 30 months, and 2.5–3.9 at 36 months (Miller, 1981); thus, by 24 months of age, most middle-class children are averaging between one and three words. Children whose MLU lags behind those of their peers and who have other evidence of delays should be referred.

Language Comprehension Skills

In assessing young children, it is important to identify both their linguistic and their non-linguistic comprehension and response strategies. Chapman (1978) provided an excellent overview of response strategies that infants and toddlers use in comprehending their envi-ronment. Early nonlinguistic strategies that are used between 8 and 12 months include looking at objects that are looked at by others, acting on objects that are noticed, and imi-tating ongoing actions. Strategies that are used in the 12- to 18-month stage typically are based on some linguistic aspect and include attending to an object that is mentioned, giv-ing evidence of notice to objects or actions, and doing what is usually done in that situa-tion (e.g., child goes to door when others do). In addition to those mentioned, strategies that are used from 18 to 24 months include acting on objects as the agent (e.g., child brushes own teeth when asked to "brush the baby's teeth") and using conventional behaviors (e.g., combing hair with comb). To help determine whether a referral is necessary, profes-sionals should ask caregivers about the kinds of gestures and words that their child will respond to and follow. Examples include whether the child responds to his or her own name or those of others, whether the child looks at an object that is named, and, for older tod-dlers, whether the child points to an object that is named or complies with simple requests (e.g., come here, give me that). By the age of 2, children should be able to respond to many object names, two-step commands, and requests to get something that is out of sight.

Parent–Child Interaction that Focuses on Communication

Given the strong influence that parents have on their children's communication and feeding development, including parent–child interaction as a key area within the assessment process has been recommended by many (Greenspan & Meisels, 1994; McLean & McCormick, 1993). The three primary means for examining parent–child interaction include using one or more formal parent–child interaction scales, using information from parent–child interaction scales to guide informal information gathering, or using evaluative judgment that is based on personal experiences and beliefs (see Mahoney, Spiker, & Boyce, 1996, for a thorough review of each method). As indicated by Mahoney and his colleagues (1996), although each approach is worthwhile, all three are influenced by problems with reliability and validity. For example, many of the parenting characteristics (e.g., enjoyment, praise, physical involvement) that are identified on parent–child interaction scales fail to be significant predictors of child functioning (Mahoney et al., 1996). In addition, across all three means of assessment, contextual issues such as the setting (e.g., home, clinic), familiarity of the observer(s), type of materials or toys that are available, type of interaction that is requested (e.g., completion of particular task, free play), and length of the observation all can affect the ways in which children and their parents interact. Moreover, sociocultural factors such as culture, ethnicity, and socioeconomic level as well as personality and interactive style strongly influence the ways in which different behaviors are exhibited and viewed; thus, the problems with reliability and validity of some parent–child assessment methods indicate a need for care in their use.

An additional dilemma in "assessing" parent–child interaction, particularly for identifying the need for communication intervention, is how to accomplish this task in a way that keeps the family at the center of the decision-making process. One method, described by Gillette (in press) and MacDonald and Gillette (1989), involves collaboration of the professionals and the family to identify current parent–child interaction practices. These practices are then related to four primary outcomes: establishing a partnership between parent and child, developing routines together, acting and communicating in progressively matched ways, and sharing enjoyment. As parents and professionals identify desired modifications to parent–child interactions, they can use the guidelines and child and parent strategies that are available to enhance their interactions through play.

Another alternative in keeping with family-centered practices is to find out first what families want from professionals (e.g., help in feeding skills, ideas for how to enhance their child's communication skills, ideas for ways to play with their child) and to begin working from the family's and child's strengths in their current interactions (Crais, 1993). Family members can be asked what they do already that helps the child communicate or eat and the conditions or situations when the child communicates or eats most effectively. Through this process, family members and professionals can build on skills and strategies that are used already and identify ways to make small refinements. In this way, professionals scaffold the type and the amount of support that is provided to parents without making all of the decisions regarding the ways in which the parent–child interactions should or could be modified (McCollum & Yates, 1994).

Finally, as a cautionary note suggested by Conti-Ramsden (1990), assessing and attempting to modify parental interactional and communicative behaviors may convey the message that the parents somehow have failed to provide what the child needed or, worse, that they may have contributed to the communication difficulties; thus, in both examining and identifying strategies for modification, professionals need to be mindful of the message that they send and respectful of the parents' own style of communicating. (Positive ideas for examining and influencing parent–child communicative interactions within a family-centered context can be found in McCollum & Yates, 1994.)

FACILITATING COMMUNICATION DEVELOPMENT IN YOUNG CHILDREN

Because communication skills are so much a part of any interaction with a child and family and because some undernourished children will also have communication difficulties, it is important for professionals who are serving these children to be knowledgeable about key principles that are related to facilitating communication development. Many of these principles guide the facilitation of feeding development in young children and, therefore, already will be familiar to some professionals. The kinds of facilitation strategies that are used by professionals and caregivers to promote communication development naturally will vary depending on the child's current levels across domains within communication, as well as the child's chronological age, overall developmental level, interests, learning style, and temperament. In addition, the caregivers' agreement with the need for and interest in communication facilitation plays a large part in successful intervention (Dunst, Trivette, & Deal, 1988); thus, in planning interventions for young children, professionals and caregivers should work together to identify the strategies that would be helpful to the young child and, most important, that will fit most naturally within the caregivers' daily routines. As indicated by the work of Dunst et al. (1988), any intervention effort that is accepted and endorsed by the child's family has the most potential for success. (Practical suggestions for gathering information about caregiver priorities, preferences, and daily routines can be found in McWilliam, Winton, & Crais, 1996.)

For professionals who are developing and instituting interventions with young children who are at risk for or evidencing communication difficulties, certain key principles of enhancing communication development can be helpful. The following principles have been drawn from the work of Crais and Roberts (1996).

Start where the child is functioning: Although this maxim seems quite obvious in the area of feeding, it is helpful to remind professionals and caregivers to match their expectations for the child's communication skills to the typical level that the child displays. It is better to underestimate than to overestimate the child's communication skills and to allow the child and/or the caregivers to indicate that the child can perform at a higher level. As described previously, questions to caregivers about the child's typical ways of communicating and comprehending can help guide the professional's interactions with the child.

Be aware of the child's cues, and respond contingently: *Readability,* or the ability of professionals and caregivers to "read" the child's cues and respond appropriately, is key to successful intervention in both feeding and communication. As the child begins to realize that the adult has "understood" the cues, the child learns to be more consistent in his or her efforts and to expand the cues to higher levels. If the adult fails to read the cues accurately and, therefore, cannot make his or her response contingent on what the child wants or needs, then a breakdown in interaction occurs. One means by which to help caregivers (and professionals) be more attentive to the child's cues is to encourage them to imitate the child, which can result in the child's being more attentive and responsive to his or her caregivers (Field, 1987; Satter, 1990). For children who are experiencing communication difficulties, imitating their nonverbal and vocalization behaviors can encourage them to continue their efforts and can help develop a game of turn taking in communication. As the "game" becomes fun for the child, he or she may be willing to imitate the adult in gestures, sounds, and, later, words or word combinations. The intent (as in facilitating feeding development) is to build a trusting relationship with the child and for the child to feel supported in his or her efforts to communicate. As the adult supports and scaffolds for the child, the child is allowed to reach progressively higher levels of development.

Another way for professionals and caregivers to be more contingent is to recognize and use pauses. As with children who are learning to eat, the importance of both responding to and providing pauses within communicative interchanges cannot be overestimated. Pausing in feeding is important for social interaction but depends on the caregiver's ability to read the child's cues to socialize (Pridham, 1990; Satter, 1990). In both feeding and communication exchanges, allowing the child at times to be the initiator of interaction also is critical and helps the child recognize the behaviors that are necessary to get attention. Helping caregivers learn how to "wait expectantly" can be a positive addition to caregiver–child communicative interactions.

Be facilitative: The literature has indicated a number of behaviors that facilitate communication, including providing models for what the child might be expected to gesture, vocalize, or say; accepting and reinforcing all of the child's communicative attempts; and providing input that is slightly higher than the child's current level (Duchan, 1989; Dunst et al., 1990). In addition, children gain more in their communication skills when caregivers and professionals use strategies such as frequently repeating important words (e.g., "Here's the ball. I have the ball"), using simpler words (e.g., "TV" versus "television") or simple sentences (e.g., "Daddy's home" versus "I think I hear Daddy coming home"), later expanding what the child says (e.g., child says, "I see a ball," and caregiver says, "I see a big ball"), and following the child's interests rather than taking a more directive approach (Duchan, 1989; Manolson, 1992). Helping families gradually become aware of and utilize some of these techniques intermixed with their current practices can facilitate the child's communication development.

SUMMARY

For children who have or who are at risk for feeding and communication difficulties, professionals and families need to recognize the multiple factors that place children at risk for these disorders and utilize positive strategies for identifying those children who are not likely to "outgrow" their early deficits. When working within an interdisciplinary approach in which family members are active decision makers, professionals and family members can utilize the strategies identified to determine whether a child is in need of a referral for evaluation for suspected communication difficulties. In addition, in becoming more aware of the many links between feeding development and communication development, professionals and families may intervene earlier when there are suspected communication deficits.

REFERENCES

Aram, D., & Hall, N. (1989). Longitudinal follow-up of preschool communication disorders: Treatment implications. *School Psychology Review, 18,* 487–501.

Barnard, K., Hammond, M., Booth, C., Bee, H., Mitchell, S., & Spieker, S. (1989). Measurement and meaning of parent–child interaction. In F. Morrison, C. Lord, & D. Keating (Eds.), *Applied developmental psychology* (Vol. 3, pp. 39–80). San Diego: Academic Press.

Barnard, K., Morisset, C., & Spieker, S. (1993). Preventive interventions: Enhancing parent–infant relationships. In C.H. Zeanah, Jr. (Ed.), *Handbook of infant mental health* (pp. 386–401). New York: Guilford Press.

Bates, E., O'Connell, B., & Shore, C. (1987). Language and communication in infancy. In J. Osofsky (Ed.), *Handbook of infant development* (2nd ed., pp. 149–203). New York: John Wiley & Sons.

Benoit, D., Zeanah, C., & Barton, M. (1989). Maternal attachment disturbances in failure to thrive. *Infant Mental Health, 10*(3), 185–202.

Berkowitz, C., & Senter, S. (1987). Characteristics of mother–infant interactions in nonorganic failure to thrive. *Journal of Family Practice, 25*(4), 377–381.

Beukelman, D.R, & Mirenda, P. (1998). *Augmentative and alternative communication: Management of severe communication disorders in children and adults* (2nd ed.). Baltimore: Paul H. Brookes Publishing Co.

Bricker, D., & Squires, J. (1989). The effectiveness of parental screening of at-risk infants: The infant monitoring questionnaires. *Topics in Early Childhood Special Education, 9,* 67–85.

Chapman, R. (1978). Comprehension strategies in children. In J. Kavanaugh & W. Strange (Eds.), *Speech and language in the laboratory, school, and clinic* (pp. 308–327). Cambridge: MIT Press.

Conti-Ramsden, G. (1990). Maternal recasts and other contingent replies to language-impaired children. *Journal of Speech and Hearing Disorders, 55,* 262–274.

Coplan, J. (1987). *Early Language Milestone Scale* (Rev. ed.). Austin, TX: PRO-ED.

Crais, E. (1993). Professionals as collaborators in assessment. *Topics in Language Disorders, 14*(1), 29–40.

Crais, E., & Roberts, J. (1996). Assessing communication skills. In M. McLean, D. Bailey, & M. Wolery (Eds.), *Assessing infants and preschoolers with special needs* (2nd ed., pp. 334–397). Upper Saddle River, NJ: Prentice-Hall.

Duchan, J. (1989). Evaluating adults' talk to children: Assessing adult attunement. *Seminars in Speech and Language, 10,* 17–27.

Dunst, C., Lowe, L., & Bartholomew, P. (1990). Contingent social responsiveness, family ecology, and infant communicative competence. *National Student Speech-Language-Hearing Journal, 17,* 39–49.

Dunst, C., Trivette, C., & Deal, A. (1988). *Enabling and empowering families.* Cambridge, MA: Brookline Books.

Fenson, L., Dale, P., Reznick, J., Bates, E., Thal, D., Hartung, J., & Reilley, J. (1990). *The MacArthur Communicative Development Inventories.* Thousand Oaks, CA: Singular Publishing.

Field, T. (1987). Affective and interactive disturbances in infants. In J. Osofsky (Ed.), *Handbook of infant development* (2nd ed., pp. 972–1005). New York: John Wiley & Sons.

Fogel, A. (1991). *Infancy* (2nd ed.). St. Paul, MN: West Publishing.

Frankenburg, W., Dodds, J., Archer, P., Bresnick, B., Maschka, P., Edelman, N., & Shapiro, H. (1990). *Denver II: Screening manual.* Denver: Denver Developmental Materials.

Gillette, Y. (in press). Collaboration with families in communication intervention. In L. Watson, T. Layton, & E. Crais (Eds.), *Handbook for early language impairment in children: Assessment and treatment.* Albany, NY: Delmar Publishers.

Glascoe, F., MacLean, W., & Stone, W. (1991). The importance of parents' concerns about their child's behavior. *Clinical Pediatrics, 30,* 8–11.

Greenspan, S. (1992). *Infancy and early childhood: The practice of clinical assessment and intervention with emotional and developmental challenges.* Madison, CT: International Universities Press.

Greenspan, S., & Meisels, S. (1994). Toward a new vision of developmental assessment of infants and young children. *Zero to Three, 16*(6), 1–8.

Kennedy, M., Sheridan, M., Radlinski, S., & Beeghly, M. (1991). Play-language relationships in young children with developmental delays: Implications for assessment. *Journal of Speech and Hearing Research, 34,* 112–122.

MacDonald, J., & Gillette, Y. (1989). *The introduction to the ECO program.* Chicago: Riverside.

Mahoney, G., Spiker, D., & Boyce, G. (1996). Clinical assessments of parent–child interactions: Are professionals ready to implement this practice? *Topics in Early Childhood Special Education, 16*(1), 26–50.

Manolson, A. (1992). *It takes two to talk* (2nd ed.). Toronto, Ontario, Canada: Hanen Early Language Resource Centre.

McCollum, J., & Yates, T. (1994). Dyad as focus, triad as means: A family-centered approach to supporting parent–child interactions. *Infants and Young Children, 6*(4), 54–63.

McCune-Nicholich, L., & Bruskin, C. (1982). Combinatorial competency in symbolic play and language. In D. Pepler & K. Rubin (Eds.), *The play of children: Current theory and research* (pp. 30–45). Basel, Switzerland: S. Karger.

McLean, M., & McCormick, K. (1993). Assessment and evaluation in early intervention. In W. Brown, S. Thurman, & L. Pearl (Eds.), *Family-centered early intervention with infants and tod-*

dlers: Innovative cross-disciplinary approaches (pp. 43–79). Baltimore: Paul H. Brookes Publishing Co.

McWilliam, P., Winton, P., & Crais, E. (1996). *Practical strategies for family-centered early intervention: Getting down to brass tacks.*Thousand Oaks, CA: Singular Publishing.

Miller, J. (1981). *Assessing language production in children: Experimental procedures.* Needham Heights, MA: Allyn & Bacon.

Paul, R. (1991). Profiles of toddlers with slow expressive language development. *Topics in Language Disorders, 11*(4), 1–13.

Paul, R., Looney, S., & Dahm, P. (1991). Communication and socialization skills at ages 2 and 3 in "late talking" young children. *Journal of Speech and Hearing Disorders, 34,* 858–865.

Polan, H., Leon, A., Kaplan, M., Kessler, D., Stern, D., & Ward, M. (1991). Disturbances of affect expression in failure to thrive. *Journal of the American Academy of Child and Adolescent Psychiatry, 30*(6), 897–903.

Pridham, K. (1990). Feeding behavior of 6- to 12-month old infants: Assessment and sources of parental information. *Journal of Pediatrics, 117,* S174–S180.

Rescorla, L. (1989). The language development survey: A screening tool for language delay in toddlers. *Journal of Speech and Hearing Disorders, 54,* 587–599.

Rescorla, L., & Ratner, N. (1996). Phonetic profiles of toddlers with expressive language impairment (SLI-E). *Journal of Speech and Hearing Research, 39,* 153–165.

Rossetti, L. (1996). *Communication intervention birth to three.* Thousand Oaks, CA: Singular Publishing.

Sameroff, A., & Fiese, B. (1990). Transactional regulation and early intervention. In S.J. Meisels & J.P. Shonkoff (Eds.), *Handbook of early childhood intervention* (pp. 119–149). Cambridge, MA: Cambridge University Press.

Satter, E. (1990). The feeding relationship: Problems and interventions. *Journal of Pediatrics, 117,* S181–S189.

Satter, E. (1992). The feeding relationship. *Zero to Three, 12*(5), 1–9.

Smith, A., Goffman, L., & Stark, R. (1995). Speech motor development. *Seminars in Speech and Language, 16*(2), 87–99.

Sternberg, R., & Powell, J. (1983). Comprehending verbal comprehension. *American Psychologist, 38,* 878–893.

Stoel-Gammon, C. (1985). Phonetic inventories, 15–24 months: A longitudinal study. *Journal of Speech and Hearing Research, 28,* 505–512.

Sturm, L., & Drotar, D. (1992). Communication strategies for working with parents of infants who fail to thrive. *Zero to Three, 12*(5), 25–28.

U.S. Department of Education. (1987). *Ninth annual report to Congress on the implementation of the Education of the Handicapped Act.* Washington, DC: Office of Special Education Programs.

Wetherby, A., & Prizant, B. (1993). *Communication and Symbolic Behavior Scales.* Chicago: Riverside.

Wetherby, A., & Prizant, B. (1996). Toward earlier identification of communication and language problems in infants and young children. In S. Meisels & E. Fenichel (Eds.), *New visions for the developmental assessment of infants and young children* (pp. 289–312). Washington, DC: National Center for Infants, Toddlers, and Their Families.

Wyley, V. (1995). *Premature infants and their families.* Thousand Oaks, CA: Singular Publishing.

Chapter 25

Nutrition Services in Early Intervention Programs

Cynthia Taft Bayerl and Karen Welford

Infants and children who are served in early intervention (birth to 3 years) programs and who have or who are at risk for developmental disabilities are at an increased nutritional risk because of feeding problems, drug and nutrient interactions, metabolic disorders, decreased mobility, and altered growth patterns. The benefits of providing nutrition services to all people, especially infants and children who have developmental disabilities, include prevention of growth retardation and/or further disability in some cases and improvement in others (American Dietetic Association, 1992).

This chapter provides an overview of early intervention programs and services with a focus on nutrition services. The role that nutrition services and nutritionists play in providing children and their families with services that assist in achieving optimum nutritional status is discussed. This chapter highlights the major nutritional concerns of children who are served in early intervention programs and provides guidance on how to integrate nutrition services in early intervention programs so that children may reach their full potential.

EARLY INTERVENTION

Services for people who have developmental disabilities have changed greatly since the mid-1970s. Since 1975, federal laws have required states to provide education programs to all children, regardless of disability, as part of their inclusion into mainstream society (McLean & Hanline, 1990; Odom & McEvoy, 1988).

In 1975, Congress passed the Education for All Handicapped Children Act (PL 94-142), which was reauthorized in 1986 (PL 99-457) and then reauthorized in 1990 and renamed the Individuals with Disabilities Education Act (IDEA) (PL 101-476). Part H of this law required each state to set up delivery systems of early intervention for children who have developmental disabilities and their families. In 1997, IDEA was reauthorized (PL 105-17) and Part H was renamed Part C. Part C emphasizes interagency collaboration and coordination of health and education services. Each state has established eligibility criteria for early intervention. They include established delays, disabilities, and conditions that have a high probability of resulting in developmental delays. In addition, some states include children who are at environmental or biological risk (Bryant & Graham, 1993). One of the key components of the legislation is the recognition of the central role of the family through the individualized family service plan (IFSP). Part C mandates that an IFSP, developed by a multidisciplinary team that includes the child's parent(s), must be written for each child and family enrolled in early intervention. The IFSP is a family-centered service plan that lists concerns, priorities, and resources that have been identified by a family to help their child reach his or her potential (McGonigel & Garland, 1988).

Early intervention programs provide a range of services to meet the identified needs of the child and the family. As eligibility is established, the child and the family participate in an assessment to determine the strengths and needs of the child. Following this assessment, the child's IFSP is developed in collaboration with the family and is reviewed and updated at regular intervals. Early intervention services are provided in as natural a setting as possible (e.g., home, community-based centers, child care programs) and may be provided individually or in groups. (See Meisels & Shonkoff, 1990, for a description of the history of early intervention and the types of service models, tools, and services.)

Early intervention programs provide a comprehensive services model that enhances the educational capacity of infants and children. Through a variety of services, including nutrition, infants and children improve or ameliorate their developmental delays. The rest of this chapter examines the role of nutritionists and nutrition services as part of early intervention.

NUTRITION SERVICES

When PL 99-457 was passed, nutrition services were mandated as part of the multidisciplinary early intervention program (Bujold, 1991). Under section 303.11 of the regulation, nutrition services are defined as

A. nutritional history and dietary intake;
B. anthropometric, biochemical, and clinical variables;
C. feeding skills and feeding problems; and
D. food habits and food preferences;
   (ii)   developing and monitoring appropriate plans to address the nutritional needs of children eligible under this part, based on the findings in paragraph (b)(7)(i) of this section; and
   (iii)   making referrals to appropriate community resources to carry out nutrition goals.

Importance of Nutrition to Children Who Have Special Health Care Needs

Nutrition is important for all children who are at critical stages of growth and development but is especially important for young infants and toddlers who have special health care needs (Dwyer, 1993). Nutritional issues have been discussed widely in the literature (Baker, Boulard-Backunas, & Davis, 1993; Bayerl & Ries, 1995; Cloud, 1993). These issues are generally grouped into five major categories: poor growth and failure to thrive, overweight and obesity, feeding problems, constipation, and drug–nutrient interactions (Bayerl & Ries, 1995; Brizee, Sophos, & McLaughlin, 1990; Ekvall, 1993; Queen & Lang, 1993). Problems within these five categories can occur when the child experiences poor oral intake, diges-tion, or absorption of calories, protein, vitamins, and/or minerals. If the child obtains ade-quate nutrition for his or her feeding needs and growth, then the child can participate in and benefit more fully from the services that are provided in early intervention programs. Inadequate nutrition can impair the child's physical and emotional development. For exam-ple, a child who has cerebral palsy may have impaired oral-motor function and, thus, inad-equate intake of liquids or foods. As a result, the child's physical development may be affected (e.g., shorter, thinner), and he or she may require a high-calorie formula or tube-feedings or both to increase calories (Breedon, 1993; Glass & Lucas, 1990; Lane & Cloud, 1988). The same child's emotional development may be affected by his or her inability to eat textured foods (e.g., pizza, French fries) as a result of his or her oral-motor impairment. When that child is present at a social gathering (e.g., birthday party), the child may be lim-ited to a puréed diet or tube-feeding and, thus, would not be able to enjoy the same foods that his or her peers without disabilities are enjoying. The child may feel left out or may be teased by his or her peers. To diminish the possible negative impact on the child's physical and emotional health, the child's nutritionist or speech or physical therapist can work with the family to plan creative ways for the child to eat under special circumstances.

Researchers have found that children who are poorly nourished experience a low energy level, limited attention span, more difficulty fighting infection, and limited stamina when participating in play groups and other preschool settings (Ault, Guy, Rues, & Noto, 1994; Ekvall, 1993). A child's eating problems (e.g., swallowing, gagging, choking) and self-feeding skills (use of cup, spoon, or fingers) can adversely affect the quantity and quality of the child's diet. A long-term reduction of calories or other nutrients can lead to poor growth (see Chapter 23).

Feeding young infants and toddlers can be difficult for parents and caregivers. When young children exert independence from caregivers, which may be manifested through food jags (irregular eating habits), picky eating, and/or tantrums during mealtimes, meeting their nutritional needs can be a challenge for even the most patient caregiver. Parents and care-givers of children who have special health care needs often face additional barriers. For example, a child who has oral-motor hypersensitivity may react negatively to having food put in or near his or her mouth (Campbell, 1988; Gleason, 1992). Other obstacles include the side effects of medications on the child's appetite. Complex medical conditions, such as a child with short gut (Ernst & Young, 1993), bronchopulmonary dysplasia (Adams, 1991), or cystic fibrosis, may require a special diet (Ekvall, 1993).

Nutritional services and treatment are important not only for children with develop-mental delays but also for children with previously diagnosed medical, emotional, or phys-ical disabilities. Proper nutrition is important for preventing or minimizing the potentially debilitating secondary effects of an existing condition such as cerebral palsy or spina bifida (Ekvall, 1993). A well-nourished child has a greater chance of remaining healthy and reaching his or her potential both physically and cognitively.

Nutrition Services Models

Screening for feeding, growth, and nutrition issues may be initiated as part of the process of eligibility for early intervention or begin as part of the assessment and evaluation phase (Bujold & Sadeghian, 1988). Many programs for infants and children have questions on feeding, growth, and diet included in the screening tools that are used to assess the needs of the child and the family (Baer, Tanaka, & Blyler, 1991; see the appendix at this end of this chapter). The information contained in these completed forms can be used to determine the nutritional needs of the child. It can also be used to assess the nutritional status and needs of the population that is served by that program and in that community. Children who are identified as being at nutritional risk should be referred to nutrition services, which may be part of the early intervention program or located within another community-based agency such as the Special Supplemental Nutrition Program for Women, Infants and Children (WIC), a community health center, or a hospital (Bayerl & Ries, 1995).

To optimize a child's nutrition while the child is enrolled in early intervention, nutritional services should be integrated into the comprehensive services model. Programs do this in a variety of ways. The following description of nutrition services and job description for a nutritionist may be helpful in designing an effective service model.

Job Description of a Nutritionist

Key areas of responsibility for the nutritionist may include participation in the IFSP process in which the nutritionist may collaborate in the following activities: conducting nutrition assessments (see Table 1), developing nutrition care plans, monitoring the child's nutritional status and reevaluating care plans as needed, initiating contact with other food and nutrition programs (e.g., WIC, primary care) to facilitate collaboration among services that are needed by the child, and providing direct nutrition counseling services as requested by families in the IFSP (Project CHANCE, 1995; Tluczek & Sondel, 1991).

The responsibilities of the nutrition services provider should be determined by the individual program's service model. The staffing options for utilizing a nutritionist in an early intervention program depend on the size of the program, the availability of qualified nutrition services providers in an area, and the goals of the program. The model that an early intervention program selects will greatly influence staff responsibilities. For example, a nutritionist who works full time would be a full team member (versus a consultant) in many programs. This usually occurs in a transdisciplinary model. A transdisciplinary model is one in which all members of the team, including parents, come to a consensus on an integrated plan for child and family (see Chapter 1). The nutritionist's responsibilities in the transdisciplinary model may include identifying and addressing a client's needs in several areas (e.g., social, education, speech) in addition to the more traditional responsibilities (screening, assessment, and monitoring the nutritional status of the child). In the transdisciplinary model, the care provider then refers the client to other staff members for more intensive specialty interventions when appropriate. In a consultant or part-time role or in an interdisciplinary team model, the role of the nutritionist may be more focused on nutrition services (Cloud, 1993; Woodruff & Hanson, 1987).

To determine the job responsibilities of a nutritionist, the characteristics of the early intervention program (e.g., type of model, number of children enrolled, scope and depth of nutritional problems, clients' diagnoses) should be assessed to determine the nutritionist's role. The nutritionist's job responsibilities should be flexible, as they may need to be modified as the program changes.

The nutritionist may also participate in the provision of education, training, and support services for parents and staff. This would involve identifying nutrition training needs; conducting parent support groups on feeding concerns for specific groups of children, such as those with Down syndrome, or on broad-scope nutrition issues (e.g., picky toddlers, healthful eating, breast-feeding); and conducting staff in-service sessions on growth, nutrition, and feeding. The nutritionist may also develop a system of referral and follow-up, which identifies community nutrition services providers; establishes communication with them; refers clients for follow-up; and provides to staff, parents, and community services providers education and training on nutritional needs of children who have special needs (Baer, Blyler, Cloud, & McCamman, 1991).

Table 1.   Nutrition assessment components

What to look for	Key area	Methodology
Medical History Diagnosis and related complications (e.g., failure to thrive, cerebral palsy, cardiac)	Review medical record; question parent, care provider, case manager, and other relevant health care providers	• Use of special formulas • Drug–nutrient interactions • Allergies/dental/fluoridation • Effect of GI or oral-motor function
Anthropometrics Length (height) Weight Head circumference	Review record for previous measurements; weigh and measure child using standardized equipment; plot on appropriate grid; adjust for gestational age	• Identify poor growth pattern • Identify problems with weight gain
Lab Work Hemoglobin or hematocrit Blood lead Other labs	Review medical record; check with health care provider or parent for most recent test	• Identify anemia • Lead poisoning concerns
Nutrition History	Complete • 24-hour recall • Food frequency • Review typical 24-hour intake or 3- to 5-day food record	• Quality and quantity of food intake • Current appetite • Changes in eating pattern • Food intolerances, aversions, or preferences • Inadequate or excessive food, vitamin, or mineral intake • Pica
Feeding Skills	Observe mealtime; question parent or caregiver and/or case manager regarding feeding concerns	• Delayed skills with use of cup, spoon, self-feed • Mealtime behavior and feeding position • Mechanical feeding problem • Uses or needs special feeding equipment • Overuse or inappropriate use of bottle • Related dental problems • Caregiver–child interaction at mealtime
Psychosocial	Question parent or caregiver, case manager, or other relevant people	• Availability of resources (e.g., food, financial, health) • Parental needs or limitations (e.g., parenting, education, food preparation) • Need for community referrals

From Bayerl, C.T., & Ries, J.D. (1995). *EARLY START: Nutrition services in early intervention programs* [Training manual], p. 3-20. Worcester, MA: Area Health Education Center; adapted by permission.

The nutritionist who works in early intervention must have the proper credentials, training, work experience, and educational skills. Part C specifies that nutrition services be provided by qualified staff. The nutrition services provider should be a registered dietitian (R.D.) of the American Dietetic Association (preferred) or a nutritionist who is not an R.D. but who has a master's degree in public health or nutrition. In addition to the appropriate degree, the early intervention nutritionist should have training and/or work experience in pediatrics and in the following areas: developmental delays, working in community settings with families of young children (birth to 3), work experience as a member of a team, and training and experience in early intervention. Also, knowledge of the following areas would enhance the nutritionist's effectiveness: early childhood development; preschool nutrition education; federal, state, and community food assistance programs; and consumer nutrition issues (Bayerl & Ries, 1995).

Financing Nutrition Services

Paying for nutritional services may be the most difficult barrier that administrators face when planning a nutrition services system. The difficulty of integrating nutrition services into early intervention programs depends on public and private sources for reimbursement of nutrition services that are available in that state ("Paying the Bills," 1992). The nutrition department within the state department of public health and the state chapter of the American Dietetic Association are very involved in reimbursement issues and can provide valuable information to providers (American Dietetic Association, 1991; American Dietetic Association & Morrison Health Care, Inc., 1996).

The EARLY START Project

An understanding of the role of nutrition and nutritionists in early intervention programs and documenting the nutritional status of children in early intervention programs was the focus of the EARLY START Project, which was funded by the Bureau of Maternal and Child Health of the U.S. Department of Health and Human Services from 1990 to 1995. The Massachusetts Department of Public Health and The Eunice Kennedy Shriver Center were the lead agencies in developing and implementing models of nutrition services to meet the needs of children who are served under Part C in Massachusetts.

The EARLY START Project studied the nutritional status of infants and children in early intervention programs in Massachusetts. The children were identified through a system of screening and referral for being at nutritional risk and in need of services. Of the 493 children in the study, 453 (92%) met at least one of the criteria for referral. Parents of 364 of the children (75%) had at least one concern or question about their child's nutritional intake, feeding skills, or growth; 287 children (59%) had a medical diagnosis or ongoing medical condition that put them at nutritional risk; 248 (50%) had one growth measurement below the 10th percentile; 43 had a weight-for-height above the 95th percentile; and 42 children had blood work that indicated possible iron deficiency anemia or high lead levels.

The EARLY START data indicated complex relationships among existing environmental and medical conditions, developmental delay, and growth. The recommendations and findings of the EARLY START project support the idea that nutritional services should be part of the comprehensive model of services for children who are at nutritional risk and who are served by early intervention. Findings from the EARLY START Project were used to develop recommendations to guide the development of nutrition services that could be fully integrated into the early intervention system. The experiences and findings from EARLY START may be similar to what occurs in other states, although, as of 1998, no additional statewide nutritional surveillance system has specifically addressed the early intervention population.

The recommendations from the EARLY START project are directed toward parents, nutritionists, program administrators, and providers who work with children under the age of 3 years. They can be adapted and used by other states as part of their system of community-based comprehensive services for children from birth to 3 years who are served by early intervention services.

1. *Involve parents and families, staff, qualified nutrition services providers, and other appropriate providers in the development and implementation of models for delivery of nutrition services in early intervention.* To increase the capacity of the early intervention program to provide quality nutrition services to clients, collaboration between families and early intervention team members—including the nutritionist—is essential. Collaboration and coordination with other community nutrition services are necessary for the development of a comprehensive, effective nutrition services delivery system.

2. *Collaborate with families of children who have special health care needs to ensure that the nutritional services meet family needs.* Provision of high-quality nutrition services should be based on a partnership with parents as providers and consumers of health care services for their children.

3. *Identify during screening and evaluation children who are at nutritional risk.* Ideally, screening for feeding, growth, and diet concerns should be completed as part of the initial intake process.

4. *Use standardized screening and evaluation methods to identify children who are at nutritional risk.* Although staff and parents can identify some children who are at nutritional risk, many will not be identified unless standardized methods are used.

5. *Develop broad-based training and education programs for families, early intervention staff, and nutrition services providers.* Nutrition knowledge and skills of early intervention staff and families should be enhanced through training, education, and support activities. Training early intervention staff in growth, nutrition, and feeding will increase the capacity of programs to provide appropriate information. Training and education programs for parents, early intervention staff, and nutrition services providers should reflect the community-based nature of early intervention programs and be both family centered and culturally appropriate. A network of trained pediatric nutrition services providers should be developed to expand the scope and quality of nutrition services that are available to children who have special health care needs.

6. *Establish a state or regional group to plan for the provision of consistent nutrition services.* Ideally, this should occur under the personnel development subcommittee of the statewide interagency coordinating council or its equivalent. Strategies and plans to integrate nutrition services within the early intervention service model should be developed by program administrators and providers. Guidelines to coordinate key players and provide nutrition services should be developed.

7. *Develop a system of referral and follow-up care among all nutrition services providers in a community to ensure comprehensive services.* A number of programs provide nutrition services to the early intervention population. Although the nature and the scope of services vary, collaboration among all nutrition services providers ensures comprehensive care without duplication of services.

8. *Include nutrition services within information and referral systems for children who have special health care needs.* Including nutrition services within information and

referral systems will help families identify quality services, forge valuable linkages, enhance collaboration between hospital and community nutrition programs, and raise awareness of the importance of nutrition among family-centered, community-based services.

9. *Develop a system to integrate nutrition surveillance data into statewide data systems.* A nutrition surveillance and monitoring system for children who have special health care needs is needed to aid policy development and program planning at state health departments and in the agency in each state that leads in the implementation of Part C.

10. *Identify mechanisms for reimbursement of nutrition services.* Nutrition services are included under federal early intervention program mandates; however, the procedures for reimbursement vary for individual programs as well as for different states. Informing policy makers, providers, and families about funding resources and gaps is an essential first step to improving coverage for nutrition services.

SUMMARY

Research has shown that many children who are served in early intervention programs are at risk for feeding or growth delays; therefore, integrating nutrition services and nutritionists into early intervention programs can provide the child and his or her family with a full range of services that will help him or her to achieve optimum health. The team of providers, including a nutritionist, can work with the family to identify feeding, growth, and nutritional issues. If the early intervention program does not provide a full range of services, then appropriate referral to a qualified nutritionist will help the family to address their issues. Provision of nutrition services by qualified providers will help the early intervention staff provide the best-quality and much-needed services within the comprehensive services model specified in the early intervention program guidelines.

REFERENCES

Adams, E. (1991). Nutrition for the young child with bronchopulmonary dysplasia (BPD). *Nutrition Focus, 6*(3), 1–6.

American Dietetic Association. (1991). *Reimbursement and insurance coverage for nutrition services.* Chicago: Author.

American Dietetic Association. (1992). Nutrition in comprehensive program planning for persons with developmental disabilities. *Journal of the American Dietetic Association, 92*(5), 613–615.

American Dietetic Association & Morrison Health Care, Inc. (1996). *Medical nutrition therapy across the continuum of care: Patient protocol.* Chicago: American Dietetic Association.

Ault, M.M., Guy, B., Rues, J., & Noto, L. (1994). Some educational implications for students with profound disabilities at risk for inadequate nutrition and the nontherapeutic effects of medication. *Mental Retardation, 12,* 200–205.

Baer, M.T., Blyler, E., Cloud, H., & McCamman, S. (1991). Providing early intervention services: Preparation of dietitians, nutritionists, and other team members. *Infants and Young Children, 3*(4), 56–66.

Baer, M.T., Tanaka, T., & Blyler, E. (1991). *Nutrition strategies for children with special needs.* Los Angeles: University of Southern California, University Affiliated Program.

Baker, S.S., Boulard-Backunas, K., & Davis, A. (1993). Common oral motor and gastrointestinal nutritional problems in children referred to early intervention programs. *Seminars in Pediatric Gastroenterology and Nutrition, 4,* 3–7.

Bayerl, C.T., & Ries, J.D. (1995). *EARLY START: Nutrition services in early intervention programs* [Training manual]. Worcester, MA: Area Health Education Center.

Breedon, C. (1993). Increasing the caloric density of infant formulas. *Nutrition Focus, 8*(6), 1–6.

Brizee, L., Sophos, C., & McLaughlin, J. (1990). Nutrition issues in developmental disabilities in young children. *Infants and Young Children, 2*(3), 10–21.

Bryant, D., & Graham, M. (1993). *Implementing early intervention: From research to effective practice.* New York: Guilford Press.

Bujold, C. (1991). Public Law 99-457: A review. *Newsletter of the Dietetics and Developmental and Psychiatric Disorders Practice Group of the American Dietetic Association, 10*(1), 1–3.

Bujold, C.R., & Sadeghian, K. (1988). *Nutrition screening for children with special needs.* Santa Fe: New Mexico Health and Environment Department.

Campbell, A. (1988). Tube feeding: Parental perspective. *Exceptional Parent, 18*(2), 36–41.

Cloud, H. (1993). Feeding problems of the child with special health care needs. In S.W. Ekvall (Ed.), *Pediatric nutrition in chronic diseases and developmental disorders: Prevention, assessment and treatment* (pp. 203–217). New York: Oxford University Press.

Dwyer, J. (1993). Early intervention: Early prevention. *Seminars in Pediatric and GI Nutrition, 4,* 11.

Education for All Handicapped Children Act of 1975, PL 94-142, 20 U.S.C. §§ 1400 *et seq.*

Education of the Handicapped Act Amendments of 1986, PL 99-457, 20 U.S.C. §§ 1400 *et seq.*

Ekvall, S. (1993). *Pediatric nutrition in chronic diseases and developmental disorders: Prevention, assessment and treatment.* New York: Oxford University Press.

Ernst, L., & Young, R. (1993). Common gastrointestinal problems in children with developmental disabilities. *Nutrition Focus, 8*(4), 1–6.

Glass, R., & Lucas, B. (1990). Making the transition from tube feeding to oral feeding. *Nutrition Focus, 5*(6), 1–8.

Gleason, C. (1992). Aaron: A view from both sides of the fence. *Nutrition Focus, 11,* 4–5.

Individuals with Disabilities Education Act (IDEA) of 1990, PL 101-476, 20 U.S.C. §§ 1400 *et seq.*

Individuals with Disabilities Education Act Amendments of 1997, PL 105-17, 20 U.S.C. §§ 1400 *et seq.*

Lane, S.J., & Cloud, H.H. (1988). Feeding problems and intervention: An interdisciplinary approach. *Topics in Clinical Nutrition, 3*(3), 23–32.

McGonigel, M., & Garland, C. (1988). Individualized family service plan and the early intervention team: Team and family issues and recommended practices. *Infants and Young Children, 1*(1), 10–21.

McLean, M., & Hanline, M. (1990). Providing early intervention services in integrated environments: Challenges and opportunities for the future. *Topics in Early Childhood Special Education, 10*(2), 62–77.

Meisels, S.J., & Shonkoff, J.P. (Eds.). (1990). *Handbook of early childhood intervention.* Cambridge, MA: Cambridge University Press.

Odom, S., & McEvoy, M. (1988). Integration of young children with handicaps and normally developing children. In S.L. Odom & M.B. Karnes (Eds.), *Early intervention for infants and children with handicaps* (pp. 241–268). Baltimore: Paul H. Brookes Publishing Co.

Paying the bills: Tips for families on financing health care for children with special needs. (1992). Boston: New England SERVE.

Project CHANCE. (1995). *A guide to feeding young children with special needs.* Phoenix: Arizona Department of Health.

Queen, P., & Lang, C. (1993). *Handbook of pediatric nutrition.* Gaithersburg, MD: Aspen Publishers.

Tluczek, A., & Sondel, S. (Eds.). (1991). *Project SPOON (Specialized Program of Oral Nutrition for Children with Special Needs).* Madison: University of Wisconsin.

Woodruff, G., & Hanson, C. (1987). *Project KAL.* Brighton, MA: Project KAL.

RECOMMENDED RESOURCES

Amorda-Spauling, K. (1997). The issues of the ketogenic diet for seizure control in children. *Nutrition Focus, 12*(3), 1–10.

Anderson, V., Dufton-Gross, N., Young, G., Piette, L., & Bartlett, M. (1984). Nutrition in an early intervention project. *Journal of the American Dietetic Association, 84*(2), 205–207.

Babbitt, L.R. (1994). Nutrition concerns for children with seizure disorders. *Nutrition Focus, 9*(4), 1–6.

Bayerl, C.T., & Ries, J.D. (1992). Nutrition services in early intervention in Massachusetts. *Zero to Three, 12*(5), 29–31.

Bayerl, C.T., Ries, J.D., Bettencourt, M.F., & Fisher, P. (1993). Nutritional issues of children in early intervention programs: Primary care team approach. *Seminars in Pediatric Gastroenterology and Nutrition 4,* 11–15.

Blyler, E.M., & Lucas, B.L. (1997). Position of the American Dietetic Association: Nutrition in comprehensive program planning for persons with developmental disabilities. *Journal of the American Dietetic Association, 97*(2), 189–193.

Brizee, L., Sophos, C., & McLaughlin, J. (1990). Nutrition issues in developmental disabilities in young children. *Infants and Young Children, 2*(3), 10–21.

Ekvall, S., Ekvall, V., & Frazier, T. (1993). Dealing with nutrition problems of children with developmental disorders. *Topics in Clinical Nutrition, 2*(4), 50–57.

Goldberg, D., Holland, M., Cunniff, P., Dwyer, J., Palmer, C., Taft Bayerl, C., & Ries, J. (1996). *Consuming concerns: Nutrition services in early intervention programs.* Boston: Frances Stern Nutrition Center.

Hines, J., Cloud, H., Carithers, T., Hickey, C., & Hinton, A. (1989). Early intervention services for children with special health care needs. *Journal of the American Dietetic Association, 89*(11), 1636–1639.

Horsely, J.W. (1994). Nutrition issues facing children with special health care needs in early intervention programs and at school. *Nutrition Focus, 9,* 1–8.

Klein, M., & Delaney, T. (1994). *Feeding and nutrition for the child with special needs.* Tucson, AZ: Therapy Skill Builders.

New England SERVE. (1989). *Enhancing quality: Standards and indicators of quality care for children with special health care needs.* Boston: Massachusetts Health Research Institute, Inc.

Palmer, C., Leung, J., & Casey, V. (1996). *Consuming cues: Helping children reach their potential through good nutrition* [Videotape and workbook]. Boston: Frances Stern Nutrition Center.

Pipes, P.L., & Glass, R.P. (1997). Nutrition and special health care needs. In C.M. Trahms & P.L. Pipes (Eds.), *Nutrition in infancy and childhood* (6th ed., pp. 378–405). New York: McGraw-Hill.

Appendix

Early Intervention Nutrition Services Screening Form
and
Early Intervention Nutrition Referral Criteria

EARLY INTERVENTION NUTRITION SERVICES SCREENING FORM

1. Screening date _____

2. Child's I.D. number _____

3. Child's gender (M = male, F = female)_____

4. Date of birth _____

5. Birth weight _____ kg OR _____ lb _____ oz

6. Birth length _____ cm OR _____ in _____ /8th

reported by caregiver_____ OR found in medical records _____

7. Gestational age _____

ANTHROPOMETRICS   PERCENTILES

8. Date of measurements _____   12. Wt/age _____ to _____ percentile

9. Weight _____ kg OR   13. Ht/age _____ to _____ percentile

_____ lb _____ oz   14. Wt/ht _____ to _____ percentile

10. Length or height _____ cm OR _____ in _____ /8th

11. How was child measured? 1 = standing, 2 = lying down _____

LAB WORK

15. Date of hemoglobin or hematocrit _____

16. Hemoglobin _____ g/100 ml   18. Date of blood lead (Pb) _____

17. Hematocrit _____ %   19. Result _____ µg/dl

20. Are you concerned about your child's growth or nutrition?   yes   mildly   no

21. Does this child have any of the following diagnoses or chronic medical conditions? (Check all that apply)

____ Down syndrome   ____ Failure to thrive   ____ Cerebral palsy   ____ Cardiac

____ Spina bifida   ____ Anemia   ____ Liver   ____ Respiratory

____ Cystic fibrosis   ____ Neuromuscular   ____ Gastrointestinal   ____ Kidney

____ Seizure disorder   ____ Poor growth   ____ Fetal alcohol syndrome

____ Other (specify)_____

From Bayerl, C.T., & Ries, J.D. (1995). *EARLY START: Nutrition services in early intervention programs* [Training manual], p. 3-22. Worcester, MA: Area Health Education Center; adapted by permission.

Ask parent or caregiver the following questions. All questions can be answered with a "yes" or "no" response. Check the appropriate box next to each question. A "yes" response indicates a possible nutritional risk. A "no" response indicates no nutritional risk in that particular area.

YES NO

22. Does your child have food allergies? ☐ ☐

23. Does your child take any medication on a regular basis (excluding vitamins, iron, fluoride, or other mineral)? ☐ ☐

    If yes, then which ones?_____

24. Does your child experience any of the following: ☐ ☐
    (Circle all that apply)   1. diarrhea   2. constipation   3. vomiting/reflux

25. Does your child use a feeding tube or other special feeding equipment? ☐ ☐

26. Do any of the following apply to your child at his or her present age? ☐ ☐

    a. Seven months of age or older and has not started using a cup yet

    b. Nine months of age or older and does not finger-feed yet

    c. Twelve months of age or older and drinks primarily from the bottle

    d. Nineteen months of age or older and does not use a spoon yet

27. Does your child experience any of the following? ☐ ☐

    a. Difficulty with sucking

    b. Difficulty with swallowing

    c. Difficulty with chewing

    d. Gagging

28. If your child uses a bottle, does he or she take the bottle to bed? ☐ ☐

29. Do you add solid food to the bottle? ☐ ☐

30. If your child is under 12 months and drinks formula, is he or she drinking less than 24 ounces per day? ☐ ☐

31. If your child is under 12 months, does he or she reject any of the following foods: ☐ ☐
    (Circle all that apply)   1. milk   2. meats   3. vegetables   4. fruits

32. Does your child do anything that upsets you at mealtimes, such as refusing to eat, excessive throwing of food or utensils, or other? ☐ ☐

    If yes, then explain _____

33. Do you ever find that you are almost out of food at the end of the month?

34. Do you have any questions or concerns about your child's nutrition and feeding? ☐ ☐

    If yes, then explain _____

35. If you are currently breast-feeding, do you have any questions or concerns? ☐ ☐

    If yes, then explain _____

Failure to Thrive and Pediatric Undernutrition: A Transdisciplinary Approach
edited by Daniel B. Kessler and Peter Dawson
© 1999 by Paul H. Brookes Publishing Co.

EARLY INTERVENTION NUTRITION REFERRAL CRITERIA

Check the "yes" column next to any nutritional risk that applies to the child.

YES

____ Weight-for-age is **below the 10th percentile**
____ Length-for-age or height-for-age is **below the 10th percentile**
____ Weight-for-length or weight-for-height is **below the 10th percentile**
____ Weight-for-length or weight-for-height is **above the 95th percentile**
____ Hemoglobin: less than 11 g/dl
____ Hematocrit: less than 34%
____ Lead (Pb): 10µg/dl or GREATER

Child has any of the following diagnoses or chronic medical conditions:

Down syndrome	Failure to thrive	Cerebral palsy	Cardiac
Spina bifida	Anemia	Liver	Respiratory
Cystic fibrosis	Neuromuscular	Gastrointestinal	Kidney
Seizure disorder	Poor growth	Fetal alcohol syndrome	

If TWO or more of the following apply, then refer child to a nutritionist/RD for further assessment.

YES

____ History of food allergies
____ Medications taken on a regular basis
____ Chronic problems with diarrhea, constipation, and/or vomiting
____ On a feeding tube or special feeding equipment
____ Seven months of age or older and has not started using a cup yet
____ Nine months of age or older and does not finger-feed yet
____ Twelve months of age or older and drinks primarily from a bottle
____ Nineteen months of age or older and does not use a spoon yet
____ Difficulties with sucking, swallowing, chewing, or gagging
____ Bottle to bed (night or naptime)
____ Solids (cereal, fruit, etc.) added to bottle
____ Formula intake is less than 24 ounces in 24 hours (for infants 0–12 months)
____ Meals regularly lack one or more of the basic food groups (meats, milk, fruits, or vegetables)
____ Mealtime behavior frustrating to parent
____ Lack of food in household to meet child's or family's needs
____ Nutrition or eating habits of child are a concern to parent or caregiver
____ Breast-feeding questions or concerns of mother

Failure to Thrive and Pediatric Undernutrition: A Transdisciplinary Approach
edited by Daniel B. Kessler and Peter Dawson
© 1999 by Paul H. Brookes Publishing Co.

Section V

Families

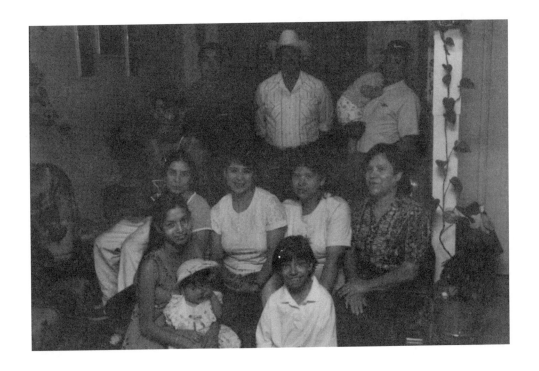

Chapter 26

Cultural Issues in Provider–Parent Relationships

Lynne Sturm and Sheila Gahagan

Cultural issues that affect relationships between providers and families of infants and toddlers have been described eloquently in the fields of early intervention (Anderson & Fenichel, 1989; Lynch & Hanson, 1998), child care (Gonzales-Mena, 1993), and pediatrics (Kinsman, Sally, & Fox, 1996; Pachter & Harwood, 1996). Cultural characteristics encompass both ethnic-cultural differences and professional–patient role differences. Provider familiarity with cultural issues is important for optimizing care because "as the cultural distance between individuals increases, the likelihood of a communication problem increases" (Pachter, 1994, p. 691).

Population projections suggest that professionals increasingly will interact with families whose cultural identities differ from their own. By the turn of the century, the non-Hispanic, White proportion of the U.S. population is expected to decrease to less than 72%; 13% of the population will be Black; 11% Hispanic; 4% Asian and Pacific Islander (API); and less than 1% American Indian, Eskimo, and Aleut (U.S. Bureau of the Census, 1995). APIs are the fastest growing ethnic minority, followed by Hispanics (Flack et al., 1995; U.S. Bureau of the Census, 1995).[1]

These demographic trends stand in stark contrast to an underrepresentation of ethnic minorities in professional training programs. For example, minorities such as Black Americans, Mexican Americans, American Indians, and Mainland Puerto Ricans made up only

The authors thank Dr. Carole Ashenberg for her thoughts and insight on working with families of undernourished children in different cultural groups, particularly Southeast Asians in Seattle. In addition, the editorial comments of Dr. Betsy Lozoff are greatly appreciated.

[1]Terminology as used by the U.S. Bureau of the Census.

9% of medical school graduates for the 1994–1995 year (Jolly & Hudley, 1996). Clearly, professionals who have a similar cultural background to that of ethnic minority families of undernourished children will continue to be in short supply.

The growing diversity of families who have children younger than 5 years and the potential clash of cultures during professional–parent encounters call for culturally sensitive care during evaluation and treatment of undernourished children. This chapter describes the concept of culture and how cultural issues can influence the quality of child nutrition and provider–parent communication and relationships. Then, steps that providers can take to improve their cultural competence in the area of undernutrition will be presented. Throughout, the focus is on practical recommendations for identifying and addressing barriers to care that can arise from culture clashes.

WHAT IS CULTURE?

Culture is the framework of beliefs and practices of a defined group of people. It encompasses religion, health, music, food, dress, work habits, style of homes, family habits, and relationships. Cultural identity may be based on common language, religion, national origin, geographical location, or historical experience. It includes shared and socially learned beliefs, values, and traditions that are transmitted from generation to generation and contribute to the learner's sense of belonging to an identified group and community (Kinsman et al., 1996). Cultural patterns may not be translated easily into words but carry normative expectations about how everyday life should be conducted. A related meaning of culture refers to the different role expectations of medical professionals and patients or parents (Pachter, 1994). Medical staff are socialized through their professional training into a Western biomedical paradigm that emphasizes disease processes and physiological malfunction as causes of illness states. In contrast, the patient (or parent) enters into a medical encounter concerned with difficulties resulting from his or her illness and may use a variety of causal explanations apart from medical ones that place the pathogen within the individual. In this socially sanctioned, asymmetrical relationship between the professional expert and the patient, power, status, and expertise traditionally have been attributed to the provider. Applying this model more broadly, when a provider and a parent meet, their communication may reflect the influence of the provider's professional culture, his or her ethnic-cultural background, the parent's lay patient role, and the parent's ethnic-cultural beliefs.

Practitioners need to exercise caution in generalizing knowledge of characteristics of a given cultural subgroup (e.g., Mexican Americans, vegetarians, Orthodox Jews, Cambodian refugees) to a specific family in a clinical situation. First, it is prudent to allow a parent to self-identify his or her cultural affiliation rather than assume an identification from family name or medical record information. This increasingly is important in light of the number of individuals whose mothers and fathers are from different racial and ethnic groups. Second, there is considerable diversity in beliefs and practices within specific cultural groups, and ethnographic summary descriptions typically describe a cultural norm or average that may not be relevant to an individual family. Providers should resist a tendency to view a family through the expectations that are derived from unintentional cultural stereotypes.

The range of heterogeneity and diversity within cultural subgroups is immense and thought to be influenced by such factors as social class, educational attainments, geographical location, and immigrant and generational status. Individuals within a cultural group differ with regard to their degree of acculturation—the adoption of cultural beliefs and behavioral patterns that are held by the mainstream U.S. culture. The challenge to immigrants is to adapt their customs to the social demands of their new country of residence (Pomerleau, Malcuit, & Sabatier, 1991). The degree to which a given individual holds acculturated or traditional beliefs has been related to such factors as place of birth (United States or foreign), educational attainment, proficiency with English, sense of ethnic identification, urban or rural background, residence in immigrant enclaves, and length of time that the family has lived in the United States (Pachter, 1994). Research indicates, however, that acculturation is a selective process (see Patel, Power, & Bhavnagri, 1996, for a review); that is, an individual may adopt behavioral patterns from the dominant culture only for particular contexts, such as those involving face-to-face interaction with members of the American culture (e.g., behavior in the workplace). Other values and customs pertaining to family, interpersonal relationships, and food practices may be maintained from the culture of origin; thus, over time, many immigrants assume characteristics of bi- and multiculturalism in that they acquire and maintain values of two or more cultures and must be able to function adaptively in each (Patel et al., 1996).

In work with families, it is important to determine which areas of health and child-rearing beliefs are acculturated, which are more traditional, and to what extent the family has achieved a successful bicultural adaptation. Within individual families, family members may differ significantly in their levels of acculturation. This can lead to intrafamily tension and conflict or to social isolation of the less acculturated family member (often the mother). The following example illustrates how such social isolation can contribute to child undernutrition:

> *An undernourished toddler presented for evaluation from a Middle Eastern family in which the father experienced a better fit with mainstream American culture than did his wife. The father was a graduate student in biochemistry at an American university, and his wife maintained a culturally traditional role at home with their toddler but without the usual social supports that she would have in her country of origin. Her resulting depression contributed to her difficulties with supporting her toddler's thrust for autonomy during meals and his inadequate caloric intake.*

Professionals always must be sensitive to the powerful experience of immigration or refugee status for a family. The greatest increases in population from 1980 to 1990 were among ethnic groups that were able to enter as refugees (Barker, 1992), such as Southeast Asians, Middle Easterners, Africans, and Eastern Europeans. Immigration under these conditions typically is associated with tremendous stress, repeated loss experiences, social isolation, and financial hardship, all of which can contribute indirectly to undernutrition in a young child, as illustrated in the following case:

> A young Laotian couple brought their emaciated 9-month-old child to medical attention. Their first-born child had died in a refugee camp shortly before the birth of this child. Hospitalized for assessment, this second infant ate voraciously and was soon approaching normal weight. The family interview revealed that the maternal grandmother had declared the baby a "spirit baby"— that is, the reincarnation of the dead child, come back to die again and thus cause further misery to the parents. In family therapy, the parents were guided in grieving their earlier loss—a process that they had not undergone in the midst of this infant's birth and the transition from camp to the United States. Furthermore, it was suggested that the child's rapid growth in the hospital indicated that the child was not a "spirit baby." The grandmother changed her assessment of the child. The child's subsequent course was very good. (Westermeyer, 1991, p. 145)

Providers need to be aware that malnutrition can develop during refugee flight because of the unavailability of a nutritious diet. Furthermore, after resettlement, some families may not provide enough fruits and vegetables to their children because they tend to be more expensive than in developing countries, whereas meat and grains are the same price or less expensive in the United States (Westermeyer, 1991).

CULTURAL ASPECTS OF FOOD

Food is central to many cultures. As families who originate from all parts of the globe are incorporated into the dominant U.S. culture, culturally typical food may be the last characteristic to be lost. Long after traditional dress, language, and even beliefs have faded into the background, people still will enjoy the foods of their culture, especially on holidays and feast days. At Christmas, people of English ancestry may enjoy roast beef and plum pudding, whereas people of French descent often celebrate with roast duck and a Yule log ("bouche de Noël"); people who have immigrated from Mexico may include tamales in their celebration.

Although certain foods often may be associated with particular cultures, it is important that providers not assume that they know what or how a family eats just because their cultural identification is known. A Navajo family living on the reservation may have a traditional diet of mutton stew and fry bread, or they may regularly eat Kentucky Fried Chicken (a favorite food on the Navajo reservation); however, it is likely that they eat some combination of traditional Navajo foods and foods of the "dominant" culture that are easily accessible. In supermarkets on the Navajo reservation, people have access to fresh fruits and vegetables that they would not have had in the past because of the terrain and climate. Traditional foods, such as huge pieces of mutton and large vats of lard, also are displayed. In essence, this is a visual representation of the bicultural nature of current life on the reservation. Similar experiences can be found in grocery stores in other ethnic enclaves across the United States.

INFANT FEEDING PRACTICES

The ways in which infants and toddlers are fed vary by culture, geography, and climate. Taste preferences may be established prenatally when the fetus is first exposed to tastes through the amniotic fluid. A culture that uses garlic and onions, for example, will have children who habituate to this taste even prenatally (Mennella, 1996; Mennella, Johnson, & Beauchamp, 1995). Breast-feeding has remained the culturally sanctioned method of infant feeding in many parts of the world and has been adapted to socioenvironmental needs of cultural groups. For example, in parts of China and Africa, grandmothers breast-feed (Richardson, 1975). By suckling her young grandchild, the grandmother lactates and can provide milk for the baby when the mother is tired or busy with another activity; however, when women immigrate to the United States, they may choose formula feeding in an effort to emulate the dominant American culture. A Navajo woman once said to her doctor (the second author of this chapter) that she was going to bottle-feed because she had never seen an "Anglo" breast-feed her infant. Other aspects of breast-feeding are culturally determined, including the frequency and length of feeding and the timing of weaning.

Although American pediatric recommendations (Barness, 1993) are to introduce solid foods at 4–6 months of age, the practices of culturally diverse groups may differ substantially. At 2–4 months of age, a Navajo mother will begin to give her infant little bits of fried bread dipped in the broth of mutton stew as well as other bits of chewed food. Chinese infants often are fed little bits of apple as early as 3 weeks of age, and egg yolk is considered a good food for a young infant. Many African American infants are given foods earlier than 4 months because of the recommendations of grandmothers and aunts, family members who often are involved in child care. Individuals from many Caucasian cultures believe that early feedings will help the infant sleep through the night.

Nutritional anthropology provides a wealth of ethnographic information about the meaning of traditional foods for specific cultural groups around the world and within the United States (Brown, 1986). Parental feeding practices reflect cultural beliefs about nutritional value of foods for different ages, prestige and status of different foods, responsibility for child intake, and presumed healing and medicinal value of foods (Zeitlin, 1996). Furthermore, the daily routines of feeding reflect deeply held values about child socialization (e.g., respect, independence) (Gonzales-Mena, 1993). Table 1 presents different dimensions of feeding beliefs and practices that can influence nutritional intake in young children.

Cultural beliefs about nutritional value of foods can underlie practices that inadvertently contribute to undernutrition. For example, in the Amele culture of New Guinea, mothers' feeding beliefs and practices accounted for the consistent drop-off in growth parameters at 4–6 months of age (Jenkins, Orr-Ewing, & Heywood, 1984). Mothers believed that breast milk improved in quality and nutritional value as the child grew older and hence met the child's nutritional requirements. Few mothers believed that they needed to introduce supplementary foods, and those that were given (e.g., liquid foods such as hot soup) led to decreased breast-milk consumption.

TODDLER FEEDING PRACTICES

Dettwyler (1989) compared cultures on a dimension of caregiver–child control of eating. At one end are cultures in which parents insist that children eat all food that is presented to them and use such practices as force feeding (e.g., holding the infant's nose and pour-

Table 1.   Cultural dimensions of feeding practices and effects on child nutrition

Dimension	Potential effect
Nutritional value of foods for different age groups	Timing of weaning and introduction of solids
Prestige and status of food types	Which foods are restricted or freely distributed in the family
Healing and medicinal value of foods	Which foods and liquids are given to children during illness
Religious significance of foods	Dietary laws for when foods can be eaten and which foods can be combined
Caregiver–child control of eating	Scheduling of meals, physical setup of mealtime, whether adults monitor intake
Prestige and status of eaters and gender	Prioritization and order of who gets fed in the family
Developmental timetable for eating behaviors	When self-feeding, utensil use, neatness, and manners are expected and encouraged
Ideal baby construct	Which eating behaviors are reinforced; preference for "chubby" or "lean" body type
Religious customs (fasting by adults)	Availability of adult models for eating behavior

ing liquid into his or her mouth) or persuasion (e.g., threats or encouragement). At the other end are societies in which parents give greater autonomy to children in deciding the timing and location of their meals and the amounts that they eat. In short, they believe that children eat when they are ready. Mothers in these cultures provide little encouragement for or insistence on eating.

Toddlerhood is a high-risk time for undernutrition around the world. In cultures with a laissez-faire attitude toward toddler eating, the child may not have a place to sit at the family table. He or she may wander around during meals, perhaps asking for food from different family members. No one may have a clear idea of what the child has eaten. Whereas the majority of children in such a culture may grow well, certain children who are at risk for undernutrition may suffer in this environment of extreme independence.

Some toddlers (1–3 years of age) who are undernourished refuse food because their drive for independence is so great that they cannot tolerate having feeding imposed on them by a caregiver. The strength of developmental and temperament-based needs for autonomy and independence varies between toddlers. Some cultures have feeding norms that accommodate this thrust for autonomy more easily than others. For toddlers who want to self-feed, it certainly is easier to prosper in a culture in which it is customary to eat with one's hands than in one in which utensil use is required. A toddler who has a strong desire for autonomy ("*I* do it!") may have difficulties in a culture that emphasizes extreme neatness and table manners. Cultural norms that insist on dependence in the feeding relationship well into the second or third years (e.g., some Chinese American and Vietnamese American families) also may be frustrating for certain toddlers.

In many societies throughout the world, toddler weaning practices unintentionally can result in "benign neglect" (Cassidy, 1980). These customs, considered harmful from the biomedical perspective, comprise society-approved ways in which the child becomes a member of his or her social group. By limiting toddler access to the food supply (e.g., through food competition with elders, siblings, and caregivers; imposition of dietary restrictions), these practices may unintentionally lead to malnutrition. Other weaning-related practices, such as forcible separation of the toddler from his or her mother or punishment for display of dependency behaviors, also can lead to malnutrition.

DEVELOPMENTAL EXPECTATIONS FOR YOUNG CHILDREN

Expectations for developmental achievements can play a role in feeding practices. Pomerleau et al. (1991) found that Vietnamese immigrants in Québec expected infant abilities such as taking the bottle alone and eating unaided to emerge at significantly later ages than did Québecois mothers. Not surprising, the ages at which these mothers introduced these activities also were significantly later. Pachter and Dworkin (1996) also found differences in developmental expectations for eating behaviors among mothers of different ethnic groups in Hartford, Connecticut. Puerto Rican mothers expected infants to be able to be fed from a spoon at a significantly later age than did African American and Caucasian mothers. Overall, Puerto Rican mothers expected personal social milestones of infants and toddlers to appear at later ages than did African American, Caucasian, or West Indian mothers.

Another set of cultural beliefs that can affect nutritional intake involves the qualities that are believed to be associated with the construct of a good infant. Most cultures appear to value greater weight and larger size as indices of health. Thinness often is considered a sign of weak health or poverty, and describing a child as underweight may be experienced by parents as insulting. For example, in the Mexican American culture, rapid weight gain in infancy is an important criterion of health. In contrast, some parents who value vegetarian feeding principles or are concerned with prevention of adult risk conditions such as atherosclerosis or obesity may view lean infants and toddlers as healthier. If parents employ nutritional practices that are suited to adults, then undernutrition may result (Dwyer, 1993). For example, Pugliese, Weyman-Daum, Moses, and Lifshitz linked the following practices, intended to ensure a "healthy diet," to undernutrition in a 20-month-old child:

> The parents of patient 5 avoided cow's milk and processed cereals to eliminate fat and processed sugar which they considered important for good health. They had adopted a partial vegetarian diet which consisted mainly of fruits, vegetables, and whole grain products, but included lean meats and dairy products. They were aware of the published benefits of breast milk as a sole source of nutrition for infants, and they extended this idea to conclude that breast milk should be a good source of nutrition for older children. Therefore, they continued to use breast milk as a major source of nutrition for this child into the second year of life. (1987, p. 179)

Cultures that value motoric development may prefer less chubby infants. For example, Yoruba women in Nigeria prefer "wiry and agile babies who learned to walk early" (Zeitlin, 1996, p. 412). Consequently, introduction of heavy staple foods such as yams is postponed until the child walks in order to prevent development of a "heavy, clumsy baby" (Zeitlin, 1996, p. 412). A "good baby" also may be defined in terms of appetite-related behavior. For instance, in Lagos, Nigeria, an area of economic scarcity, mothers evaluated their children's social development by the children's ability to control expressions of hunger (i.e., not whine for or request food). One mother said, "He is a good baby, he never demands food unless he really needs to eat" (Zeitlin, 1996, p. 423).

Food customs also play an important part in religious practices. For example, a complex set of rules guides dietary planning (keeping Kosher) in Orthodox Jewish households. In some cultures, religious practices related to fasting can indirectly alter household routines in ways that jeopardize child nutrition. Najib, Laraque, and Leung (1996) described a 33-month-old male Muslim child of a Gambian mother living in New York City who experienced poor weight gain during the month of Ramadan for each of his first 3 years. Adults past the age of puberty of Muslim faith fast all day for the month of Ramadan. During this time, the feeding of the toddler occurred mainly at night when adults were breaking their fasts.

Significantly, even in developing countries with widespread economic scarcity, non-nutritional influences on nutrient intake have been identified in the domains of cultural norms and caregiver beliefs (Engle, Zeitlin, Medrano, & Garcia, 1996). Cultural issues that are important for service delivery for undernutrition include cultural beliefs and practices that are related to feeding of young children, child health and illness conditions, and behavioral expectations for the provider–patient relationship.

GUIDELINES FOR PROVIDERS: INTERVIEWING

Pachter (1994) outlined characteristics of culturally sensitive health care that are relevant broadly for early childhood services for undernutrition. Service providers should be accessible, flexible in acknowledging that health and illness are influenced by cultural issues, respectful of the patient's cultural lifestyle, and careful to avoid stereotyping patients on the basis of a cultural label. Importantly, the culturally constructed meaning of illness should be valued by the provider in addition to biomedical aspects of illness. Such care is implicitly multicultural in its support of and respect for many different cultural perspectives (Kinsman et al., 1996).

Comfort in talking with parents about family nutritional practices is key to working with parents of undernourished children. The following questions should be asked:

- What do they eat every day?
- What do they eat when they are celebrating?
- What do they eat when they are in a hurry?
- What do their children eat?
- Does the undernourished child eat what other family members eat?
- What might the child eat if the family were living in their country of origin?
- What do the parents think that the child should eat?
- What do relatives (e.g., grandparents) think that the child should eat?
- What are the structural and environmental feeding practices (e.g., mealtime environment, timing of meals, adult involvement in child intake), and how do these fit with the child's unique temperamental and developmental needs?

To plan effective interventions, then, it is crucial first to identify the feeding practices of a family. Providers should take time to explore the cultural meaning of foods and feeding practices to determine which practices are amenable to alteration and how to present and explain any suggested changes. When planning how to increase high-calorie foods for a child, the provider should explore collaboratively the cultural taste preferences. For example, some foods that are enjoyed in one culture may be considered disgusting in another culture. One Asian mother told her doctor (a colleague of the second author) that cheese on rice would be like soy sauce on ice cream!

When parents are asked to change their customary ways of interacting with children around feeding, practitioners must remember that they may be asking the parents to revise their notions of what is culturally competent parenting. As Pomerleau et al. observed, "a competent mother will be competent only within her own culture" (1991, pp. 45–46). For example, in many cultures, mothers chew their young infants' food before giving it to them. Many health care providers are quick to condemn such a practice, especially when the child is undernourished; however, this practice is culturally acceptable for many groups and certainly predates commercially prepared baby foods. When the health care provider can view such a practice nonjudgmentally, it becomes clear that the issue is *how much* food the infant is ingesting rather than that the mother is chewing it for the infant. It is important to focus on issues of importance to the child's nutritional status, not on extraneous, albeit interesting, issues that may be culturally important to the family. If the clinician counsels this family not to chew food for the infant, then there could be adverse effects on the provider–family relationship and, ultimately, on the infant's health status. For example, the family might feel alienated or insulted or may decide that the provider knows very little about child care. In either case, the family may react by avoiding any further contact with the provider. The family also may feel conflict between the physician's expectation to discontinue the practice of chewing food for the infant and the cultural belief that this is proper care for the infant. If the mother discontinues this practice, then she may be judged as incompetent or uncaring by other family members.

HEALTH BELIEFS AND PRACTICES

Cultural groups differ widely in their beliefs and practices that are related to health and illness (Hellman, 1990). In particular, a wide variety of explanatory models (i.e., cognitive interpretations) of malnutrition and its causes have been documented in developing countries (Bentley et al., 1991); however, less is known about parental explanatory models of mild to moderate undernutrition in the United States. Explanatory models encompass the parents' concepts of undernutrition: symptom presentation, causes, course of illness and projected consequences, and optimum treatment (Sturm & Drotar, 1992; Sturm, Drotar, Laing, & Zimet, 1997).

Encounters between provider and parent involve transactions between two explanatory models (Kleinman, Eisenberg, & Good, 1978) that can result in communication and relationship problems. For example, providers predictably feel frustrated when their concern about the potential seriousness of a child's undernutrition is not immediately appreciated by a parent who reacts with, "Everyone in our family is small," or, "All of my children were small as babies, and then they grew very well. My 16-year-old is taller than me."

Pachter (1994) noted that "folk illnesses" represent the most striking example of cultural differences in the area of health. A *folk illness* is defined as an interpretation of illness within a cultural group whose explanatory model may clash with biomedical explanations. To care for "folk illnesses," parents may make use of multiple sources of care for a child's condition, such as folk and religious healers, home remedies, and physicians. Harwood (1981) noted that physicians need to be aware of potential dual regimens (folk or popular remedies and biomedical treatments) in order to assess their potential interactions and impact on the child's health. In a case report, Pachter (1994) described collaboration between a traditional healer and a physician in treating a Puerto Rican child who experienced undernutrition, which the family attributed to a folk illness, **empacho.** This case also illustrated the value of incorporating traditional healers into interventions (Bentley et al., 1991; Pachter, 1994).

Provider familiarity with culturally based health beliefs and practices also is crucial to optimizing family follow-through or compliance with recommended treatments for undernutrition. The construct of compliance derives from the authority–subordinate model of medical practice in which the provider gives the family a program with the expectation that the family will follow it without question. With culturally dissimilar clients, Kinsman et al. proposed that problems with compliance be reframed as "the physician's difficulty in supplying appropriate care that suits the patient's beliefs and lifestyle" (1996, p. 352). Health-related noncompliance then can be viewed as a shared responsibility between provider and parent (Liptak, 1996), an attitude that can further the parent's therapeutic alliance with the provider.

In health care settings, judgments are frequently made about parental competence based on whether there is adequate follow-through or compliance with provider recommendations for treating undernutrition. Magana and Clark (1995) noted that folk-healing interventions with Mexican Americans may be misconstrued by providers as parental ignorance, superstition, or abuse and neglect if they are used in place of provider recommendations. Involvement with folk healing should always be explored when attempting to understand a family's lack of follow-through with provider recommendations. For example, a pediatrician made a home visit to the Hmong family of an undernourished 17-month-old. The family then consulted a folk healer, who told them that the child was afraid of the "man with the beard"; they subsequently stopped attending pediatric appointments. In this case, the folk healer's appraisal of the child's comfort with the physician probably played a role in the family's decision about which help-seeking steps were in the best interest of their child (P. Dawson, personal communication, 1997).

Undernutrition in young children is a condition that lends itself to a "blame-focused view of illness" (Finerman & Bennett, 1995, p. 2) because poor growth still is dichotomized by some providers as "organic" (translated as not the parent's fault) or "nonorganic" (translated as the parent's fault). Medical anthropology, however, challenges such automatic attributions of psychopathology and neglect to parents. Finerman (1995) hypothesized that many parents who are viewed as incompetent or neglectful are interested in their child's health and struggle to cope with health needs of an individual child within the context of the global household unit. Many perceived costs can limit health-related decisions, such as financial costs for implementing a recommended intervention, time away from other siblings, and loyalty binds (e.g., when a recommended intervention clashes with beliefs of other family members).

Traditional cultural values and practices (e.g., folk healing) have typically been viewed by providers as potential barriers to successful treatment; however, the protective function of a traditional cultural orientation is increasingly receiving attention (Bagley, Angel, Dilworth-Anerson, Liu, & Schinke, 1995). For example, religiosity and spirituality in Mexican American immigrant women has been proposed as a possible protective factor (Magana & Clark, 1995). Women who more strongly identified themselves as connected to their subgroup culture and country of origin were less likely to have a low birth weight infant. Another example of a potential strength that may be misinterpreted as a sign of family instability involves informal adoption and fosterage during times of family stress in African American families (Stack, 1974). With respect to child undernutrition, providers should take the time to evaluate potential strengths of the traditional cultural beliefs and practices of the families with whom they work. Whenever possible, some of the solutions to a child's eating problem should be sought from within the culture.

ROLE EXPECTATIONS IN PROVIDER–PARENT RELATIONSHIPS

Culture enters into the role expectations that families bring to their relationships with authority figures such as physicians and teachers. Role customs encompass such aspects of interaction as timing of disclosure of personal information, appropriate communication style with different age groups, behavior toward individuals of different status, and criteria for professional competence. It is important to understand what parents expect culturally from their physicians and early intervention providers to achieve an effective working relationship. It is always prudent to ask parents how they would like to be addressed rather than assume that mainstream American customs will be acceptable. Following are some recommendations for culturally sensitive introductions by providers to parents:

- Introduce yourself slowly.
- Shake hands if appropriate in your own culture.
- Use a formal address (e.g., Mr., Mrs.).
- Ask what the family's cultural background is.
- Admit to little knowledge of their culture.
- Express interest in their culture.

To maximize collaboration, providers may need to alter their typical interaction style with patients to accommodate different cultural preferences. For example, people from many Latino cultures look to the physician for authority. When patients come to pediatric care with this expectation, a doctor who provides them with many treatment choices may leave the family confused and anxious. It may appear that the physician does not know what is wrong or what needs to be done. When working with cultural groups with this expectation, it is prudent to begin the physician–parent relationship with a teaching style that is intended to allow the family to learn the competence of the physician and the extent of his or her knowledge. (This would not be necessary for a primary care physician who has a long-standing relationship with the family.) After a relationship is formed, the physician may begin to offer choices. The physician then is viewed as understanding yet continues to be the authority.

Harwood (1981) recommended that mainstream medical providers sometimes incorporate aspects of the interpersonal style of traditional healers to help families feel comfortable and to enhance compliance. An example of the usefulness of this approach occurred when the second author of this chapter was practicing on the Navajo reservation. She noticed that parents who were accustomed to going to a medicine man to find out what was wrong were more comfortable when the Caucasian physician reversed the usual pediatric sequence and examined the child before taking a detailed medical history. These parents often looked with suspicion on a doctor who expected them to have all of the answers, and open-ended questions often were met with short, inadequate responses. After examining the patient, she would explain her findings and then ask about the family's concerns. Another approach that was helpful was to sit quietly in the exam room and write her notes, during which time the families would appreciate the silence and offer more information.

Parents also respond according to cultural customs to clinician questions. For example, some cultures place a high value on courtesy. Parents from such a culture may try to say what they think the doctor wants to hear because of a cultural proscription against expressing negative thoughts or to allow the doctor to save face. For example, a physician advised a family to begin feeding their infant in a highchair. Every time the infant was placed in the highchair, he screamed; so the family was unable to follow the doctor's recommendations. When the family returned to the doctor, they reported that the child sat in the highchair to eat. In their view, this saved everyone the embarrassment of acknowledging that the doctor's advice was not helpful.

It also is important to be mindful of differing concepts of time and schedule to prevent labeling families as disorganized or lazy. For example, the accuracy of historical information may carry different meaning to physician and parent. When working with undernourished children, the clinician typically pays meticulous attention to the times and details of the child's eating and sleeping schedule; however, if the family comes from a culture that does not embrace the dominant American culture's notion of time, then the family may be confused by such attention to exact temporal details of daily schedule. Similarly, cultural expectations of efficiency and time management may clash with the family's need to become comfortable and get to know the provider before embarking on a collaborative relationship that involves the well-being of their child.

DEVELOPING CULTURAL COMPETENCE

Cushner and Brislin (1996) proposed that intercultural communication training prior to working in an unfamiliar country is invaluable because trained individuals can handle unfamiliar situations in the host country with more confidence, can interpret difficult situations using a more complex frame of reference, and are less likely to make ethnocentric attributions about the reasons for actions by individuals from the host culture. Training in cultural competence for providers who work with undernutrition in the United States can achieve similar results.

Cultural competence can be viewed as three interrelated challenges. First, providers should deepen self-awareness about their own cultural backgrounds and how their cultural value systems (both professional and personal) influence their professional practices with families, especially how they perceive and judge families of undernourished children

(Kinsman et al., 1996). Second, providers benefit from having some general knowledge of culture-specific information, such as folk diseases that potentially affect the child's health. Third, providers need to develop a set of communication skills for learning about a given family's specific cultural beliefs and practices as they affect the child's undernutrition. As a component of communicating effectively, providers need to learn how to employ translation services that allow families to communicate in their native language.

Provider Self-Awareness

Strategies for increasing provider cultural competence range from self-reflection exercises (Derman-Sparks, 1995) to organized curricula for cultural sensitivity training for early intervention and child welfare personnel (Rauch & Curtiss, 1992). Self-reflection activities can be used individually or adapted to agency continuing education programs. These include standardized procedures such as the Self–Other Insight Interview (Mac Kune-Karrer & Taylor, 1995), which can be used to explore how a provider's own cultural experiences are similar to and different from those of a patient's family. This can deepen the provider's awareness of how his or her own cultural history may color his or her experience of a family in a clinical situation. Sometimes a provider will overidentify with a family member, either the parents or the child, based on perceived similarities that relate to cultural history. For example, the second author of this chapter supervised a resident who related very closely with a boy who was the same age when his family immigrated to the United States as the resident was when he immigrated. Such overidentification with one member of the family may result in a concomitant failure to understand and work effectively with the other family members.

In another self-reflection activity, providers can consider specific child care practices that are embedded in cultural values. These include co-sleeping for young children (versus separate sleeping arrangements from parents) and allowing infants to cry (versus quickly picking them up). The goal of this activity is that providers begin to recognize their own culture-bound judgments that certain practices are healthy or adaptive and that others are unhealthy or maladaptive. They then can begin to consider how concepts of normality, optimum practice, and risk necessarily are cultural constructions (Nugent, 1994).

Culture-Specific Information

There is a wealth of review articles and cultural summaries about specific ethnic-cultural groups (e.g., Cambodian refugees, Gypsies, Puerto Rican immigrants) that can familiarize providers with beliefs and practices that are related to illness, communication style, and disability that may affect family relationships with providers (Barker, 1992; Birrer, 1987; Harry, 1992; Lynch & Hanson, 1998). The chief advantage of learning specific cultural practices of a cultural group is that practitioners can avoid judgmental questions or comments that would negatively affect the provider–parent relationship (Kinsman et al., 1996). The danger of prepackaged summaries is that providers may make assumptions about an individual family and neglect to discuss with the family its unique cultural-familial patterns.

In addition to ethnographic readings, agencies can organize in-service sessions and continuing education programs for staff about the most common cultural groups in their communities. For example, at Oakland Children's Hospital, which is located in one of the most culturally diverse areas of the United States, the Department of Pediatrics has implemented an ongoing cultural curriculum for all members of the faculty as well as residents (Tervalon, 1995). A monthly seminar is presented on one of the cultural groups that they serve and involves the patient community to ensure community input into the program. One of the keys to the success of this program is that it has been mainstreamed, meaning that everyone is expected to attend, including faculty, and it is considered important for the professional functioning of all members of the department, not just the interested.

Another useful strategy for developing cultural competence is for programs that serve families of undernourished children (e.g., multidisciplinary undernutrition clinics, early intervention centers, public health departments, Special Supplemental Nutrition Program for Women, Infants and Children [WIC]) to hire an individual from a key representative cultural subgroup for their program. These individuals can serve as "interpreters of culture" with whom other staff members can talk about intercultural communication issues and culture-specific practices. For example, in a Phoenix pediatric residency program, as part of a primary care training grant, a community health worker was hired to be part of the health care team for the residents' continuity clinic. This woman was Spanish-speaking and of Mexican heritage. Her job was to be a translator not only of language but also of culture. She accompanied the residents into the room when they saw their patients and often spent time with the patient before and after the physician's visit. She observed the family for signs of cultural beliefs such as a *mal de ojo* bracelet, a talisman often worn by infants to ward off the evil eye. This "interpreter of culture" was hired to teach the physicians-in-training about their patients' health beliefs and how they could develop cultural competence in their dealings with patients. Of course, she was not an expert in all Latino cultures, so she asked the patients about their beliefs and modeled this process for the residents. As a result, the residents became more aware of the diversity of health beliefs in their patients and learned that they must respect these beliefs in order to work as a team with the family to help the child. For example, they came to learn that if the family would like to give the infant some manzanilla tea to treat the infant's diarrhea, then it was prudent to address the issue of volume of tea rather than to proscribe its use.

Hiring staff whose personal cultural background matches that of the patients can provide a wealth of information when mainstream culture staff seek out their expertise. Other strategies include developing relationships with community centers and organizations that help immigrants and refugees to relocate. Respected members of the community, such as traditional healers or spiritual leaders, also can provide valuable background information about the historical and economic experiences of a cultural subgroup that settled in a particular geographical region. Becoming familiar with stages of acculturation (Karrer, 1987) can help providers understand the adjustments that a given patient's family faces.

Communication Skills

The interpersonal skills that are needed to communicate sensitively with families go beyond the obvious need for translation services when a family speaks a language other than English. Providers need skills for interviewing, negotiating cultural disagreements, and accessing quality translators.

Learning About a Family's Culture

Providers need to become comfortable with talking directly with families about cultural beliefs and practices. Lieberman (1995) suggested asking parents about their child-rearing and family practices by explaining that the provider knows that people from different countries bring up their children in different ways and that he or she would like to better understand how they do things. This nonjudgmental expression of genuine interest can help further trust and a sense of working together.

Kleinman et al. (1978) recommended that physicians learn to elicit from their patients the explanatory model of an illness, whether they come from a cultural subgroup or from the physician's own culture. This can be accomplished with simple and direct questions that include the subjective "illness" experience. These involve cause for the presenting problem, why the patient thinks that it started when it did, what the sickness does to the patient, how it works, severity of the sickness, long or short course, type of treatment that the patient believes that he or she should receive, the most important results that the patient hopes to receive from treatment, the life problems that the sickness has caused for the patient, and the biggest fear about the sickness.

Drotar and Sturm (1988) developed questions to explore an individual parent's health beliefs about undernutrition. It also is useful to inquire about the health beliefs of other individuals in the family network in order to understand the sociocultural pressures on the parents, including beliefs of less and more acculturated family members. To explore the possibility of a folk illness, an introduction such as that offered by Pachter can be helpful:

> Some of my patients have told me that there is an illness called ___ that doctors don't know about but that people get. Have you ever heard of ___? (If yes:) Do you think that . . . your child may have ___ now? (1994, p. 693)

Negotiating Provider-Parent Conflict

Sometimes cultures clash despite the best intentions of both parties. Cultural differences can result in disagreement between providers and parents about one or more aspects of the child's undernutrition and its treatment (Drotar & Sturm, 1988). Developing skills for negotiating with parents can improve communication and prevent relationship problems that interfere with the child's recovery. A model of clinical negotiation (Katon & Kleinman, 1981; Kleinman et al., 1978) has proved to be well suited to family-centered intervention with undernutrition because parents are treated as therapeutic allies and members of the treatment team.

Using this clinical negotiation model, a clinician actively discusses with the parents the child's condition, treatment, and expected outcomes. When discrepancies in interpretation occur (folk illness models), differences of opinion should be identified openly, discussed, and negotiated. The potential negative effect of a cultural practice on patient care should be assessed. Cultural practices that do not interfere with treatment should not be challenged, and providers should not attempt to talk parents out of their beliefs. Instead, efforts should focus on educating the family about the usefulness of adding the biomedical therapy to the folk method. Pachter (1994) suggested that this approach places the biomedical treatment within the cultural context of the parent and, hence, may foster trust in the provider and better follow-through.

Conversely, ethnomedical practices that could have serious negative consequences should be discouraged and replaced with an alternative that is congruent with the family's cultural system. A treatment that the family considers to be culturally inappropriate can be reframed in more acceptable terms, or the provider's recommended treatment can be replaced with an alternative, equivalent, but culturally acceptable intervention. For example, Shawyer, Gani, Punufimana, and Seuseu (1996) concluded that Thai villagers believed strongly that *su* (diarrhea in children younger than 1 year) was not an illness that required treatment such as an oral rehydration solution (ORS). To increase use of ORS, health planners could consider reframing *su* as a developmental time when a child needs strengthening and then introduce ORS as a way to meet this need.

Phillips and Cooper (1992) warned against "recipe solutions" to intercultural conflicts about child care practices. They advised that staff and parents design temporary resolutions with follow-up evaluation, review, and modification of the conflict resolution. It also is useful to remember that it is not always necessary that providers and parents come to agreement, even about the definition of a child's problem, to successfully intervene (Drotar & Sturm, 1988). For example, in working with families of undernourished children, the second author of this chapter and a social work colleague (Karen Gray) explored the relationship between parental concern about growth and the ensuing response to intervention. In a study done at Maricopa Medical Center in Phoenix, Arizona, they found that 17 of 54 mothers were not concerned about the undernutrition and that mothers and fathers agreed in all but one case. The children whose parents were not concerned about their undernutrition responded as well to the interventions as did the children whose parents expressed concern in a standardized interview.

Translation Services

Language is an important part of both culture and the provider–parent relationship. Certain feelings and ideas expressed in one language will be difficult to express in another, and many technical medical concepts may not have clear equivalents. This creates great difficulties when providers deal with diverse cultures that speak languages other than English. The United States, with more than 30 million people whose first language is not English, is progressing toward increasing multiculturalism.

The use of nonprofessional, nontrained translators clearly is inadequate. Informally asking an agency employee to translate fails to protect patient confidentiality and does not ensure that the translator has adequate educational training to accurately translate technical medical information. In contrast, trained translators are educated to interpret word for word as much as possible and do not extrapolate or condense information from either the provider or the parent. When working on the Navajo reservation, the second author of this chapter found that it was not uncommon to use nurses or nurse's aides as translators. A frequent occurrence was a lengthy response by a patient to a physician's query, followed by the following translation by the nurse: "He said, 'No.'" Obviously the patient's answer was rich and full of detail that would be important to the physician working diagnostically or therapeutically. Another common practice is using relatives or family members to translate, which places an undue burden on both the relative and the parent, who may not feel comfortable with discussing relevant issues in front of the relative. Many of the family members who are bilingual and therefore capable of translating are children, yet the expectation that children will be able to serve as a conduit for complex medical information is unrealistic, may be culturally unacceptable to parents, and places an emotional burden on the child.

How can the needs for translating be addressed in a conscientious, cost-effective way? In environments in which the majority of patients speak a language other than English (e.g., Spanish in many city hospitals in the southwestern United States), it is essential to have trained professional interpreters for most patient interactions. These institutions should hire bilingual staff whenever possible and provide formal training for professional interpreting. This principle also can work for smaller clinics and private practices. Staff also can be offered intensive training in other languages, but the limitations of the staff's resulting proficiency are such that complicated and controversial medical issues will not be able to be addressed with families.

Another option is the "Language Line," a telephone interpreting service to which a professional gains access by telephone (see the section "Selected Resources on Cultural Issues" at the end of this chapter). The patient and provider sit together both holding telephones. The provider speaks into the telephone, and the interpreter interprets to the patient over the telephone. This procedure is superior to an untrained translator, including the use of a family member; however, there are minor disadvantages, such as the impersonal feeling of using the telephone and the cost of the service.

Trained translators translate either simultaneously or sequentially. For medical translating, nonsimultaneous translation is considered superior for several reasons. Although the time involved is longer, it is preferable to have the patient looking at and listening to the English-speaking provider when he or she is talking, even if the patient does not understand the words. The patient will understand the feeling and the tone of the information, whether it is the bad news of a difficult diagnosis or stressing the importance of a particular therapy. The patient then listens to the same information being given in his or her own language. This slows the communication process in a way that may give the patient time to comprehend the information and ask questions. In contrast, simultaneous translating addresses only the words that are communicated by the provider.

Patients who have hearing impairments also have a distinct culture and require interpreters, in accordance with the Americans with Disabilities Act (ADA) of 1990 (PL 101-336). There are many interpreters who are trained in American Sign Language (ASL). With some planning, one can accompany a family to an appointment.

Guidelines for Providers: Translating

1. Use trained interpreters whenever possible.
2. When trained interpreters are not available, involve the parents in the decision regarding whom to use for an interpreter. For example, a male family member may be an inappropriate interpreter for a gynecological problem. Avoid using children as interpreters.
3. Be liberal in the use of interpreters. A parent may have some conversational ability in English and still not have an adequate knowledge of medical issues to fully understand explanations or instructions.
4. Speak to the parent, not to the interpreter.
5. Look at the parent when the interpreter is translating your words.
6. Look at the parent when the parent is speaking to you. You may position the interpreter just behind your shoulder so that the parent sees both the physician and the interpreter at the same time.
7. Pace your speech so that you stop after every thought. Do not give a lengthy explanation and expect the interpreter to remember everything that you have said.
8. If you are working with an interpreter for the first time, then explain what you expect from the interpreter—for example, that you expect word-for-word translation without "interpretation" including additions or subtractions. An example introduction is, "I am Dr. X. May I explain the way that I like to work with an interpreter? I prefer that you translate word for word or idea for idea everything that I say. I would prefer that you do not leave out anything at all. If the patient asks you to explain something, then please repeat the question to me and allow me to do this. I will stop for interpreting after each thought. If you need me to change the pace of my presentation, then please let me know. Thank you so much for your help."

EXAMPLES OF UNDERNUTRITION FROM DIFFERENT AMERICAN CULTURES

This section provides case examples of undernutrition from different cultural groups in an attempt to show how cultural approaches to feeding interrelate to other issues that affect a child's nutritional well-being, such as health, financial situation, and the psychological well-being of the mother and the family. It is important to remember the heterogeneity of people from within cultural groups and not to generalize broadly from these examples. These scenarios are not necessarily "typical" of their cultures, yet they can provide learning experiences and help providers become more open minded as they work with diverse populations.

African American

A.H. is an 18-month-old African American girl who lives in an urban area. She was born 3 months early and weighed only 700 grams (1½ pounds) at birth. She was hospitalized for chronic lung disease (bronchopulmonary dysplasia) until she was 5 months old. After discharge from the hospital, A.H. lived with her single, 19-year-old mother and her family of origin. At pediatric visits, there was concern about A.H.'s slow weight gain; however, her mother showed excellent responsibility in bringing her to doctor's visits and obviously was proud of her daughter. Her weight was monitored carefully, and the slow weight gain was attributed to increased caloric needs from her lung disease. When A.H. was 13 months old, her mother was murdered on the streets of her neighborhood. After her mother's death, A.H. continued to live with her maternal grandparents and their three living children, ages 8–16 years. Many African American families are accustomed to independent eating by toddlers. This was the case in A.H.'s family: She was expected to self-feed an adequate amount of food with minimal caregiver direction. As is the case in many African American households in the 1990s, the feeding of A.H. involved the extended family: All family members shared in her feeding. There were multiple demands on both grandparents, and the grandmother, who might have been expected to assume the role of primary feeder, worked outside the home. The child's growth velocity worsened.

This example of a child with multifactorial undernutrition reveals how normally adaptive cultural factors can become detrimental to the child in the face of unusual stress or circumstances. One of the cultural factors that contributed to this child's undernutrition was this family's comfort with a great deal of independence in toddler feeding and a non-directive feeding style. The second cultural factor was the involvement of all of the family members in A.H.'s feeding. In the context of the profound sense of loss and depression, which affected all members of the family after A.H.'s mother's death, no family member took charge of her overall feeding. No one monitored her progress or daily overall food intake. Cultural practices, child temperament, and child biological risk (increased caloric need) interacted synergistically to produce undernutrition.

Independence in toddler feeding is a practice that is seen in American families of varying cultural backgrounds, including African American families, Caucasian American families, and Mexican American families. The African American emphasis on independence in toddler feeding can be considered part of a cultural emphasis on self-reliance. The involvement of extended family, especially grandmothers, in child care is a unique strength in many African American families. Infant feeding in African American families in the 1990s often involves the extended family; therefore, the parents receive advice and help from other family members in feeding their children. Most African American women choose to formula feed their infants, although there is a resurgence of breast-feeding in some areas (Black, Blair, Jones, & Durant, 1990; Solem, Norr, & Gallo, 1992). Solid foods are introduced at a young age in many African American families, often in the first 2 months of life (Parraga, Weber, Engel, Reeb, & Lerner, 1988). Because of the comfort with feeding independence in this culture, one is less likely to find power struggles over food.

In this example, there are two cultures of which to be mindful. In addition to the African American culture, there is the culture of life in American inner cities, which includes a culture of violence. The mortality statistics alone cannot paint the full picture of the ripple effect of violence on the well-being of the children and the families who live in these environments.

Navajo

J.B. is a 15-month-old Navajo boy who was a full-term infant with no perinatal complications. He was breast-fed successfully and grew along the 75th percentile until 6 months of age. At 9 months of age, his growth began to falter. At his 15-month evaluation, his mother reported that J.B. had not taken to any solid food. He was almost exclusively breast-fed, refusing table food and crying to be breast-fed frequently. J.B.'s mother is 18 years old and has no younger siblings. This is her first baby, and she lives with her parents and several other family members. J.B.'s maternal grandmother is quite ill, with complications of diabetes mellitus.

What are the cultural components of this case? Most Navajo children are breast-fed, and prolonged breast-feeding into the second or third year of life is culturally acceptable (Van Duzen, Carter, & VanderZwagg, 1969, 1976). During the third or fourth month of life, it is common for babies to receive small quantities of broth and soft food, sometimes chewed by their mother. Once an infant can sit up and reach, he or she commonly receives modified table food and is allowed great independence in feeding. Adequate caloric intake during extended breast-feeding requires supplementation with solid foods. The cultural practice of breast-feeding toddlers becomes more problematic when risk factors in either the family or the child result in the toddler's refusal of solids.

In the case of J.B., his mother was young and inexperienced and lacked younger siblings who would have provided a context from which to learn appropriate infant and toddler feeding methods. Maternal depression also may have played a role in her reluctance to work with her son on tolerating solids. As in African American families, there usually is a significant involvement of the extended family in infant feeding because most Navajos continue to live in extended family groups. The grandmother's illness prevented her from participating directly in J.B.'s feeding or modeling ways for her daughter to encourage J.B.'s exploration and enjoyment of solid foods; thus, the usual cultural-familial social supports that buttress the cultural practices of independent toddler self-feeding and prolonged breast-feeding were unavailable. The nutritional outcome of this case was excellent once J.B. was weaned from breast-feeding and he began to take adequate oral feeding. It is interesting to consider whether there may have been other culturally appropriate treatment options. For example, perhaps allowing another family member to care for J.B. for portions of the day would have allowed him to begin to eat and to reduce the dependence on breast-feeding.

Since the late 1980s, it has been common for many Navajo mothers to breast-feed with formula supplementation from the WIC program. Prolonged use of the bottle was common even for breast-fed infants until the 1980s when the Indian Health Service began a campaign to discourage baby-bottle tooth decay.

The Navajo culture allows great independence in toddler feeding; in general, children are allowed to be quite self-directed as Navajos have respect for the autonomy and destiny of each individual (Kluckhohn & Leighton, 1974). Undernutrition is uncommon in Navajo infants and toddlers, a change from the mid-1970s. WIC had a major effect in eradicating undernutrition in young children in this population. Rare cases of undernutrition are seen in instances of prolonged unsupplemented breast-feeding and in families who live in severe poverty or social disruption, such as that caused by alcoholism.

Mexican American

P.J. is a 6-month-old Mexican American girl who presented to the pediatrician with a 20% weight loss over 6 weeks. Her physical examination was consistent with protein-energy malnutrition (PEM). Her history revealed that she had developed diarrhea 6 weeks before and that the doctor had prescribed an oral rehydration solution (ORS). Because P.J.'s bowel movements had not become normal in consistency, her mother had continued to feed her only the rehydration solution for the entire 6-week period.

Mexican American adults are accustomed to treating diarrhea with rice water, which is a type of ORS. Their belief is that it cures the diarrhea; however, the medical goal was not to eradicate the diarrhea but to treat and prevent dehydration. If ORS is used for a prolonged period of time, then the child may develop starvation diarrhea. In this case, a well-meaning mother armed with a cultural belief that rice water cures diarrhea inadvertently exposed her child to starvation and PEM. This could have been avoided by specific instructions by the doctor about the importance of continuing nutritional intake such as formula and food along with the rehydration solution. Although cultural attitudes played a role in P.J.'s malnutrition, this course of events could happen in many different cultural contexts if physicians do not communicate clearly about the length and goal of treatment.

In the 1990s, many Mexican American women have given up breast-feeding in favor of emulating the dominant culture: Many believe that it is more "American" to bottle-feed. Fat babies are highly valued, and feeding of solids often begins before 4 months of age. Mashed rice, fruits, and vegetables are common first foods. During the toddler period, independence is allowed and children are given great choice about the foods that they eat. Although undernutrition is unusual in this population, the availability of and preference for snack foods may predispose these children to other forms of malnutrition, such as obesity or micronutrient deficiencies. This is an important area for research and nutritional counseling and guidance. It is worth mentioning that as health care becomes more restricted for undocumented aliens, children who are citizens (born in the United States) may be at risk for poor medical care if their parents fear seeking timely care because of their own immigration status.

Vietnamese Refugee

N.D. is a 2-year-old Vietnamese boy with poor growth. His family came to the United States after spending 6 months in a refugee camp in the Philippines. He had been fed from birth with formula from Russia. His parents could not read the preparation instructions in Russian, so they mixed the formula to taste. Solids were introduced at 4 months in the form of rice flour mixed with formula or mashed rice and broth mixed together. In the refugee camp, at the age of 10 months, he was given canned milk once every evening and rice broth with meat and vegetables twice per day. The family arrived in Seattle when N.D. was 1 year of age, at which time he was started on a standard infant formula by a pediatric care provider. The parents again could not read the preparation instructions and continued to mix his formula to taste. They continued to offer him broth with rice and vegetables twice per day.

This example illustrates the impact of removing cultural supports and putting young parents in a situation in which they cannot feed their infant according to cultural norms. Without the basis of knowledge provided by a cultural practice, mistakes are inevitable.

The feeding history also highlights the conditions of scarcity in refugee camps in which infant and toddler refugees must attempt to maintain adequate growth. In the context of inadequate formula and food scarcity, the cultural norms for first solid foods for infants also may have contributed to the risk for undernutrition.

In Vietnam, women almost always breast-feed their infants; yet after immigrating to America, 90% of these women choose to bottle-feed, reporting reasons of convenience and avoidance of embarrassment (Romero-Gwynn, 1989; Tuttle & Dewey, 1994). Introduction of solid foods occurs between 3 and 6 months. Premasticated food has been a common way to offer infants their first solid feeding; boiled and mashed rice is a common first food. Meals are not necessarily scheduled because families are expected to respond unconditionally to an infant's demands. Early self-feeding is uncommon in this culture, and even 4-year-olds often are spoon-fed by their mother. These children are not reported to object or to insist on feeding themselves.

FINAL COMMENTS

The 1990 U.S. Census identified more than 60 countries of origin for immigrants (Eliades & Suitor, 1994). No one can be expected to be expert in all cultures. The challenge for providers who care for undernourished children is to become sensitized to how their professional and personal cultural backgrounds influence their work with families. In an increasingly multicultural United States, clinicians are compelled to become familiar with the socioeconomic and cultural issues that may either influence the provider–parent relationship or play a role in the development, treatment, and recovery of the child from undernutrition. Providers would be wise to expect that their explanatory models will differ from those held by parents. This may reduce the clinician's anxiety and frustration when he or she is faced with inevitable clashes of culture.

Providers routinely should ask families from mainstream American cultures (e.g., Caucasians of Western European heritage) as well as nonmainstream cultural subgroups about their beliefs and practices related to feeding, illness and growth, and help-seeking behavior. With many parents, a respectful inquiry into the parents' perceptions and experiences will have the added benefit of fostering the therapeutic relationship between provider and family. With a strong foundation in place for provider–parent collaboration, the match or mismatch between the family's way of doing things and their child's individual developmental and temperament-based needs can be assessed. Parents should be asked directly about relevant folk illnesses that may play a role in the parents' understanding of the undernutrition or its developmental and behavioral sequelae. Guidelines from the model of clinical negotiation can help the provider and the parent to develop an action plan to help the child.

REFERENCES

Americans with Disabilities Act (ADA) of 1990, PL 101-336, 42 U.S.C. §§ 12101 *et seq.*

Anderson, P.P., & Fenichel, E.S. (1989). *Serving culturally diverse families of infants and toddlers with disabilities.* Washington, DC: National Center for Clinical Infant Programs.

Bagley, S., Angel, R., Dilworth-Anerson, P., Liu, W., & Schinke, S. (1995). Panel V: Adaptive health behaviors among ethnic minorities. *Health Psychology, 14,* 632–640.

Barker, J. (1992). Cultural diversity: Changing the context of medical practice. *Western Journal of Medicine, 157,* 248–254.

Barness, L.A. (Ed.). (1993). *Pediatric nutrition handbook* (3rd ed.). Elk Grove Village, IL: American Academy of Pediatrics, Committee on Nutrition.

Bentley, M.E., Dickin, K.L., Mebrahtu, S., Kayode, B., Oni, G.A., Verzosa, C.C., Brown, K.H., & Idowu, J.R. (1991). Development of a nutritionally adequate and culturally appropriate weaning food in Kwaru State, Nigeria: An interdisciplinary approach. *Social Science and Medicine, 33,* 1103–1111.

Birrer, R.B. (Ed.). (1987). *Urban family medicine.* London: Springer-Verlag.

Black, R.F., Blair, J.P., Jones, V.N., & Durant, R.H. (1990). Infant feeding decisions among pregnant women from a WIC population in Georgia. *Journal of the American Dietetic Association, 90,* 255–259.

Brown, A.B. (1986). Nutritional anthropology: The community focus. In S.A. Quandt & C. Ritenbaugh (Eds.), *Training manual in nutritional anthropology* (No. 20, pp. 41–59). Washington, DC: American Anthropological Association.

Cassidy, C. (1980). Benign neglect and toddler malnutrition. In L.S. Greene (Ed.), *Social and biological predictors of nutritional status, physical growth and neurological development* (pp. 109–139). San Diego: Academic Press.

Cushner, K., & Brislin, R.W. (1996). *Intercultural interactions: A practical guide* (2nd ed.). Thousand Oaks, CA: Sage Publications.

Derman-Sparks, L. (1995). Developing culturally responsive caretaking practices: Acknowledge, ask and adapt. In P.L. Mangione (Ed.), *Infant/toddler caregiving: A guide to culturally sensitive care* (pp. 40–63). Sacramento: California Department of Education.

Dettwyler, K.A. (1989). Styles of infant feeding: Parental/caretaker control of food consumption in young children. *American Anthropologist, 91,* 696–703.

Drotar, D., & Sturm, L. (1988). Parent–practitioner communication in the management of nonorganic failure to thrive. *Family Systems Medicine, 6,* 304–316.

Dwyer, J.T. (1993). Vegetarianism in children. In P.M. Queen & C.E. Lang (Eds.), *Handbook of pediatric nutrition* (pp. 171–186). Gaithersburg, MD: Aspen Publishers.

Eliades, D.C., & Suitor, C.W. (1994). *Celebrating diversity: Approaching families through their food.* Arlington, VA: National Center for Education in Maternal and Child Health.

Engle, P.L., Zeitlin, M., Medrano, Y., & Garcia, M.L. (1996). Growth consequences of low-income Nicaraguan mothers' theories about feeding 1-year-olds. In S. Harkness & C.M. Super (Eds.), *Parents' cultural belief systems: Their origins, expressions, and consequences* (pp. 428–446). New York: Guilford Press.

Finerman, R. (1995). "Parental incompetence" and "selective neglect": Blaming the victim in child survival. *Social Science and Medicine, 40,* 5–13.

Finerman, R., & Bennett, L.A. (1995). Overview: Guilt, blame and shame in sickness. *Social Science and Medicine, 40,* 1–3.

Flack, J.M., Amaro, H., Jenkins, W., Junitz, S., Levy, J., Mixon, M., & Yu, E. (1995). Panel I: Epidemiology of minority health. *Health Psychology, 14,* 592–600.

Gonzales-Mena, J. (1993). *Multicultural issues in child care.* Mountain View, CA: Mayfield Publishing Co.

Harry, B. (1992). Developing cultural self-awareness: The first step in values clarification for early interventionists. *Topics in Early Childhood Special Education, 12,* 330–350.

Harwood, A. (1981). Guidelines for culturally appropriate health care. In A. Harwood (Ed.), *Ethnicity and medical care* (pp. 482–507). Cambridge, MA: Harvard University Press.

Hellman, C.G. (1990). *Culture, health and illness: An introduction for health professionals.* London: Wright.

Jenkins, C.L., Orr-Ewing, A.K., & Heywood, P.F. (1984). Cultural aspects of early childhood growth and nutrition among the Amele of lowland Papua New Guinea. *Ecology of Food and Nutrition, 14,* 261–275.

Jolly, P., & Hudley, D. (1996). *AAMC data book statistical information related to medical education.* Washington, DC: Association of American Medical Colleges.

Karrer, B.M. (1987). Families of Mexican descent: A contextual approach. In R. Birrer (Ed.), *Urban family medicine* (pp. 228–232). London: Springer-Verlag.

Katon, W., & Kleinman, A. (1981). Doctor–patient negotiation and other social science strategies in patient care. In L. Eisenberg & A. Kleinman (Eds.), *The relevance of social science for medicine* (pp. 253–279). Boston: D. Reidel.

Kinsman, S.B., Sally, M., & Fox, K. (1996). Multicultural issues in pediatric practice. *Pediatrics in Review, 17,* 349–354.

Kleinman, A., Eisenberg, L., & Good, B. (1978). Culture, illness, and care: Clinical lessons from anthropologic and cross-cultural research. *Annals of Internal Medicine, 88,* 251–258.

Kluckhohn, C., & Leighton, D. (1974). *The Navajo.* Cambridge, MA: Harvard University Press.

Lieberman, A.F. (1995). Concerns of immigrant families. In P.L. Mangione (Ed.), *Infant/toddler caregiving: A guide to culturally sensitive care* (pp. 28–37). Sacramento: California Department of Education.

Liptak, G.S. (1996). Enhancing patient compliance in pediatrics. *Pediatrics in Review, 17,* 128–134.

Lynch, E.W., & Hanson, M.J. (Eds.). (1998). *Developing cross-cultural competence: A guide for working with young children and their families* (2nd ed.). Baltimore: Paul H. Brookes Publishing Co.

Mac Kune-Karrer, B., & Taylor, E.H. (1995). Toward multiculturality: Implications for the pediatrician. *Pediatric Clinics of North America, 42,* 21–30.

Magana, A., & Clark, N.M. (1995). Examining a paradox: Does religiosity contribute to positive birth outcomes in Mexican American populations? *Health Education Quarterly, 22,* 96–109.

Mennella, J.A. (1996). The flavor world of infants: A cross-cultural perspective. *Pediatric Basics, 77,* 2–8.

Mennella, J.A., Johnson, A., & Beauchamp, G.K. (1995). Garlic ingestion by pregnant women alters the odor of amniotic fluid. *Chemical Senses, 20,* 207–209.

Najib, N., Laraque, D., & Leung, J. (1996). Failure to thrive during Ramadan: A patient report. *Clinical Pediatrics, 35,* 323–326.

Nugent, J.K. (1994). Cross cultural studies of child development: Implications for clinicians. *Zero to Three, 15,* 1–8.

Pachter, L.M. (1994). Culture and clinical care: Folk illness beliefs and behaviors and their implications for health care delivery. *Journal of the American Medical Association, 271,* 690–694.

Pachter, L.M., & Dworkin, P.H. (1996, April). *Cultural beliefs and maternal expectations regarding normal infant development.* Paper presented at the International Conference on Infant Studies, Providence, RI.

Pachter, L.M., & Harwood, R. (1996). Culture and child behavior and psychosocial development. *Developmental and Behavioral Pediatrics, 17,* 191–198.

Parraga, I.M., Weber, M.A., Engel, A., Reeb, K.G., & Lerner, E. (1988). Feeding patterns of urban black infants. *Journal of the American Dietetic Association, 88,* 796–800.

Patel, N., Power, T.G., & Bhavnagri, N.P. (1996). Socialization values and practices of Indian immigrant parents: Correlates of modernity and acculturation. *Child Development, 67,* 302–313.

Phillips, D.B., & Cooper, R.M. (1992). Cultural dimensions of feeding relationships. *Zero to Three, 12,* 10–13.

Pomerleau, A., Malcuit, G., & Sabatier, C. (1991). Child-rearing practices and parental beliefs in three cultural groups of Montreal: Quebecois, Vietnamese, Haitian. In M.H. Bornstein (Ed.), *Cultural approaches to parenting* (pp. 45–68). Mahwah, NJ: Lawrence Erlbaum Associates.

Pugliese, M.T., Weyman-Daum, M., Moses, N., & Lifshitz, F. (1987). Parental health beliefs as a cause of nonorganic failure to thrive. *Pediatrics, 80,* 175–182.

Rauch, J.B., & Curtiss, C.R. (1992). *Taking a family health/genetic history: An ethnocultural learning guide and handbook.* Baltimore: University of Maryland at Baltimore School of Social Work.

Richardson, B.D. (1975). Lactation in grandmothers. *South African Medical Journal, 49,* 20–28.

Romero-Gwynn, E. (1989). Breast feeding pattern among Indochinese immigrants in northern California. *American Journal of Diseases of Children, 143,* 804–808.

Shawyer, R., Gani, A., Punufimana, A.N., & Seuseu, N.K.F. (1996). The role of clinical vignettes in rapid ethnographic research: A folk taxonomy of diarrhoea in Thailand. *Social Science and Medicine, 42,* 111–123.

Solem, B.J., Norr, K.F., & Gallo, A.M. (1992). Infant feeding practices of low-income mothers. *Journal of Pediatric Health Care, 6,* 54–59.

Stack, C. (1974). *All our kin: Strategies for survival in a black community.* New York: HarperCollins.

Sturm, L., & Drotar, D. (1992). Communication strategies for working with parents of infants who fail to thrive. *Zero to Three, 12,* 25–28.

Sturm, L., Drotar, D., Laing, K., & Zimet, G. (1997). Mothers' beliefs about causes of infant growth deficiency: Is there attributional bias? *Journal of Pediatric Psychology, 22,* 329–344.

Tervalon, M.M. (1995, May). *The multicultural project at Children's Hospital Oakland, 1994–1995: Origin, content, process, structure and lessons for other health care institutions.* Paper presented at the annual meeting of the Ambulatory Pediatric Association, San Diego.

Tuttle, C.R., & Dewey, K.G. (1994). Determinants of infant feeding choices among southeast Asian immigrants in northern California. *Journal of the American Dietetic Association, 94,* 282–286.

U.S. Bureau of the Census. (1995). *Population profile of the United States: 1995* (Current Population Reports, Series P23-189). Washington, DC: U.S. Government Printing Office.

Van Duzen, J., Carter, J.P., & VanderZwagg, R. (1969). Protein and calorie malnutrition among preschool Navajo Indian children. *American Journal of Clinical Nutrition, 22,* 1362–1370.

Van Duzen, J., Carter, J.P., & VanderZwagg, R. (1976). Protein and calorie malnutrition among preschool Navajo Indian children, a followup. *American Journal of Clinical Nutrition, 29,* 657–662.

Westermeyer, J. (1991). Psychiatric services for refugee children: An overview. In F.L. Ahearn, Jr., & J.L. Athey (Eds.), *Refugee children: Theory, research, and services* (pp. 127–162). Baltimore: The Johns Hopkins University Press.

Zeitlin, M. (1996). My child is my crown: Yoruba parental theories and practices in early childhood. In S. Harkness & C.M. Super (Eds.), *Parents' cultural belief systems* (pp. 407–427). New York: Guilford Press.

SELECTED RESOURCES ON CULTURAL ISSUES

Food and Nutrition Service and Public Health Service. (1990). *Cross-cultural counseling: A guide for nutrition and health counselors.* Washington, DC: U.S. Department of Agriculture and U.S. Department of Health and Human Services. (Available from National Maternal & Child Health Clearinghouse, 2070 Chain Bridge Road, Suite 450, Vienna, VA 22182; [703] 356-1964)

National Center for Education in Maternal and Child Health. (1996). *Celebrating diversity: Approaching families through their food* [Annotated resource list]. Arlington, VA: Author. (Available from NCEMCH, 2000 15th Street North, Suite 701, Arlington, VA 22201-2617; [703] 524-7802)

AT&T Language Line: offers interpreting in 140 languages, 7 days per week, 24 hours per day. Contact Marketing Department: (800) 752-0093.

American Sign Language: for access to interpreters, contact the local state office serving Deaf and hard-of-hearing individuals.

HEALTH ASSOCIATIONS FOR SPECIFIC CULTURAL SUBGROUPS

American Indian Health Care Association
245 E. Sixth Street
Suite 499
St. Paul, MN 55101
(612) 293-0233

Asian and Pacific Islander American Health Forum
116 New Montgomery
Suite 531
San Francisco, CA 94105
(415) 541-0866

National Coalition of Hispanic Health and Human Services Organizations (COSSMHO)
1030 15th Street, NW
10th Floor
Washington, DC 20005
(202) 371-2100

National Migrant Resource Program
1515 Capital of Texas Highway South
Suite 220
Austin, TX 78746
(512) 328-7682

Chapter 27

Family Routines and the Feeding Process

H. Lorrie Yoos, Harriet Kitzman, and Robert Cole

Sustenance, stimulation, and support are important elements that enable young children to thrive (Bradley, 1995). For these elements to achieve maximum benefit, they need to be organized into meaningful patterns. A child care system that provides regular routines that are somewhat structured around the child's own biological rhythms promotes better outcomes for the child (Keltner, 1990, 1992; Thomas, 1995). Assessing the routines of daily family life may give health care providers and other professionals an important insight into young children's nutrition and general well-being as well as provide a basis for intervention strategies.

FAMILY ROUTINES

Family routines are a critical aspect of structuring the child's environment to provide predictable and stable features to the day (Norton, 1993). Routines are the day-to-day repetitive activities that occur within the family unit in a predictable manner (Boyce, Jensen, James, & Peacock, 1983; Denham, 1995; Keltner, Keltner, & Farran, 1990). Not only do routines give temporal anchors to the day for child and parent, but they also afford opportunities for social interaction and promote the regulation of biological rhythms (Klinnert & Bingham, 1994). One of the important tasks for an infant in the first months of life is behavioral organization (Minde, Barr, & Benoit, 1995). Neurobehavioral development in young children involves, in part, the ability of the child to coordinate internal biological clocks, which have recurring body signals, such as hunger, with periodic environmental cues, such as the light–dark cycle, and regularly scheduled periods of social interaction (Sadeh & Anders, 1993). Some infants and young children have more difficulty regulating their biological states and needs. For these children in particular, Minde et al. (1995) proposed that parents help with external regulation. Routines that take into consideration the child's rhythms and needs afford such an opportunity.

Two important activities in the young child's life around which routines evolve are mealtime and bedtime. Mealtime and bedtime routines for the infant and young child often are interrelated. Sadeh and Anders (1993) proposed that inconsistent feedings may reflect general inconsistency in parenting, which in turn influences the consolidation of sleep–wake patterns. According to Johnson (1993), following a regular, predictable daily routine is the single most important measure that parents can take to help their infants with sleep regulation.

In addition to promoting biological rhythms, mealtimes are an important opportunity for interaction between children and caregivers. Food and feeding have immense cultural and social importance; much of family life revolves around meals (Mackenzie, 1995). Appropriate feeding is a metaphor for the nurturing relationship, and mealtime routines and rituals play a central role in human connectedness in most cultures (Mackenzie, 1995). Clear variations exist across families and cultures in the balance of parent–child control over meal timing, frequency of meals, control of meal size, and food selection.

There is some preliminary evidence that a predictable environment acts as a stabilizing force for the child, even in the presence of other stressors and disadvantages (Keltner et al., 1990; Werner & Smith, 1982). The Kauai study (Werner & Smith, 1982) of 698 children identified several characteristics that are associated with stress resistance and competence. A central component of coping with stressors was believed to be the child's feeling of confidence that his or her environment was predictable and understandable.

Factors that Influence Family Routines

A number of child, family, and broader contextual factors influence the development of routines that are associated with caregiving and feeding. Child characteristics that may influence the development of and response to routines include age, general health, and temperament of the child. The specific type of feeding difficulty often varies as a function of the age of the child (Sanders, Rinu, LeGrice, & Shepherd, 1993). A number of mealtime behaviors are influenced by child temperament. Low-intensity infants who have a reduced level of response may not signal their hunger needs effectively. Distractible children who are diverted readily by extraneous stimuli may be drawn away from the table by siblings or television (Chess & Thomas, 1977). How early in life the child develops a regular feeding schedule, how long the child will stay at the dinner table, the approach to new foods and textures, and the desire for meals at a certain time all are affected by temperament (Zuckerman, 1995).

Maternal and family characteristics that have been implicated in feeding disorders include parental depression, social isolation, substance abuse, family conflict and other stressors, and parental knowledge and beliefs about nutrition and ideal weight (Drotar, 1991; Sanders et al., 1993). Depression may jeopardize caregiving routines through the parent's sense of helplessness and loss of control. For the isolated mother, there may be few role models who have meaningful structure to their day.

The social context potentially affects the development of pediatric undernutrition in diverse ways. A number of aspects of contemporary life make the development of family and mealtime routines challenging. Barriers may range from poverty, with its impact on material and emotional resources, to the lack of opportunities for meaningful structure in the life of an adolescent mother who attends neither school nor work. Dual-income homes with multiple, competing demands and complex schedules also may find family time and family routines undermined. Twenty-four–hour availability of prepared or prepackaged fast foods makes mealtime preparation less central to the life of the family; thus, the time that each individual may eat becomes more flexible. Individual family members may eat on the way to a variety of activities without sharing a meal with other family members or indeed being aware of their meals. Having multiple caregivers within the household or in alternative child care settings makes the possibility of consistent feeding practices for children more difficult.

The contribution of family routines to adequate caregiving and nutrition has not been studied extensively. Denham (1995) suggested that research and clinical practice should incorporate consideration of family routines when there is concern about the health status of an individual. These child, family, and contextual factors may function directly to affect nutrition, or they may affect it indirectly by impairing the family's ability to adopt useful routines of caregiving. Interventions that are related to helping families achieve functional daily routines may, in this model, foster positive outcomes, even in the presence of adverse interactional and contextual factors. Figure 1 summarizes the proposed model.

Effective Mealtime Routines

Health care professionals generally counsel parents about appropriate nutrition for children at various developmental stages. Advice about how to structure mealtimes is an important component of anticipatory guidance.

Infants

Across cultures and throughout history, the prevailing approach to infant feeding has been to allow the infant to take the lead in determining the timing of meals and to feed on demand. A notable exception to this view was the strict scheduling of infant feedings in the United States in the 1920s and 1930s. Over time, there has been a return to on-demand feedings for the infant (Birch & Fisher, 1995). From a strictly physiological perspective, breast-fed infants usually empty the stomach in 2–3 hours, whereas bottle-fed infants may require 3–4 hours or longer. This provides some guidance in terms of appropriate feeding intervals.

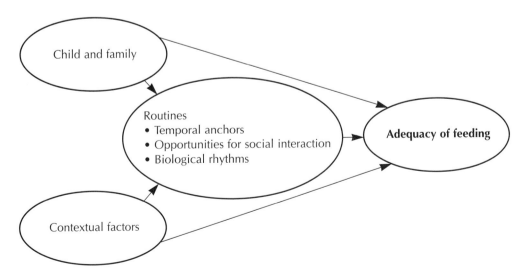

Figure 1.   Factors that influence the development of caregiving and feeding.

Many child development specialists and health care providers believe that encouraging infants to develop patterns of behavior in response to their own needs is essential for optimum infant growth and development and for the evolution of **contingency interactions** between caregivers and infants (Blackburn, 1983). This type of interaction enables children to recognize that there is a connection between their actions and the resulting response by the caregiver. The supportive mother modulates infant arousal by responding promptly to hunger cues and organizes the infant by responding to his or her schedule, regulation of amounts, and feeding abilities. By responding appropriately to their infants' needs yet providing stable routines, caregivers help them to modulate physiological tension and support their development of physiological regulation (Cicchetti, 1996).

The type of feeding routine also affects the development of **circadian rhythms** and cycles that approximate a 24-hour period (Thomas, 1995). Because most adult caregivers organize their own lives according to a 24-hour clock, this is an important achievement for the infant. Contrary to concerns about spoiling the infant, on-demand feeding reinforces the infant's developing sleep–wake rhythm and actually is related to movement of the longest sleep interval to nighttime hours (Hellbrugge, Lange, Rutenfranz, & Stehr, 1964). Infants who are fed on a strict schedule that does not attend to their own biological rhythms are denied opportunities to develop patterns of behavior that provide hunger cues to their caregivers (Saunders, Friedman, & Stramoski, 1991). Fomon (1993) submitted that allowing the infant to control the timing and the size of feedings also is conducive to establishing habits of eating in moderation.

Whether all parents are capable of determining what a particular infant wants at a given point in time is an important consideration for the health care provider, as is the infant who gives few or very subtle hunger cues. There is considerable variation both in children's ability to communicate their needs with clarity and in parents' abilities to read and respond to cues. Feeding on demand risks that some parents will feed at all signs of infant distress or discomfort rather than evaluate other needs and attempt other interventions such as stimulation. Conversely, low-intensity infants may, in some households, be underfed because they fail to communicate their needs. Wolke, Skuse, and Mathisen (1990) found that infants who are experiencing failure to thrive vocalize less and use low-level, undifferentiated communication signals. For these infants, health care providers may need to make recommendations about the maximum amount of time that is permissible between feedings and, in fact, establish an appropriate schedule. As mentioned previously, some infants require more external structuring than others in terms of neurobehavioral organization.

Silver, Kempe, Bruyn, and Fulginiti (1987) proposed that neither strict adherence to a time schedule nor feeding whenever the infant cries is necessary for successful feeding. For most parents and infants, a flexible schedule with reasonable regularity probably is most satisfactory. In some cases, however, professionals may need to help families reduce or increase their temporal structuring of feedings. Systematic studies that have investigated the effects of on-demand versus scheduled feedings on infants' physical growth are not available (Birch & Fisher, 1995; Fomon, 1993).

Toddlers and Preschoolers

Whereas the infant benefits from routines that are developed in response to infant needs, the toddler and older child benefit from adult help in structuring the day. As infants become older, they begin to be socialized into the temporal patterns of meals for their culture, and their control over the timing of their meals generally becomes more limited (Birch & Fisher, 1995). *Hunger* as a biological phenomenon and *appetite* as a learned response that is associated with past experiences with food begin to be differentiated. Toddlers, unlike newborns, do not benefit from being fed on demand (see Chapter 7). To mature optimally, toddlers need the structure of regularly scheduled meals and snacks with restriction of food handouts between these scheduled times. Toomey (1994) found that toddlers who are offered structured meals and snacks and who are not allowed food or caloric beverages between these times eat as much as 50% more than those who are allowed to snack at will. They come to the table hungry and are willing to approach the food there, and they are able to eat with concentration and focus until they are full. Frank (1995) recommended that young children eat often but not constantly. Similarly, Birch and Fisher (1995) recommended that while they allow children control over how much is eaten, parents should work toward shaping the timing of the child's meals to the adult pattern of the culture by imposing some control over meal intervals. The American Academy of Pediatrics, Committee on Nutrition (1993) recommended three meals and two snacks per day for this age group.

Recommendations for older children include that adults provide structured, nutritious meals and snacks, including breakfast, and limit eating between those times (Satter, 1995). Parental control over the amount and the type of snacks by older children also is recommended by the American Academy of Pediatrics, Committee on Nutrition (1993). Table 1 summarizes recommendations that are related to mealtime routines for young children.

Other Routines in the Young Child's Life

Lack of mealtime routines may reflect a more generalized disorganization within the household that also affects other caregiving behaviors. Not infrequently, mealtime and bedtime routines are interrelated, and intervention in both caregiving activities is mutually beneficial. Helping families to develop manageable strategies in relationship to this very specific content area may promote cooperation, satisfaction, and cohesiveness in other areas of family life and caregiving. Sprunger, Boyce, and Gaines (1985) found that families who had higher scores on the Family Routines Inventory (Boyce et al., 1983) had

Table 1.   Effective mealtime routines

Infants:
- Provide "demand" feeding for newborns.
  1. Feed promptly when the infant is hungry.
  2. Feed on the infant's schedule, but provide stable routines.
  3. Let the infant set the tempo.

Toddlers and older children:
- Feed young children often (three meals and two snacks per day) but not constantly ("grazing").
- Control the menu, and structure the eating time.
- Provide a variety of healthful foods at regularly scheduled meals, but allow children to determine what and how much they will eat.
- Resist children's demands for specific foods at odd times ("food begging").
- Have at least one shared family meal per day.
- Monitor the quality and timing of snacks of the older child.
- Discourage snacking and eating during television viewing.

Overall:
- If other family members or child care providers are feeding the child, then talk about which foods are being given and when.
- Try to organize work and child care so that as few people as possible are feeding and caring for the child.
- Separate meals, as much as possible, from the stresses of the day.

higher scores on perceived maternal competence and overall family adjustment. Mealtime and bedtime patterns are readily amenable to concrete suggestions and focused interventions, much more so than factors such as maternal depression, relational issues, and poverty. Interventions may be particularly useful in high-risk groups such as single adolescent mothers who may not have family routines.

Achieving regularity in the timing of daily functions such as eating and sleeping is an important part of early socialization. For the parents, developing a reliable day–night pattern is important as the infant becomes connected with the family. For the infant, there likely are physiological benefits associated with organized sleep that may be related to growth hormone or **cortisol** levels (Gunnar, 1989). Environmental cues such as light and dark, noise and quiet help to synchronize the infant's behavior. Providing structure and repetition creates a predictable, recurrent pattern of events so that the infant can anticipate the next activity (Froese-Fretz & Keefe, 1997).

For older children, when activities such as eating, sleeping, and playing are unpredictable or do not correspond to the child's biological rhythms, the child is under stress from unmet biological needs. Stress that is associated with hunger and sleep deprivation interferes with the self-regulation of behaviors and is often expressed through irritability, aggression, and/or difficulty attending to tasks (Blum & Carey, 1996). Mealtime and bedtime routines help children to understand the cyclical nature of time and provide important anchors of predictability within their day. Following is a brief discussion of bedtime routines and appropriate sleep hygiene for the infant and young child.

Sleep problems may be divided into two broad categories: bedtime struggles and night awakenings. Bedtime struggles involve difficulties and resistance on the part of the child with initially being put to bed; night awakening involves a request for interaction after child and parent have had a period of sleep. At times, the two sleep problems coexist. The process for establishing useful bedtime routines for both parent and child should begin in the earliest months of life. Probably the single most important strategy is to put the infant to bed while he or she is drowsy but still awake. This teaches the infant self-soothing skills, which may also be used for middle-of-the-night awakening (Blum & Carey, 1996; Ferber, 1992). Establishing physical environments that are conducive to sleep as well as consistent, predictable, relaxing bedtime routines is important for good sleep hygiene. Table 2 summarizes these activities.

Toni is a 17-month-old girl who has been brought to the doctor for a well-child visit. She was last seen at the age of 11 months and is behind in immunizations. Toni was born at term to an 18-year-old mother and weighed 3,850 grams (75th percentile) and measured 50 centimeters in length (50th percentile). Prenatal history was negative for problems, and her health has been good, according to her mother. At Toni's last visit, her height and weight were at the 50th percentile. Today, Toni weighs 9,400 grams (20th percentile) and is 79 centimeters tall (40th percentile) (weight-for-height 10th percentile). Development, according to her mother, is normal, although her language skills are delayed—she has only a five-word vocabulary. Toni's mother describes Toni as busy, always on the go. The family history for medical problems is negative. Toni's mother is 5 feet, 5 inches tall and weighs 130 pounds. Her father is reported to be about 6 feet tall. He is not in the household.

There have been no significant illnesses since the 11-month visit. The physical exam as well as screening laboratory tests are essentially negative except for a mild anemia.

Table 2.   Effective bedtime routines

Infants: Average amount of sleep is 16½ hours per day at 1 week of age and 14 hours per day at 1 year of age (Blum & Carey, 1996).

- Put the infant to bed drowsy but awake from the beginning to promote the development of self-soothing skills.
- Taper then discontinue night feedings after about 6 months of age.
- Introduce transitional objects (objects [e.g., special blankets, teddy bears] that help the child work through the challenges of separation and individuation) at around 6 months of age.
- Regularize both daytime and nighttime routines to help establish circadian rhythms (Ferber, 1992).

Toddlers and older children: Average amount of sleep is 12–13 hours per day.

- Communicate to the older infant that nighttime is neither a mealtime nor a playtime.
- Limit nap length to ensure that the child is tired at bedtime.
- Provide transitional objects such as a favorite blanket or a stuffed animal at bedtime.
- Leave the child's room at the end of the bedtime routine, and do not succumb to tantrums or pleading for further interaction.

All ages:

- Establish and maintain a relaxing and consistent bedtime routine.
- Provide quiet and sufficient darkness (a nightlight may be useful).
- Normal sleep cycles for all ages include brief nighttime awakening. Young children need to learn to make the transition to sleep by themselves.
- Remember that chronic sleep deprivation serves neither the parent nor the child.

Toni's mother has recently (within the past 4 months) returned to work as a waitress. She has pieced together a patchwork of child care: The child is cared for by a variety of family members. She has indicated that she is afraid of using strangers. She has a difficult time giving a feeding history because multiple providers feed Toni. Toni falls asleep in front of the television every night and generally awakens too late for breakfast at home prior to rushing out in order to accommodate her mother's work schedule.

METHODS OF ASSESSMENT

Information about the feeding interactions and routines within a household may be gathered by a variety of means including interviews, diaries and logs, and home observations (see Figure 2 and Appendix F). The clinician needs a feel for how the family is structured and who provides material and social support. Asking the parent to describe a typical day in the life of the child may give data that alerts the health care provider to potential problem areas. Possible questions include what and how much is eaten, who feeds the child, and when and where meals and snacks are consumed. In addition to patterns that are related to the child's eating, it is useful to ask about other routines for the child as well as routines for the entire family. Does the family eat together as a unit on a regular basis? Does the family eat at the same time most nights? What are the parents' work schedules? What are the bedtime patterns? Who cares for the child when the parents are unavailable?

Scheduling conflicts and demands that may affect meals should be elicited. Further important information about meals may be gathered through a 24-hour dietary recall for a typical day and a mealtime log for a 2- to 3-day period. A direct observation of feeding, ideally in the child's home, is often extraordinarily helpful.

MEALTIME LOG

Date	Time of day	Where	Food eaten (what and how much)	Adult present

Figure 2. Mealtime log.

Toni's mother is unable to give an adequate 24-hour food recall because Toni is fed by a variety of caregivers who apparently do not communicate with one another about her intake. Mealtimes and rules about eating vary from household to household as do other routines, such as naps and bedtime. Toni's mother's meals also are erratic, and the two rarely eat a meal together.

Toni's mother is instructed to obtain a 2- to 3-day food log from the various child care providers in order to capture a total 24-hour intake for several days. She is startled by how minimal the actual intake is when the log is reviewed with the health care provider and calories are calculated.

Interventions with Toni's mother included specific instructions with regard to nutritional requirements for a toddler as well as recommendations about mealtime and bedtime routines. An iron supplement was given to treat Toni's anemia. The proposed daily schedule was shared with all of Toni's child care providers, and Toni's mother has actually visited several child care centers as she evaluates what would offer the best overall child care situation within her financial means. A community health nurse is working with her on nutritional and parenting issues.

CONCLUSION

Specific management strategies should be tailored to the needs of the individual child and family. The interview and food log provide a basis for improving the diet and mealtime and bedtime routines. Other interventions may include education about the importance of regularity and predictability in the young child's life and helping the family to work out child care and work schedules. Care of the family that includes a child who is experiencing growth deficiency often is a long-term intervention. Home visiting is a mainstay of treatment and affords useful diagnostic information as well as the opportunity for ongoing teaching, counseling, and monitoring. Interventions that are related to establishing family routines are readily taught and potentially have the power to influence a wide range of child outcomes.

REFERENCES

American Academy of Pediatrics, Committee on Nutrition. (1993). *Pediatric nutrition handbook.* Elk Grove Village, IL: Author.

Birch, L.L., & Fisher, J.A. (1995). Appetite and eating behavior in children. *Pediatric Clinics of North America, 42,* 931–953.

Blackburn, S. (1983). Fostering behavioral development of high-risk infants. *Journal of Obstetric, Gynecologic & Neonatal Nursing, 12,* 76S–86S.

Blum, N.J., & Carey, W.B. (1996). Sleep problems among infants and young children. *Pediatrics in Review, 17,* 87–92.

Boyce, W.T., Jensen, E.W., James, S.A., & Peacock, J.L. (1983). The Family Routines Inventory: Theoretical origins. *Social Science & Medicine, 17,* 193–200.

Bradley, R. (1995). Environment and parenting. In M. Bornstein (Ed.), *Handbook of parenting* (Vol. 2, pp. 235–661). Mahwah, NJ: Lawrence Erlbaum Associates.

Chess, A., & Thomas, A. (1977). Temperament and the parent–child interaction. *Pediatric Annals, 6,* 574–582.

Cicchetti, D. (1996). Child maltreatment: Implications for developmental theory and research. *Human Development, 39,* 18–39.

Denham, S.A. (1995). Family routines: A construct for considering family health. *Holistic Nursing Practice, 9,* 11–23.

Drotar, D. (1991). The family context of nonorganic failure to thrive. *American Journal of Orthopsychiatry, 61,* 23–34.

Ferber, R. (1992). Sleep disorders. In M.D. Levine, W.B. Carey, & A.C. Crocker (Eds.), *Developmental-behavioral pediatrics* (2nd ed., pp. 398–406). Philadelphia: W.B. Saunders.

Fomon, S.J. (1993). *Nutrition of normal infants.* St. Louis: Mosby Year Book.

Frank, D. (1994). Failure to thrive. In S. Parker & B.S. Zuckerman (Eds.), *Behavioral and developmental pediatrics: A handbook for primary care* (pp. 134–140). Boston: Little, Brown.

Froese-Fretz, A., & Keefe, M. (1997). The irritable infant. A model for helping families cope. *Advance for Nurse Practitioners, 5*(2), 63–66.

Gunnar, M. (1989). Studies of the human infant's adrenocortical response to potentially stressful events. In M. Lewis & J. Worobey (Eds.), *Infant stress and coping* (pp. 3–18). San Francisco: Jossey-Bass.

Hellbrugge, T., Lange, J.E., Rutenfranz, J., & Stehr, K. (1964). Circadian periodicity of physiological functions in different stages of infancy and childhood. *Annals of the New York Academy of Science, 117,* 361–373.

Johnson, D. (1993). Helping infants learn to sleep. *Pediatric Basics, 65,* 10–15.

Keltner, B. (1990). Family characteristics of preschool social competence among black children in a Head Start program. *Child Psychiatry and Human Development, 21,* 95–108.

Keltner, B. (1992). Family influences on child health. *Pediatric Nursing, 18,* 128–131.

Keltner, B., Keltner, N., & Farran, E. (1990). Family routines and conduct disorders in adolescent girls. *Western Journal of Nursing Research, 12,* 161–174.

Klinnert, M.D., & Bingham, R.D. (1994). The organizing effects of early relationships. *Psychiatry, 57,* 1–10.

Mackenzie, M. (1995). The feeding relationship: An anthropological perspective on meals. *Pediatric Basics, 74,* 10–15.

Minde, S., Barr, R.G., & Benoit, D. (Speakers). (1995). *Infant psychiatry: Crying, feeding and sleeping problems* (Cassette Recording Vol. 16, No. 11). Port Washington, NY: Medical Information Systems, Inc.

Norton, D. (1993). Diversity, early socialization, and temporal development: The dual perspective revisited. *Social Work, 38,* 82–89.

Sadeh, A., & Anders, T. (1993). Sleep disorders. In C.H. Zeanah, Jr. (Ed.), *Handbook of infant mental health* (pp. 305–316). New York: Guilford Press.

Sanders, M.R., Rinu, K., LeGrice, B., & Shepherd, R.W. (1993). Children with persistent feeding difficulties: An observational analysis of feeding interactions of problem and non-problem eaters. *Health Psychology, 12,* 64–73.

Satter, E. (1995, July–August). Feeding dynamics: Helping children to eat well. *Journal of Pediatric Health Care,* 178–184.

Saunders, R.B., Friedman, C.B., & Stramoski, P.R. (1991). Feeding pre-term infants: Schedule or demand. *Journal of Obstetric, Gynecologic & Neonatal Nursing, 20,* 212–218.

Silver, H.K., Kempe, C.H., Bruyn, H.B., & Fulginiti, V.A. (1987). *Handbook of pediatrics.* Norwalk, CT: Appleton and Lange.

Sprunger, L.W., Boyce, W.T., & Gaines, J.A. (1985). Family–infant congruence: Routines and rhythmicity in family adaptations to a young infant. *Child Development, 56,* 564–572.

Thomas, K. (1995). Biorhythms in infants and role of the care environment. *Journal of Perinatal and Neonatal Nursing, 9,* 61–75.

Toomey, K.A. (1994). [Caloric intake of toddlers fed structured meals and snacks vs. on demand]. Unpublished raw data.

Werner, E., & Smith, R. (1982). *Vulnerable but invincible: A study of resilient children and youth.* New York: McGraw-Hill.

Wolke, D., Skuse, D., & Mathisen, B. (1990). Behavioral style in failure-to-thrive infants: A preliminary conversation. *Journal of Pediatric Psychology, 15,* 237–255.

Zuckerman, B. (1995). Healthy parenting choices: Children's temperament styles and parent expectations. *Pediatric Basics, 74,* 2–7.

RESOURCES FOR PARENTS

Cuthbertson, J., & Schevill, S. (1985). *Helping your child sleep through the night.* New York: Doubleday and Company.

Ferber, R. (1985). *Solve your child's sleep problem.* New York: Simon & Schuster.

Schmitt, B.D. (1991). *Your child's health* (2nd ed.). New York: Bantam Books.

Chapter 28

Home-Visiting Intervention for Families of Children Who Experience Growth Delay

Maureen M. Black,
Julie Berenson-Howard, and Pamela L. Cureton

Home-visiting programs to prevent low birth weight and to promote children's health have attracted national attention and have been introduced into many communities throughout the United States (Carnegie Task Force on Meeting the Needs of Young Children, 1994; U.S. General Accounting Office, 1990). Although there is limited evidence on the effectiveness of home-visiting programs in reducing growth delay, there are many lessons to be learned from home-visiting programs regarding the basic skills that families may need. This chapter reviews several home-visiting programs that have been targeted toward families with children who are experiencing growth delay, provides general recommendations for home visiting, and outlines the curriculum of one home-visiting program.

STUDIES OF HOME-VISITING PROGRAMS

Growth delay is an early marker of children's vulnerability, whether it occurs prenatally and leads to low birth weight or occurs postnatally and leads to failure to thrive (FTT). In either case, children who do not grow according to age and gender expectations are at increased risk for long-term academic and behavior problems (Aylward, Peiffer, Wright, &

Support for this chapter was provided partially by grants from the Maternal and Child Health Research Program (Title V, Social Security Act), Health Resources and Services Administration, Department of Health and Human Services, and from Share Our Strength, Inc.

Verhulst, 1989; McCormick, 1989; Oates, Peacock, & Forrest, 1984). Home-visiting programs have been developed to promote children's growth and cognitive development and to support families in their mission to provide protection and nurturance to their young children (Guralnick, 1996).

Growth

Reports of home-visiting programs that are directed toward reductions in postnatal growth delay suggest that, for the most part, home-visiting programs have been unsuccessful in altering children's rate of growth (Black, Dubowitz, Hutcheson, Berenson-Howard, & Starr, 1995; Casey et al., 1994; Drotar & Sturm, 1988, 1989; Grantham-McGregor, Powell, Walker, Chang, & Fletcher, 1994; Meyer et al., 1994). A 3-year home-visiting program for children from very-low-income families who had been hospitalized in Jamaica for malnutrition did document a slight, though significant, increase in height (1 centimeter) but no weight gain (Grantham-McGregor et al., 1994; Grantham-McGregor, Schofield, & Powell, 1987). It is unclear why home-visiting programs have had so little impact on growth, but it is possible that the children required a nutrition intervention or that the curricula did not address the specific feeding behaviors that are associated with growth delay.

Cognitive Development

Home-visiting programs that are directed toward children with growth delay also have attempted to ameliorate the decline in cognitive development that is often experienced among children with growth delay; however, the impact of home-visiting programs on children's development has been inconclusive. Two studies that implemented home visiting among children who had been hospitalized for growth delay reported no benefits in children's growth or development. One group (Haynes, Cutler, Gray, & Kempe, 1984) conducted a 6-month lay home–visitor intervention and found no differences when they compared outcomes over a period of 3 years with those of families who did not receive intervention. Drotar and Sturm (1988, 1989) compared a home-visiting program (home visitors were trained in social work, nursing, or psychology) with two less extensive types of intervention. There were no effects when the intervention ended or up to 3 years later during follow-up.

Black and colleagues (1995) conducted a randomized clinical trial of home intervention among 130 children with growth delay who were recruited from pediatric primary care clinics. They reported that at the end of the intervention, infants of mothers in the home intervention group obtained better cognitive development scores when compared with infants of mothers who received only a clinic-based intervention, although toddlers did not show a similar pattern. The home intervention also had a beneficial impact on language development and on the child-centeredness of the home among both infants and toddlers. At age 4, approximately 2 years after the home intervention ended, the children who had received the home intervention had better motor development, and those whose mothers were not depressed, anxious, or hostile had better cognitive development and behavior during play (Hutcheson et al., 1997).

Casey and colleagues (1994) examined changes in cognitive development among 180 children with FTT who participated in the Infant Health and Development Project, an eight-site randomized clinical trial of home- and center-based intervention among infants who were either born preterm or had low birth weight (less than 2,500 grams). They found that children in the intervention and control groups were equally likely to experience FTT; however, when other variables were controlled, treatment groups contributed significantly to the model for IQ scores and scores on the Home Observation for the Measurement of the Environment (HOME) inventory (Bradley & Caldwell, 1978) at 36 months. In addition, children with FTT who attended the child development center more than 250 days had more favorable IQ scores, behavior ratings, and lengths than children who attended for fewer than 250 days.

Meyer and colleagues (1994) conducted a family-based care program for 34 preterm infants who were randomized into intervention and control groups. Mothers in the intervention group reported less stress and depression and were more nurturing during interactions with their infants. Meyer and colleagues did not report differences in infant growth or development.

A report from the 8-year evaluation of the overall Infant Health and Development Project found no group differences in children's cognitive development and behavior (McCarton et al., 1997); however, children in the heavier birth weight group (2,001–2,500 grams) who received intervention obtained higher full-scale IQ scores (4.4 points), higher verbal IQ scores (4.2 points), higher performance IQ scores (3.9 points), higher mathematics achievement scores (4.8 points), and higher receptive language scores (6.7 points) than children in the control group. These differences are relatively modest (less than 0.5 standard deviation), suggesting the need to consider alternative strategies for early intervention among premature, low birth weight infants. There were no significant differences among children in the lighter birth weight group (less than 2,000 grams).

These findings suggest caution before adopting universal programs of home visiting to promote growth and development among children with growth delay. In addition, much of the research on home-visiting programs is difficult to interpret because home visiting refers to a general service delivery strategy rather than a well-defined intervention (Halpern, 1984; Powell, 1990). Goals, curricula, and procedures vary among home-visiting programs. Even the training of home visitors is controversial because some programs employ lay home visitors and others employ highly trained professionals (Musick & Stott, 1990).

HOME-VISITING RECOMMENDATIONS

Long-term evaluations of first-time mothers from low-income, semi-rural families have revealed that home visiting was effective in reducing subsequent pregnancies, welfare use, child abuse and neglect, and criminal behavior (Olds et al., 1997). Analyses of successful home-visiting programs have yielded several recommendations. The recommendations begin with a family-focused intervention framework and address the relationship between the home visitor and the family, the strategies that are useful in promoting effective parenting, the need to consider individual characteristics of the child and the family, and the importance of support.

Family-Focused Intervention

Family-focused intervention is based on the theory that children's development occurs within a multilevel social context, beginning with the family. Intervention programs should be comprehensive and include family members as partners to promote effective parenting and a nurturing, child-oriented home. Because growth delay is conceptualized as a psychosocial or family problem (Black, 1995; Drotar, 1991) rather than merely as a nutritional problem, family-focused home intervention may be an optimum strategy to promote health, growth, and development.

Home-visiting programs often utilize principles from ecological and family systems theory as they encourage primary caregivers to look to family, neighbors, and community members for support and cooperation (Bronfenbrenner, 1993). For example, adolescent mothers frequently remain in their family of origin and share caregiving with the baby's grandmother rather than marry the baby's father and move to their own household as has been done in the past. Although grandmothers often provide support, nurturing, and social, financial, and legal stability, multigenerational caregiving introduces new challenges as adolescent girls assume parenting roles (Black & Nitz, 1996). When home visitors are able to form relationships with both the mother and the grandmother, they can facilitate the negotiation of roles between mothers and grandmothers as they decide, for example, who assumes responsibility for shopping, cooking, feeding, and other caregiving tasks (Black & Bentley, 1996).

Relationship Between the Visitor and the Family

A primary recommendation for home intervention is that it be an ongoing, supportive, therapeutic alliance between the child's primary caregiver and the home visitor (Klass, 1997). Home visiting is part of many disciplines: nursing, social work, public health, medicine, and physical and occupational therapy, to name a few. In addition, there are many lay home visitors who do not have a professional degree but have participated in community-oriented training programs or supervision to learn how principles of support and intervention can be introduced in a home environment. Lay home visitors have been effective in family-focused interventions (Black et al., 1995; Sia & Breakey, 1985), their familiarity with the culture may enable them to establish relationships easily (Musick & Stott, 1990), and they may be cost-effective (Bailey & Simeonsson, 1988); however, lay home visitors may require more supervision than professionally trained home visitors.

Regardless of their training, home visitors should be selected for their experience with children and families, their interpersonal skills, their knowledge of the community, and their commitment to building on family's strengths through home visitation. Home visitors also require basic information on the goals and procedures of the program, together with ongoing supervision.

Home visiting is often seen as a negotiated partnership between families and interventionists. In contrast with earlier programs in which families were regarded as deficient or disadvantaged, families are viewed as resourceful and able to influence the services that they receive. This philosophy is consistent with the Individuals with Disabilities Education Act Amendments of 1997 (PL 105-17) in which families are included as active participants in planning and implementing services. Information flows from the home visitor to the family and from the family to the home visitor; the home visitor serves as a liaison rather than as a teacher. Home visitors begin by asking families about their strengths, needs, and priorities and then work with them to develop an individualized program.

Strategies for Effective Parenting

Modeling is an active strategy that is used to help families promote optimum growth and development among their children; however, modeling alone could lead to dependence if families are not given opportunities to practice what they have observed. Therefore, active strategies, such as shopping trips, meal preparation, and shared meals, are also used to help parents gain additional competence and confidence in using new skills.

Another example of an active strategy is a family notebook, used in a home intervention with families of children with growth delay to help mothers organize their lives (Black et al., 1995). During the initial home visit, parents put together a personalized notebook, containing a photograph of their child, a calendar to record appointments and important events, handouts describing normal child development and age-appropriate activities, and pages and pockets for a journal and personal mementos. Notebooks also include pages for recording meals and mealtimes. Parents are encouraged to use the notebook to remind themselves of upcoming appointments and events, and the home visitor periodically provides handouts that could be inserted into the notebook.

Individual Characteristics

Children's individual characteristics, such as development and temperament, are important considerations in home-visiting programs because they influence children's feeding skills and mealtime behavior. Children with growth delay are at increased risk for experiencing both developmental delays and difficult temperaments (Drotar, Eckerle, Satola, Pallotta, & Wyatt, 1990; Polan et al., 1991). Parents who do not consider their children's individual characteristics may precipitate feeding challenges that are frustrating and that lead to behavior problems (see Chapter 8). Through home observations, interventionists can observe children as they eat and help parents select foods and mealtime settings that are developmentally and temperamentally appropriate. Strategies that are effective for one developmental level (e.g., grinding table foods for the child to eat with his or her hands while seated in a highchair) may not necessarily be effective at other developmental levels. It is unlikely that one intervention strategy will be successful for all families, but incorporating children's individual characteristics into an intervention should increase the likelihood of success.

Support

A number of successful home-visiting programs have been designed to provide support to the family (Barrera, Cunningham, & Rosenbaum, 1986; Dawson, Van Doorninck, & Robinson, 1989). Parents who feel supported often have better interactions with their young children and are better able to cope with the challenges of children's health or developmental problems (Crnic, Greenberg, Ragozin, Robinson, & Basham, 1983). Because home intervention provides access to the informal activities of families, support is an important component of the relationship between the home visitor and the parent. An observant home visitor notices subtle changes in the parent, child, or household that provide opportunities for support. For example, Klass described the "shared delight in the child" (1996, p. 28) that serves as a bond between the home visitor and the parent and enables the home visitor to support the parent in his or her role.

HOME-VISITING CURRICULUM

The use of a curriculum in home-visiting programs is controversial. Although a curriculum provides the structure and criteria for evaluation, thus ensuring that important areas are addressed and that successful programs can be replicated, it must be flexible enough to enable home visitors to provide individualized support to families when crises occur. The authors of this chapter have combined individualized support with general recommendations of basic skills.

The following curriculum was developed by the authors of this chapter for low-income families of children who are experiencing growth delay. Because many families lack basic skills in meal planning and preparation, the curriculum is skill oriented and focuses on the caregiver's role in planning the child's meals. There are eight topics: shopping, food preparation, nutrition, mealtime scheduling, mealtime setting, feeding context, children's behavior, and access to services.

Intervention begins with an assessment of each family's strengths and needs, including basic skills that are associated with children's nutritional needs (Black, 1995). Topics that are relevant to each family are introduced and incorporated into the intervention in the context of a supportive relationship.

Shopping

A family's ability to buy healthful food can be hampered by the lack of supermarkets in low-income neighborhoods, by transportation, or by economic limitations (Wiecha & Palombo, 1989). Many families must rely on nearby convenience stores, which normally stock expensive, prepared foods.

The home visitor may work with the family to develop strategies for economical shopping, such as taking advantage of sales and coupons, evaluating unit pricing, and buying lower-priced cuts of meat. The home visitor may also help the family identify the best grocery stores in the area, find transportation, plan meals, and make economical purchases. By accompanying the family on shopping trips to a grocery store, the home visitor can evaluate each family's skill level and make recommendations that are tailored to the individual family's needs. Shopping trips can be used to purchase food that is then used in other components of the intervention, such as mealtime setting, feeding, nutrition, and food preparation. Shopping trips later in the intervention can serve as an evaluation of the success of the shopping intervention. For example, the home visitor may record the food that was purchased by the family and, together with a nutritionist, rate the nutritional and economic value of the purchases (e.g., low value for prepackaged, sweetened drinks).

Food Preparation

Along with familiarity with nutritional information, some families lack understanding of safe and healthful food preparation. Lack of attention to food handling and storage may result in the dangerous growth of bacteria, resulting in the possibility of food poisoning, and may lead to contamination from insects and rodents. Unhealthful food preparation may also increase the risk of long-term health problems, such as obesity or problems associated with high fat or cholesterol.

Appropriate methods of food handling, preparation, and storage can prevent spoilage and can encourage nutritious methods of cooking. By cooking together with families, home visitors can show families how to protect the vitamin content in food, decrease the use of fat in cooking, store food safely, and ensure more economical use of the food budget.

Nutrition

To provide children with nutritious meals, parents must have some familiarity with nutritional guidelines. One precipitating factor of growth delay is parental misconceptions regarding nutrition (see Chapter 6). For example, many parents do not realize that many low-cost drinks are not juice and that these drinks only serve to satisfy hunger without providing any nutritional benefits. Incorrect preparation of formula can contribute to serious lack of nourishment and can endanger infant health. For other parents, an eagerness to eliminate fat and cholesterol from their children's diets can result in inadequate nutrients (Pugliese, Weyman-Daum, Moses, & Lifshitz, 1987).

Through active involvement in meal selection and preparation, home visitors can dispel misconceptions and help families learn about their children's nutritional needs. Parents who eat unhealthful foods themselves (e.g., low-nutrient snack foods) or eat meals on an irregular schedule set negative examples for their children. Just as clinicians encourage parents to model for children, home visitors can model for parents by helping them recognize their children's nutritional needs and children's desire to eat what they see their parents eat. One option that works with some families is to ask them to keep a nutrition diary to record their meal plans, which may be included in their individualized notebook. The home visitor provides weekly feedback regarding the adequacy of the meals and offers recommendations for alternatives.

Mealtime Scheduling

Children benefit from regular scheduling of meals and structured mealtime routines because they learn when to expect food (see Chapter 27). If children snack throughout the day, then they will not be hungry during meals. If children regularly sleep through breakfast, then they will lack nutrients during an important part of the day. If meals are available at different times each day, then children become anxious and confused about when it is time to eat. Undependable mealtimes make it difficult to learn about hunger and satiety cues.

The home visitor can work with families not only to develop meal plans but also to organize their daily schedule so that mealtimes are incorporated on a consistent basis. Attention to planning can also help families develop alternatives for when mealtimes are disrupted. For example, families could pack a lunch or a snack for their child if they have an appointment that will disrupt lunch. One way to evaluate mealtime scheduling is to ask families to record mealtimes in their individualized notebooks. The home visitor reviews the logs and helps families reorganize when mealtimes are missed or disrupted.

Mealtime Setting

Increasing parental awareness of appropriate mealtime settings can optimize opportunities for successful feeding (see Chapters 7 and 8). To assess the mealtime setting accurately, it is best for the home visitor to observe children as they eat in their home. Some families do not have child-oriented materials, such as highchairs, sippy cups, and child-size utensils. Some children have to kneel on adult-size chairs, and many children eat alone or in front of the television. Other children continue to be fed by a parent even when they are old enough to begin self-feeding.

The home visitor and the parent work together to identify specific needs and allocate family allowance money for necessary equipment. Materials such as highchairs and child-size equipment enable children to participate more independently in feeding. An important advantage to home-visiting programs is that they help families learn how to use new equipment. For example, children who are not used to sitting in a highchair may resist until they get used to it. Reducing environmental distractions, such as turning off the television or radio, putting away toys, and avoiding family conflict during mealtime, can help families focus on mealtime and encourage self-feeding among their children.

Feeding Context

Growth delay in infants commonly involves insufficient food intake, often related to behavior problems (see Chapter 8). Infants who experience growth delay may present with food refusal behaviors such as spitting out food, turning away, and refusing to swallow. Unresponsive, rigid behavior on the part of the parent contributes to unsuccessful feeding. Effective feeding is dependent on sensitive, appropriate, and pleasant offers of food from the parent. Mealtimes that consist of battles, force feeding, and threats serve to reinforce a dangerous pattern of unpleasant struggles around food.

The home visitor helps families put the principles of dividing mealtime responsibility into practice. Families are responsible for providing healthful food according to a predictable schedule in a pleasant environment, and children are responsible for determining how much they will eat (see Chapter 7). Sharing meals with families enables the home visitor to model the division of responsibilities and communication in a supportive context. For example, parents who attend, listen, demonstrate empathy, and respond to their children promptly are less likely to misinterpret their children's signals and more likely to communicate their own messages clearly. Viewing videotapes of mealtime behavior is another effective strategy for improving mealtime communication (see Chapter 8).

Children's Behavior

Feeding behavior problems are not uncommon among children who experience growth delay (see Chapter 8). Although some families require the assistance of a professional therapist to understand the dynamics of their relationship with their child, particularly when the behavior disturbances extend beyond mealtimes, many families can benefit from basic behavior management principles that are suggested by a home visitor. In some cases, problems emerge because parents are unaware of normative child development and have unrealistic expectations of their children (e.g., expecting children to be neat and not make a mess while learning to eat independently). In other cases, parents exacerbate their children's behavior problems with their own inconsistent responses (e.g., ignoring food refusal in one instance and punishing the child in another instance). Through their informal observations in the home, home visitors may observe unreasonable expectations or parental inconsistencies. They can intervene through modeling to help parents modify their expectations or recognize how they maintain their children's behavior problems by not providing clear and consistent consequences. Similarly, the home visitor can help parents increase children's appropriate behavior through reinforcement and limit their attention to the child during times of inappropriate behavior.

Access to Services

A challenge in helping families meet their children's nutritional needs involves increasing awareness of available resources. Low-income families may be eligible to receive services such as from the Special Supplemental Nutrition Program for Women, Infants and Children (WIC) and food stamps, and they may have access to soup kitchens and food pantries; however, families cannot benefit from such services if they are unaware of their availability or do not know how to gain access to them (see Chapter 36).

To be effective in helping families gain access to services, home visitors often have to be aware of the services that are available in the community. They can share information with the family regarding specific sources of assistance and provide methods for gathering information and gaining access to these resources. Although families are encouraged to advocate for themselves, it may sometimes be necessary for the home visitor to take the family to the service provider, at least for an initial visit.

IMPLICATIONS

This curriculum illustrates the process of using home visitors in a supportive context to help families acquire basic skills to promote healthy growth among children. It is specific because it identifies eight target areas to be addressed, but it is flexible because the home visitor attempts to build on individual family strengths in each area. Feedback from families has been positive: Most have welcomed the home visitors and have developed additional skills in managing their children's meals.

CONCLUSION

Home-visiting programs for families of children who have or who are at risk for growth delay offer cautious optimism. They highlight the importance of including families in the planning process and building on family strengths by ensuring that families have the skills that are necessary for providing nutritious, developmentally appropriate meals to their children. Although home visiting may be useful in promoting child development and a nurturing home environment, it does not satisfy all of the needs of vulnerable families (Chamberlain, 1989). Home visiting is most effective when it is integrated with other nutritional, medical, educational, and family services (Ramey, Bryant, & Suarez, 1985).

REFERENCES

Ayleward, G.P., Peiffer, S.I., Wright, A., & Verhulst, S.J. (1989). Outcome studies of low birth weight infants published in the last decade: A meta-analysis. *Journal of Pediatrics, 115,* 515–520.

Bailey, D.B., & Simeonsson, R.J. (1988). *Family assessment in early intervention.* Columbus, OH: Charles E. Merrill.

Barrera, M.E., Cunningham, C.E., & Rosenbaum, P.L. (1986). Low birth weight and home intervention strategies: Preterm infants. *Journal of Developmental and Behavioral Pediatrics, 7,* 361–366.

Black, M.M. (1995). Failure to thrive: Strategies for evaluation and intervention. *School Psychology Review, 24,* 171–185.

Black, M.M., & Bentley, M.E. (1996). Adolescent parenthood: A family-centered, culturally-based perspective. *Pediatric Basics, 73,* 2–9.

Black, M.M., Dubowitz, H., Hutcheson, J., Berenson-Howard, J., & Starr, R.H. (1995). A randomized clinical trial of home intervention for children with failure to thrive. *Pediatrics, 95,* 807–814.

Black, M.M., & Nitz, K. (1996). Grandmother co-residence, parenting, and child development among low income, urban teen mothers. *Journal of Adolescent Health, 18,* 218–226.

Bradley, R.H., & Caldwell, B.M. (1978). Screening the environment. *American Journal of Orthopsychiatry, 48,* 114–130.

Bronfenbrenner, U. (1993). Ecological systems theory. In R. Wozniak & K. Fisher (Eds.), *Specific environments: Thinking in contexts* (pp. 3–44). Mahwah, NJ: Lawrence Erlbaum Associates.

Carnegie Task Force on Meeting the Needs of Young Children. (1994). *Starting points: Meeting the needs of our youngest children.* New York: Author.

Casey, P.H., Kelleher, K.J., Bradley, R.H., Kellogg, K.W., Kirby, R.S., & Whiteside, L. (1994). A multifaceted intervention for infants with failure to thrive: A prospective study. *Archives of Pediatric and Adolescent Medicine, 148,* 1071–1077.

Chamberlain, R.W. (1989). Home visiting: A necessary but not in itself sufficient program component for promoting the health and development of families and children. *Pediatrics, 84,* 178–179.

Crnic, K.A., Greenberg, M.T., Ragozin, A.S., Robinson, N.M., & Basham, R.B. (1983). Effects of stress and social support on mothers and premature and full-term infants. *Child Development, 54,* 209–217.

Dawson, P.M., van Doorninck, W.J., & Robinson, J.L. (1989). Effects of home-based, informal social support on child health. *Journal of Developmental and Behavioral Pediatrics, 10,* 63–67.

Drotar, D. (1991). The family context of nonorganic failure to thrive. *American Journal of Orthopsychiatry, 61,* 23–34.

Drotar, D., Eckerle, D., Satola, J., Pallotta, J., & Wyatt, B. (1990). Maternal interactional behavior with nonorganic failure-to-thrive infants: A case comparison study. *Child Abuse and Neglect, 14,* 41–51.

Drotar, D., & Sturm, L. (1988). Prediction of intellectual outcome in children with early histories of failure-to-thrive. *Journal of Pediatric Psychology, 13,* 281–295.

Drotar, D., & Sturm, L. (1989). Influences on the home environment of preschool children with early histories of nonorganic failure-to-thrive. *Journal of Developmental and Behavioral Pediatrics, 10,* 229–235.

Grantham-McGregor, S., Powell, C., Walker, S., Chang, S., & Fletcher, P. (1994). The long-term follow-up of severely malnourished children who participated in an intervention program. *Child Development, 65,* 428–439.

Grantham-McGregor, S., Schofield, W., & Powell, C. (1987). Development of severely malnourished children who received psychosocial stimulation: Six-year follow-up. *Pediatrics, 79,* 247–254.

Grantham-McGregor, S.M., Walker, S.P., Chang, S.M., & Powell, C.A. (1997). Effects of early childhood supplementation with and without stimulation on later development in stunted Jamaican children. *American Journal of Clinical Nutrition, 66,* 247–253.

Guralnick, M.J. (1996). Second-generation research in the field of early intervention. In M.J. Guralnick (Ed.), *The effectiveness of early intervention* (pp. 3–22). Baltimore: Paul H. Brookes Publishing Co.

Halpern, R. (1984). Lack of effects for home-based early intervention? Some possible explanations. *American Journal of Orthopsychiatry, 54,* 33–42.

Haynes, C.F., Cutler, C., Gray, J., & Kempe, R.S. (1984). Hospitalized cases of failure to thrive: The scope of the problem and short-term lay health visitor intervention. *Child Abuse and Neglect, 8,* 229–242.

Hutcheson, J., Black, M., Talley, M., Dubowitz, H., Berenson-Howard, J., Starr, R.H., & Thompson, B.S. (1997). Risk status and home intervention among children with failure to thrive: Follow-up at age 4. *Journal of Pediatric Psychology, 22,* 651–668.

Individuals with Disabilities Education Act Amendments of 1997, PL 105-17, 20 U.S.C. §§ 1400 *et seq.*

Klass, C.S. (1996). *Home visiting: Promoting healthy parent and child development.* Baltimore: Paul H. Brookes Publishing Co.

Klass, C.S. (1997). The home visitor–parent relationship: The linchpin of home visiting. *Zero to Three, 17*(4), 1–9.

McCarton, C.M., Brooks-Gunn, J., Wallace, I.F., Bauer, C.R., Bennett, F.C., Bernbaum, J.C., Broyles, R.S., Casey, P.H., McCormick, M.C., Scott, D.T., Tyson, J., Tonascia, J., & Meinert, C.L. (1997). Results at age 8 years of early intervention for low-birth-weight premature infants. *Journal of the American Medical Association, 277,* 126–132.

Meyer, E.C., Coll, C.T., Lester, B.M., Boukydis, C.F., McDonough, S.M., & Oh, W. (1994). Family-based intervention improved maternal psychological well-being and feeding interaction of preterm infants. *Pediatrics, 93,* 241–246.

Musick, J.S., & Stott, F.M. (1990). Paraprofessionals, parenting, and child development: Understanding the problems and seeking solutions. In S.J. Meisels & J.P. Shonkoff (Eds.), *Handbook of early childhood intervention* (pp. 651–667). Cambridge, MA: Cambridge University Press.

Oates, R.R., Peacock, A., & Forrest, D. (1984). Long-term effects of nonorganic failure to thrive. *Pediatrics, 75,* 36–40.

Olds, D.L., Eckenrode, J., Henderson, C.R., Kitzman, H., Powers, J., Cole, R., Sidora, K., Morris, P., Pettitt, L.M., & Luckey, D. (1997). Long-term effects of home visitation on maternal life course and child abuse and neglect. *Journal of the American Medical Association, 278,* 637–643.

Polan, H.J., Leon, A., Kaplan, M.D., Kessler, D.B., Stern, D.N., & Ward, M.J. (1991). Disturbances of affect expression in failure-to-thrive. *Journal of the American Academy of Child and Adolescent Psychiatry, 30,* 897–903.

Powell, D.R. (1990). Home visiting in the early years: Policy and program design decisions. *Young Children, 3,* 65–72.

Pugliese, M.T., Weyman-Daum, M., Moses, N., & Lifshitz, F. (1987). Parental health beliefs as a cause of nonorganic failure to thrive. *Pediatrics, 80,* 175–182.

Ramey, C.T., Bryant, D.M., & Suarez, T.M. (1985). Preschool compensatory education and the modifiability of intelligence: A critical review. In D. Detterman (Ed.), *Current topics in human intelligence* (pp. 247–256). Norwood, NJ: Ablex.

Sia, C.J., & Breakey, G.F. (1985). The role of the medical home visitor in child abuse prevention and positive child development. *Hawaii Medical Journal, 44,* 242–243.

U.S. General Accounting Office. (1990). *Home visiting: A promising early intervention strategy for at-risk families.* Washington, DC: U.S. Government Printing Office. (Report No. GAO/HRD-90-83)

Wiecha, J., & Palombo, R. (1989). Multiple program participation: Comparison of nutrition and food assistance program benefits with food costs in Boston, Massachusetts. *American Journal of Public Health, 79,* 591–595.

Chapter 29

Psychological Issues and Infant–Parent Psychotherapy

Marian Birch

In any case of pediatric undernutrition, it is important to evaluate psychosocial factors carefully from the beginning. Research has consistently shown associations between undernutrition and many psychosocial factors (see Chapter 30). Clinical work shows that the factors that contribute to undernutrition may be complex, multiple, and often relatively subtle, and they may vary greatly from one case to another.

It may be difficult for staff in medical and nutritional services to detect psychosocial issues because staff are not trained in these domains and because of time pressures. Furthermore, studies have linked undernutrition to neglect, which may make health care providers reluctant to consider a psychological component in families whom they perceive as concerned and loving because they associate psychological factors with neglect. Instead, they may provide more and more testing, monitoring, and advice.

This chapter presents indications for referral for mental health services and a framework for understanding dysfunctions in the feeding relationship. A model of intervention—infant–parent psychotherapy—is described for treating these dysfunctions and other disturbances in infant–parent relationships. Also described is the role of mental health professionals in consulting with other providers.

LEVELS OF INTERVENTION

Following a diagnosis of undernutrition, initial interventions usually are about medical or nutritional issues or about feeding. In many instances, one or more of these modes of intervention will be successful, leading to resumed growth and improved nutritional status; however, that may not always be the case.

Medical intervention focuses on identifying and treating any physical or metabolic condition that contributes to or results from the child's poor nutritional status. The success of such interventions depends not only on accurate diagnosis and appropriate treatment but also on the family's ability and willingness to comply with treatment recommendations. Although this often is taken for granted by physicians, compliance may be made difficult by misunderstanding, stress, inadequate parental skills, psychological conflict, or mental disorder in the parent.

Nutritional interventions, simply stated, focus on reviewing the child's diet for nutritional adequacy and providing suggestions for improvement. Again, success depends to a significant degree on the family's ability to work with the nutritionist and follow through with his or her suggestions. Efforts to improve feeding provide the family with pertinent information about child development and the feeding relationship. They may include specific techniques for feeding, such as behavioral programs, or exercises prescribed by occupational therapists or speech-language pathologists to enhance the child's oral-motor skills. Such educational interventions may help the parents understand their child's difficulties and developmental challenges. For example, a parent who has been battling for control with a toddler may be helped enormously by being taught the importance of self-feeding experiences for the child at this age.

These approaches depend on parents' changing their behavior through education. Professionals provide information and advice, and parents follow through; yet, despite professionals' best efforts, some families fail to respond. They are unable to use the information and advice that they are given. They insist that they are complying, yet the child does not gain weight. They have a seemingly endless list of reasons and excuses for being unable to follow treatment recommendations. Professionals worry, and with good reason. Cases such as these can stir up frustration, anger, and a sense of desperate urgency even in normally calm and controlled professional staff. The sections that follow explore the idea that such "unprofessional" feelings may be one of the more reliable indicators that a case would benefit from mental health intervention.

PSYCHOLOGICAL DISORDERS IN FAMILIES OF UNDERNOURISHED CHILDREN

The relationship between pediatric undernutrition and familial psychological disorder calls for much further investigation. For an excellent review of the research, see Benoit (1993). The picture that emerges from the literature presents overwhelming support for the idea that pediatric undernutrition is very frequently accompanied by some kind of psychological dysfunction in the family; however, the specifics of this relationship remain far from clear. Studies have shown pediatric undernutrition to be associated with a wide range of disorders. These include increased rates of child abuse, of insecure and disorganized attachment (as measured by the Strange Situation Procedure), of marital distress, of maternal depression and suicide, of addiction, and of social isolation and parental affective disorders. Pediatric undernutrition also has been linked statistically to infant apathy, irritability, hyperactivity, hypervigilance, anger, gaze aversion, and resistance to physical contact. Because of generally small sample sizes, inconsistent diagnostic criteria, and differing methodologies, it is difficult to draw broad conclusions, yet the overall trend seems very clear: Pediatric undernutrition, with or without medical etiology, is often linked to some form of psychological disorder.

These disturbances fall roughly into three broad and overlapping categories. First, pediatric undernutrition frequently coexists with family stressors such as trauma, loss, and marital conflict. Second, a diagnosed psychiatric disorder in the caregiver seems to contribute to increased risk of pediatric undernutrition. This includes depression, anxiety, personality disorders, and psychosis. Third, pediatric undernutrition is a common symptom of a disturbance in the infant–parent relationship. The first two categories—family stress and parental psychiatric disorder—both may contribute to the third category—a disturbance in the infant–parent relationship. Following a brief discussion of family stressors and psychiatric disorders of parents, disturbances in infant–parent relationships are discussed in detail.

Family Stressors

Family stressors such as loss, marital conflict, financial insecurity, and cultural dislocation may impair the feeding relationship. For example, parents who have marital problems may battle over the proper way, time, or amount to feed the infant, or a recently arrived immigrant mother may be unable to integrate her internal model of how to feed an infant, brought from her culture of origin, with the expectations and resources that are common to American families (see Chapter 26). Stress may make parents tense and preoccupied and, consequently, less sensitive and responsive interpreters of their infant's cues for hunger, satiety, and social interaction.

Psychiatric Disorders of Parents

Some parents experience psychiatric disorders, such as depression, anxiety, personality disorder, and thought disorders. All of these psychiatric disorders are characterized by difficulties in forming and sustaining healthy, mutually satisfying relationships. These difficulties may carry over to the infant–parent relationship and, frequently, to feeding interactions. For example, a depressed parent is often out of touch with his or her own body's nutritional needs, as well as emotionally withdrawn and inexpressive. Such a parent is at increased risk for missing hunger signals from the infant and has fewer emotional resources to engage the resistant, distractible infant. A parent who has psychotic symptoms may have difficulty distinguishing the real infant from his or her projections (as with one mother who exclaimed with delight, "Look at that smile!" as her 7-month-old screamed, purple-faced, in rage). Although education and guidance can be helpful in such cases, it is most effectively delivered by someone who understands the nature of the parent's mental and emotional challenges and can make needed accommodation to them.

Disturbances in Infant–Parent Relationships

In the previous sections, the common denominator is the presence of disturbance in the infant–parent relationship. Feeding is such an important medium for infant–parent communication and mutual adaptation that any problems in the relationship are likely to be reflected in feeding. Conversely, disturbances in feeding threaten the security and mutual pleasure in relatedness that characterize healthy relationships.

Since the mid-1970s, there has been great expansion in the understanding of the richness, complexity, and importance of the early infant–parent relationship and its central role in the unfolding psychological structuring of the child's personality (Brazelton, 1992; Emde, 1989; Greenspan, 1997; Stern, 1985). Interactions around feeding are one of the major arenas in which the infant–parent relationship evolves and takes shape during the first 2 or 3 years of life.

Infant and parent move together through the developmental and caregiving challenges of the first 2 years of life. The first 3 months are a time when infant and parent learn to acclimate to the infant's life outside the womb. They establish the first patterns and routines for soothing, stimulating, sleeping, and, of course, feeding. From about the third to the eighth month, infant and parent develop an increasingly rich and complex repertoire of interactive "games," which enable them to communicate and connect nonverbally. Toward the end of the first year of life, the infant begins to function more autonomously, and the parents must adjust their caregiving accordingly, for example, by monitoring the now-mobile child or by permitting some self-feeding. In addition to becoming more autonomous, toddlers are learning to cope with separations and to retain an internal, psychological security about being cared for, even when the caregiver is not present.

Disturbances in the infant–parent relationship may occur at any point along the developmental trajectory, and such disturbances may either center on or be reflected in the infant's feeding behavior. For example, during the neonatal period, there may be difficulties in the successful coordination of nursing, whereas in the middle of the first year, disturbances around weaning are common. In the second year, struggles over control of the feeding process are frequent. Whereas transient feeding disturbances are universal, severe and protracted disruptions of feeding often signal a disturbance in the relationship between child and parent.

Comparing the feeding interaction to a dance, these infants and their caregivers are out of step, treading on each other's toes and dancing to different music. The following are a few observations that illustrate this lack of synchrony:

- A mother continues to spoon cereal into the mouth of her infant, who appears to have fallen asleep.
- A large slab of ham is placed in front of a 14-month-old in his highchair. No one notices that it is too big for him to handle.
- A mother feels rejected by her distractible infant's squirming in her arms and cannot help the infant settle down to nurse.
- A father repeatedly teases his infant by snatching away her bottle just as she reaches for it.
- An infant's hands are slapped each time she reaches for the spoon that her mother holds.
- Feeding is mechanical and rushed, without eye contact or vocalization between infant and mother.

The common theme in these observations is that parent and infant are not sending clear signals to each other or are not reading each other's signals accurately. The finely tuned mutuality, reciprocity, and pleasure that characterize healthy relationships are notably absent. Sometimes a particular infant is difficult to read. He or she may use weak or confusing signals or may have a nervous system that is disorganized easily by social stimulation. Often, the parent has deeply ingrained, emotionally charged preconceptions about what infants are or should be like, which cause him or her to distort the meaning of the infant's behavior. Most common, the disturbance is the product of distorting influences from both parent and infant; that is, a particular infant has a temperament and a behavior style that is discordant with the parent's expectations, sensitivities, and emotional strengths. This explains the common observation that not all of the children in a given family have the same problems. (For an excellent review of available instruments for evaluating parent–infant interaction, see Clark, Paulson, & Conlin, 1993, and Appendixes B, C, D, and E.)

The kinds of disturbances that are examined here may or may not coexist with insecure attachment as measured by the Strange Situation Procedure (Ainsworth, Bell, &

Stayton, 1974), but they are not, in themselves, evidence of insecure attachment. Nor do they reliably predict insecure attachment, although some studies (Valenzuela, 1990; Ward, Kessler, & Altman, 1993) show dramatically increased risk.

The attachment disorder classification system proposed by Zeanah, Mammen, and Lieberman (1993) is useful clinically and provides behavioral criteria for assessing disturbance. It has the limitation of focusing exclusively on the disturbance in the child rather than locating the disorder in the parent–infant relationship. (This is consistent with the *Diagnostic and Statistical Manual of Mental Disorders, Fourth Edition* [DSM-IV] [American Psychiatric Association, 1994], in which diagnoses belong to individuals, not to relationships.)

Within the attachment relationship, whether it is secure or insecure, maladaptive patterns may develop in how the parent and the infant jointly coordinate particular activities, such as eating, sleeping, or expressing feelings. Following is an examination of the normal developmental stages in this joint regulation of infant–parent interaction, illustrated by clinical examples of how dysfunctional patterns may affect the feeding interaction. (See Brazelton, 1992; Greenspan, 1997; Mahler, 1975; and Sander, 1964, for descriptions of the developmental issues that are negotiated by the parent–infant dyad in the first 2–3 years of life.)

Homeostasis

The first developmental challenge to be negotiated by the parent–infant dyad is the attainment of regulatory homeostasis. In the first days and weeks of life, the infant's need for regulation of body temperature, blood sugar, sleep, arousal, and quieting come to depend not on the mother's womb but on behavioral coordination between parent and infant, two physically distinct individuals. Patterns of holding, cuddling, vocalizing, nursing, and touching replace the placental tie and are needed to help the infant cope with massive quantities of novel stimulations from light, gravity, air, sound, and, most important, people. Difficulties in making these tremendous adjustments are often reflected in problems with nursing or bottle-feeding. These may include weak sucking, apparent lack of interest in or rejection of the nipple, excessive gagging or spitting up, sore and painful breasts, and so forth. All of these problems may have simple educational solutions. The clinician also should be alert to the possibility that the mother–infant dyad is floundering for psychological reasons as well. If there is too much discrepancy between the infant's temperament and behavior and the mother's expectations, if the mother is conflicted about closeness and nurturing, if the mother is frightened by the infant's helplessness and utter dependence, or if the mother identifies the infant with hurtful people in her past, then the successful mutual adaptation that is necessary for establishing stable daily rhythms in feeding and in other areas of infant care can be compromised.

Jane, age 38, was a successful artist who spent much of her time alone in her studio. Her husband, a 50-year-old businessman, traveled frequently. Jane and her husband never ate at home; in fact, they owned no cooking utensils other than a toaster and a coffee maker. They socialized mainly with professional colleagues and had little contact with their families of origin. Jane had not much wanted children; but, giving in to her husband's urging and to the ticking of her "biological clock," she became pregnant and gave birth to Thomas. She thought that breast-feeding would tie her down too much, so she opted for bottle-feeding. Thomas was a quiet, somewhat passive baby. As a newborn, he spit up frequently and was distracted easily from sucking by visual or auditory stimulation. Jane, whose own discomfort with physical intimacy caused her to hold Thomas awkwardly and tensely during bottle-feeding, interpreted his spitting up and his turning away to look at something as signals that he was full and that he did not want to be held or offered more food. Being very visually oriented herself, she positioned him during feedings so that he had interesting things to look at, which increased his distractibility. Because of his low-key temperament, Thomas fussed only mildly when put down. Jane did not attribute the fussing to hunger; instead, she attributed to Thomas her own dislike of intimacy and resentment of intrusion and believed that he wanted to be left alone, as she often did. Not surprisingly, Thomas's poor weight gain and growth soon aroused the concern of Thomas's pediatrician. Because of Jane's psychological issues and because she had an infant who gave weak, somewhat unclear signals, she was not successful at following her pediatrician's instructions for more effective feeding. Thomas was hospitalized and quickly gained weight when fed by nurses.

Focalization of Attachment

Occurring roughly between 3 and 8 months, focalization of attachment is ushered in by the first social smiling that is directed preferentially at the caregiver. It culminates with the infant's perceiving the parent as a consistent, intimately known source of security, which is indicated by the common resistance to strangers and to separations that is characteristic of the last third of the first year of life. During this period, parent and infant build an increasingly rich and highly personal repertoire of mutually regulated, patterned interactions around the routines of caregiving, the expression of feeling, the sharing of experiences, comforting, and playing.

The infant and the parent come to know each other's ways and moods. They come to have shared expectations and to anticipate one another's responses. Greenspan and Lieberman (1980) identified two distinct patterns of parental dysfunction that may disrupt this process, which they called noncontingent and anticontingent responsiveness. The term *noncontingent* refers to parental behavior that appears unrelated to infant signals or needs, apparently deriving instead from the parent's own presuppositions and agenda. *Anticontingent* behavior, by contrast, is related to what the infant is doing and feeling but in a rejecting, punitive way. The noncontingent parent, for environmental or psychological reasons, does not provide consistent and predictable responses to the infant's signals. In the feeding situation, for example, food may be offered or taken away without apparent reference to the infant's state or nutritional needs. Parent response to infant initiatives may be absent, erratic, or bizarre. Lieberman and Birch (1985) identified noncontingent responding as characteristic of parents who are suffering from thought disorder or depression or of extremely chaotic families in which there is no clearly defined person or persons in charge of caregiving. In the anticontingent pattern, the parent is consistent, even rigidly so, in his or her structuring of the feeding interaction, but this is in response to his or her own agenda and to his or her need to control the infant. Infant initiatives are ignored or rebuffed, sometimes harshly; thus, the infant who reaches for the bottle may have his or her hands restrained, or the bottle may be removed from an actively sucking infant when a certain number of ounces have been consumed. Following are two case studies. The first demonstrates noncontingent parenting; the second demonstrates anticontingent parenting.

Jamal was diagnosed with pediatric undernutrition when he was 6 months old. In the year between diagnosis and referral for infant–parent psychotherapy,

Jamal's pediatrician had conducted a comprehensive series of medical tests, which ruled out any known organic cause for Jamal's failure to grow. In finally making the referral to mental health services, the pediatrician expressed his misgivings at doing so by emphasizing that Jamal's parents were very loving and that Jamal appeared to be very attached to them. That was quite true, but a mental health evaluation uncovered that Jamal's mother was an extremely passive woman with a marked thought disorder, initially masked by her polite reserve. She seldom took the initiative in interacting with Jamal and did very little to structure his life. There were no routines for feeding or any other aspect of his daily experience. Jamal's mother often did not notice behaviors that required prompt intervention, such as Jamal's climbing on a stool to reach a toy. The father was more aware and appropriate, but he was often away from home and his comings and goings were rather sudden and unexplained. Although both of Jamal's parents cherished Jamal, they led a very unstructured lifestyle in which the connections between things were often obscure. Nobody in the family ate regular meals, and nobody seemed to keep track of whether or how much Jamal had eaten. He sometimes was encouraged to help himself from the refrigerator and sometimes scolded for doing so. On one occasion, his mother tried to feed him oatmeal that was scorching hot; another time, Jamal was given a huge slab of ham, uncut, which he tried to nibble, unsuccessfully. Jamal adapted to this chaotic, unstructured environment with a precocious investment in feverish motor activity. He seemed literally to bounce off the walls to get his feedback about where he began and ended. Naturally, this did not help him to eat properly.

Claude was diagnosed with pediatric undernutrition when he failed to resume adequate weight gain and growth following a hospitalization at 6 months for a gastrointestinal obstruction. His mother, a single parent with little social support, responded to his increased anxiety and clinginess with sullen anger and withdrawal. She pushed him away when he tried to pull himself up to her lap, and she put him alone in his crib when he protested being put down. When he reached for his bottle, she held it out of his reach and told him to "stop being a baby." Claude soon adapted to this by angrily rejecting the few overtures that his mother made, for instance to comfort him after a fall. His mother applauded this behavior as evidence of toughness, which she considered a valuable trait in a harsh, unpredictable world.

Infant characteristics may either exacerbate or ameliorate the effects of such parental lack of contingency. If parental behaviors evoke angry or withdrawn behavior in the infant, then the result may be a breakdown in feeding. More resilient, "rewarding" infants who vigorously reinforce parents with big smiles and cuddles may train noncontingent parents to take better care of them. Such was the case with a pair of infants, born to two teenage sisters in a household in which eight adults who led very chaotic lifestyles shared their care.

One infant, nicknamed "Bruiser," was a healthy, strapping boy who responded intensely and positively to the casual, haphazard, but mostly benevolent attention that he received. The other infant, a quiet, unresponsive boy with chronic gastrointestinal problems, was diagnosed with pediatric undernutrition. It was clear that his family found him far less rewarding to feed than "Bruiser" and frequently ended feedings prematurely.

Separation and Individuation

In the last part of the first year of life and the first part of the second year, the focus of the parent–infant dyad shifts to accommodating the infant's emergent capacities for initiative and exploration and balancing these with his or her ongoing dependence and need for a secure base. Feeding problems that originate during this period often coincide with weaning, the introduction of new foods, and self-feeding. The toddler's active exploration of the environment requires the parent to watch, help, and, inevitably, interfere with infant initiatives. Ideally, the parent is able to accommodate by permitting some self-feeding, tolerating infant food preferences, and allowing some exploratory manipulation while continuing to provide appropriate structure for mealtimes. This phase makes very complex demands on the caregiver, who must remain emotionally available while also setting limits and supporting and tolerating increasing self-direction by the infant. Importantly, as the infant becomes mobile, the dyad must rely increasingly on distal modes of communication (speech and visual signaling) rather than on physical contact. Parents who feel rejected by their infants' increased autonomy or burdened by the infants' more focused demands often have difficulty during this phase.

> Candy, a good-tempered, easygoing infant of 11 months, was described by her mother as "into everything." Candy's mother felt overwhelmed by the new need to monitor Candy and seemed unaware of the possibility of "child-proofing" the environment. Instead, she kept Candy almost continuously in a walker, which allowed her to travel around the apartment but not to touch anything. Candy's mother was very controlling of feedings, chastising Candy for using her left hand or getting food on her dress. She fed Candy in the walker and actually appeared relieved when, as usually happened, Candy propelled herself away from the tense, uncongenial feeding interaction. Candy's mother was unable to adapt to Candy's need to explore and to have more control of her feeding. Candy, rather than engage in protracted power struggles or submit, chose to avoid both mother and food.

Finally, for the older toddler, the central developmental challenge is the establishment of internal object constancy (Fraiberg, 1969; Mahler, 1975). This is the capacity to sustain feelings of loving and being loved by one's parent, even when the parent is physically absent or is frustrating the child's wishes. During this period, eating and other issues of body management increasingly emerge from the parent–infant orbit into the realm of autonomous function. Behaviors, particularly social negotiations, seem guided by what Brazelton and Cramer (1990) have called the "I am not you" principle. The stage is characterized by ambivalence as the toddler struggles with balancing his or her drive for autonomy with the ongoing need for care and nurturing. The caregiver is called upon to model, in the frequent control struggles, firm but nonviolent boundaries and modes of dispute resolution. This is difficult for all parents but particularly so for those who themselves have unresolved issues about control and about anger management. Following are two case studies. The first demonstrates difficulties with object constancy; the second demonstrates difficulties with autonomy.

> Duncan, who had gained weight adequately during his first 18 months, experienced a sudden weight loss and increasingly refused food after his family

moved to another city, leaving behind the grandmother who had been his principal caregiver during the day. His mother, also dislocated by the move, felt hurt and rejected that Duncan refused to eat for her. She was unable to understand and help him with his grief and bewilderment over the disappearance of a beloved caregiver as well as his entire familiar environment. Careful observation of his behavior with food suggested that he was trying to work through questions about how things disappear. He would taste things repeatedly and spit them out, hide food under his plate, and keep food in his mouth for hours. When the infant–parent therapist helped his mother to understand both Duncan's grief and her own, the feeding difficulties resolved fairly quickly.

Eva, born with mild neurological abnormalities, had long-standing difficulty with solid foods because of a hyperactive gag reflex. She had maintained adequate growth and nutrition during her first 2 years on a high-calorie formula, which she took readily from a bottle. When she was 25 months old, her mother believed that it was time to wean her from the bottle and, consequently, threw out all of the bottles in the house, presenting Eva with a fait accompli. Eva retaliated with a full-fledged hunger strike, refusing to take anything by mouth except water. The more she was pressured to eat, the more vehemently she resisted. She repeatedly pulled out the tube that was inserted for nasogastric feeding. After 2 months and an 8-pound weight loss, she had to be surgically fitted with a "peg," which allowed direct delivery of a formula by syringe to her stomach.

At each developmental phase, the feeding relationship can be affected negatively by difficulties with achieving harmonious reciprocity between parent and infant. This disharmony, or conflict, may be mirrored in the family's relationships with service providers. A service provider's feelings of intense discomfort with and aversion to a family are very good indications that the family needs skilled psychotherapeutic intervention. Patients tend to impose or project onto their relationships with doctors or therapists personal expectations and anxieties that are rooted in their own early experiences of receiving or not receiving needed help and care. Such projections, which normally operate outside conscious awareness, are called *transference.* The patient who is experiencing transference feelings toward a provider typically behaves, in subtle and not-so-subtle ways, in a manner that actually evokes the expected response from the helping professional (Sandler, 1976). For example, a patient who expects to be judged, criticized, and treated punitively may be late repeatedly or fail to make appointments, frequently provoking the expected critical attitude and punitive responses from clinical staff. When a child's parents elicit strong feelings of frustration, irritation, or despair in providers, these can be useful clues that the parents may not be able to relate to others in a direct and mutually satisfying way. In fact, there often are illuminating parallels between the parents' refusal or inability to take in what the providers have to offer and the infant's or toddler's refusal or inability to take in adequate nutrition, as well as parallels between the provider's feelings of frustration and incompetence and the parents' similar sense of failure and anger at the child's failure to grow.

Of course, in making such judgments, providers first must examine carefully their own motives and behavior to ensure that their responses truly are countertransference—that is, evoked by the client's transference—and not displaced reactions to other common personal and professional stresses, such as overwork, inadequate or shaky funding, personnel conflicts, or personal problems.

INFANT–PARENT PSYCHOTHERAPY

When a child's poor nutritional status does appear to be affected by his or her family relationships, infant–parent psychotherapy may be an appropriate intervention strategy.

The Program

Infant–parent psychotherapy was originally developed by the late Selma Fraiberg and subsequently refined and developed by her colleagues at the Infant–Parent Program of San Francisco (Fraiberg, Lieberman, Pekarsky, & Pawl, 1981a, 1981b). The program works with families who face severely compromising and challenging situations, including poor nutrition. The treatment approach has five distinctive features: 1) extended assessment; 2) focus on infant–parent relationship; 3) support, guidance, and insight; 4) relationship with the therapist; and 5) home-visiting model.

Extended Assessment

Each treatment begins with a careful five- to eight-session evaluation to ensure time to establish a working alliance and a sufficient, detailed understanding of the particulars of a given family's situation so that intervention can be tailored to meet their needs, strengths, and vulnerabilities. This process cannot be hurried or standardized as relationship building between therapist and family is the cornerstone of this approach and requires time.

Focus on Infant–Parent Relationship

The focus of treatment is on the relationship between the infant and his or her parents rather than on symptoms or pathology of one partner or the other. In most instances, the therapist does little hands-on work with the infant. Parent and infant are seen together, and the therapist works to understand the psychological obstacles that impede the parent from responding to the infant in an appropriate, sensitively attuned way. For the therapist to work directly with the infant and to "succeed" where the parent has failed would represent a defeat for the parent and a blow to any emergent trust in the therapist as a supportive ally.

Support, Guidance, and Insight

The infant–parent psychotherapist combines three therapeutic modalities: support, guidance, and insight. The first two are common to many early intervention programs. Support includes both concrete, physical help, such as providing transportation to medical appointments or showing parents how to apply for low-income housing. It includes providing emotional support, such as recognizing and praising family strengths and responding empathically to family difficulties. Developmental guidance is offered in a client-centered way. That is, the infant–parent psychotherapist explores and empathically responds to the parents' own beliefs and feelings about developmental issues, as a prelude to offering information that may expand the parents' options. For example, an infant–parent psychotherapist would listen to and sympathize with a parent's concerns about cleanliness and hygiene before advising that the parent allow more self-feeding.

Insight, the third component of infant–parent psychotherapy, results when the therapist helps the parents to understand, explore, and exorcise what Fraiberg so evocatively called "the ghosts in the nursery" (Fraiberg, Adelson, & Shapiro, 1975). The infant–parent psychotherapist is alert to the fact that parents frequently repeat in their relationships with their infants the painful and often unacknowledged inadequacies in their own early lives. Buried feelings and expectations from the parent's childhood may be unconsciously projected onto the relationship with the infant, with disastrous results.

Parents whose early histories are characterized by abandonment, lack of emotional support, harsh discipline, or unresponsiveness to dependency needs will have difficulty tolerating and responding to their own infants' needs for security, comforting, cuddling, and emotionally contingent responsiveness because of the defensive strategies that they developed as children to cope with neglect and abuse. When these buried feelings can be explored and traced to their origins and when the parent's own early suffering can be shared in a supportive, therapeutic context, the freeing up of the impasse in the present-day parent–infant relationship can be dramatic. A case in point is a father who simply could not endure the sound of his daughter's crying. It disturbed him to the point that he felt that if he did not leave the house, then he would suffocate her. With the help of the infant–parent psychotherapist, he was able to connect this response to his own severe battering as a child, which he initially dismissed as "water under the bridge—it doesn't bother me." The following case study also illustrates how these factors may come into play in feeding disorders.

Reuben, the 2¹/₂-year-old son of two pediatricians, refused to eat and weighed only 25 pounds. His mother exhibited a level of frustration and helplessness with Reuben that seemed incongruent with both her sophisticated knowledge of child development and Reuben's fairly placid, cooperative temperament. Exploration of her history uncovered that as a little girl, she had been made responsible for watching out for her brother, who was 15 months older than she, who had a severe emotional disturbance, and whose strength, size, and utter unpredictability thwarted her valiant efforts to keep him out of trouble. She had never allowed herself to know how profoundly she had resented and wished to be rid of her brother. Many of these disavowed feelings were projected onto her son, whose normal infantile and toddler unpredictability and impulsivity reminded her of her brother's behavior. Her attempts to feed Reuben were both anxiously intrusive and hypersensitive to his perceived disinterest or rebuffs. This behavior evoked both her feelings of helplessness and her buried anger about the early experience with her brother. When her relationship with her brother and with the parents who neglected them both was explored and she was helped to locate these feelings in their appropriate historical context, her relationship with Reuben improved dramatically and his growth and nutritional status returned to normal without further intervention.

Relationship with the Therapist

A distinctive feature of infant–parent psychotherapy is that the therapist is alert to the ways that "ghosts in the nursery" can affect not only the relationship between parent and infant but also that between parent and helping professional. Parents whose early histories are characterized by a lack of emotional support, by unmet dependency needs, or by harsh, rejecting caregivers will tend to anticipate similar insensitivity and rejection from helping professionals, who are perceived as quasi-parental figures. If such expectations are automatic, operating outside of conscious awareness, and deeply ingrained, then it often is not enough simply to demonstrate that one truly is kind, concerned, nonpunitive, and dependable, although this obviously is an essential first step. It may also be necessary to anticipate and label the often unconscious link that the parent is making between the therapist and his or her own early caregivers, saying, for example, "It's probably hard for you to believe that I'll do what I said I would when your own mom kept disappointing you," to a mother whose own mother had rarely appeared for scheduled visits when the client was in foster care. Frequently, such acknowledgments that the client has legitimate reasons for being suspicious and guarded are disarming and serve as openings for further exploration. Paradoxically, it may be the infant–parent psychotherapist's very willingness to understand and empathize with the client's distrust and suspicions that may set her apart from other would-be helpers and lay the foundation for a trusting working alliance.

Building trust with parents who have these kinds of difficulties is a prerequisite for all other interventions. It cannot be done quickly; time and dependability over time are essential components of the work.

An important variant of this kind of work with the client's transference feelings involves working with clients' generic transference to social services providers (Seligman & Pawl, 1984). Many families have lifelong histories of contact with social workers, nurses, doctors, teachers, case managers, protective services workers, parole officers, police, truant officers, and so forth, all offering services often against the client's will and often of a different socioeconomic and ethnic origin from the client's. All too often, these experiences have not been helpful and have felt intrusive and demeaning. Any new professional who is hoping to help such families must be prepared to be perceived initially as just like all of his or her predecessors. Again, in addition to demonstrating concern, tact, and reliability, frank acknowledgment of the inadequacy of one's own and one's predecessors' ability to help and the awkwardness and potential shame and anger that commonly accompany being in the position of needing help from strangers is a standard part of the infant–parent psychotherapeutic approach.

Home-Visiting Model

Infant–parent psychotherapy is usually conducted in the client's home. Home visits may be essential to reach overburdened, disorganized, or resistant clients. In addition, the opportunity to observe parent–infant interaction in its natural setting provides a wealth of information and insight that ordinarily is not available in a clinic or an office. Home visiting, in the case of pediatric undernutrition, provides opportunities to observe naturalistic feeding interactions, to learn about the whole family's eating patterns, and to observe firsthand in the environment the distractions and pressures that affect the feeding relationship. One mother's insistence on feeding her therapist enormous meals, at whatever time of day that she visited, provided an insight into the driven, noncontingent nature of her feeding behavior, which would not have emerged in a conventional clinic interview. It also offered a nonthreatening context in which to discuss her anxieties about being a good provider and how these affected her efforts to feed her child.

As this vignette suggests, home visiting calls for considerable tact, flexibility, and creativity on the part of the therapist. Being in someone's home requires careful sensitivity to issues of intrusion and overexposure. Professional boundaries, such as those around disclosing personal information or participating in extratherapeutic activities with the client, are considerably more fluid but no less important than in conventional, office-based psychotherapy. One must be prepared to deal with any number of unanticipated circumstances, ranging from the presence of other visitors to visiting in the dark because the power has been shut off.

The following extended case description illustrates the way in which the model of treatment offers careful assessment and a flexible mix of concrete support, developmental guidance, and psychodynamically informed interventions that are focused on observed psychological impediments to the infant–parent relationship.

Annie and her parents were referred for assessment and infant–parent psychotherapy by a pediatric gastroenterologist when Annie was 11 months old.

Annie had received almost all of her nourishment through a nasogastric tube since she was 8 months old. Prior to using the tube, her parents had reported great difficulty in feeding her and frequent vomiting dating back to a few days after birth. She had been dangerously underweight but had gained well on nasogastric feeding and was now plump and robust looking; however, she took almost no food by mouth, with the exception of frequent but very brief breast-feeding.

By the time of the referral, Annie's parents and doctors were thoroughly frustrated and angry with each other. Medical staff felt beleaguered by the parents' continuous demand for further medical tests (a great many had been done) and their insistence that there must be a physical cause for Annie's problems. They were frustrated by what they saw as the parents' pathologizing a healthy child and the parents' evident inability to follow through with guidance on how to feed Annie. Annie's parents felt misunderstood and not listened to by doctors, who seemed to be indifferent to the grave threat to Annie's growth and health. They also felt criticized and condemned as incompetent parents who were to blame for their daughter's difficulties.

The first home visit to the family's tiny apartment revealed an immaculate, colorful, and comfortable environment with many attractive and appropriate playthings for Annie. Annie's mother, who had immigrated to the United States to marry her American husband, spoke to Annie in her native language and offered the therapist a delicious snack from her native cuisine. When she offered Annie the same snack, she placed the food (a savory pastry that was cut into bite-size pieces, easily manageable by an 11-month-old) on a brightly colored plate in front of Annie, who was seated in her highchair. She gave Annie an appealing "airplane spoon" and coaxed, "Make it fly into your mouth like the plane goes to the airport." When Annie instead mashed the food with her hands, threw some on the floor, and began to try to climb down from her highchair, her mother sighed helplessly and let her down. Her other interactions with her very active toddler likewise were characterized by warmth, imagination, and the lack of clear, firm boundaries and expectations. Annie's father was vocally critical of his wife's efforts but made no attempt to intervene himself. Annie was observed to become more provocative and attention seeking when her father reproved her mother; however, at this point, the therapist kept these observations to herself and focused on drawing out Annie's parents on the subject of their difficulties and empathizing with how frustrated and worried they must feel, and she noted supportively the many positive features of their relationship with their daughter, which were readily observable. It is an important part of this approach to find ways to support and validate parents and to avoid the temptation to dive in and succeed with the child where the parents have failed.

As the therapist came to know the family better in subsequent home visits, she became aware of multiple stresses that affected the family and indirectly impaired their ability to feed their child. Most important, it became clear that the parents argued during almost every feeding about how Annie should be fed and that each blamed the other when she refused to eat or when she threw up. Annie's avoidance and opposition around eating seemed linked directly to this ongoing marital tension. The therapist was able to say to the parents, "Because she loves you both, it feels like you're fighting inside her tummy."

Both parents disclosed histories of having parents who had been and continued to be intrusive and controlling. The paternal grandparents, who lived nearby, expected daily reports on their grandchild's progress and did not hes-

itate to second-guess and give advice. Annie's mother resented this intensely, and Annie's father felt that her resentment was immature and ungrateful. The maternal grandparents had had an angry, often violent relationship. The grandfather, an alcoholic, had been prone to violent rages, and the grandmother was extremely controlling. Annie's mother recalled as a child being seated in a row at the kitchen table with her five brothers and sisters, all very close in age, and being spoon-fed en masse with near military precision. When Annie's mother had taken Annie the previous summer to visit her parents, the maternal grandmother had appropriated Annie and force-fed her cream, butter, and other rich foods, accusing Annie's mother of starving her grandchild.

In addition to these family and historic pressures, Annie's mother was very isolated and lonely. She felt out of place in this culture, and, although she believed that it was best for Annie that she stay home with her, she had no network of friends or other young mothers to give her adult contact. Her husband, who worked 6 days per week on variable shifts at a juvenile detention center, had little interest or energy for socializing outside of his family.

During the first month, the therapist mainly listened empathically to the parents' concerns, gathered information from the gastroenterologist, nutritionist, and occupational therapist who had worked with the family, and observed closely the interactions between Annie and her parents. The central focus in this phase was on building a treatment alliance by focusing on how frightening it is to have an infant who will not eat and how angry and humiliated the parents felt when others, especially authority figures such as doctors, appeared to blame them for their child's condition. Gentle inquiry about how powerless Annie's mother felt when Annie did not accept her invitations to eat elicited the memories of how overpowering the maternal grandmother had been and how fervently she wished to spare Annie similar experiences. Indeed, it seemed to the therapist that part of the problem resulted from Annie's mother's extreme reluctance to pressure Annie in any way, so Annie was quite unclear about her expectations and limits. As the memories and feelings about her own childhood were explored and responded to empathically, Annie's mother became less entreating, tentative, and apologetic in her handling of feeding. Annie responded positively to her mother's increased confidence and decreased anxiety.

As the family's trust and comfort with the therapist increased, it was possible to focus attention on the tension and mutual recrimination between the parents and the way that it seemed to heighten Annie's resistance to eating and vulnerability to vomiting. A phase that was very much like conventional marriage counseling ensued, except that Annie was always present and her responses to the fluctuating emotional tone of the discussion were a recurrent focus of attention. For example, when her father's voice became tense and angry, Annie had a way of getting herself into a predicament that required immediate rescuing, like standing up on the rocking chair. Although there was little direct discussion of feeding, by the end of this phase, which lasted between 3 and 4 months, Annie was eating well enough to discontinue the nasogastric feedings completely.

The therapist helped Annie's parents resolve the discrepancy between their ideal of having the mother stay at home with Annie and the reality of the financial constraint, social isolation (for Annie's mother), and exhaustion (for Annie's father) that resulted from this choice. Annie's mother chose to work part time and was helped to find appropriate child care. As her depression lifted, her interactions with Annie around feeding and other areas became livelier, more engaged, and more effective.

In this case, a child's feeding disorder was resolved successfully by building a therapeutic relationship within which both the parents' early histories and their marital relationship could be examined for their impact on their daughter's eating.

Effectiveness

Fraiberg and her colleagues (Fraiberg et al., 1981a, 1981b) performed a 6-year study to assess the outcomes of infant–parent psychotherapy with high-risk dyads. Close to 80% of the sample of 35 extended treatment cases showed measurable improvement in affective and social functioning, adaptive modes, and parenting. Lieberman, Weston, and Pawl (1991) subsequently demonstrated the effectiveness of infant–parent psychotherapy for increasing security of attachment in a sample of anxiously attached infants and their mothers. Both of these outcome studies reflect work with the kinds of clients who often are difficult to reach: poor, poorly educated, culturally diverse, multiproblem families with little trust in helping professionals and a history of unsuccessful interventions.

Mental Health Consultation

Unfortunately, in these times of harsh budgetary constraints, funding and adequately trained personnel seldom are available for the kind of intensive, relatively long-term treatment that infant–parent psychotherapy entails. When this is the case, the services of a mental health consultant can be very helpful. The ideal consultant will be a specialist in early parent–infant relationships, with a solid background in the assessment and treatment of adult psychiatric disorders as well. The presence of a mental health consultant at regular staffings of patients can alert service providers to potential psychosocial factors and transference–countertransference issues both in the infant–parent relationship and in the parent–provider relationship. Such consultation can do much to help providers become more effective in building treatment alliances and in finding more palatable ways to present advice and services to resistant, hard-to-reach families. Consultation can also help staff develop a cognitive framework for understanding inevitable treatment failures and can contribute to a clearer understanding of both the strengths and the limits of available treatment resources. Although many intervention programs for pediatric undernutrition may be unsuccessful in helping parents who have borderline personality disorder, for example, a mental health perspective can reduce the stress and reactive punitiveness that such failures can produce in staff when the failure is not understood in the context of the client's mental health issues. An excellent resource for such consultation is ZERO TO THREE: National Center for Infants, Toddlers and Families, a clearinghouse for early intervention programs. A critical insight from the work of Fraiberg and her colleagues for those working with pediatric undernutrition is that an infant's difficulties with taking in adequate nutrition frequently are reflections of his or her parents' difficulties with "taking in" nurturance, social support, and advice. Addressing the latter can be an effective means of improving the former. Consultation also can help providers become comfortable in lowering their goals to what they realistically can expect to achieve. Understanding this link between infant undernutrition and parental psychological need can be a fruitful avenue into successful intervention with these often hard-to-reach families.

REFERENCES

Ainsworth, M., Bell, S.M., & Stayton, D. (1974). Infant–mother attachment and social development: Socialization as a product of reciprocal responsiveness to signals. In M. Richard (Ed.), *The inte-*

gration of the child into a social world (pp. 99–135). Cambridge, England: Cambridge University Press.

American Psychiatric Association. (1994). *Diagnostic and statistical manual of mental disorders* (4th ed.). Washington, DC: Author.

Benoit, D. (1993). Failure to thrive and eating disorders. In C.H. Zeanah, Jr. (Ed.), *Handbook of infant mental health* (pp. 317–331). New York: Guilford Press.

Brazelton, T.B. (1992). *Touchpoints: Your child's emotional and behavioral development.* Reading, MA: Addison Wesley Longman Inc.

Brazelton, T.B., & Cramer, B.G. (1990). *The earliest relationship.* Reading, MA: Addison Wesley Longman Inc.

Clark, R., Paulson, A., & Conlin, S. (1993). Assessment of developmental status and parent–infant relationships: The therapeutic process of evaluation. In C.H. Zeanah, Jr. (Ed.), *Handbook of infant mental health* (pp. 191–209). New York: Guilford Press.

Emde, R.N. (1989). The infant's relationship experience: Developmental and affective aspects. In A.J. Sameroff & R.N. Emde (Eds.), *Relationship disturbances in early childhood* (pp. 33–51). New York: Basic Books.

Fraiberg, S. (1969). Libidinal object constancy and mental representation. *Psychoanalytic Study of the Child, 24,* 9–47.

Fraiberg, S., Adelson, E., & Shapiro, V. (1975). Ghosts in the nursery: A psychoanalytic approach to the problem of impaired infant–mother relationship. *American Academy of Child Psychiatry, 14,* 387–421.

Fraiberg, S., Lieberman, A., Pekarsky, J., & Pawl, J. (1981a). Treatment and outcome in an infant psychiatry program: Part 1. *Journal of Preventive Psychiatry, 1,* 89–111.

Fraiberg, S., Lieberman, A., Pekarsky, J., & Pawl, J. (1981b). Treatment and outcome in an infant psychiatry program: Part 2. *Journal of Preventive Psychiatry, 1,* 143–165.

Greenspan, S.I. (1997). *The growth of the mind and the endangered origins of intelligence.* Reading, MA: Addison Wesley Longman Inc.

Greenspan, S.I., & Lieberman, A.F. (1980). Infants, mothers, and their interaction. In S.I. Greenspan (Ed.), *The course of life: Vol. 1. Infancy and early childhood* (pp. 271–312). Washington, DC: U.S. Department of Health.

Lieberman, A.F., & Birch, M. (1985). The etiology of failure-to-thrive: An interactional developmental approach. In D. Drotar (Ed.), *New directions in failure to thrive: Implications for research and practice* (pp. 259–277). New York: Plenum.

Lieberman, A.F., Weston, D., & Pawl, J.H. (1991). Preventive intervention and outcome with anxiously attached dyads. *Child Development, 62,* 199–209.

Mahler, M. (1975). *The psychological birth of the human infant.* New York: Basic Books.

Sander, L.W. (1964). Adaptive relationships in early mother–child interaction. *Journal of the American Academy of Child Psychiatry, 3,* 231–264.

Sandler, J. (1976). Countertransference and role-responsiveness. *International Review of Psycho-Analysis, 3,* 43–47.

Seligman, S., & Pawl, J. (1984). Impediments to the formation of the working alliance in infant–parent psychotherapy. In J. Call, E. Galenson, & R.L. Tyson (Eds.), *Frontiers of infant psychiatry* (Vol. 2, pp. 232–237). New York: Basic Books.

Stern, D. (1985). *The interpersonal world of the infant: A view from psychoanalysis and developmental psychology.* New York: Basic Books.

Valenzuela, M. (1990). Attachment in chronically underweight young children. *Child Development, 61,* 1984–1986.

Ward, M.J., Kessler, D.B., & Altman, S.C. (1993). Infant–mother attachment in children with failure to thrive. *Infant Mental Health Journal, 14,* 208–220.

Zeanah, C.H., Jr., Mammen, O.K., & Lieberman, A. (1993). Disorders of attachment. In C.H. Zeanah, Jr. (Ed.), *Handbook of infant mental health* (pp. 332–349). New York: Guilford Press.

Chapter 30

Toward Understanding the Role of Attachment in Malnutrition

Mary J. Ward, T. Berry Brazelton, & Marlene Wüst

Failure to thrive (FTT) is the term that has traditionally been used to describe a syndrome of impaired growth in young children. Among researchers, a variety of standards were used to classify children as experiencing FTT until the mid-1980s, when the consensus of a panel of experts recommended classification based on anthropometric criteria alone (Drotar et al., 1985). In this chapter, the term *FTT* is used to describe children with weights below the 5th percentile on standardized norms for age and gender and children who show significant failure to gain weight over time (falling back 2 or more standard deviations in 6 months or less). It is important to note that the degree of weight deficit that is labeled "FTT" in the United States and other Western nations is identical to the degree of deficit that is endemic in developing countries and simply called malnutrition; thus, FTT is perhaps more accurately called "malnutrition in the first world."

FTT is a diagnosis with a long history of imprecise definition (see Chapter 1). Beliefs, often not supported by evidence, sometimes guide clinical practice and appraisal of data. For example, it was long believed that FTT was linked inexorably with later developmental delay. Indeed, in many studies, current developmental delay was used as a necessary criterion for inclusion; however, when children with FTT are selected for study on the

Work on this chapter was supported by Grant No. R01-HD27261 from the National Institute of Child Health and Human Development and in part by award No. M01-RR06020 from the General Clinical Research Centers Program, National Center for Research Resources, National Institutes of Health.

The authors thank Rosalie Bastone, Jacqueline Brathwaite, Luisa Escolar, Shelley Lee, Evelyn Lipper, Helen Maloney, Lauren Marcus, Catherine Monk, Rica Vizarra, Marie Whiteside, and Mei Wong for invaluable assistance. Special gratitude belongs to the families who shared their lives with us in support of this work.

basis of anthropometric criteria alone, the occurrence of developmental problems is less pervasive (Frank & Zeisel, 1988).

Similarly, it is common to find scientists and clinicians who hold a belief that malnutrition that is accompanied by another disease ("organic FTT") is different in etiology and maintenance than malnutrition that is not accompanied by other disease ("nonorganic FTT"). By the 1980s, writers were rejecting that dichotomy as spurious and unproductive (Woolston, 1985); however, it is not uncommon for researchers today to report excluding from their studies children with any illness known to co-occur with FTT. For example, cleft palate and gastroesophageal reflux may be used as exclusion criteria, although neither of these conditions leads necessarily or even with undue frequency to FTT.

Ward, Kessler, and Altman (1993) provided the first data from a sample of children who were selected solely with anthropometric criteria that when "organic" influences were quantified objectively (using the Woolston, 1985, criteria), organic and nonorganic FTT groups did not differ in the frequency with which stressful lives and disrupted attachments were observed, although both FTT groups differed from a sample of normally growing children (Ward et al., 1993) on those factors.

For most children, FTT describes the endpoint of a process that involves medical and nutritional (i.e., biological) as well as psychological and social (i.e., environmental) influences (Drotar et al., 1985). There is evidence of an association between malnutrition and stressors in the family environment and in parent–child interaction (cf. Ward et al., 1993), although some researchers have urged careful review of this evidence. For example, Wolke (1996) reported that fewer than 20% of a cohort of British infants who had weights below the 3rd percentile were referred for evaluation, leading him to question the representativeness of many samples from which data have been published. Drotar and colleagues (1985) suggested that disrupted relationships are the crucial factor in the development of FTT, as challenged relationships fail to buffer these families from the stressful experiences that they report.

JOINT INFLUENCES ON MALNUTRITION

Recognizing the *inter*dependence of mind and body in malnutrition, it is possible to define strategies for understanding the physiological and psychological processes that serve to maintain growth failure.

Cravioto and DeLicardie (1976) noted that in impoverished communities where limited access to resources and other macroenvironmental factors lead to high risk of malnutrition in children, the prevalence of severe protein-energy malnutrition (PEM) rarely is greater than 10%, in part because of the high mortality that is associated with severe malnutrition and in part because only some children seem to manifest the disorder. These investigators used data from a longitudinal study of malnutrition in a Mexican village. Macroenvironmental variables (e.g., socioeconomic status, family size, parents' weights) were not useful in distinguishing children who experienced severe malnutrition from those who were growing normally. In contrast, measures of home stimulation, maternal sensitivity, and the mother's active engagement with the child during a test distinguished the two groups, with little overlap in the ranges of scores. Thus, it was in process-oriented measures of children's close relationships that malnourished and thriving children differed most, even in an environment where access to food was limited.

In an article that was largely unrecognized among those researching disordered growth, Hepner and Maiden (1971) advocated attention to mother–child relationships as "controlling factors" in the emergence of malnutrition among children at risk. Using data from a large study of impoverished American children, these authors presented evidence that harmonious mother–child relationships were protective of good nutritional outcome even for children with poor diets, and disharmonious relationships were precipitating of malnutrition even for children with good dietary intake. In other words, an exclusive focus on either nutritional intake or mother–child relationships would not provide sufficient prediction. It was only with simultaneous focus that the predictions emerged clearly.

Hepner and Maiden's work went unrecognized in part because it was published by a researcher in nutrition at a time when psychoanalytic approaches dominated the literature on FTT. When the psychodynamic approach was misinterpreted or misapplied as mother blaming, it was rejected by writers who favored an environmental stress model for explaining the genesis of malnutrition. During the 1980s, in a move to obtain greater objectivity, clinicians placed increasing emphasis on medical, nutritional, and oral-motor factors (viz, Frank & Zeisel, 1988), which may have led to an unfortunate tendency for relationship issues to be reduced to observing behavioral contingencies in evaluations of malnourished children (Monk, 1997). This chapter suggests that 1) careful and objective attention to relationships is crucial in treating malnourished children and 2) giving attention to relationships will not lay blame for children's problems on mothers but will benefit families.

ATTACHMENT THEORY

The concept of attachment has dominated the study of parent–child relationships since the mid-1970s. Three central concepts in attachment theory, all derived from Bowlby's (1969, 1973, 1980) writings, are described. These concepts are security, internal working model, and sensitivity. Although many readers are familiar with some or all of these concepts, they are discussed in some detail to ensure a common set of definitions for the discussion that follows.

Security

Security is the core concept of attachment theory. Bowlby (1969, 1973, 1980) used the term *attachment* to refer to a relationship between an infant and a specific adult. Bowlby emphasized that attachments are significant for their endurance over time and space (i.e., they continue to exist beyond infancy and despite separation). He also described that an attachment cannot be observed directly; its characteristics can be inferred only from observed behavior.

In his writings, Bowlby contributed three important insights about infant attachment. First, the infant–parent relationship is a genuine attachment, not merely an infantile precursor to adult love relationships. Second, infants' reactions to separation and loss are much more than merely tears and wails. Instead, infants' reactions to separation and loss reflect the same process of grief and mourning that is experienced by adults. Finally, qualities of infants' attachments reflect their actual experiences, not merely fantasies that are based in aggressive instincts.

In Bowlby's writings, the term *attachment* also refers to a system of behavior that is seen in all human beings. Bowlby proposed that infants' behavior with their caregivers is determined by an inborn, biologically determined attachment behavior system. This system has a biological significance that is equivalent to other behavioral systems, such as feeding, and is not merely important because it becomes associated with provision of food.

The attachment behavioral system involves multiple behaviors—clinging, crying, following, reaching, and so forth. The system functions to maintain a balance between attachment (attempts to seek proximity) and exploration of the world. Bowlby explained that the attachment system assumed importance in evolution because it afforded infants protection from environmental hazards, ensuring that they would remain within the protection of adults. Given the helplessness of human infants, it is essential for infants' very survival that they remain in proximity to adults.

Bowlby (1969) described four stages in the development of attachment:

1. *Undiscriminating social responsiveness.* In the phase from birth to 3 months, inborn reflexive behaviors—such as crying, rooting, grasping, and turning toward—serve to increase the time that caregivers spend with infants. These reflex patterns initially serve a number of nonattachment functions but become organized through interactions with caregivers. Bowlby emphasized that attachment arises out of interactions rather than emerging fully formed. Specifically, attachment is the product of both experience and typical learning abilities.

2. *Focus on one or a few figures.* During this phase, 3- to 6-month-old infants exhibit differential responsiveness to others and focus attachment behaviors on one or a few caregivers with whom they have extensive experience. The average expectable environment consisting of an available and responsive caregiver is necessary for the emergence of typical infant attachment behavior.

3. *Emergence of secure base behavior.* Starting at 6 or 7 months and certainly by 12 months, a typical infant comes to use the caregiver as a secure base from which to explore and as a haven of safety. Confidence in the availability of the caregiver makes children less fearful of novelty and more competent in exploration. This "secure base phenomenon" is a central feature of the organization of emotion, thought, and behavior in close relationships across the life span.

4. *Transformation of secure base behavior into a goal-corrected partnership.* Bowlby described how, beginning in the preschool years, a child is increasingly able to take into account the caregiver's goals and activities when attachment is active; that is, by the age of 3 or 4 years, overt attachment behaviors are somewhat less evident, although the relationship itself does not attenuate. In other words, attachment does not decline along with separation protest.

According to Bowlby, infants are born with a set of behaviors that serve to elicit care from the adults around them because adults have an inborn set of caregiving behaviors that are complementary to infants' attachment behaviors. For example, most adults experience discomfort and a desire to help a crying infant; similarly, a common reaction when an infant nestles into an adult's neck is to hold the infant closer.

Social development is expected to follow a normal course when a child experiences the reliable and predictable care that is typical of humans. In normal human development, children move from dependence on caregivers in the first year toward greater autonomy in the second year because experiences of reliable care have led to expectations of safety and protection in the caregiver's presence—or what Bowlby called *security.*

When the rearing environment departs from the expected and caregivers are unavailable physically or psychologically, anomalies in social development occur. Children who do not experience safe and reliable care are, according to Bowlby, *anxious* (or insecure) about protection that is afforded them and, thus, are hampered in normal social and emotional development. Bowlby's formulation makes it obvious that Harlow's (Harlow & Harlow, 1962) isolation-reared monkeys (with their self-abuse and stereotypical behavior), institution-reared infants (with their inability to form focused attachments [cf. Rutter, 1996]), and abused children (with their varied maladaptive behavior) all had something in common: They experienced unexpected environments and, as a result, showed atypical social development.

Beyond these extreme examples of inadequate care, Bowlby was interested in the repercussions of his theory for normal-range variations in development. His colleagues and students have produced abundant evidence of the value of his theory for understanding variations in children's and adults' attachments.

Ainsworth, a colleague of Bowlby, used his theory to examine individual differences in security and anxiety among normal children. In her extensive observational research, Ainsworth developed a method, the Strange Situation (SS) (Ainsworth, Bell, & Stayton, 1971), a research paradigm to assess in a standardized way attachment behavior in 12- to 18-month-old infants. The episodes in the SS approximate situations that most children from industrialized countries encounter in their everyday lives (e.g., meeting an unfamiliar adult, undergoing brief separations from mother). The sequence of episodes in the SS allows observation of the degree to which the infant shows a balance between proximity-seeking and exploratory behaviors. Although the infant's behavior is the focus of the SS, abundant evidence supports the idea that SS measures fundamental characteristics of the mother–child relationship (Sroufe, 1983).

Security in infant–mother attachment is assessed in the SS on the basis of infant behavior, primarily in reunions after brief separations. Four patterns can be observed (Ainsworth, Blehar, Waters, & Wall, 1978; Main, Kaplan, & Cassidy, 1985):

1. *Secure (Group B) attachment,* characterized by a balance between attachment and exploration, is the most common pattern observed among infants (50%–70% of most samples [Ainsworth et al., 1978]). In an unfamiliar room, a secure infant separates readily to play with toys. When a stranger enters, a secure infant may interrupt play momentarily to take note. Soon, though, the infant warms up and may even become quite sociable to the stranger—maybe even giving more attention and smiles to the stranger than to the mother. When the mother leaves, a secure infant will take note—he or she may or may not cry, but his or her play certainly becomes more subdued. In any case, when the mother returns, a secure infant responds actively—greeting her and interacting with her or, if distressed, seeking and maintaining contact. When a securely attached infant is upset, only an attachment figure will do—the mother is preferred to a stranger, and the mother is the only one who can really comfort the child.

2. *Anxious-avoidant (Group A) attachment* is seen in approximately 10%–25% of most samples (Ainsworth et al., 1978). This pattern is characterized by adequate exploration *and* active avoidance of the mother, especially when distress is present. An avoidant infant reacts to separation with *de*tachment, giving the impression of indifference to the mother's presence. These infants play well but without sharing pleasure with the mother. On reunion, they actively avoid the mother: They turn away, crawl away, look away, or ignore her altogether; or they may begin to approach, only to abort the approach before getting close to the mother. When distressed, sometimes these infants are settled more readily by a stranger than by the mother. These infants are not just precociously independent: Their avoidance is accompanied by physiological signals (e.g., rapid heart-rate accelerations) that belie their apparent detachment. Furthermore, as preschoolers, these children are highly *de*pendent (e.g., clingy) on teachers (Sroufe, 1983).

3. *Anxious-resistant (Group C) attachment* is seen in approximately 5%–20% (Ainsworth et al., 1978) of most samples. This pattern is characterized by incompetence in

exploration, wariness about novelty, and anger. These infants are ambivalent on reunion with mothers. A resistant infant's anger is mixed with an apparent desire for contact, so the child both rejects contact *and* seeks to be close to the attachment figure. Contact with the mother is woefully ineffective in calming these infants—their angry distress is nearly unreachable. Characteristically, these infants show strong wariness of the unfamiliar room, impoverished exploration, and difficulty separating even when stress is low. These are the most clearly anxious infants.

4. *Anxious-disorganized or disoriented (Group D) attachment* (Main et al., 1985) is characterized by fearfulness or *lack* of strategy in attachment, in contrast to avoidant and resistant infants, whose patterns of behavior clearly are strategic. Disorganized infants may mix strong avoidance with strong resistance, may show frank fear on reunion, or may exhibit stereotypies or freezing of movement. Children who experience abuse and the children of parents who have bipolar disorder are likely to fall into this category, suggesting that it may be a sign of clinical significance.

It is important to reemphasize that avoidant, resistant, and disorganized infants all are anxious. They have in common a lack of the balance between attachment and exploration seen in secure infants. It is also important to emphasize that with attachment theory, the question is *not* whether a child is attached versus nonattached but what the quality of that attachment is. All normal human infants form attachments to caregivers with whom they have regular interactions. That fact of attachment is based in biology, whereas variations in quality of attachment are based in experience.

The major clinical limitation of the SS is that it is assumed to measure variations within the normal range of development. Anxious attachment, as observed in the SS, is seen as nonoptimum adaptation but not as psychopathology. Adopting a perspective that examines adaptation changes the focus from pathologizing nonoptimum patterns to understanding the resistance of established patterns to change. Further research will have to specify the developmental repercussions of disorganized attachment to determine whether its presence indicates long-term maladaptation. Current intervention is most prudently focused on recognizing evidence of disorganization in relationships and instituting treatment to reduce atypical patterns of coping.

Internal Working Model

In his later work, Bowlby (1980) described the mechanism through which early attachment experiences affect later competence and later parenting. Working models are mental representations—ideas in the mind—about relationships. In the beginning of life, they represent expectations about the availability or nonavailability of caregivers, developed from the infant's actual experiences. These representations are thought to be the mechanism through which qualities of attachment affect behavior throughout life.

Bowlby described that working models of the self develop in tandem with working models of caregivers; thus, responsive care leads an infant to feel confidence in the caregiver plus confidence in him- or herself or a sense that "I am loved" and "I am worthy of love." A child who experiences unresponsive or rejecting care, conversely, is likely to form a representation of self as unworthy or unacceptable and to expect denial of attachment needs.

Mental representations that are established in infancy and childhood are assumed to affect later social and emotional development because, once established, working models tend to remain stable. Although a person's working model can be amended by later experience, such as therapy or new relationships, these changes do not occur easily after infancy. As a result, Bowlby predicted, parents who raise secure children are those with secure working models. Such parents not only give responsive and supportive care to their children, he postulated, but also tend to engage in frank communication about their own working models and, as a result, indicate to the child that thoughts and memories about close relationships (i.e., working models) are open to questioning and revision.

Bowlby's predictions about the intergenerational transmission of attachment led Main and her students (Main et al., 1985) to develop a method to classify parents' internal working models: the Adult Attachment Interview (AAI). The AAI is a standardized research interview protocol that probes for general descriptions and specific memories of childhood relationships. The adult is asked to describe early relationships and to reflect on the influence of past relationships on current personality and parenting.

In coding the AAI, the adult's language is the focus, as motor and affective behavior are the focus of SS coding. Two major features of discourse are coded: 1) the adult's actual experiences—of love, rejection, role reversal, neglect, and pressure to achieve—in early relationships, as inferred from memories reported, and 2) current state of mind with respect to attachment, including coherence of discourse, use of idealization, expression of anger, claims of lack of memory, and evidence of lapses of reasoning.

Main et al. (1985) described four patterns of adult working models observed in adults' descriptions of and reflections on their childhood experiences. The characteristics of discourse and behavior that differentiate secure from insecure relationships appear to be robust across social class and maternal age (Ward & Carlson, 1995). These four categories correspond to the four patterns of infant–mother attachment described previously:

1. *Autonomous* adults value attachments freely and show objective and continuing evaluation of particular relationships (i.e., they balance recognition of the importance of close relationships with a capacity for objective appraisal of experience, just as secure children show a balance between attachment and autonomous exploration). Autonomous adults' discourse is coherent and often shows new insight. They acknowledge the effects of childhood—positive or negative—in consistent and believable ways and often use humor effectively in evaluating the impact of early experience on the self.
2. *Dismissing* adults are cut off from attachments, as avoidant infants adopt a strategy of cutting themselves off from attachment cues. Their childhood experiences generally were characterized by rejection and a lack of closeness, leading these adults to limit the influence of attachments. They may idealize early relationships strongly, even while claiming to have no memories of childhood; they may dismiss and devalue the importance of relationships, actively denying the impact of attachments on the self. These adults sometimes emphasize extraordinary self-reliance. They often provide episodic memories that contradict their general descriptions of early experience, apparently without recognizing the contradiction.
3. *Preoccupied* adults are overwhelmed by early experiences, as resistant infants are overwhelmed by novelty. These adults describe childhoods characterized by a lack of love and by role reversal. They are not objective about these childhood experiences; they may be incoherent and confused in their descriptions of early experience; and they often are caught up in current anger toward parents, unable to evaluate the impact of early relationships on current feelings. Psychological jargon and nonsense often are seen in the discourse of these adults in unconvincing ways as they discuss early relationships.

4. *Unresolved* adults have experienced trauma that is related to attachment and have not yet reconciled the loss or trauma with their present emotional experience. They are left with vaguely fearful, guilt-ridden, even irrational thoughts and feelings about childhood experiences, such as blaming themselves for abuse or for a death. Their discourse reveals extraordinary lapses in reasoning or logic as they discuss childhood loss or trauma. The adult's anomalous resolution of trauma or loss is reflected in the fearful, odd, or contradictory behavior of the disorganized infant.

As with the three anxious patterns of infant attachment, all three of the nonautonomous adult working models have a common characteristic: a lack of integration between current feelings and memories of past experiences that are relevant to attachment. Autonomous parents provide coherent, clear, and consistent discourse about the qualities and effects of childhood relationships, whether experience was positive or negative. For these individuals, in other words, current emotions and past experiences are integrated. In contrast, adults in the three nonautonomous groups all demonstrate a lack of integration between current feelings and past experiences that are relevant to attachment, albeit in distinctive ways. Indeed, Main et al. (1985) have defined the presence of such integration as the hallmark of security in adulthood.

A critical test of the value of Main et al.'s (1985) description of adult attachment is its correlation with infant attachment. In studies of attachment across two generations (e.g., Ward & Carlson, 1995), researchers have demonstrated strong continuity between patterns of infant attachment behavior and patterns of mothers' discourse about early attachments and their effects, in the ways predicted by theory.

Sensitivity

The concept of sensitivity was described by Ainsworth and her students (Ainsworth et al., 1978). It is used to characterize individual differences in caregiving that promote the development of secure attachment and later competence in children. Across social classes and cultures, maternal sensitivity is a central component of effective parenting.

Sensitivity to a child's signals involves a number of components: 1) being aware to receive signals or acting as though infant behavior is meaningful and indicates specific needs to be met by caregivers; 2) interpreting signals accurately; 3) formulating an appropriate response, based on an accurate interpretation of the infant's behaviors; and 4) responding in a timely way so that the infant can perceive the contingency of caregiver response and develop expectations. In contrast, insensitive caregiving may involve not noticing signals; misinterpreting signals when noticed; and responding late, inappropriately, or not at all. Sensitivity implies responsiveness to a *particular* infant, so there are no absolute definitions of what is appropriate or inappropriate caregiving; thus, this construct is well suited for measuring caregiver behavior with children of different ages and temperaments.

In a number of studies around the world (cf. Bretherton & Waters, 1985), researchers have confirmed Ainsworth's (Ainsworth et al., 1971) original findings about the association between sensitivity and security of attachment. In these studies, high sensitivity early in the first year was associated with secure attachments; low sensitivity, with anxious attachments.

In Ainsworth's studies (e.g., Ainsworth et al., 1971), sensitive mothers showed behavior that was much alike, probably because it is typical behavior for humans. Insensitive mothers, conversely, showed a variety of patterns. Ainsworth et al. (1971) found that patterns of insensitivity combined three basic characteristics: 1) *rejecting* behaviors, 2) *ignoring* behaviors, and 3) *interfering* behaviors. Rejecting behaviors included aversion to close contact and flat affect. This pattern was seen most often in parents of avoidant children. Ignoring behaviors involved neglectful and unavailable caregiving. This pattern was seen most often in parents of resistant children. Interfering behaviors included intrusiveness and interrupting. This pattern was seen in the parents of avoidant and resistant children.

In home observations, Belsky and colleagues (e.g., Isabella & Belsky, 1991) have confirmed Ainsworth's initial observations about maternal sensitivity and later attachment. In their studies, when infants were 3 and 9 months old, mothers of resistant infants engaged in little interaction with their children. In contrast, mothers of avoidant children showed very high levels of interaction, leading them to be overstimulating. Mothers of children who were secure showed moderate levels of interaction, implying an approach that was more adapted to the infants' level of engagement.

Main and colleagues (1985) suggested that mothers' mental integration about attachments may account for differences in maternal sensitivity. A secure mother, who has integrated memories of attachments with current emotions, can be consistent in using her attention to interpret and respond to infant behavior. In contrast, when a parent's memories and feelings are not integrated, restrictions are placed on attention. These restrictions are apparent in parents' discourse about early relationships as incoherences and contradictions and in maternal behavior as insensitivity. Indeed, Ward and colleagues (e.g., Ward & Carlson, 1995) have demonstrated an association between mothers' AAI classifications and their sensitivity. Autonomous mothers provided significantly more sensitive care than mothers who were dismissive, preoccupied, or unresolved.

From the standpoint of intervention, sensitivity may be the most unappreciated concept within attachment theory and is the aspect of mother–infant relationships that is most available to change. In this regard, it is wise to note Greenspan's (e.g., 1981) caveat: Although infant behavior may affect caregiver responses, there is relatively little opportunity for infants to consciously change their behavior. In contrast, caregiving behaviors offer multiple opportunities to effect change.

ASSOCIATIONS BETWEEN ATTACHMENT AND MALNUTRITION

There is strong evidence from three controlled studies, using current criteria for coding attachment, that malnutrition is associated with a particular pattern of anxious infant–mother attachment—disorganized, disoriented (Valenzuela, 1990; Ward et al., 1993; Ward et al., 1997). Ward and her colleagues (e.g., Ward et al., 1993) included in their studies children whose malnutrition is accompanied by other illnesses (excluding genetic and familial growth impairment and several life-threatening diseases). Furthermore, they have made strong efforts (see Ward et al., 1997) to include in their study enrollments all children in their clinics who meet definitions of FTT based on anthropometrics alone, in an effort to acquire as representative a sample of malnourished children as possible (cf. concerns of Wolke, 1996). Finally, neither the staff who run study procedures nor those who code behavior are aware of children's nutritional status, so expectations about qualities of relationships among children with FTT do not intrude on data.

With these precautions, Ward and her colleagues have found high rates of anxious, disorganized attachment among children with FTT (Ward et al., 1993; Ward et al., 1997). In their most recent findings (Ward et al., 1997), children with FTT ($n = 48$) showed secure attachment at nearly half the rate of the 82 normally growing children observed (36% versus 64%). In contrast, children with FTT were more than twice as likely as controls to

show anxious, disorganized attachment (48% versus 20%). Two points must be emphasized: First, one third of the malnourished children showed secure attachment, emphasizing the diversity that exists among children with malnutrition and the opportunities for
clinicians to build on strengths in relationships. Second, these findings demonstrate only
that malnutrition and disorganized attachment co-occur; strong inferences cannot be made
about causation from these data. Given the high rates of a pattern of behavior (i.e., disorganized attachment) that is known to have negative developmental sequelae, however, malnourished children clearly are a group at risk for relationship disturbance. Gunnar and
colleagues (Gunnar, Broderson, Nachmias, Buss, & Rigatuso, 1996) posited that secure
attachment serves as a coping resource for young children in their adaptation to stressors
in the environment, suggesting that a central vulnerability of children with FTT may be the
lack of a focal coping resource.

The rates of anxious attachment in Ward et al.'s studies are confirmed by the observations of Valenzuela (1990), who found that nutritionally compromised children were
more susceptible to the stresses of severe poverty. She found an extreme elevation (93%)
in the rate of anxious attachment among very poor and malnourished children ($n = 42$) in
Chile. In contrast, in a group of equally poor but adequately nourished children ($n = 43$),
anxious attachments were much less common (50%). Similarly, Goldberg (1988) found
that anxiously attached children with cystic fibrosis showed much poorer nutritional status
than securely attached children with the same disease; thus, there may be a direct link
between caloric intake and qualities of mother–child relationships.

Indeed, data link children's malnutrition to mothers' mental representation about their
own early relationships (Lee, Polan, & Ward, 1997), confirming an earlier study by Benoit,
Zeanah, and Barton (1989). In a subsample of 60 mothers, Main et al.'s (1985) AAI was
administered and coded by people who were blind to the child's nutritional status (Lee
et al., 1997). AAI classifications and SS classifications agreed in 74% of families. In addition, mother's AAI classification was related significantly to the child's nutritional status.
Mothers of children who had FTT were more than twice as likely as controls (56% versus
24%) to use discourse that indicated unresolved loss or trauma. In contrast, mothers of the
malnourished children were dramatically less likely to show autonomous (secure) discourse than mothers of well-nourished children (17% versus 59%). These findings provide
further evidence of the value of relationship constructs in distinguishing between malnourished children and those who are growing normally, highlighting the promise of
understanding the dynamics of mothers' representations of their own relationships in their
children's growth.

A ROLE FOR ATTACHMENT IN THE TREATMENT OF UNDERNUTRITION

From the perspective of attachment theory, current infant–mother attachments are seen
as products of actual interactions and experiences and, thus, are amenable to change.
The possibility of change, however, is seen in the light of expectations held by the mother
that have developed out of her own relationships. Parents' representations of attachments, although complex constructions of reality, also are seen as amenable to change,
perhaps especially so with the onset of parenting (Juffer, vanIJzendoorn, & Bakermans-
Kranenburg, 1997).

Recommendations for interventions with undernourished children—especially
changes in feeding interactions—must be made with recognition of what a parent has
experienced and what he or she is capable of acknowledging and changing. More important, it is crucial that clinicians be sensitive to the *meaning* of recommended interventions
and the meaning of infant behavior in light of parents' own relationship histories.

Most clinicians have been impressed with how the same intervention sometimes is effective and sometimes is not. The authors of this chapter suggest that the missing variable in predicting effectiveness in interventions for undernutrition is parents' working models of attachments. With attachment theory, parents are seen as products of their own attachment experiences. Each parent's reactions to clinicians are viewed as a logical outcome of his or her expectations about the likelihood that others will be trustworthy and provide useful help. Not only will the parent's expectations affect the degree of success that the parent will experience in complying with therapies, but those expectations also will alter the parent's likelihood of trusting the clinician in further therapy, especially if noncompliance with recommendations leads to frustration among clinicians. Thus, a parent's own experiences in relationships are given a central role in understanding current interactions. Understanding the parent's behavior as a product of the parent's own experience functions in a very crucial way to remove blame from him or her.

The authors of this chapter first collaborated in discussing issues of mothers' needs that affect the course of treatment of undernutrition in children. In their conversations, they recognized several features of some families of children with FTT. First, in many cases, malnourished children had been vulnerable newborns who were born into stressed families, where a cycle of "ill-fitting" interaction began at birth. For example, an infant with neonatal feeding difficulties and later FTT had a mother whose history included early loss of a parent. This mother felt enormous guilt about her infant's feeding and growth problems because she felt unable to protect her child, just as she had not been protected in childhood. Eliciting this history of mismatched interaction and mother's loss was a crucial first step in formulating a treatment plan for this dyad—a plan that included emphasis on the ways in which the mother had succeeded in protecting her child.

Second, in some cases, the role of inadequate caloric intake as a source of undernutrition is obscured by relationship issues, as when clinicians battle with parents about what appear to be sound and reasonable treatment plans. This was the case when efforts to increase caloric intake and institute treatment for reflux were ineffective with a mother who was attempting to protect her vulnerable child from what she perceived as painful procedures and foul-tasting medicine. She remembered her own parents as weak and neglectful, leaving her to cope alone with challenges that she faced in childhood, and she was determined not to abandon her own child in a similar way.

Decreased caloric intake often is linked with issues of caregiver–child interaction. Causal statements concerning the primacy of inadequate intake, infant vulnerability, or disordered interaction are not needed to acknowledge and work with the recognition of that connection; but a parent's behavior with his or her infant is not simply a matter of behavioral contingencies or availability of food. Recognizing the contribution of a mother's relationship history along with medical factors to a child's food refusal does not constitute blaming the mother or alleging maternal deprivation. Instead, knowledge of a mother's own experiences of inadequate care leads to recognition of the mother as a victim of a previous family system and suggests that care of the mother will benefit the infant. It is important to note that infant–parent psychotherapy addresses many similar issues, although many people do not have such resources available to them.

IMPLICATIONS FOR EVALUATION AND INTERVENTION

Although procedures such as the SS and the AAI are not practical in clinical settings, findings from research that is based on these instruments provide direction for assessments and treatments of undernourished children. Several implications for clinical approaches to undernutrition emerge (see also Chapters 7 and 29).

First, psychological and medical factors must be considered in tandem, requiring the *simultaneous* examination of relationship factors and physiological factors. No one factor can be said to take precedence. History about the earliest mother–infant interactions and about parents' relationships in childhood can provide critical information. Sometimes clinicians do not know the answers about psychological distress in the parents of their patients until they ask the relevant questions. Until all of the facts are known, there is the distinct possibility that growth problems are merely the most apparent symptom of relationship disorder in a family (Lieberman & Birch, 1985).

Second, assisting children with growth deficits requires that the parents' relationships with staff members be a focus of treatment. Parental history of troubled attachments and personality disorder co-occurs with FTT (Lee et al., 1997; Polan et al., 1991), implying that these are not just any parents with whom to establish alliances (see Chapters 4 and 29). Parents of children with FTT may be challenging in many ways, placing what may be undue demands on clinicians.

Finally, including consideration of attachment in assessing children's malnutrition provides opportunities for parents to receive supportive therapy. When presented as a support for a parent who is caring for an ill child and as an asset to the child, a recommendation for adult mental health services can be perceived by the parent as a caring gesture.

REFERENCES

Ainsworth, M.D.S., Bell, S.M., & Stayton, D. (1971). Individual differences in Strange Situation behavior of one-year-olds. In H.R. Schaffer (Ed.), *The origins of human social relations* (pp. 17–57). London: Academic Press.

Ainsworth, M.D.S., Blehar, M., Waters, E., & Wall, S. (1978). *Patterns of attachment.* Mahwah, NJ: Lawrence Erlbaum Associates.

Benoit, D., Zeanah, C.H., & Barton, M.L. (1989). Maternal attachment disturbances in failure-to-thrive. *Infant Mental Health Journal, 10,* 185–202.

Bowlby, J. (1969). *Attachment and loss: Vol. 1. Attachment.* New York: Basic Books.

Bowlby, J. (1973). *Attachment and loss: Vol. 2. Separation.* New York: Basic Books.

Bowlby, J. (1980). *Attachment and loss: Vol. 3. Loss, sadness, and depression.* New York: Basic Books.

Bretherton, I., & Waters, E. (1985). Growing points in attachment theory and research. *Monographs of the Society for Research in Child Development, 50*(Serial No. 209).

Cravioto, J., & DeLicardie, E.R. (1976). Microenvironmental factors in severe protein calorie malnutrition. In N.S. Scrimshaw & M. Behar (Eds.), *Nutrition and agricultural development.* New York: Plenum.

Drotar, D., Malone, C.A., Devost, L., Brickell, C., Mantz-Clumpner, J., Negray, J., Wallace, M., Woychik, J., Wyatt, B., Eckerle, D., Bush, M., Finlon, M., El-Amin, D., Nowak, M., Satola, J., & Pallotta, J. (1985). Early preventive intervention in failure-to-thrive. In D. Drotar (Ed.), *New directions in failure-to-thrive* (pp. 119–138). New York: Plenum.

Frank, D., & Zeisel, S. (1988). Failure-to-thrive. *Pediatric Clinics of North America, 35,* 1187–1201.

Goldberg, S. (1988). Risk factors in attachment. *Canadian Journal of Psychology, 42,* 173–188.

Greenspan, S. (1981). *Psychopathology and adaptation in infancy and early childhood: Principles of clinical diagnosis and preventive intervention.* Madison, CT: International Universities Press.

Gunnar, M.R., Broderson, L., Nachmias, M., Buss, K., & Rigatuso, R. (1996). Stress reactivity and attachment security. *Developmental Psychobiology, 29,* 10–36.

Harlow, H.F., & Harlow, M.K. (1962). Social deprivation in monkeys. *Scientific American, 207,* 136.

Hepner, R., & Maiden, N.C. (1971). Growth rate, nutrient intake, and "mothering" as determinants of malnutrition in disadvantaged children. *Nutrition Reviews, 29,* 219–223.

Isabella, R.A., & Belsky, J. (1991). Interactional synchrony and the origins of infant–mother attachment: A replication study. *Child Development, 62,* 373–384.

Juffer, F., vanIJzendoorn, M., & Bakermans-Kranenburg, M.J. (1997). Intervention in transmission of insecure attachment: A case study. *Psychological Reports, 80,* 531–543.

Lee, S., Polan, H.J., & Ward, M.J. (1997). *Attachment, psychopathology, and failure-to-thrive.* Manuscript submitted for publication.

Lieberman, A., & Birch, M. (1985). The etiology of failure-to-thrive: An interactional developmental approach. In D. Drotar (Ed.), *New directions in failure to thrive: Implications for research and practice* (pp. 259–278). New York: Plenum.

Main, M., Kaplan, N., & Cassidy, J. (1985). Security in infancy, childhood, and adulthood: A move to the level of representation. In I. Bretherton & E. Waters (Eds.), Growing points in attachment theory and research. *Monographs of the Society for Research in Child Development, 50*(1–2, Serial No. 209).

Monk, C. (1997). *Representational content and quality of mothers whose children are failing to thrive.* Unpublished doctoral dissertation, City University of New York, New York.

Polan, H.J., Kaplan, M., Kessler, D., Shindledecker, R., Newmark, M., Stern, D., & Ward, M.J. (1991). Psychopathology in mothers of children with FTT. *Infant Mental Health Journal, 12,* 55–64.

Rutter, M. (1996, April). *Profound early deprivation and later social relationships in early adoptees from Romanian orphanages followed at age 4.* Invited address at the International Conference on Infant Studies, Providence, RI.

Sroufe, L.A. (1983). Infant–caregiver attachment and patterns of adaptation in preschool: The roots of maladaptation and competence. In M. Perlmutter (Ed.), *Minnesota symposia on child psychology* (Vol. 16, pp. 41–81). Mahwah, NJ: Lawrence Erlbaum Associates.

Valenzuela, M. (1990). Attachment in underweight children. *Child Development, 61,* 1984–1996.

Ward, M.J., & Carlson, E.A. (1995). Associations among adult attachment representations, maternal sensitivity, and infant–mother attachment in a sample of adolescent mothers. *Child Development, 66,* 69–79.

Ward, M.J., Kessler, D.B., & Altman, S.C. (1993). Infant–mother attachment in children with failure to thrive. *Infant Mental Health Journal, 14,* 208–220.

Ward, M.J., Maloney, H.A., Brathwaite, J., Lee, S., Polan, H.J., & Lipper, E.G. (1997). *Infant–mother attachment and failure-to-thrive: Malnutrition AND disorganized relationships.* Unpublished manuscript.

Wolke, D. (1996, July–December). Failure-to-thrive: The myth of maternal deprivation. *The Signal: Newsletter of the World Association for Infant Mental Health, 4,* 1–6.

Woolston, J. (1985). Diagnostic classification. In D. Drotar (Ed.), *New directions in failure-to-thrive* (pp. 225–234). New York: Plenum.

RECOMMENDED READING

Karen, R. (1995). *Becoming attached: Unfolding the mystery of the infant–mother bond and its impact on later life.* New York: Warner Books.

Chapter 31

Child Protective Services

Nick Claxton and Andrew P. Sirotnak

There is a presumption in the United States that parents have the right and responsibility to raise their children as they see fit without interference from others. This assumes that the parents have their children's best interests at heart. There is another presumption that children have the right to be brought up in a safe and nurturing environment and to have their basic needs met. Ideally, there should be no conflict between the rights and interests of the children and those of the parents; however, in cases of abuse and neglect, parents' and children's rights conflict and the law provides protection for the child. The primary goal of child protective services is to keep children safe.

REPORTING LAWS

All 50 states have in place laws to guarantee for children some degree of protection from abuse and neglect. They differ in wording, emphasis, and definitions, but they provide minimum criteria to ensure that a mechanism exists for reporting and investigating alleged child maltreatment, that services can be offered to prevent further maltreatment, and that standard legal procedure guides the entire process to its conclusion. State intervention in the sensitive area of family life must be "guided by the legal base for action, strong philosophical underpinnings, and sound professional standards for practice" (U.S. Department of Health and Human Services, National Clearinghouse on Child Abuse and Neglect, 1996, p. 1).

With respect to pediatric undernutrition, only seven states specifically refer to "failure to thrive" in their child protection laws: Alaska, Arkansas, California, Colorado, Hawaii, Idaho, and Montana. The laws of Connecticut, West Virginia, and Wyoming refer, respectively, to malnutrition, nutritional deprivation, and substantial malnutrition (U.S. Department of Health and Human Services, National Clearinghouse on Child Abuse and Neglect, 1996). Undernutrition in the other states falls under the general definition of neglect, which refers to failure to meet the child's basic needs, such as adequate food, medical attention, shelter, protection, or education.

REPORTING CASES

Every state has civil laws that mandate the reporting of suspected child abuse and neglect. The people who are mandated to report vary by state but include primarily those who have professional contact with children. Most states also have immunity from prosecution provisions for professionals who report in good faith. Even with these laws, reporting of pediatric undernutrition is not uniform. Generally, pediatric undernutrition should be reported to child protective services when there is reason to suspect that it is due to neglect. Reasons for suspecting neglect could include failure of the parents to follow through with a treatment plan and social or family risk factors for maltreatment (see basic assessment questions later in this chapter). If the child is growing poorly and one does not suspect neglect, then one need not report. Deciding whether to report requires clinical judgment.

Service providers may be reluctant to report cases for many reasons: fear of losing a relationship with the family, fear of losing control of the case, fear of court involvement, and reluctance to believe that the parents have maltreated the child. This reluctance must be balanced by concern for the child's welfare and the realization that families may find the reporting and intervention helpful. In some cases, reporting helps the family gain access to social work or other services, such as subsidized child care. Before reporting, one should be honest with the family about the concerns and about the requirement to report the case.

When the report is received from either a mandated reporter, a family member, or even an anonymous reporter, the county agency will screen the call and make an initial risk assessment. An intake worker will ask whether there is evidence of abuse or imminent danger, such as bruises, burns, fractures, abusive head trauma in an infant, sexual abuse or assault with a potential perpetrator in the home, pediatric death under investigation as a possible child abuse fatality with other children at risk in the home, severe malnutrition, or a hospitalized child with multiple injuries. Other risk factors that may require prompt investigation are violence in the home, substance abuse, a drug-exposed newborn, homelessness, and mental illness.

Most agencies will assign cases as guided by risk assessment policies, and a worker will contact the family, child, and reporter, if necessary, to begin investigating the report. Not every case must or should be assigned to a worker (e.g., a child's undernutrition is mild, and the parents are willing to take advice, or a case is more appropriately handled by a physician or another agency). Mandated reporters subsequently may express frustration that a case is not investigated. Reviewing the case with a supervisor in the agency may be helpful.

In some communities, child protective services staff may be available to professionals and other reporters to discuss cases, without using the child's or the family's names, before a formal report is made. If such consultation leads to a recommendation that the case should be reported, then the professional should make the report after informing the family. Consulting with child protective services staff before reporting helps potential reporters make better judgments, and the child protective services staff may receive more appropriate reports.

COMPREHENSIVE INITIAL ASSESSMENT

Much emphasis has been placed on the diagnosis of "organic failure to thrive" with medical reason for poor growth versus "nonorganic failure to thrive" with no apparent primary medical cause of poor growth (see Chapters 1 and 19). This dichotomy is no longer con-sidered useful. The focus should be on the undernutrition and what has led to the child's current condition. When a case of pediatric undernutrition seems to be due to neglect, a comprehensive initial assessment of the family situation is warranted. This is often diffi-cult because the undernutrition may not be severe and its evaluation requires the parents' cooperation. Very few children in the United States reach fatal malnutrition by means of deliberate neglect.

Because a diagnosis of pediatric undernutrition involves much medical and nutri-tional information, the initial data gathering must be focused in this area. Information that should be collected includes past medical history, birth records, growth records, including all plotted curves; and data from programs, such as the Special Supplemental Nutrition Program for Women, Infants and Children (WIC), and professionals, such as visiting nurses, social workers, occupational therapists, and speech-language pathologists (see Chapter 9). The basic nutrition evaluation, including feeding observation and record of food intake, is also very important (see Chapters 6 and 8).

Although in this era of managed care few infants and children are admitted for under-nutrition, inpatient hospital records often will contain a wealth of information regarding the child–parent interaction and family dynamics. Hospital social workers, nurses, thera-pists, residents, medical students, and child abuse physicians may have documented valu-able information.

During the data-gathering stage, the following basic assessment questions may help guide the investigation:

- How severe is the undernutrition? What do the data reveal to the medical care providers?
- Are there signs of physical abuse, sexual abuse, or chronic neglect apart from the undernutrition?
- Does the family understand the growth deficiency, other medical diagnoses, and the reasons for concern that have been expressed by medical care providers?
- Has the family been cooperative, compliant, and concerned; or are they uncooperative, difficult, and distant? Do not accept descriptions such as "appropriate" and "inappro-priate." What exactly do the care providers mean by this?
- Do the parents have the correct knowledge about proper diet, age-appropriate food, and the importance of nutrition?
- Is there structure to the family routine around meals, infant feeding, and snacking, or do they occur at unpredictable and chaotic times? (See Chapter 27.)
- Is there parent–child conflict over feeding? (See Chapter 8.)
- Is there enough food in the home? Does the family have the money to buy food? Are they aware of resources to supplement food for the infant, child, or family?
- Does the family have adequate provisions in the home: clean kitchen space, cooking utensils, baby bottles, clean or potable water, a table and chairs?
- Can the parents read (e.g., for instructions for formula, medicine prescriptions, feeding schedules, cooking instructions, nutrition content of foods, telling time)?
- Can the parents write (e.g., for food diary, supplemental assistance and Medicaid forms, job applications)?
- How do the parents communicate (language, mental illness and thought disorders, brain injury)? Are interpreters or bilingual workers needed?
- Are there any religious, social, or cultural factors influencing the feeding or parenting (e.g., unusual diets or feeding practice; folk medicines; fasting; roles of the mother, father, and family members in the household)? (See Chapter 26.)

- How does the family function (e.g., daily routines, mental illness, depression, substance abuse, violence, physical disabilities, chronic illness, overwhelmed by daily living responsibilities or other children)?
- Do the parents understand the basics of child development and age-appropriate expectations for development and discipline (e.g., rolling, crawling, standing, walking, talking, bowel and bladder habits, sleep and wake cycles, teething, fever, temperament, colic, toilet training, language, safe child care arrangements, feeding)?
- Are there any domestic issues that have not been addressed (e.g., substance abuse, alcoholism, child sexual abuse or incest, child physical abuse, violence, spousal or partner abuse, mental illness, eating disorder in parent, marital conflict, divorce, criminal records for any of the caregivers in the home)?
- Are the parents overwhelmed by internal or external factors (e.g., economic, relatives, other children, illnesses, unemployment)?
- What does the family understand about the intervention of the child protective services agency? Do they have prior involvement with the agency? If so, then was this perceived as a bad or a helpful experience? Was there prior court involvement? Was the treatment plan completed? What about other counties, states, countries, and military or federal family services agency involvement (e.g., Native American family services for children living on reservations)?
- Were there criminal investigations, prosecution, or conviction for any crime but especially child abuse, domestic violence, assault, sexual assault or sexual abuse of a child, or drug offense?

Ideally, such an extended evaluation would include many visits to the family home by both the child protective services worker and the outreach workers or visiting nurse if they are involved. A single visit is not adequate to obtain the necessary or helpful information. Seeing a family in their own environment may provide much more information than interviews in a hospital or an office.

Signed releases of information from parents are helpful. Obtaining legal assistance from the child protective services attorney or county attorney for release of records can be planned at the outset in anticipation of any difficulty with family, medical personnel, or other agencies refusing to release records. It is important to know how local civil laws detail confidentiality and access to information when investigating possible child abuse.

CHILD PROTECTIVE SERVICES INTERVENTION

Intervention by child protective services is needed in cases of undernutrition in which the primary problems are neglect and family dysfunction, as in a case with social stressors and with a complex medical diagnosis. If it is determined that maltreatment has occurred or that there is substantial risk that it will occur, then the child protective services worker must determine whether it is safe for the child (and siblings) to remain in the home. The increasing emphasis on keeping families together has led to the provision of services not to the child alone but to the child in the context of his or her family. The general recognition here is that the child fares better when raised and cared for by the family of origin. If the state needs to intervene to ensure the safety of a child, then that intervention should be the least intrusive and disruptive possible. For example, child protective services may monitor a family for a short period to assess whether the incident that brought the family to its attention was either an isolated occurrence or part of a pattern or a more deeply rooted problem. The next step is to request that the family voluntarily accept services to address the problems that led to the abuse or neglect.

Placement of a Child

If these voluntary services are not accepted, are unable to reduce the risk of future maltreatment, or cannot remedy specific problems, then the child and siblings should be removed and placed out of the home. Placement ideally is sought with appropriate relatives. Specific requests by the family for nonrelative placement (e.g., friends, neighbor, co-worker) may be considered, but strict policy and procedure should guide the approval of such placement. It should be emphasized that out-of-home placement in foster care or relative care does not in itself ensure the continued safety of the child, as maltreatment can occur in those settings as well.

While the child is in placement, services are provided to the child and the family to achieve the goals of maintaining the safety of the child and working toward family reunification. The case is followed in civil court, and the agency delineates the nature of the maltreatment, the problems within the family, and the concerns of the agency. The court then will adjudicate a treatment plan that addresses each problem. If it is determined that it is impossible to keep the child safe from maltreatment or if the family demonstrates a continued unwillingness to accept court-ordered treatment plans, then adoption should be considered. The termination of parental rights is a very serious and final step in this process. Adoption can be considered only after termination of parental rights.

Child Protective Services' Goals for the Child and the Family

When intervention by child protective services has been made with a family in which a child is diagnosed as experiencing malnutrition, multiple goals may be set forth from many disciplines. Strong emphasis should be placed at the onset of the agency intervention on the common goal of establishing improved nutrition, growth, and development of the child in the context of the family. The specific infant or child goals may be more complex than simply to gain weight and grow. Although success is often described in terms of growth (see Chapter 10), the related goals of the intervention may be just as important for continued success of the child. These include keeping medical appointments, following the feeding regimen or diet, participating in therapies with the infant or child, and accepting the support and monitoring of either the voluntary or the court-ordered treatment plan.

The intervention plan should involve supportive counseling, education, referral, and case management. The plan should include concrete support: Look for the available child care and encourage community leaders to advocate for it as well; help transport the client to supplemental food sources; search for the resources to provide the table, highchair, pots, and bottles; place a case aide or homemaker in the home to teach, monitor, and supervise the care of the child and the running of the household; and check the visiting nurse's impression of the parents' progress as well as the weight gain of the child. "Poverty is the greatest single risk factor for failure to thrive" (Frank & Drotar, 1994, p. 298); and, although it may not be completely eliminated as a risk factor, carefully monitored concrete provisions can improve the health of the child in a low-income environment (see Chapter 28).

A particularly important goal for the infant or very young child is maintaining a healthy attachment to the parent or caregiver. Assessment of the parent–child relationship early on may guide treatment and make reunification less difficult (see Chapters 29 and 30). Assuming that the ultimate goal is reunification, the family must remain central in the intervention process even if the child is placed out of the home. The family of origin can be excluded only if parental rights have been terminated.

Working with the Family

Engaging the parents from the outset by recognizing that the child's best interests are their foremost concern is both eminently practical and professionally courteous. That is the starting point of the initial assessment, the ongoing involvement of the family, and the coordinated treatment plan. Family members are often disregarded by professionals who presume that involvement with child protective services equates somehow with the family's inability to contribute to the child's further care. The manner in which professionals interact with such families—statements, attitudes, demeanor, and body language—will convey to them either a genuine, concerned effort to help the child and the family or a disdainful mistrust of their ability to participate in a treatment plan.

The initial involvement by the child protective services worker may be at the often unavoidable time of disagreement between the professionals and the family regarding the growth of a child and usually after there has been much effort made with the family to address the growth deficiency. The question of what is normal growth for the child, what constitutes a medical emergency, or what medical intervention is required may be a point of considerable conflict between parents and professionals. Establishing communication and collaboration with all of the professionals who are involved may not be an easy task in the context of such conflict; however, the initial resistance may be overcome by skilled workers who engage the family respectfully. "Start where the client is," and easier service planning will follow. The treatment plan should become mutually acceptable to both the family and the child protective services agency.

TEAMWORK IN CHILD PROTECTION

Treatment of undernourished, neglected children requires work in several areas, including nutrition, medicine, social services, and mental health (Frank & Drotar, 1994). This involves multiple professionals and invites the formation of a team (see Chapters 9 and 22). The team may be internal to an institution or comprise professionals from different agencies (see Chapter 35). Each team member should have a defined role and should understand the others' roles. Team members should commit enough time to the case so that they can have regular ongoing meetings for case review. The most advanced form of collaboration is transdisciplinary, in which professionals learn to share their roles (see Chapter 1). Shared goals, well-defined procedures, diligent collaboration, and open communication all are important for the team's success.

Communication between the agency worker and the other professionals should address the specific nature of the growth and development problems, medical care needs, and necessary follow-up plan of care. The medical passport system developed by many state agencies can be used for this purpose. This can detail who is involved with the child's care, the diagnoses and plan of care, and when follow-up is needed for each part of the plan (Simms, 1991; Simms & Kelly, 1991).

Communication between the family or foster caregivers and the agency should be in concert with the medical and other service providers so that everyone involved in the case is on the same page. For example, the worker needs to know the latest growth measurements, the foster parent needs to know the contact person from each agency, and the physician and the dietitian must give consistent advice.

The child protective services worker should expect the medical provider to convey information in clear layman's terms to both the family and the worker. For example, a physician could state, "This is a 13-month-old child whose weight is average for a 6-month-old and whose length is average for a 9-month-old. His weight is very low relative to his height." This conveys the picture of a very small and thin child who is well below his potential growth.

An obvious value of such an approach is the availability of the expertise of many disciplines in the coordination of a treatment plan and the supervision of a family. The child protective services worker can share confidential information in order to discuss ongoing treatment if consent is obtained from the family. A sometimes inevitable disadvantage is the possibility of professional difference of opinion and conflict. A team leader or chair should be conversant with most disciplines and be prepared to offer a final decision to resolve conflict and preserve the team. Realizing the existing different personal values and opinions, accepting the expert input of each professional, and respecting each member as a colleague in child welfare are good foundations for any such team.

The following case examples demonstrate success because of the team approach and a failure because of its absence.

A family who was referred to social services presented with a complex situation including two undernourished young children, suspected sexual abuse of a child by a grandparent, and poor housing conditions. The mother had little family support, appeared to have difficulty understanding the nature of the children's poor growth and medical problems, and was later diagnosed with depression. After months of social work and nursing intervention, one child continued to do poorly and was placed in foster care, where she began to gain weight. Sexual abuse was ruled out by further assessment and medical examination.

Child protective services considered placing the other child because of continued poor growth. After further medical testing, this child was diagnosed and treated for gastroesophageal reflux. The child was put in child care, ensuring two daily meals. These interventions plus an eventual move to better housing and improved support from extended family allowed the child to remain in the home. To attain this success, collaboration was required among the child protective services worker, physician, child care worker, dietitian, and psychotherapist.

The foregoing case demonstrates the need for continuous case assessment and how ongoing communication with involved disciplines brings about good outcomes.

A child who was unresponsive and in the advanced stages of starvation was admitted to the hospital after being brought to the emergency room by ambulance. Although he was 2 years, 8 months old, his weight was that of an average 7-month-old, and he was covered with abrasions and bruises. He remained in intensive care in critical condition for 1 week. Global developmental delays, seizures, anemia, and poor skin and hair growth related to vitamin deficiency all were diagnosed subsequently. His 5-week hospitalization involved multiple consultants, physical therapy, psychological and developmental testing, and teaching the child how to eat.

The child and his three siblings had been placed abruptly with a maternal relative by child protective services because the mother had developed an incapacitating medical condition. One month after placement, the child's growth chart began to show a drastic decline in weight and height. This maternal relative gave birth to her third child after the toddler was placed in her care and was overwhelmed by the care of the five children.

Multiple care providers had been involved in the case, but there was no effective case management, and communication among professionals was poor. An ongoing caseworker had failed to keep contact with the family, and an outreach worker from an early intervention program had failed to transfer the case to a new worker. The child had been lost to medical care once the relative's infant was born. A physician had told the family that the child was depressed and not eating well because of this and would eventually gain weight.

The siblings were immediately placed in foster care, as was the child upon hospital discharge. One of the older siblings subsequently disclosed that the malnourished child had indeed been a target of maltreatment in the home. Parental rights were terminated, and the child was adopted by another family.

This case shows the nearly disastrous effects of lack of follow-up and a failure to address the initial diagnosis of pediatric undernutrition with a team approach.

CONCLUSION

In some cases, a child's family fails to meet the child's basic need for nutrition. The child, whose development is at risk, deserves protection. Reporting of such cases and action by child protective services, in collaboration with professionals and agencies in the community, may be necessary. The unique role of the social worker and of the team in ensuring the health and safety of children may be of critical importance. With pediatric undernutrition, this role may be most clearly understood and valued in the context of a team approach.

REFERENCES

Frank, D.A., & Drotar, D. (1994). Failure to thrive. In R.M. Reece (Ed.), *Child abuse: Medical diagnosis and management* (pp. 298–324). Philadelphia: Lea and Febiger.

Simms, M.D. (1991). Foster children and the foster care system: Part II. Impact on the child. *Current Problems in Pediatrics, 21*(8), 345–369.

Simms, M.D., & Kelly, R.W. (1991). Pediatricians and foster children. *Child Welfare, 70*(4), 451–461.

U.S. Department of Health and Human Services, National Clearinghouse on Child Abuse and Neglect. (1996). *State Statute Series, No. 1: Reporting Laws.* Washington, DC: Author.

RESOURCES

Bross, D.C., Krugman, R.D., Lenherr, M.R., Rosenberg, D.A., & Schmitt, B.D. (1988). *The new child protection team handbook.* New York: Garland Publishing.

Fahlberg, V.I. (1991). *A child's journey through placement.* Indianapolis, IN: Perspective Press.

Filip, J., McDaniel, N., & Schene, P. (Eds.). (1992). *Helping in child protective services: A competency based casework handbook.* Englewood, CO: American Humane Association.

Frank, D.A., Silva, M., & Needlman, R. (1993, February). Failure to thrive: Mystery, myth, and method. *Contemporary Pediatrics,* 114–133.

Harper, G., & Irvin, E. (1985). Alliance formation with parents: Limit-setting and the effect of mandated reporting. *American Journal of Orthopsychiatry, 55,* 550–560.

Iwaniec, D., Herbert, M., & McNeish, A.S. (1985). Social work with failure to thrive children and their families. *British Journal of Social Work, 15,* 243–259.

Pardeck, J.T. (1996). *Social work practice: An ecological approach.* Westport, CT: Greenwood Publishing Group.

Pawl, J. (1984). Strategies of intervention. *Child Abuse and Neglect, 8*(2), 261–270.

Schmitt, B.D. (1988). Failure to thrive: The medical evaluation. In D.C. Bross, R.D. Krugman, M.R. Lenherr, D.A. Rosenberg, & B.D. Schmitt (Eds.), *The new child protection team handbook* (pp. 82–101). New York: Garland Publishing.

Schor, E.L. (1982). The foster care system and the health status of foster children. *Pediatrics, 69,* 521–528.

Schor, E.L. (1988). Foster care. *Pediatrics in Review, 35,* 1241–1252.

Schor, E.L. (1989). Foster care. *Pediatrics in Review, 10,* 209–215.

U.S. Department of Health and Human Services. (1994). *Public health service, Clinician's handbook of preventive services.* Washington, DC: U.S. Government Printing Office.

U.S. Department of Health and Human Services. (1997). *National Center on Child Abuse and Neglect, Child Maltreatment 1995: Reports from the states to the National Child Abuse and Neglect Data System.* Washington, DC: U.S. Government Printing Office.

U.S. General Accounting Office. (1995). *Child welfare: Complex needs strain capacity to provide services.* Washington, DC: Author.

Section VI

Community Services

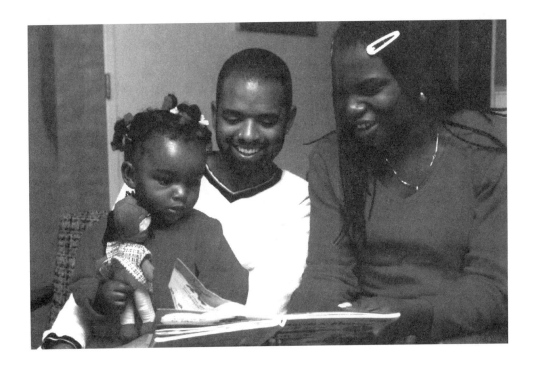

Chapter 32

Nutrition in Child Care

Donna Wittmer

A delicious bottle of milk, a hearty bowl of soup, or a nutritious vegetable or fruit makes the day seem brighter and healthier for young children. Child care providers, both in child care centers and in homes, have a crucial role to play in meeting the nutritional needs of children younger than 3 years. Caregivers must work hard to provide nutritious, delicious meals and snacks in an atmosphere that is caring and responsive. Infants and toddlers thrive, both physically and emotionally, when caregivers pay attention to quality—in food, preparation, presentation, interactions with children, and relationships with families. Happy mealtimes for young children promote good nutrition habits, positive social interactions, and opportunities to learn. Positive relationships with families ensure that there will be continuity for infants and toddlers across time, space, and settings and that family preferences are respected.

WHAT IS QUALITY? STANDARDS FOR
MEETING YOUNG CHILDREN'S NUTRITIONAL NEEDS

Quality in child care programs is the key to nutritional success with infants and toddlers. What is quality in relation to nutrition, and how is it determined? Several organizations provide standards for health and safety for out-of-home child care programs. Child care providers can use these organizations' publications to obtain information and improve nutrition for very young children.

National Academy of Early Childhood Programs

The National Academy of Early Childhood Programs is a division of the National Association for the Education of Young Children (NAEYC). This professionally sponsored, national, voluntary accrediting system for early childhood programs identifies 10 indicators of quality programs. Both the Administrator's Report and the Early Childhood Program Description sections include a "Nutrition and Food Service" component. Items on the

Administrator's Report include the following (National Academy of Early Childhood Programs, 1998):

- Meals and/or snacks are planned to meet the child's nutritional requirements in proportion to the amount of time the child is in the program each day, as recommended by the Child Care Food Program of the U.S. Department of Agriculture. (p. 16)
- Written menus are provided for parents. (p. 16)
- Feeding times and food consumption information is provided to parents of infants and toddlers at the end of each day. (p. 16)
- Foods indicative of children's cultural backgrounds are served periodically. (p. 16)
- Food brought from home is stored appropriately until consumed. (p. 16)
- Where food is prepared on the premises, the center is in compliance with legal requirements for food preparation and service. Food may be prepared at an approved facility and transported to the program in appropriate sanitary containers and at appropriate temperatures. (p. 17)

The Early Childhood Program Description form includes identical standards for the director and the external validator to rate as not met, partially met, or fully met.

ZERO TO THREE: National Center for Infants, Toddlers and Families

ZERO TO THREE: National Center for Infants, Toddlers and Families (previously known as ZERO TO THREE: National Center for Clinical Infant Programs) has created a document, *Caring for Infants & Toddlers in Groups: Developmentally Appropriate Practice* (Lally et al., 1995), that provides guidelines for high-quality group care for infants and toddlers. The component of quality infant-toddler child care that is discussed first is "Promoting Health and Safety":

> A basic challenge in the group care of infants and toddlers is creating a safe and sanitary environment that is interesting to the children and can be maintained efficiently so that caregivers have enough time for intimate, responsive interaction with each infant and toddler. (Lally et al., 1995, p. 29)

Appropriate practice for infants includes holding young infants for feeding and sitting mobile infants in small chairs with arms for support. Highchairs should be cleaned, folded, and put away when they are not in use. Caregivers need to have comfortable seating while they are sitting with infants during mealtimes. Care providers should label infant food and store it in individual bins in the refrigerator. Labeled bibs hang individually on hooks near the eating area. Dishes, utensils, and bottles are not shared and are washed after each use. Inappropriate practice includes

- Strapping infants in seats and propping their bottles
- Allowing older infants to crawl or toddle around with their bottles
- Leaving highchairs out, which take up a great deal of floor space
- Providing no place for adults to sit with mobile infants
- Piling food in the refrigerator
- Leaving bottles out on counters
- Not labeling anything (Lally et al., 1995)

Toddlers need small tables for a small group with individual place mats. Toddlers should help set, clear, and clean the table. Caregivers should sit with their special group of children and join in conversations with toddlers (Lally et al., 1995).

These guidelines for appropriate and inappropriate care describe the kind of equipment to provide for infants and toddlers and also the kind of adult–child interactions that help young children thrive physically and emotionally.

American Public Health Association and the American Academy of Pediatrics

The result of the collaboration between two national organizations (American Public Health Association & American Academy of Pediatrics, 1992) is a thorough book: *Caring for Our Children: National Health and Safety Performance Standards—Guidelines for Out-of-Home Child Care Programs.* Chapter 4, Nutrition and Food Service, highlights general requirements for nutrition for infants, toddlers, preschoolers, school-age children, and children with special needs. Topics covered in depth include staffing, meal service, seating, supervision, food brought from home, kitchen and equipment, access to the kitchen, food safety, maintenance, and nutritional experiences. The book provides standards, rationale, and interesting comments on each topic to help providers in family child care homes and centers provide nourishing, attractive, and safe meals and snacks.

Food and Nutrition Service of the U.S. Department of Agriculture

The Child and Adult Care Food Program (U.S. Department of Agriculture, Food and Nutrition Service, 1990) specifies nutritional standards and serving size ratios for children who attend child care. The Food Guide Pyramid (U.S. Department of Agriculture, 1992) and child care meal planning charts are available (see Chapter 6). For child care programs that qualify, there is government reimbursement for food costs. Contact your local public health department for more information concerning subsidized meals and meal planning menus.

HEALTH AND SAFETY ISSUES

Families entrust child care providers to keep their infants and toddlers healthy and safe while family members work outside the home. Table 1 provides a summary of health and safety issues for infants and toddlers. Of course, not all health and safety tips are listed, but the table provides a child care provider with information concerning the major issues and further resources to consider.

IT IS MORE THAN JUST FOOD

Food meets more than the nutritional needs of young children. Children feel worthy, satisfied, pleased, content, and fulfilled when they are fed in a loving environment. Eating and feelings mix together: When positive, they nourish physical, emotional, social, and cognitive development; when negative, they result in "emotional malnutrition" (Brazelton & Cramer, 1990). Relationships develop, trust is established, and children learn that they are worthy of love and positive care through responsive, sensitive caregiving around feeding and eating.

Developing Warm Relationships Through Feeding

Eating is a social experience. A caring relationship develops between infant and caregiver when a caregiver feeds an infant a spoonful of cereal, waits patiently for the infant to mush the food around in his or her mouth, and then offers another spoonful when the infant opens his or her mouth. Toddlers enjoy eating when a caregiver sits with a small group, responds to their needs, comments on the delicious food, and connects with them emo-

Table 1.   Health and safety tips

Infants (birth to 18 months)	Toddlers (18 months to 3 years)	Both infants and toddlers
Do not hold infants flat when giving them their bottle, as they may choke.	Toddlers should be seated when eating to reduce the risk of aspiration.[a]	Adults should not have hot liquids (e.g., coffee, tea) around young children. A hot spill could be disastrous.[a]
Microwaving bottles of milk can result in uneven heating and burning of the infant.	To prevent choking, watch for toddlers who eat too fast, stuff food, or do not chew their food.	Serve food on plates or other materials that can be disinfected easily.[a]
Always hold infants for bottle-feeding. To prevent choking and tooth decay, never prop a bottle to feed infants.[d]	To prevent choking, cut foods into small pieces ($\frac{1}{2}$" cubes).[a]	Adults should stay near and on the child's level. Never leave young children by themselves.[b, c]
Never add cereal to a baby bottle. The nipple can clog, or choking can occur.[d]	To prevent choking, do not let a toddler eat when he or she is having a tantrum; however, stay near to provide emotional support. Acknowledge a toddler's feelings.	Do not offer foods that are round, hard, small, thick, sticky, smooth, or slippery.[a]
Watch for "squirreling" of several pieces of food in the mouth. This can lead to choking in infants who are just beginning to eat solid foods or feed themselves.[a]		Food brought from home is labeled and stored appropriately until the infant or toddler eats it.[a, b]
Cut foods into small pieces ($\frac{1}{4}$" cubes) to prevent choking.[a]		Handwashing is imperative to prevent the spread of infection.[a, b, c]
Serve baby food and well-puréed foods.[a]		There should be a plan in place and training for responding to emergencies.[a]
Pacifiers must be of adequate size to prevent choking. Ensure that the nipple will withstand 2 pounds of force to prevent dislocation from the base.[d]		Do not serve honey to infants or toddlers. Honey may contain botulism spores, a type of bacteria.[a]

[a]American Public Health Association & American Academy of Pediatrics (1992). (See Chapter 7.)
[b]National Academy of Early Childhood Programs (1998).
[c]Lally et al. (1995).
[d]Edelstein (1995).

tionally. Warm relationships that develop through eating and feeding are crucial for young children's sense of well-being. Caring relationships are important for the development of well-adjusted, emotionally secure, happy children as well as of a sense of identity as a loved, loving, and capable person (Lally, 1994, 1995).

Meeting Emotional Needs

Children need a healthy sense of control. They learn to trust themselves to decide when they are hungry and how much to eat. They learn to regulate themselves and learn self-control. Child care providers decide which types of food to serve; infants and toddlers decide how much they can eat at one sitting. When child care providers give young children this type of control, food battles disappear and infants and toddlers feel a sense of self-worth.

> *A caregiver at a child care center routinely made all of the toddlers sit with folded hands at the beginning of lunch until every toddler in the group had not moved for several minutes. Only then could the toddlers begin to eat. Of course, it was too difficult for a group of seven toddlers to sit and wait, with the food sitting in front of them on a plate. Each one in turn moved or twitched or reached for food. The caregiver then made all of the toddlers start over again to wait. Tears and tantrums erupted from the toddlers while the caregiver tried harder and harder to maintain control.*

These toddlers were learning that mealtime was one of the most unpleasant times in the center. They also were learning that they had no control, that adults thought that they were naughty because they could not wait, and that their caregiver was a person to distrust. These toddlers' emotional needs obviously were not being met.

Caregivers meet young children's emotional needs when they understand the relationship between healthy emotional development and positive eating times. Infants and toddlers feel regarded, appreciated, and esteemed when infants' rhythms for eating fast or slowly are respected, mobile infants in highchairs are given finger foods to eat or are fed with a spoon and a smile, and toddlers are allowed to start with utensils but lapse into eating with fingers when they become tired.

MEALTIMES CAN BE FUN AND EASY

Mealtimes made fun and easy? Anyone who has worked in a child care center or a family child care home knows that mealtimes can be messy, confusing, disorganized, unhappy, and distressing times. Infants and toddlers may fuss, cry, refuse to eat, eat too fast, fall asleep, complain, whine, and protest. Conversely, mealtimes can be happy events that are comfortable and fun for infants, toddlers, and caregivers. How can feeding and eating times become happy, fun times *most* of the time? Preparing carefully; planning deliberately and thoughtfully when, where, and how to eat; and providing responsive adult care help create eager, enthusiastic eaters and mealtimes that are easier and enjoyable for all.

Making Handwashing Fun

Because handwashing is the best way to prevent infection and disease, both adults and children must wash their hands frequently. With infants, care providers can describe what is happening as they use a warm cloth and soap to wash infants' hands. Prepare an infant rather than surprise him or her with a wet cloth. Talk about the cloth as you get it wet. Then say, "I'm going to wash your hands. Here we go." *Wait,* see whether the infant will hold out his or her hands to you, then say, "First, I'm washing your little finger. Then, I'm washing your ring finger." Infants may not only enjoy the handwashing time but also learn language. Sinks that are used for handwashing must be separate from sinks that are used for food preparation (American Public Health Association & American Academy of Pediatrics, 1992). Small, safe steps for toddlers to climb up to a sink are important if toddlers are to wash their hands by themselves. Low towel racks will encourage toddlers to develop autonomy as they learn to enjoy the handwashing routine. Towels should be washed frequently. Be sure to check the temperature of the water to prevent scalding sensitive infant and toddler hands.

Involving Young Children in Meal Preparation and Cleanup

Young children begin to develop motor skills and a sense of responsibility for themselves and others when they help in meal preparation and cleanup. Infants, with a caregiver's hand over theirs, can help to stir their first puréed food that they eat. Toddlers can help set the table with unbreakable dishes. Providing for each toddler a special place mat with his or her name on it helps children begin to learn the letters in their names. With caregivers chanting the numbers, 2- and 3-year-olds can help count the spoons and cups. Preparation tasks that toddlers can do include stirring, mixing, spreading margarine or peanut butter, carrying unbreakable objects, or breaking bread or crackers into smaller pieces. Cleanup responsibilities for toddlers involve wiping their place mats and chairs with big sponges (disinfected often), dumping uneaten food into a container, and putting bibs or aprons away. Involving infants and toddlers in meal preparation and cleanup leads to children's sense of competence, even though care providers will have to do the final cleanup of tables and chairs.

When to Eat

Infants need to eat on demand, and toddlers need to eat frequently. When care providers respond to cues of hunger, infants learn to eat when and how much they need. Care providers, in collaboration with families, can work toward a schedule, but it is important to realize that infants and toddlers may eat more or less on one day than on the next. Their health, amount of sleep, and activity level can differ and affect their nutritional needs. Toddlers' stomachs are small, and toddlers need to be offered nutritious foods at scheduled and frequent times. Often, toddlers are asked to wait too long; they may become irritable or fall asleep by the time the noon meal is served. If this begins to happen, then serve lunch and have nap time earlier in the morning.

How and Where to Eat

Young infants need to be held for feeding (Lally et al., 1995). A comfortable rocking chair or plush chair provides relief to the care provider while meeting infants' needs for holding and feeding. It is inappropriate to strap infants into infant seats with their bottles propped (Lally et al., 1995). This not only can cause the infant to choke, but it also does not meet the social and emotional needs of infants. Older infants who are capable of sitting and who are eating finger food or who are being fed solid food by a caregiver can sit in small chairs with arms (Lally et al., 1995). Caregivers need to have comfortable seating, also, so that they can sit with mobile infants to talk, smile, and eat with them (see Figure 1).

For mobile infants and toddlers to be comfortably seated, the table should be between the waist and mid-chest level and allow the child's feet to rest firmly on the floor (American Public Health Association & American Academy of Pediatrics, 1992). Encourage toddlers to hold and drink from a cup and use a spoon, but be patient—these skills are difficult to learn. Care providers should sit *with* toddlers for snacks or meals to model eating skills, encourage language, and prevent problem behavior. The American Public Health Association and American Academy of Pediatrics (1992) recommend one caregiver to three children to prevent the cross-contamination of infection or disease among children

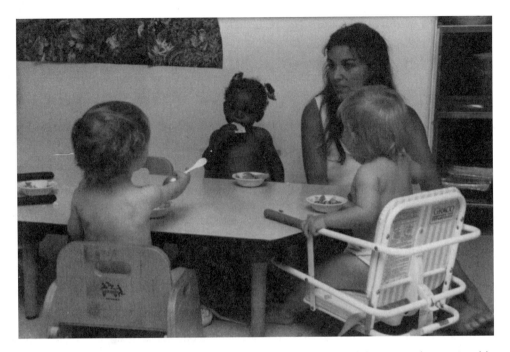

Figure 1. The caregiver sits and eats with three children and makes a meal an enjoyable experience.

who are being fed simultaneously by one adult. Caregivers *cannot* meet the social and special needs of children when there is a high ratio of children to caregivers. "Mealtime should be a socializing occasion. If more than three children are being fed at the same time, feeding resembles an impersonal production line" (American Public Health Association & American Academy of Pediatrics, 1992, p. 125).

Responsive Caregiving

Responsive caregivers are in tune with children's individual developmental levels, support development, encourage young children to make choices, are sensitive to children's needs, and avoid control issues. Responsive caregivers work closely with families to meet infants' nutritional and emotional needs.

Respect Developmental Levels and Note Developmental Progress

When infants begin to use a raking motion with their hands, they usually are ready to begin to pick up soft foods with their fingers. When older infants are able to sit securely, they are ready to sit at a small table and eat lunch with a group. When care providers are observant of these developmental milestones, expectations do not exceed developmental capabilities. Charting the development of young children, when done in collaboration with parents, will help caregivers provide developmentally appropriate experiences, materials, and challenges and develop realistic expectations of children.

Charting development provides valuable information about all children, including those who are identified as having a disability. When developmental levels are understood, adaptations can be made that allow all children to succeed in the child care setting. (For more information concerning nutrition policies and the Americans with Disabilities Act [ADA] of 1990 [PL 101-336], see Rab & Wood, 1995, p. 74.)

Support Children's Language, Cognitive, and Fine Motor Development

Use mealtimes as opportunities to develop young children's knowledge and skills. Talk with children about the names, colors, shapes, sizes, textures, and tastes of foods. Do not bombard children with questions such as, "What's this?" or, "What's this called?" Most children do not like being drilled with questions for which the caregiver already knows the answers. For children who are not speaking yet, use many one-word labels and point to what it is that you are naming. As children learn more words, follow their lead, and use one or more words per sentence than they do to provide a model while staying in tune with their language development. Cognitively, children will begin to classify foods according to color and taste, for example. Toddlers might put foods in order on their plates according to height or width. Give infants and toddlers the opportunity to feed themselves, help prepare the meals, and assist in clean-up activities so that the fine motor skills in their hands and eyes will develop.

Encourage Choices

Giving toddlers choices within reasonable nutritious boundaries gives children a feeling of control over their eating and helps caregivers avoid food battles. Asking toddlers, "Do you want orange juice or grape juice?" usually results in the child's choosing one and drinking juice. Choice questions are perfect for toddlers because they offer the domain of the answer and they give children an opportunity to develop a sense of autonomy and mastery (Honig & Wittmer, 1982). Offer choices only when there are true choices. Also, offer a choice between two similar foods in a food group, thus ensuring that the child's diet meets nutritional standards.

Respond in Sensitive Ways

When caregivers respond to infants and toddlers in sensitive ways, exciting things begin to happen for the child and the caregiver. Children flourish nutritionally and emotionally, develop trust in adults as caring, helpful people, and believe in themselves as deserving positive care. Adults also benefit from providing sensitive care. It is very satisfying emotionally to adults who satisfy children's hunger and emotional needs and help them learn about foods and how to feed themselves. Children are calmer, are easier to comfort, learn more quickly, and enjoy the adult–child interactions.

Primary care and continuity of care help caregivers prepare a responsive environment and interactions with young children. *Primary care* refers to the concept of providing infants and toddlers with a caregiver who has the primary responsibility for building a relationship with that child. Whereas all caregivers in a room care for an infant or toddler at various times, a primary caregiver assumes the role of primary nurturer and responder to the infant or toddler's needs.

Continuity of care is a concept that delineates the role of time (across months and years) that an infant spends with a caregiver. The goal of continuity of care is to develop a healthy caregiver–child attachment. When infants (10–38 months of age) could continue with their primary caregiver for more than 1 year, 91% had secure attachments. When infants spent 9–12 months with a caregiver, 67% had secure attachments. When infants spent only 5–8 months with a caregiver, only 50% were securely attached to a caregiver (Raikes, 1993). The time spent with teacher had a significant and positive relation to security of attachment in infant child care. Allow infants to develop a relationship with a teacher over time. The infant–teacher relationship, then, becomes more defined, predictable, and functional in creating a secure base for the infant.

Avoid Control Issues

Do not use food as a reward or a punishment. Do not force children to eat. Even though you are worried about a child who does not eat much, forcing will only make the child dislike eating or use eating as a control issue. You may feel that you are not a good caregiver if the children in your care do not eat well; however, forcing children or using food as a reward or a punishment will not work in the long run. Use your positive caregiving skills to entice children to eat healthful foods. (See Table 2 for some suggestions for curbing challenging eating behaviors; see also Chapter 8.)

Families and Child Care: Working Together

Child care providers and families must work out differences and find ways to communicate about nutrition, feeding infants, and toddlers' eating. Written menus should be provided for parents so that they can plan at home meals that complement the foods that are served in child care. Provide at the end of each day feeding times and food consumption information for parents of infants and toddlers. "The facility shall inform the parents of the nutritional requirements established by the facility and suggest ways to meet them. The facility shall have food available to supplement a child's food brought from home if it is deficient in meeting the child's nutrition requirements" (American Public Health Associa-

Table 2.   Feeding and eating challenges

Challenging behavior	Special caregiving	Environment
Child will not eat; child will not try new foods.	Never force a child to eat. Build trust, problem-solve with families, and entice child with delicious foods. Offer small amounts frequently, and increase amounts as the child begins to eat more. Allow children to take part in food preparation. Explain why certain foods are good to eat.	Create a pleasant atmosphere. Infants: Use rocking chairs for special one-to-one feeding with bottles. Set highchairs so that a caregiver can feed no more than two infants at a time and so that infants can see one another. Create small groups of toddlers at tables with their special caregiver.
Child eats too much; child always wants to eat.	Meet children's emotional needs with responsive, loving caregiving. Provide nutritious foods often. Check with the child's family and physician to determine whether the child has any health problems.	Feed infants less food more frequently. With toddlers, eat together with a small group and a primary caregiver. Provide utensils, small pitchers, and so forth so that toddlers can be involved with serving themselves and others.
Child cries, has tantrums, or is sad (generally unpleasant at mealtime).	Respect rhythms. A child may not like to be hurried or to wait. Respect a child's schedule. A child may need to eat more frequently. Assure a child who is having a tantrum that you are there for him or her, and help him or her begin to use words.	Eat together with a small group and a primary caregiver. Provide utensils, small pitchers, and so forth so that the child can be involved with serving him- or herself and others.

(continued)

Table 2.   (*continued*)

Challenging behavior	Special caregiving	Environment
Child plays with food; child starts food fights; child throws food.	Sing songs with the children when you are waiting for food. Observe toddlers carefully during eating. When they are finished, let them play or nap or have a special reading time. Never keep toddlers at the table for extended periods of time. Waiting before eating or after eating is very difficult for toddlers. Caregivers should sit and eat *with* mobile infants and toddlers rather than rush around serving food and wiping faces.	Provide comfortable highchairs for infants and toddler seats for toddlers. Toddlers' feet need to touch the floor. Provide special nonslip mats under the plates. Provide special cups and utensils that promote toddler self-feeding.
Child has trouble with weaning from breast or bottle.	Proceed very slowly by removing one bottle- or breast-feeding at a time over several months. Rock, sing, and play with the infant or toddler more often to provide comfort to him or her. Work closely with the family to be consistent.	Use special cups that make drinking from a cup easier for an infant who is being weaned.[a]
Child uses pacifier excessively.	Be patient. Some infants have more sucking needs than others. After the first 6 months, when sucking needs are the strongest, pacifiers can be taken away slowly. Rock, sing, and play with the infant or toddler more often to provide comfort to him or her. Work closely with the family to be consistent.	Pacifiers must be of adequate size to prevent choking. The nipple must withstand 2 pounds of force to prevent dislocation from the base. As children grow, continually check the safety of the pacifier.
Child has disabilities.	Observe for developmental strengths and challenges. Work closely with the family to be consistent.	Use special cups, adapted eating utensils, nonskid plates, and so forth.[a]

Note: Always work with families. To rule out an eating disorder, encourage referral to a physician, a mental health provider, or a dietitian if a problem persists.

[a]Special cups are available from Flaghouse (800) 793-7900.

tion & American Academy of Pediatrics, 1992, p. 126). If parents are negligent in their feeding practices, then the child care provider has a responsibility to provide nutritious foods to meet the daily requirements and refer the family to a nutrition specialist or to the family's primary provider of health care.

Early childhood standards (National Academy of Early Childhood Programs, 1985) as well as National Health and Safety Performance Standards (American Public Health & American Academy of Pediatrics, 1992) detail how child care programs can respond sensitively to a family's cultural preferences. "Foods indicative of the children's cultural backgrounds are served periodically" (National Academy of Early Childhood Programs, 1998, p. 63). "Children shall be offered familiar foods that are typical of the children's culture" (American Public Health & American Academy of Pediatrics, 1992, p. 124). (See also Chapter 26.)

Figure 2 provides an easy-to-use checklist for families of infants and toddlers to use when observing a child care center or family child care home. Caregivers are also encouraged to use this checklist to monitor their nutritional standards.

FEEDING AND EATING CHECKLIST FOR PARENTS AND CAREGIVERS

Types of Food Served
___ Nutritious, tasty foods are attractively presented to children.
___ The recommended dietary allowance (RDA) requirements and the recommendations of the Child Care Food Program are followed closely.
___ The child care center or family child care home provides a written nutrition plan that includes what, when, where, and how children are fed.
___ For children under 2, whole milk or infant formula is given.

Communication with Families
___ Families are asked about their cultural and family preferences for the child's eating habits, needs, and food preferences.
___ Family preferences for types of food are honored (unless these preferences are negligent of infant or toddler needs).
___ The child care provider gives daily information to families concerning how, when, and what the child ate.
___ The child care provider respects the mother's wish to breast-feed, encourages regular visits to the center or child care home, and provides a private place for breast-feeding to occur.
___ Educational programs, newsletters, and literature related to nutrition are offered to families.

Safety Issues
___ Toddlers are seated at small tables in chairs that allow their feet to touch the floor.
___ Food is given to children on plates that can be disinfected.
___ Infants or toddlers are not given foods that could make them choke.
___ All health and safety standards are followed.

Responsive Caregiving
___ Infants are held by caregivers for bottle-feeding. Infants need to be held for feeding to ensure safety and to meet infants' emotional needs.
___ Child care providers work closely with families on issues that are related to weaning from the breast or the bottle.
___ Caregivers are seated with toddlers rather than hovering above or running around waiting on the toddlers.
___ Caregivers speak to the children in a soft, kind, friendly, gentle, encouraging, and positive way.
___ Caregivers name foods; use words that describe the color, shape, size, texture, and taste of foods; and talk about pleasant events while feeding and eating with the children.
___ Caregivers respond to young children's requests and comments while feeding and eating with the children.
___ Caregivers respect children when they indicate that they are satisfied or want to stop eating.
___ Caregivers respond when infants or toddlers indicate that they are hungry or want more food.

Figure 2. Feeding and eating checklist for caregivers and parents.

CONCLUSION

Meeting children's nutritional needs in a child care setting is a challenging and complex task; however, providing for infants' and toddlers' nutritional needs while meeting their emotional and social needs may be one of the most important tasks that a caregiver does. When young children are fed nutritious foods in a family-sensitive, emotionally supportive environment, both care providers and children thrive, children demonstrate fewer behavioral problems, and families feel respected.

REFERENCES

American Public Health Association & American Academy of Pediatrics. (1992). *Caring for our children: National health and safety performance standards. Guidelines for out-of-home child care programs.* Ann Arbor, MI: Edwards Brothers.

Americans with Disabilities Act (ADA) of 1990, PL 101-336, 42 U.S.C. §§ 12101 *et seq.*

Brazelton, T.B., & Cramer, B.G. (1990). *The earliest relationship.* Reading, MA: Addison Wesley Longman Inc.

Edelstein, S. (1995). *The healthy young child.* Minneapolis, MN: West Publishing Company.

Honig, A.S., & Wittmer, D. (1982). Teacher questions to male and female toddlers. *Early Childhood Development and Care, 9,* 19–32.

Lally, J.R., Griffin, A., Fenichel, E., Segal, M., Szanton, E., & Weissbourd, B. (1995). *Caring for infants and toddlers in groups: Developmentally appropriate practice.* Washington, DC: ZERO TO THREE: National Center for Infants, Toddlers and Families.

Lally, R. (1994). Caring for infants and toddlers in groups: Necessary considerations for emotional, social, and cognitive development. *Zero to Three, 14*(5), 1–8.

Lally, R. (1995). The impact of child care policies and practices on infant/toddler identity formation. *Young Children, 51,* 58–67.

Marotz, L., Rush, J., & Cross, M. (1993). *Health, safety, and nutrition for the young child* (3rd ed.). Albany, NY: Delmar Publishers.

National Academy of Early Childhood Programs. (1998). *Guide to accreditation.* Washington, DC: National Association for the Education of Young Children.

Rab, V., & Wood, K. (1995). *Child care and the ADA: A handbook for inclusive programs.* Baltimore: Paul H. Brookes Publishing Co.

Raikes, H. (1993). Relationship duration in infant care: Time with a high-ability teacher and infant–teacher attachment. *Early Childhood Research Quarterly, 8,* 309–325.

U.S. Department of Agriculture. (1992). *Food guide pyramid.* Hyattsville, MD: Author.

U.S. Department of Agriculture, Food and Nutrition Service. (1990). *Food buying for child nutrition programs.* Washington, DC: U.S. Government Printing Office.

RESOURCES

Endres, J.B., & Rockwell, R.E. (1993). *Food, nutrition, and the young child* (4th ed.). New York: Merrill.

Graves, D.E., Suitor, C.W., & Holt, K.A. (1997). *Making food healthy and safe for children: How to meet the National Health and Safety Performance Standards. Guidelines for out-of-home child care programs.* Vienna, VA: National Maternal and Child Health Clearing House. (Available from National Maternal and Child Health Clearing House, 2070 Chain Bridge Road, Suite 450, Vienna, VA 22182; [703] 356-1964.)

National Resource Center for Health and Safety in Child Care. (1997). *Stepping stones to caring for our children.* Denver: University of Colorado, Health Sciences Center. (Available from University of Colorado, 4200 E. Ninth Avenue, Denver, CO 80220; [800] 598-KIDS; http://hrc.uchsc.edu.)

Satter, E. (1987). *How to get your kid to eat . . . but not too much.* Palo Alto, CA: Bull Publishing. (Available from Bull Publishing, 110 Gilbert Avenue, Menlo Park, CA 94025; [800] 676-2855.)

Satter, E. (1991). *Child of mine: Feeding with love and good sense.* Palo Alto, CA: Bull Publishing. (Available from Bull Publishing, 110 Gilbert Avenue, Menlo Park, CA 94025; [800] 676-2855.)

Satter, E. (1989). *Feeding with love and good sense* [Videotapes]. Palo Alto, CA: Bull Publishing. (The four 15-minute videotapes demonstrate to parents and child care providers how to understand feeding from the child's perspective and how adult behaviors influence the behaviors of the child. Available from Bull Publishing, 110 Gilbert Avenue, Menlo Park, CA 94025; [800] 676-2855.)

Warren, J. (1992). *Super snacks.* Everett, WA: Warren Publishing House.

National Association for the Education of Young Children (NAEYC), 1509 16th Street, NW, Washington, DC 20036-1426; (800) 424-2460 or (202) 232-8777; http://www.naeyc.org/naeyc

Pamphlets from the American Academy of Pediatrics:
- Choking and First Aid for Infants and Toddlers
- Feeding Kids Right Isn't Always Easy: Tips for Preventing Food Hassles
- Right from the Start: ABC's of Good Nutrition for Young Children
- What's to Eat? Healthy Foods for Hungry Children
- Growing up Healthy—Fat, Cholesterol, and More

(Available from American Academy of Pediatrics, 141 Northwest Point Boulevard, Elk Grove Village, IL 60007-1098; [800] 433-9016.)

Chapter 33

Community Food and Nutrition Programs

Marion Taylor Baer

Community food and nutrition programs are part of the national system to promote security and preserve the health and well-being of all Americans. Food programs may provide cash assistance or actual food or both. Nutrition programs, often in conjunction with food assistance programs, focus on improving nutritional status through individual counseling or group education.

Professionals who work with families of children who are demonstrating inadequate growth must consider *food insecurity,* defined as a lack of assured access at all times to enough food to promote an active and healthy life, as one of the possible environmental factors related to the etiology of the condition. This is especially important in the late 1990s. In 1996, 5.5 million children—nearly one quarter of those younger than 6 years—lived in poverty; 63% of these lived in families with at least one employed adult (Community Nutrition Institute, 1998g). Professionals must also be knowledgeable about the community-based food and nutrition programs that exist to provide assistance to families in need and be able to coordinate their services with those programs.

This chapter provides an overview of the food and nutrition programs that focus on infants and young children, including children with special health care needs. Although these are federally funded programs, there are variations from state to state in administration as well as in implementation (or even availability) at the local level.

HISTORY OF U.S. FOOD AND NUTRITION PROGRAMS FOR CHILDREN

Federal health and nutrition services for mothers and children in the United States began in 1912 with the creation of the Children's Bureau (Schmidt & Wallace, 1994). In those early years, there was a growing recognition of the importance of food and nutrition to health, beginning with the relationship between contaminated milk and the diarrhea-induced deaths of infants and children and reinforced by the explosion in the discovery of vitamins in the 1920s.

The Great Depression and the devastation that American families faced during those years led to the passage of the Social Security Act of 1935 (PL 74-271), which included Title V, the legislative authority for the programs of today's Maternal and Child Health Bureau, then the Children's Bureau. Thirty years later, in the 1960s, the acknowledgment that poverty and hunger existed on a large scale in the United States was one of the factors that led to the social reforms of the Great Society, which included many programs that were aimed at eliminating hunger.

The Personal Responsibility and Work Opportunity Reconciliation Act of 1996 (PL 104-193) represents a philosophical shift in the approach to providing basic security for Americans, devolving to the states much of the responsibility for the welfare of citizens. This has major implications for the complementary food and nutrition programs that have evolved during this century. The repeal of Aid to Families with Dependent Children (AFDC) and its replacement with the Temporary Assistance for Needy Families (TANF) block grants (Title I), with frozen funding through fiscal year (FY) 2002, effectively reduced the amount of money that needy families have to spend on food. Title II, which tightened Supplemental Security Income (SSI) eligibility for children, shifted the burden of their care back to families, again effectively reducing the total income of those families. Title VII instituted restrictive changes to the child nutrition programs, and Title VIII made across-the-board cuts to food stamps, both directly and by redefining eligibility criteria (California Food Policy Advocates, personal communication, 1996).

MAJOR GOVERNMENTAL AGENCIES THAT ARE RESPONSIBLE FOR FOOD AND NUTRITION PROGRAMS FOR CHILDREN

The following sections provide brief descriptions of the federal agencies that are mandated to implement and oversee the food and nutrition programs that are most important to young children and their families. Because these programs began largely as a result of an effort to support farmers and their products, major responsibility for both food and nutrition programs was given to the United States Department of Agriculture (USDA). This situation had been maintained in spite of the increasing realization of the importance of food to the health of the population. The Department of Health and Human Services (DHHS) has been responsible for the development and integration of nutrition services into the public health system.

DEPARTMENT OF HEALTH AND HUMAN SERVICES

There are several agencies within the DHHS that have responsibility for financing nutrition services or otherwise ensuring their provision through programmatic or training services. Most important are the Bureau of Maternal and Child Health (MCHB) under the Health Resources and Services Administration (HRSA), the Indian Health Service (IHS), the Health Care Financing Administration (HCFA), and the Administration on Children and Families (ACF). The U.S. Department of Education also plays a role as do its counterparts at the state level, which often are mandated to implement federal child nutrition programs at the state level.

Health Resources and Services Administration

Under the United States Public Health Service of DHHS, HRSA has the mission to provide leadership and direction to programs and activities that are designed to improve health services for all Americans. HRSA funds community and migrant health centers, the Primary Health Care Block Grants to the states, rural health services, AIDS education, and training for health professions.

Part of HRSA, MCHB has statutory responsibility for the Maternal and Child Health Block Grant, funded at $683 million in FY 1998, which aids states to build the infrastructure to deliver services to all mothers and children, including those with special health care needs, particularly those who are of low income or in isolated locations and who otherwise have limited access to care (MCHB, 1994). A portion of the Block Grant (15%, or $102.5 million in FY 1998) is used to fund Special Projects of Regional and National Significance (SPRANS), which include research and demonstration activities that often focus on improving nutritional status and/or services for this population. MCHB also provides federal moneys for training nutritionists in public health, pediatric, and maternal nutrition.

Indian Health Service

The IHS provides health services to federally recognized American Indians and Alaskan Natives based on the special relationship between the federal government and the tribes, which has been defined and developed through treaties, laws, executive orders, and certain provisions of the Constitution. Nutrition services to any given tribe may include hospital-based dietitians, dietitians in outpatient clinics, or public health nutritionists who provide community-based services and home visiting. The IHS also provides nutrition training to health professionals and paraprofessionals who work with the native programs. Since the passage of PL 94-638, a law that allows tribes to choose to be self-governing, the IHS no longer provides services to all tribes.[1]

Health Care Financing Administration

The HCFA was created in 1977 to oversee and administer the Medicaid (and Medicare) programs. Early and Periodic Screening, Diagnosis and Treatment (EPSDT) is Medicaid's federally mandated child health program, part of the 1967 amendments to the Social Security Act of 1935 whose final regulations, effective in 1972, provided comprehensive and preventive health services to eligible children in partnership with the states.

United States Department of Agriculture

The Food and Consumer Service (FCS) of the USDA administers, at the federal level, food assistance through nine programs that are classified as child nutrition programs, including School Lunch, School Breakfast, Child and Adult Care Food Program, Summer Food Program, and Special Milk Program, as well as commodity distribution programs and the Special Supplemental Nutrition Program for Women, Infants and Children (WIC). At the state level, these programs are administered through the departments of education in the case of the child nutrition programs and, usually, by the departments of health in the case of WIC. The FCS also administers the Food Stamp Program (FSP) and The Emergency

---

[1]For information about the situation of a given group, contact the Office of the Director at (301) 443-1083.

Food Assistance Program (TEFAP), which may be delegated to a variety of agencies at the state level, including the Department of Social Services.

The Expanded Food and Nutrition Education Program (EFNEP), administered through the Extension Service of the Science and Education Administration of the USDA, operates in the states through the State Cooperative Extension Service. (For a description of EFNEP, see "Expanded Food and Nutrition Education Program" on pp. 461–462.)

PUBLICLY FUNDED FOOD PROGRAMS FOR YOUNG CHILDREN AND FAMILIES

The federal government spends approximately $40 billion each year on many types of food assistance (Community Nutrition Institute, 1998e). Although nongovernmental organizations (NGOs) also provide emergency food for needy children and families, the federal government has primary responsibility for this function. Following are descriptions of the major United States food distribution programs.

Food Stamp Program

The FSP originated in the 1930s during the Great Depression with the commodity distribution programs that served to support farm prices (and farmers) and reduce commodity surpluses by government purchase of the commodities to distribute to the needy. It became a permanent program with the Food Stamp Act of 1964 (PL 88-525). All states were required to serve those who were eligible, making the FSP an entitlement program.

The purpose of the FSP is to ensure a basic level of nutrition through the provision of coupons to cover part of the food budget of low-income households. In 1994, it accounted for 70% of the total funding of the food assistance programs that were administered through the USDA (Community Nutrition Institute, 1994).

Structure and Eligibility

The FCS of the USDA administers the FSP, printing coupons and distributing them to welfare agencies, approving and overseeing participation by food stores, and conducting periodic state program reviews. Eligibility is determined on the basis of the financial status of the household (income and resources) and nonfinancial requirements (citizenship, social security number, and work requirements). The welfare reform law, the Personal Responsibility and Work Opportunity Reconciliation Act of 1996 (PL 104-193), cut $27.7 billion from the FSP over 6 years (1996–2002); that is one half of the total savings to be realized by welfare reform (California Food Policy Advocates, personal communication, 1996). The entitlement for legal aliens was removed in 1996 and partially restored in 1998 (Community Nutrition Institute, 1998i). According to the law, the states have a limited amount of money for food stamps and make decisions regarding the determination of eligibility for them.

Services and Benefits

The coupon allotment is based on the Thrifty Food Plan that was formulated by USDA nutritionists to provide a nutritionally adequate diet. It assumes that the participants have adequate cooking facilities, can shop at large supermarkets rather than at more expensive local stores, and can buy food in bulk quantities; however, poor people often lack transportation, refrigeration, and/or storage. The basis for allotment levels has been decreased by the welfare reform law from 103% to 100% of poverty (California Food Policy Advocates, personal communication, 1996); 45% of the cuts will come from across-the-board benefit reductions, which will equal 20% by the year 2002. Another way of looking at it is that the benefit will fall from 80 cents per person per meal to 66 cents. Participation in the FSP in November 1997 was 20.6 million people at a cost of $1.5 billion (Community Nutrition Institute, 1998d). This represents 4 million fewer participants than in November 1996 and a $280-million reduction in cost; however, many of those who are no longer receiving food stamps are hungry and malnourished (Community Nutrition Institute, 1998h).

Policy

Financial eligibility is 130% of poverty-level income, which eliminates many people who are in need of assistance. There also are indications that the allotment is not sufficient for recipients; 79% of those who use food banks report that food stamps do not last the month (Community Nutrition Institute, 1998f). Attempts in Congress in 1991 to raise the poverty line, had they been successful, would have brought the total number of eligible people to 25% of the U.S. population (U.S. House of Representatives, 1991). In 1997, the poverty line, which is adjusted annually, for a family of four in the 48 contiguous states was $16,050 (Community Nutrition Institute, 1997c).

An electronic benefits transfer (EBT) and automation system has been introduced in some parts of the country as pilot projects. The participant is issued an electronic card that is imprinted with the total value of the coupons for a certain time period. At the point of purchase, the amount spent is deducted automatically from the "account." Use of this system results in cost savings and reduction in fraud as well as removes the stigma that is attached to using coupons. PL 104-193 requires that EBT be implemented in every state by October 1, 2002, unless the state receives a waiver. As of 1997, 16 states had operational on-line food stamp systems; 5 were running EBT systems statewide (Community Nutrition Institute, 1997d).

The Emergency Food Assistance Program

The Temporary Emergency Food Assistance Program was established in 1981 by executive order as a temporary response to the hunger crisis that was caused by the economic recession of the early 1980s. It still exists, although in 1990 "temporary" was removed from the title. Its original purpose was to distribute surplus commodities to needy Americans while reducing government inventories and storage costs. The Hunger Prevention Act of 1988 (PL 100-435) required the USDA to purchase food in addition to commodities for TEFAP and created the Soup Kitchen/Food Bank Donation Program to provide commodities to congregate feeding sites. PL 104-193 now combines the two programs in the "new TEFAP," which is authorized at $100 million annually in mandated food purchases and another $50 million in administrative costs.

Structure and Eligibility

States are allocated surplus and purchased commodities according to a formula that is based 60% on the numbers of persons below the poverty level and 40% on the number of persons unemployed. The USDA also provides administrative funds, 40% of which must go to local agencies. Each state establishes its own financial criteria for eligibility; typically the rate is less than 130% of poverty. The agency that administers the program varies by state, and more than 95% of the local providers are private, nonprofit organizations (Second Harvest, 1997).

Services and Benefits

The commodities are generally distributed through warehouses called food banks. These, in turn, supply food pantries, which distribute bags of food, or soup kitchens, which serve meals. The food banks use the TEFAP surpluses and commodities to leverage food donations from the private sector (see "Food Pantries and Banks" on p. 464). Surplus foods include flour, cheese, nonfat dry milk, butter, cornmeal, rice, and honey. Purchased foods include canned and dried fruits, canned vegetables and meats, and peanut butter.

Policy

Surplus commodities are decreasing as a result of changes in farm supports. Many people, including the homeless, may not be served because of difficulties in establishing eligibility. Distribution problems arise in rural areas and because of federal cuts to administrative funds, which are needed to ensure distribution. Finally, with the $27.7-billion cut in food stamp funding as a result of welfare reform, it is unlikely that TEFAP or the other sources of donated food will be able to respond to the anticipated increased need for emergency food (Cook & Brown, 1997). Budgetary and legislative proposals have been made to increase federal funding to help support food banks, help communities recover wasted food for the hungry, and increase TEFAP.

Child and Adult Care Food Program

The Child Care Food Program was established in 1965 as part of the "special food service programs" created under the amendments to the National School Lunch Act (PL 87-823). It received separate authorization in 1975 and permanent authorization in 1978. Its purpose is to provide nutritious meals and snacks to low-income children in public or private nonprofit child care programs, including Head Start, who otherwise would not have access to food programs. It is funded through the USDA and has been expanded to cover adults; the official name is now the Child and Adult Care Food Program (CACFP).

Structure and Eligibility

Family day care homes, Head Start programs, and other centers are approved or licensed to participate in the CACFP according to local, state, or federal regulations. Prior to 1996, all preschool children in licensed child care facilities were eligible to participate. PL 104-193 created a two-tier reimbursement structure, beginning July 1, 1997, whereby family day care homes serving children at or below 185% of poverty generally will be reimbursed at current rates, whereas others will receive a lower rate (95 cents for lunch and supper; 27 cents for breakfast; 13 cents for snack) (California Food Policy Advocates, personal communication, 1996). Rates will be readjusted each year, and the effects of these new regulations will be reported to Congress.

Services and Benefits

Assistance is in the form of reimbursement for meals based on the number served and the family income of the children as well as donated foods and technical assistance. There are federal requirements that child care providers who participate in CACFP be given information and ongoing training in child health and development and the nutritional needs of young children. An option to serve an additional meal or snack to children who are in child care centers for more than 8 hours has been eliminated under PL 104-193 (California Food Policy Advocates, personal communication, 1996). In February 1997, 66 million meals were served in participating centers (Community Nutrition Institute, 1998d).

Policy

CACFP provides a major incentive for family day care homes to become licensed, making it an important regulatory link to those homes (Community Nutrition Institute, 1997e). In fact, the number of licensed family day care providers tripled between 1978 and 1983, when the means test (income eligibility requirement) for CACFP was dropped. Those providers now include more middle-income homes, which is the main rationale for the new requirement for means testing (Community Nutrition Institute, 1997e); however, there is concern that the additional administrative burden that has resulted from means testing will not reduce costs and may increase for providers the disincentives that already result from lengthy paperwork and detailed rules for participation.

PUBLICLY FUNDED NUTRITION OR FOOD AND NUTRITION PROGRAMS FOR YOUNG CHILDREN AND FAMILIES

In addition to food distribution programs, the federal government sponsors programs that provide nutrition or nutrition education services. Some of these programs, such as WIC and Head Start, also distribute either vouchers for food (WIC) or meals (Head Start).

Special Supplemental Food Program for Women, Infants and Children

In 1962, as part of a national effort to improve health care for high-risk mothers, the Department of Health, Education, and Welfare (DHEW), Division of Maternal and Child Health (MCH) staff began discussions with the USDA Food Distribution Division staff to explore increasing the allotments of selected food commodities for needy expectant mothers (Egan & Oglesby, 1990). This was followed by 10 years of joint efforts, including a 2-year pilot program that was launched by the USDA for low-income groups that are vulnerable to malnutrition—the Special Supplemental Food Program for Women, Infants and Children. In 1972, WIC was authorized to continue for 2 years under the Child Nutrition Act (PL 92-433). By 1974, WIC was serving 88,000 participants at a cost of $10.5 million. At the beginning of 1997, there were 7.5 million participants; the budget was $310 million, $241 million of which was food costs (Community Nutrition Institute, 1997b).

WIC was renamed in 1994 the Special Supplemental *Nutrition* Program for Women, Infants and Children. The purpose of WIC is to prevent health problems and to improve the health status of program participants during critical times of growth and development.

Structure and Eligibility

Funding for WIC is through the USDA, although it is usually administered through state health departments. The states then funnel the money to the local level, where the actual programs are run by both public and private nonprofit agencies. Typically, a WIC agency has several community-based sites where participants are served.

WIC serves pregnant, lactating, and postpartum women and their infants and children up to the age of 5. It is not an entitlement program, and the individual states set their priorities as to which participants to serve. Criteria for eligibility include 1) income below 133% of the federal poverty level (with state-determined option to cover up to 185%), 2) poor nutritional status (based on dietary, biochemical, and anthropometric risk criteria), and 3) poor health or health history. Because not all of the women who are eligible to participate can be served, recommendations for changes in the nutrition risk criteria have been proposed (Committee on Scientific Evaluation of WIC Nutrition Risk Criteria, Food and Nutrition Board, Institute of Medicine, 1996) with the goal of increasing the "yield of benefit" by enabling the programs to better select those who are most at risk and also most likely to benefit from the intervention.

Under PL 104-193, states have the option to deny benefits to undocumented individuals and certain legal immigrant categories. The bill also makes technical changes, such as eliminating (but not disallowing) the requirements for outreach for providing materials in other languages as well as information about other food assistance programs (California Food Policy Advocates, personal communication, 1996).

Services

Although WIC provides supplemental food by way of vouchers, it differs from the FSP in that the types of food are limited to those that provide nutrients that are known to be both insufficient in the diets of poor women and children and important to prenatal and post-natal development. It also differs from the FSP in that the program aims to improve the overall health of the population by also providing nutrition education and linkages to other health services.

Supplemental Food

Vouchers for USDA-authorized supplemental foods (rich in iron, protein, calcium, and vitamin C) are issued monthly by the local agencies; different packages are geared toward the varied needs of participants. Vendors can cash the vouchers like checks to be paid by the State Treasurer's office through local banks.

The USDA has made policy decisions that improve access to special formulas for children in need. For example, its definition of *allowable formulas* includes formulas that are designed for oral consumption, even if administered by tube (USDA, 1994). Also, increased amounts of formula are allowed for infants with special needs (USDA, 1990). The USDA also has recommended WIC policies that ensure that participants with medical conditions receive the most appropriate foods to address their unique dietary needs (USDA, 1994). Individual states, such as California, have established processes for approving, on an individual basis, provision of special formulas to infants not otherwise covered through Title V, Medicaid, Developmental Disabilities funds, or private insurance (California Department of Health Services WIC Supplemental Nutrition Branch, 1995).

The WIC Farmers' Market Nutrition Act of 1992 (PL 102-314) formally established the Farmers' Market Nutrition Program (FMNP); in 1995, 30 states participated. The goals are to 1) provide WIC participants with fresh produce and 2) expand awareness and use of farmers' markets. Federal funds pay 70% of the costs for those states that initiated their programs before FY 1995 when funding was frozen. Not all WIC clients receive FMNP benefits, which cannot exceed $20 per client per year and are given in addition to the regular coupons. Because of the limited funding, state WIC agencies may choose to use them as incentives (e.g., to encourage breast-feeding) or to target certain areas (e.g., those close to farmers' markets). The coupons may be used only for fresh fruits and vegetables. Farmers redeem them through the market or the FMNP administration or deposit them as checks (Alexander, 1996). As of 1998, there were more than 1 million WIC participants who received these benefits at 8,200 markets nationwide. For FY 1998, the budget for the FMNP was increased substantially: $12 million in grants was awarded to 32 states, two Indian Tribal Organizations, and the District of Columbia (Community Nutrition Institute, 1998c).

Nutrition Education

According to a 1978 amendment to the Child Nutrition Act, at least one sixth of the state's WIC funds are to be spent on nutrition education. Educational goals are to 1) emphasize individual needs, 2) improve health status and eating habits, and 3) encourage breast-feeding. The last has received more of an emphasis in recent years. By 1989, each local agency had a breast-feeding coordinator; in 1994, there was an augmentation in funds that were earmarked for efforts to increase breast-feeding.

Linkage with Health Care Services

There is a federal requirement that WIC be coordinated with Medicaid. Medicaid participation is accepted as proof of WIC eligibility; individuals in a family of a Medicaid participant are usually income-eligible for WIC. Conversely, WIC agencies are required to refer to Medicaid women and children who appear to be income-eligible. Recent initiatives have the goal of ensuring that women who are in Medicaid managed care be referred to WIC and that certain data be collected for purposes of quality assurance.

Participation requires documentation of ongoing health care to increase the likelihood that pregnant woman will receive prenatal care. This also improves the possibility of linkages with other sectors of the health care and social services network. WIC sites, for example, have been used for immunization as well as voter registration campaigns.

Nutrition Services

Clinical nutrition services are *not* mandated by WIC; this tends to be a major source of confusion among health care providers who think of WIC as a resource for nutrition services as well as food. Although some WIC clinics may be colocated with community clinics where nutrition services are provided and some WIC agencies may have gained access to additional funding streams (usually Title V or the Individuals with Disabilities Education Act [IDEA]) such that public health services are also provided, most do not provide clinical nutrition services. Nor are all WIC "nutritionists" qualified providers of nutrition services (i.e., registered dietitians [RDs]). Some WIC programs may extend the time allotted per participant to allow for more counseling, and some will schedule the visit with an RD for high-risk women and children; however, WIC usually is not an appropriate resource for nutrition referral.

Policy

Formula vendors now bid for WIC contracts in many states. For the exclusive right to sell formula to WIC participants in the state, the vendor agrees to rebate a certain amount of the price. The additional funds allow WIC agencies to increase participant enrollment and/or the number of WIC sites and have become a major strategy for cost containment. This policy has been under attack in Congress; however, its elimination was not included in PL 104-193.

To make WIC more accessible to families, many agencies are colocating WIC sites with other programs. This strategy has been used successfully as outreach to early intervention programs and migrant health centers, for example, and should be encouraged. However, the assumption that WIC is fully funded at 7.5 million participants because only 80% of those who are eligible will participate is limiting enrollment in some states (Community Nutrition Institute, 1998b).

Other WIC policy initiatives that should enhance the importance of WIC for families of infants at risk include expanded lists of high-risk conditions, training of "high risk" nutritionists (RDs who spend additional time with women or children who are identified as at high risk), general staff training in disabilities and chronic conditions, establishing liaisons with state Children with Special Health Care Needs Programs, and participation in the development of Medicaid managed care requests for bids.

Head Start

The Head Start program was funded in 1964 in response to the recognition that part of the legacy of poverty is a population of young children who are not ready to benefit from school because of a variety of deficits in their early environment. The purpose of Head Start is to deliver a comprehensive child development program, including educational, health, and social services, to low-income preschool-age children and their families and to involve families in the program. It began as an 8-week summer experience but today operates year-round.

The program was strengthened in 1992 when Congress passed the Head Start Improvement Act of 1992 (PL 102-401). This legislation allowed grantees to provide health care to siblings of Head Start children and required them to provide or arrange for parent literacy and education services. In 1995, an expansion of the program was added, on a pilot basis, called Early Head Start, whereby services begin at birth.

Structure and Eligibility

Head Start is a federal program, administered through the DHHS, Administration for Children, Youth and Families, by the Head Start Bureau. States have only an advisory role. Grants are awarded by the DHHS Regional Offices to a variety of public agencies, private nonprofit organizations, and public school systems. These grantees may run the actual programs and/or they may have delegate agencies that run programs.

The Head Start statute requires that at least 90% of the children who are served by the program be from families with incomes at or below the federal poverty level or receiving TANF. It is not an entitlement program, and it has been estimated that less than half of the eligible low-income children participate. Almost 15 million children and their families have been served since the mid-1960s.

In FY 1993, more than 700,000 children were served at a cost of $2.78 billion in federal funds (Aron, Loprest, & Steuerle, 1996). Grantees are required to provide matching funds (20%), which may be cash or in-kind services and which may be waived under certain conditions.

Head Start was mandated in 1974 to accept and integrate into the program children with special needs and disabilities, 10% in each state. By 1984, the requirement was that 10% of the children served by each grantee have a certifiable disability. By a large margin, the most common of these disabilities (nearly 70%) is speech impairment, although the numbers of children with severe or multiple disabling conditions being integrated into classrooms are growing.

Services and Benefits

All Head Start programs must offer five major components: education, health services (including medical, nutritional, dental, and mental health), social services, parent involvement, and special needs. Children with disabilities also receive special education and related services. Head Start programs are required to be payers of last resort whenever possible, so most Head Start children receive medical, nutritional, and dental services, for example, paid for by Medicaid or EPSDT.

Nutrition services are planned and carried out in conjunction with the health component coordinator or, in larger programs, with the nutrition coordinator. In any case, a qualified nutritionist or dietitian, as defined in the Head Start guidance material, must provide direction. The services include nutrition screening and referral, food service, and nutrition education.

Nutrition Screening and Referral

As part of the complete physical exam that is required for enrollment in Head Start, the nutritional status and needs of the child and the family are assessed. Data include height, weight, and hemoglobin or hematocrit; information about the family's habits and needs; and information about the major community nutrition programs.

Food Service

Head Start agencies participate in the CACFP. Depending on the length of time that a child spends in the program, he or she receives one third to two thirds of the daily nutrient needs at appropriate intervals in accordance with performance standards. The food service contributes to the overall development and socialization of the children by providing a variety of foods from different cultural groups and by providing appropriate serving sizes, utensils, and time to eat in a relaxed and family-style atmosphere where children are encouraged to take part in the meal service.

Nutrition Education

A nutrition education program for staff, parents, and children is planned and integrated into the total education program with the goal of creating sound eating practices. For example, foods are used for conceptual, sensory, and vocabulary development. Food-related activities include planting gardens, feeding pets, role-playing as a grocer, and so forth.

Policy

Head Start has proved to be a very successful approach to combating the effects of poverty, both for the children and for their parents. The program should be supported and expanded; Early Head Start, beginning at birth, is a promising policy initiative that deserves full funding.

Individuals with Disabilities Education Act

The Individuals with Disabilities Education Act (IDEA) of 1990 (PL 101-476) (formerly the Education for All Handicapped Children Act of 1975 [PL 94-142]) and its amendments of 1991 (PL 102-119) and 1997 (PL 105-17) are the main form of federal government educational assistance to children with disabilities. (The nutrition implications of this program are discussed in Chapter 25.)

Expanded Food and Nutrition Education Program

In 1968, following the recognition of the extent of poverty and hunger in the United States and the need for an effective nutrition education program for low-income families, the USDA provided a $10 million grant to initiate pilot education projects under the EFNEP. Two years later, Congress authorized funds for EFNEP under the Department of Agriculture and Related Agencies Appropriations Act, which also increased its budget to $50 million. By 1977, the budget had reached $60 million, and the Food and Agriculture Act of that year also required that EFNEP be expanded to include food stamp recipients. In the 1980s, EFNEP survived attempts to cut its budget as well as to eliminate the program.

The purpose of EFNEP is to aid families and youth with low incomes to improve their diets by improving their knowledge, attitudes, and behaviors with regard to the choice and preparation of foods as well as cooking and sanitary practices. It is the largest federally funded nutrition education program; however, EFNEP reaches only some of those eligible (about 1 million per year) because of budget restrictions.

Structure

EFNEP is administered by the Extension Service of the Science and Education Administration of the USDA. At the state and county levels, services are delivered through the State

Cooperative Extension Service, the state-level educational arm of the USDA Extension Service. Cooperative Extension Services are based at 52 land-grant colleges and have staff in nearly all U.S. counties. Although not mandated to do so, many states and counties provide additional funding.

Management at the state level is provided by program coordinators; food and nutrition specialists develop training and resource materials to meet the needs of the counties. At the county level, professional home economists supervise a staff of paraprofessionals and volunteers who are indigenous to the community and who relate to and work directly with the low-income families and youth.

Services

EFNEP comprises two components. The Youth EFNEP component provides nutrition education in low-income areas. Trained leaders work directly with young people using a variety of program delivery methods. The Adult EFNEP component targets low-income homemakers on a one-to-one or, more often, a group basis to teach principles of food and nutrition and homemaking skills. Originally, a "learn by doing" approach was used in the home. Since the 1980s, alternative techniques such as radio advertisements, newspapers, and group meetings have been added to reach more participants at a lower cost. Evaluations have shown both approaches to be effective.

Policy

Because there has been no increase in funding for the program, the increase in the proportion of families with children living in poverty, and the implications of PL 104-193, EFNEP is inadequately prepared to serve its target population. The EFNEP staff, with respect to the numbers of persons served, is now at about one third of its original level. This program should be supported fully and even better integrated with the FSP to enhance its benefits.

Title V Programs

Title V of the Social Security Act of 1935 established a federal–state partnership to support a range of core program functions, including needs assessment; program planning and development; service delivery, coordination, and financing; standard setting and monitoring; technical assistance, information and education; and reporting (Bureau of Maternal and Child Health, 1994). States are required to match each $4 of federal funds with $3 in cash or in-kind contributions.

Maternal and Child Health

By 1920, nearly every state had a division of maternal and child health (MCH). Plans developed by the Children's Bureau became the foundations of the child health section of Title V. In 1967, the Children's Bureau was dismantled and the health component was transferred to the Public Health Service under what is now known as the MCHB. MCH programs are located in the department of health in every state.

Nutrition has always played a central role in MCH activities, beginning with the milk stations in the early 1900s, which provided safe milk for infants and children. Nutritionists were among the first professionals to be appointed to local and state public health programs, with the Children's Bureau providing much of the impetus (Egan & Oglesby, 1990). Today, all states and many localities have nutritionists with responsibilities in their health department's MCH programs.

Structure and Eligibility

MCH programs focus on the health of underserved children and adolescents, mothers, and families. Eligibility criteria, where they exist, vary according to the program.

Services

Nutritionists' activities range from program planning and evaluation (populations and systems focus) to consultation and training for other health professionals to nutrition education of groups to provision of direct services (individual or client focus), depending on the position and the health department. Most often, there is a mix of responsibilities.

Policy

Although MCH survives, Congress has provided level or decreased funding for the MCH Block Grants in the past few years (American Association of Maternal and Child Health Programs, 1996). This has effectively caused downsizing and/or elimination of some programs. This has important implications for nutrition services because MCHB is a major source of funding both for training public health nutritionists and for the services that they provide.

Children with Special Health Care Needs

As part of Title V of the Social Security Act of 1935, federal grants were made to states for "Crippled Children's Services," which included prevention activities and an entire array of medical and social services. Today, Children with Special Health Care Needs (CSHCN) programs exist, in one form or another, in all states, funded through federal MCH Block Grants (Part C, or approximately one third of the total moneys). Most are administered by state health departments; nine are administered by other state agencies, including human services or education agencies, or universities.

Structure and Eligibility

Eligibility for services varies according to the state but usually involves means testing as well as medical criteria. The federal definition of *children with special health care needs* is very broad and focuses on emotional and behavioral aspects of the condition as well as the need for extended or unusual medical services. In practice, states that are faced with limited financial resources tend to determine eligibility based on a list of categorical diagnoses.

Services

In some states, the CSHCN program is largely a system of payment; in others, medical and allied health and social services are also organized and/or provided. The scope of the services provided or paid for also varies from state to state. Usually, there is a nutrition consultant at the state level who, if not directly responsible for service provision in the CSHCN program, is paid through Title V funds and is knowledgeable about the benefits in that state. Nutrition is a focus of all prevention activities and services; the latter are often provided in tertiary care settings as part of those of a multidisciplinary team that is trained to work with children who have special needs and their families. These clinical services are often organized categorically, according to the child's medical condition (e.g., cardiac, gastrointestinal, neuromuscular), and are provided by pediatric subspecialists. Nutrition services generally are covered when the problem is related to the eligible condition.

Policy

In addition to issues related to level funding of the MCH Block Grants, CSHCN programs face new challenges in ensuring appropriate services under managed care. The specialty and allied health (including nutrition) services that are required by many children who have special health care needs are not available in all medical settings, and there is concern that the quality of their care be maintained in the current atmosphere of cost containment.

NONGOVERNMENTAL FOOD PROGRAMS AND NUTRITION SERVICES

Food donations from the private sector have always played an important role in alleviating hunger and food insecurity. During the 1990s, especially with the cutbacks of the welfare reform act, this role has become increasingly important. Approximately 12%, or 12 million, of the households in the United States experienced food insecurity during 1995; almost 1% experienced severe hunger, according to USDA data (Community Nutrition Institute, 1997g). Food insecurity was most prevalent among households with children younger than 6 years (14%) and especially among Hispanic (24%) and black (20%) households with children younger than 6 years. In 1997, 26 million people in the United States turned to food banks (Second Harvest, 1997). Of those, 8 million (31%) were children, and 46% of those were younger than 5 years.

Food Pantries and Banks

Most large communities have some privately organized food pantries and banks that help to sustain needy families. Whereas some are local, others have a larger scope. The Second Harvest Network, for example, is the nation's largest distributor of donated food to private charitable emergency food providers. It distributed food to 183 food banks serving 42,000 community agencies with over 69,000 local food programs in 1992 (Van Amburg Group, 1993). Donations are categorized as "salvage" items, which are damaged but edible goods, or as "caselot" items. The latter typically are not damaged and simply are surplus or unpopular items that are donated in bulk by companies or other organizations. Food banks also obtain donations from food drives, often held in conjunction with other agencies, such as the Salvation Army. They also serve as warehouse and distribution centers for USDA Commodity Foods.

World SHARE (Self-Help and Resource Exchange) is a nonprofit organization with an approach to providing affordable food based on volunteerism. SHARE has 25 United States affiliates in 20 states, most of which are along the eastern seaboard or in the midwest. The affiliates, through 7,500 community-based organizations such as schools and churches, offer a monthly food package, which has a retail value of about $30, in exchange for 2 hours of volunteer work and $14 in cash or food stamps. The SHARE participants themselves, who number 350,000, decide on the nature of the volunteer work based on their knowledge of the community's needs.[2]

Dietitians in Hospitals or Health Maintenance Organizations

Dietitians who work in community-based hospitals or health maintenance organizations may or may not have experience with the variety of pediatric conditions that may lead to growth failure. Dietitians who are located in tertiary care centers or in children's hospitals should have pediatric and, ideally, interdisciplinary training. Dietitians who are employed

---

[2]World SHARE's national toll-free information hot line, (888) 742-7372, will automatically route the caller to the nearest SHARE program.

by CSHCN programs, where these programs provide direct services, would have such training.

Nutrition Consultants in Private Practice

Nutritionists who are qualified to work with children who have special needs may be in private practice or be associated with groups of pediatricians through consultant agreements. The nutritionist must not only be a registered dietitian but also be trained to serve this population. The American Dietetic Association (ADA) and its state affiliates often have hot lines for use in locating appropriate nutrition services.[3] In addition, ADA operates a consulting service where consumers can reach a dietitian.[4] The ADA practice groups that would be able to provide assistance are Dietitians in Pediatric Practice and Dietetics in Developmental and Psychiatric Disorders.[5]

FINANCING NUTRITION SERVICES

In spite of the importance of nutrition to the growth and development of children, particularly young children, nutrition services for those who need them are not always readily accessible outside the hospital setting. Nor is payment for nutrition services, delivered by a qualified nutritionist or RD, routinely reimbursable. Summarized next are examples of funding sources that do exist.

Title XIX: Medicaid and the Early and Periodic Screening, Diagnosis and Treatment Program

Low-income families who receive cash assistance from the TANF program are automatically eligible for Medicaid. Since the mid-1980s, Medicaid eligibility for children that is unrelated to AFDC (now TANF) has been greatly expanded, both as mandates to the states and as options. Some of the major expansions in coverage required include all women, infants, and children younger than 6 years in families with income under 133% of poverty; all children between ages 6 and 19 born after September 30, 1983, in families with income under 100% of poverty; and an additional 12 months of coverage for families who lose TANF benefits as a result of increased earnings. In addition, children may qualify for Medicaid if their medical expenses are large, even if the family income is too high through the "medically needy" programs that are established at the option of the state. In 1997, Congress authorized approximately $4 billion per year in grants to the states for health insurance for uninsured children, the State Child Health Insurance Programs (SCHIP). The funds may be used to expand Medicaid, create new state programs for children's health insurance, or both.

Medicaid and SCHIP provide a variety of services for children, which may or may not include nutrition services, depending on the state. In addition, the EPSDT program requires that states periodically provide general health screening, which includes nutrition screening, for Medicaid recipients who are younger than 21 years. According to the mandate of the Omnibus Budget Reconciliation Act of 1989, any services that are necessary to treat illnesses or conditions that are identified by screening and that are covered (manda-

---

[3]The number for ADA's referral network is (800) 366-1655. ADA also has a home page (www. eatright.org) through which dietitians can be located by specialty and by state.

[4]The service operates between 9 A.M. and 4 P.M. (Central Standard Time) Monday through Friday. The number is (900) 225-5367; the charge as of 1998 is $1.95 for the first minute and $.95 for each additional minute.

[5]ADA practice groups can be contacted through ADA's Practice Team at (312) 899-0040.

tory or optional) under federal Medicaid regulations must be provided by a state even if the services are not normally covered by the state's Medicaid program.

Under the Home and Community-Based Services (HCBS) waiver program, which some states have, additional services that are not regularly funded by Medicaid may be provided, again depending on the state. These services may include nutrition counseling and home-delivered meals and, although usually aimed at the elderly, may be available to children, especially those who have disabilities.

Title V

Title V funds are an important source of payment for children with medically eligible conditions. (For a discussion of the program, see "Title V Programs" under the section "Publicly Funded Nutrition or Food and Nutrition Programs for Young Children and Families.")

Hospitals and Health Maintenance Organizations

Hospitals and health maintenance organizations (HMOs) that are EPSDT providers can be reimbursed for outpatient nutrition services that are covered under this program. Prior authorization by the state Medicaid agency may be required. Some HMOs and other managed care organizations (MCOs) may have a qualified nutritionist or RD on staff. With the emphasis on cost containment characteristic of managed care, many plans are recognizing that timely nutrition intervention can be cost-effective.

Private Insurance

Some private insurance plans will pay for nutrition services, particularly if they are provided under the signature of a physician; however, this is not by any means guaranteed. The dietetics profession, led by the ADA and its state affiliates, is working toward more widespread recognition of the legitimate need for "medical nutrition therapy" as well as its reimbursement.

CONCLUSIONS

Because, in spite of the nation's wealth, one of every five children in the United States lives in poverty (Community Nutrition Institute, 1997f), it is important that the clinical team routinely consider family food insecurity when presented with a child who is failing to grow optimally. It is equally important that the team be able to refer families to the food assistance programs that are outlined in this chapter, which exist to combat food insecurity, and that all clinicians be aware of the nutrition components of other early childhood programs, such as IDEA or Head Start, in order to counsel families.

Nutrition services are neither universally available nor routinely reimbursable; there is a clear need for broader advocacy in this regard. Moreover, even when nutrition services are available and reimbursable, they are underutilized because both professionals and families are unaware of their importance and their existence. It is hoped that the information in this chapter will help to increase that awareness and thereby contribute to the provision of comprehensive and coordinated services for young children and their families.

REFERENCES

Alexander, J. (1996). *Strengthening WIC farmers' markets.* Medford, MA: Tufts University, Center on Hunger, Poverty and Nutrition Policy.

American Association of Maternal and Child Health Programs. (1996, October 15). Fiscal '97 funding approved by Congress and signed by President. *Interim Legislative Updates, 4*(2), 1.

Aron, L.Y., Loprest, P.J., & Steuerle, C.E. (1996). *Serving children with disabilities: A systematic look at the programs.* Washington, DC: Urban Institute Press.

Bureau of Maternal and Child Health, Health Resources and Services Administration, and Department of Health and Human Services. (1994, October). *Fact pack.* Washington, DC: Bureau of Maternal and Child Health.

California Department of Health Services WIC Supplemental Nutrition Branch. (1995, October 1). *WIC program manual.* Sacramento, CA: Special Supplemental Nutrition Program for Women, Infants and Children.

Committee on Scientific Evaluation of WIC Nutrition Risk Criteria, Food and Nutrition Board, Institute of Medicine. (1996). *WIC nutrition risk criteria: A scientific assessment.* Washington, DC: National Academy Press.

Community Nutrition Institute. (1994, July 22). Senate passes $40 billion food appropriations bill. *Nutrition Week,* 6.

Community Nutrition Institute. (1997a, March 7). Food stamp participation takes another downturn. *Nutrition Week,* 8.

Community Nutrition Institute. (1997b, March 7). House lawmakers grill agriculture officials about WIC program management. *Nutrition Week,* 1.

Community Nutrition Institute. (1997c, March 14). Briefly noted: Poverty line. *Nutrition Week,* 7.

Community Nutrition Institute. (1997d, March 28). States continue to develop separate EBT systems as interoperability is debated. *Nutrition Week,* 1.

Community Nutrition Institute. (1997e, March 28). Welfare law jeopardizes child care food program. *Nutrition Week,* 3.

Community Nutrition Institute. (1997f, May 23). Improvements in poverty and income in 1995 tempered by troubling long-term trends. *Nutrition Week,* 4.

Community Nutrition Institute. (1997g, September 19). USDA: 12 million U.S. households are food insecure. *Nutrition Week,* 4.

Community Nutrition Institute. (1998a, February 6). Clinton requests increase for WIC program. *Nutrition Week,* 2.

Community Nutrition Institute. (1998b, February 13). Scrutiny of WIC likely in the year ahead. *Nutrition Week,* 2.

Community Nutrition Institute. (1998c, February 27). New states will participate in farmers market. *Nutrition Week,* 6.

Community Nutrition Institute. (1998d, March 6). Food stamp participation falls by 4 million in a year. *Nutrition Week,* 8.

Community Nutrition Institute. (1998e, March 6). Government releases plan to cut hunger in half. *Nutrition Week,* 3.

Community Nutrition Institute. (1998f, March 13). Nearly 26 million people turned to food banks in 1997. *Nutrition Week,* 1.

Community Nutrition Institute. (1998g, March 20). Nearly 6 million young children live in poverty. *Nutrition Week,* 2.

Community Nutrition Institute. (1998h, April 24). One in 13 persons is served by food stamps. *Nutrition Week,* 2.

Community Nutrition Institute. (1998i, July 17). The federal food stamp restoration for legal immigrants. *Nutrition Week,* 4.

Cook, J.T., & Brown, J.L. (1997). *Analysis of the capacity of the Second Harvest Network to cover the federal food stamp shortfall from 1997 to 2002.* Medford, MA: Tufts University, School of Nutrition Sciences and Policy, Center on Hunger, Poverty and Nutrition Policy.

Education for All Handicapped Children Act of 1975, PL 94-142, 20 U.S.C. §§ 1400 *et seq.*

Egan, M., & Oglesby, A.C. (1990). Nutrition services in the Maternal and Child Health Program: A historical perspective. In C.O. Sharbaugh (Ed.), *Call to action: Better nutrition for mothers, children, and families* (pp. 73–92). Washington, DC: National Center for Education in Maternal and Child Health.

Food Stamp Act of 1964, PL 88-525, 7 U.S.C. §§ 2011 *et seq.*

Individuals with Disabilities Education Act (IDEA) of 1990, PL 101-476, 20 U.S.C. §§ 1400 *et seq.*

Individuals with Disabilities Education Act Amendments of 1991, PL 102-119, 20 U.S.C. §§ 1400 *et seq.*

Individuals with Disabilities Education Act Amendments of 1997, PL 105-17, 20 U.S.C. §§ 1400 *et seq.*

Personal Responsibility and Work Opportunity Reconciliation Act of 1996, PL 104-193, 8 U.S.C. §§ 1621 *et seq.*

Schmidt, W.M., & Wallace, H.M. (1994). The development of health services for mothers and children in the United States. In H.M. Wallace, R.P. Nelson, & P.J. Sweeney (Eds.), *Maternal and child health practices* (pp. 103–119). Oakland, CA: Third Party Publishing.

Second Harvest. (1997). *The Second Harvest rapid response file: TEFAP.* Chicago: Author.

Social Security Act of 1935, PL 74-271, 42 U.S.C. §§ 301 *et seq.*

United States Department of Agriculture. (1990). *Maximum monthly formula allowances in WIC food packages, WRO Policy Memo 804D.* San Francisco: United States Department of Agriculture Food and Nutrition Service, Western Region.

United States Department of Agriculture. (1994). *All States Memorandum 94–142: Oral feeding issues related to WIC-eligible formulas under Food Package III.* San Francisco: United States Department of Agriculture Food and Nutrition Service, Western Region.

United States House of Representatives. (1991). *Redrawing the poverty line: Implications for fighting hunger and poverty in America.* Washington, DC: U.S. Government Printing Office.

Van Amburg Group. (1993). *Second Harvest 1993 national research study.* Erie, PA: Author.

WIC Farmers' Market Nutrition Act of 1992, PL 102-314, 106 Stat. 280.

Chapter 34

Program Evaluation

Laura Taylor

Program evaluation is "the systematic collection and analysis of information about a health-service program to guide judgments and decisions about that program" (Health Services Research Group, 1992, p. 1301). There are many things that a program that serves undernourished children might like to know: Who are the active cases? What are they like? Who referred them? Is the program operating as planned? Are the patients satisfied with their care? Are the children benefiting? Programs may use evaluation findings to improve services, report to funding agencies, and learn what works best. All programs that serve children and families can benefit from some amount of evaluation (National Center for Clinical Infant Programs, 1987). The aim of this chapter is to describe basic approaches to program evaluation. Research is discussed elsewhere (see Chapter 5).

AREAS OF PROGRAM EVALUATION

Program evaluation involves planning. This planning can be divided into needs assessment, program goals and objectives, population served, and program monitoring and process evaluation.

Needs Assessment

Needs assessment asks which kinds of services and policies the children and families of a community really need. Service delivery programs should be designed to meet identified needs in a target population and should be evaluated on how well they meet those needs; thus, needs assessment leads to program design and evaluation.

An example of needs assessment is the process of determining the need for services for childhood undernutrition in Tulsa, Oklahoma. A task force of interested community leaders met to consider the following questions: Are there large numbers of undernourished young children in Tulsa? Who is already serving them? Is there need for additional services?

According to data from the Special Supplemental Nutrition Program for Women, Infants and Children (WIC) (Oklahoma Department of Health, 1995), approximately 500 children in the Tulsa area were at risk for childhood undernutrition as defined by being at or below the 5th percentile of weight-for-height. A survey of two university clinics and four emergency rooms was completed, using as a criterion for undernutrition weight-for-age at or below the 85th percentile of median. (Although weight-for-age alone is not the best indicator of undernutrition [see Chapter 10], it was consistently available on emergency room and clinic charts.) These data demonstrated that 10%–20% of the children were low in weight-for-age and likely to be undernourished. Through the process of asking and answering these questions, it was determined that the Tulsa area could benefit from the multidisciplinary services that were being considered but that were not then available.

Program Goals and Objectives

Program goals often include activities such as opening services in a new site, increasing the dietitian's time with clients, or serving a certain number of patients per year. In Tulsa, the goals developed were to establish a multidisciplinary team to assess and treat pediatric undernutrition, increase identification of undernourished children in the area, and maintain a network with other community agencies that were serving children who were nutritionally at risk.

Goals are broad; specific objectives are measurable. Examples of specific objectives are to see 80 children per year, to increase by 25% the number of cases that are identified and referred within the WIC caseload, or to increase from 15 to 25 the number of children who are successfully referred to early intervention programs. Measurable objectives are desirable because they provide greater accountability. One of the most challenging parts of program evaluation is establishing objectives. Doing so takes time and hard thought, but it enables a program to focus more clearly on what it really wants to accomplish.

Population Served

Once services are initiated, the staff of a program will need basic information on the population whom they serve: How old are the children at entry to the program? Are they bottle- or breast-fed? Were they low birth weight? How severe is their undernutrition? Are they participating in WIC?

Characteristics of families and the community also are important. How old are the parents? Are they living in poverty? How many are single mothers? What is the families' mode of transportation to the clinic? Which other helping agencies are involved? Have child protective services been involved? Is there a history of domestic violence?

In Tulsa, the team found that the majority of families had two parents and were Caucasian. The children were on Medicaid or managed care and were referred mainly by urban physicians and health departments. The median age at which children were referred was 27 months—an older age than some clinics see and an age when weight gain may be harder to accomplish.

Program Monitoring and Process Evaluation

Program monitoring provides a description of the process of service. It helps one know what the program is doing: How many patients are seen and how many clinical visits of various types (e.g., developmental assessment, nutritional assessment, social services assessment, home visit) are accomplished? It is also important to have a means of keeping track of a program's active patients or clients. Table 1 provides examples of items that may be used to evaluate the process of service; Table 2 provides nutritional quality assurance criteria for chart reviews.

Table 1.   Program monitoring

Population served	**Service statistics**
Age	Number of visits
Newborn status	Patterns of use
• Low birth weight	• Referral source
• Preterm	• Show rate
Gender	• Delay from referral to initial evaluation
Ethnicity	Length of treatment
Basic demographics of family	**Completeness of service provision**
Economic status	Social services
• Receiving WIC	Nutrition
• Receiving TANF	Physician
Educational level of parents	Child development specialist
Annual income of household, percent of federal poverty line	Subspecialist (e.g., psychiatry, gastroenterology)
Household composition	Laboratory tests obtained
• Biological or foster	Hospitalization
• Single parent, multigenerational, two parents	Home visits
Presence of domestic violence	**Outcomes**
Protective services involvement	Evidence of improved growth
	Increased access to community programs
	• Early intervention
	• WIC

Adapted from Joint Commission on Accreditation of Health Care Organizations (1994).

In the process evaluation of the Tulsa Growth and Nutrition Clinic, the staff developed the goal that children would wait no longer than 2 weeks between referral and initial evaluation. An analysis of the time between referral and first evaluation showed that the average was 17 days. Further analysis revealed that the delay most commonly was due to 1) families' being unable to obtain transportation or 2) a poor understanding of the reason for the referral and failure to show for the first scheduled appointment. Using this information, it was determined that two improvements needed to be made: 1) help families with transportation and 2) help referring physicians stress the importance of and reasons for referral.

Medical practitioners can benefit from a review of evaluations in primary care (Yano, Fink, Hirsch, Robbins, & Rubenstein, 1995). The reviewers found in other studies that several strategies were effective in enhancing quality and economy: computer-generated appointment reminders, use of protocols by nurses, telephone management, multidisciplinary teams, and regional organization of practices.

OUTCOME EVALUATION

Outcome (summative) evaluation assesses a program's results or effects on health status, child development, or family function; it also may measure improvements in children's growth. Little is known about the proportion of children who may be expected to gain weight or the amount that they may be expected to gain, but growth seen in one multidisciplinary clinic has been described (Bithoney et al., 1989; see Chapter 9), and growth seen

Table 2. Nutritional quality assurance criteria

Criteria	Critical time
1. Nutrition screening is completed according to established protocol, including weight-for-age, length- or height-for-age, and weight-for-length or -height. (Process)	Each clinic visit
2. Nutrition screening is completed according to established protocol, including 1) evaluation of nutrition intake or feeding history, 2) anthropometric data and growth history, 3) biochemical data, 4) clinical data, and 5) caregiver–child interaction. (Process)	Initial evaluation period and as indicated in nutrition care plan
3. Child progresses toward or achieves body weight for stature between 5th and 95th percentiles. (Outcome)	Duration of treatment
4. Child maintains or exceeds own established growth curve for height or length when measurement is plotted on NCHS growth chart. (Initial length or height may be used as baseline when previous growth data are unavailable) (Exception: acute illness) (Outcome)	Duration of treatment
5. Nutrition care plan is developed, based on assessment data and psychosocial data. (Process)	Within 24 hours of completion of nutrition assessment
6. Nutrition care plan is implemented as written or revised. (Process)	Duration of treatment
7. Parent or caregiver and child display appropriate interaction during feeding time or mealtime according to established protocol. (Outcome)	When care plan is implemented or revised
8. Parent or caregiver is able to state rationale for prescribed diet. (Outcome)	When care plan is implemented or revised
9. Parent or caregiver states appropriate feeding plan. (Outcome)	At each clinic visit
10. Parent or caregiver reports correct techniques for preparation of formula or nutritional supplements. (Exception: child not on formula or nutritional supplements) (Outcome)	When care plan is implemented or revised
11. Family and child are referred to community food and nutrition resources based on identified need. (Process)	Within 1 week of need identification

© 1990, the American Dietetic Association. *Quality Assurance Criteria for Pediatric Nutrition Conditions: A Model.* Adapted by permission.

in a group of clinics has been published in a program report (Anderson et al., 1993). The latter looked at differential growth according to degree of height and weight impairment before treatment.

Most growth and nutrition programs measure weight gain. Child and family variables are likely to be more important than treatment in influencing the outcome. Weight gain may be associated with younger age, greater cooperation by parents, and simpler problems to solve (e.g., mixing formula); therefore, it may be risky to attribute weight gain or lack of it to the program alone, and it may be more helpful to look at within-group effects of which children in which families and with which treatments gain weight well. (See Chapter 10 for measuring catch-up growth.)

To simplify measurement of some outcome data, one can count completed referrals as outcome results. Completed referrals to early intervention programs may be counted as positive effects on child development and referrals for food stamps as positive effects on family income.

Special Studies

Special questions that deserve answers may arise. For example, one clinic made an objective of asking the parents of 80% of the children whether they had food stamps and provided referrals for those who did not. The Tulsa Growth and Nutrition Program, for another example, examined children's developmental assessments, which are done at regular intervals. The results showed less than expected developmental progress in 35% of the children. Those children were then specifically reviewed. Seventy-one percent were identified as having a known reason for less than expected developmental attainment (e.g., cerebral palsy, chromosomal anomaly). Further focus for problem solving was then directed to the children who did not have a known reason for delay. Those appeared to be children from families who were attaining little benefit from intervention. For those families, the staff made referrals for extra services, such as comprehensive family support and intensive in-home therapy.

TYPES OF DATA

Most programs should use a mixture of quantitative and qualitative data.

Quantitative Data

All programs should have a system for compiling basic data about participating children so that data can be reviewed at regular intervals. The system can list names, birth dates, parents' names, and names of care coordinators. "With appropriate advance planning, the very same data collection system that enables a program to monitor the provision of services to clients can be expanded to form an evaluation-related data collection system" (Card, Greeno, & Peterson, 1992, p. 77). It can easily provide basic descriptive data such as demographics and family income.

Quantitative methods involve counts and measurements. One may count numbers of children seen or clinic visits. Parent–child interaction measures may be quantitative (see Appendixes B, C, and D). A number of useful computer programs are available for analysis of data. Epi Info (USD, Inc., 1995) is one such program that combines data entry and descriptive and analytic statistics. It also calculates percentiles, percents of median, and z-scores for height, weight, and weight-for-height.

Qualitative Data

In growth and nutrition programs, understanding the uniqueness of particular situations or individuals is as important as elucidating general tenets about a population (Murray, 1992). The ability to study real clients in a real environment makes the observational approach very compelling (Selby, 1994). The individualized treatment and outcome expectation for each case may be impossible to capture with standard measures.

Case studies may be presented to funding agencies to bring attention to particular issues by illustrating concerns. Cases can be presented in writing, with photographs, or by videotape. Following is a case study from the Tulsa Growth and Nutrition Clinic.

> Immanuelle, 5¹/₂ years old, was accompanied to the Growth and Nutrition Clinic by Maxi, her foster mother of 2 years. Maxi was very concerned about Immanuelle's eating habits: She had always eaten slowly and had a strong preference for sweets. Recently, Maxi had discovered that Immanuelle was telling her that she was eating at Head Start and telling her Head Start teacher that she was eating at home. Maxi had noticed that Immanuelle was gagging herself following eating. Maxi, in desperation, had required Immanuelle to sit at the table for 1–2 hours to complete a meal. Maxi was employed as a cook and placed strong emphasis on appropriate nutrition in her home.
>
> The speech-language pathologist, alerted by the history of gagging, found that Immanuelle had mild oral-motor dysfunction (see Chapter 23). This required advice about feeding.
>
> Maxi, though well-intentioned, had actually intensified Immanuelle's eating problem by attempting to control and force Immanuelle's intake. Maxi also had not allowed Immanuelle to participate in meal planning and preparation. She needed guidance and support in allowing Immanuelle to eat on her own. She learned to let Immanuelle have sweets in moderation and not as a reward.
>
> Immanuelle's biological mother and George, another member of the family, were to return to the community in 3 months, and Immanuelle then would be returned to her biological home. She was alleged to have experienced sexual abuse by George. A psychiatry consult was obtained. This revealed Immanuelle to be experiencing post-traumatic stress disorder with features of depression and anxiety precipitated by the knowledge of George and her mother's return. Immanuelle's child protective services case manager was notified of this concern, and it was arranged that George would not be in the home.
>
> Of course, a primary goal for the Growth and Nutrition Clinic was to correct Immanuelle's undernutrition. To accomplish that, however, a number of other issues had to be addressed. This required the coordinated efforts of Maxi and the multidisciplinary team: the dietitian, the nurse, the child development specialist, the psychiatrist, and the speech-language pathologist. The team also worked with Immanuelle's child protective services worker and her school teacher.
>
> Immanuelle has recovered from her undernutrition. She enjoys planning, preparing, and eating meals with Maxi. The transition to living with her family is proceeding in planned steps. She no longer exhibits depression or anxiety.

The case of Immanuelle demonstrates several issues: 1) the contribution of mild oral-motor dysfunction to eating difficulties, 2) the need for access to subspecialty services, 3) the need to communicate with other service agencies, and 4) the need to help children who have a history of trauma. This information helped the funding agency understand the complexity and individuality of cases while also demonstrating some common themes for families who are receiving services.

HOW MUCH EVALUATION

Program evaluation requires some commitment of time and effort. Each program must assess how much evaluation is appropriate to address its needs. Every program will want basic descriptions of the children and families served and basic service statistics. Every program should establish goals and, preferably, measurable objectives and should evaluate its success in meeting them.

Evaluation should pose and answer questions that will be useful for those who are working in the program, funding agencies, and others who may be interested. Beyond that, several questions must be answered to decide which level of evaluation will be pertinent to a program: What do we want to know? What are our options, given our budget and the size and expertise of our staff? Where can I go for consulting help? (See Joint Commission on Accreditation of Health Care Organizations, 1994, and National Center for Clinical Infant Programs, 1987, for further information on evaluation.)

REFERENCES

Anderson, E., Casey, V., Fisher, P., Peterson, K.E., Polhamus, B., & Wiecha, J.L. (1993). *Catching up: Report of the Massachusetts growth and nutrition clinics FY1985–FY1989.* Boston: Massachusetts Department of Public Health.

Bithoney, W.G., McJunkin, J., Michalek, J., Egan, H., Snyder, J., & Munier, A. (1989). Prospective evaluation of weight gain in both nonorganic and organic failure-to-thrive children: An outpatient trial of a multidisciplinary team intervention strategy. *Journal of Developmental and Behavioral Pediatrics, 10,* 27–31.

Card, J., Greeno, C., & Peterson, J. (1992). Planning an evaluation and estimating its cost. *Evaluation and the Health Professions, 15,* 75–89.

Health Services Research Group. (1992). Program evaluation in health care. *Canadian Medical Association Journal, 146,* 1301–1304.

Joint Commission on Accreditation of Health Care Organizations. (1994). *Assessing and improving community health care delivery.* Oakbrook Terrace, IL: Author.

Murray, A.D. (1992, April). Early intervention program evaluation: Numbers or narratives? *Infants and Young Children, 4,* 77–88.

National Center for Clinical Infant Programs. (1987). *Charting change in infants, families and services: A guide to program evaluation for administrators and practitioners.* Washington, DC: Author.

Oklahoma Department of Health. (1995). *Oklahoma pediatric nutrition surveillance system report.* Oklahoma City: Author.

Selby, J. (1994). Case-control evaluations of treatment and program efficacy. *Epidemiologic Reviews, 16,* 90–101.

USD, Inc. (1995). Epi Info [Computer program]. Stone Mountain, GA: Author.

Wooldridge, N.H. (Ed.). (1988). *Quality assurance criteria for pediatric nutrition conditions: A model.* Washington, DC: American Dietetic Association.

Yano, E., Fink, A., Hirsch, S., Robbins, A., & Rubenstein, L. (1995). Helping practices reach primary care goals: Lessons from the literature. *Archives of Internal Medicine, 155,* 1146–1156.

Chapter 35

Coordination of Services

P.J. McWilliam

The number and the complexity of factors that may be associated with pediatric under-nutrition require that a multidisciplinary or a transdisciplinary approach to intervention be used (see Chapters 1, 9, and 22). Especially for children living in poverty, intervention efforts not only must be multidisciplinary but also must go beyond the health and feeding of the child to facilitate other aspects of child development and to support the entire family system (Black, Dubowitz, Hutcheson, Berenson-Howard, & Starr, 1995; Parker, Greer, & Zuckerman, 1988). This typically requires gaining access to services from a variety of agencies.

DIFFICULTIES IN COORDINATING SERVICES

The fragmented service delivery system found in most communities can be confusing and frustrating for parents and professionals alike (McWilliam et al., 1995; Meisels, Harbin, Modigliana, & Olson, 1988; Melaville, Blank, & Asayesh, 1993; Roberts, Behl, & Akers, 1996). When piecing together needed services, contact with numerous agencies is often required, each in a different location and each with its own application procedures and eligibility requirements. Families may have to spend large amounts of time scheduling appointments with various agencies, traveling to and from appointments, and sitting in clinic waiting rooms. Because professionals from different agencies rarely sit down at the table together to engage in joint planning, the information and help that families receive from agencies may not always meet their needs or may not be consistent with other agencies' advice. Given this state of affairs, is it really a surprise when a young mother of three children who lives on welfare and has to rely on public transportation does not follow through on making and keeping her child's appointments? The costs of doing so may far exceed the actual or perceived benefits.

Although the need for improved service coordination has long been recognized (Strickland & McPherson, 1994), movement toward this goal has been slow and extremely limited. Studies of service coordination that is specific to pediatric undernutrition appear not to be available; however, studies of service coordination for children and families who are served under Part C early intervention programs as mandated by the Individuals with Disabilities Education Act Amendments of 1997 (PL 105-17) (see Chapter 25) provide some useful information. For example, a national survey of 193 Part C home-visiting programs, all of which were recognized for their successful use of home visits to integrate services (Roberts, Akers, & Behl, 1996; Roberts, Behl, et al., 1996), showed that the primary model that was used for service coordination was a "linked services" model (63% of programs), wherein home visiting is used to coordinate services and link families to other agencies. In this model, there may be little or no interaction between agencies at the administrative level. Even less coordination was reported by 12% of the programs surveyed, whose primary model of coordination with other local programs was "limited communication." Using this model, families are responsible for contacting other agencies to obtain services, and there is little, if any, communication between professionals who work in different agencies. Only 8% of surveyed programs reported their predominant service model as "one-stop shopping," which would include strategies such as shared intake and eligibility determination across agencies and the colocation of services. In this same survey, Roberts, Akers, et al. (1996) also found that a significant portion of programs neither provided nor linked families to general health care services (11%), professional mental health counseling (8%), financial assistance (10%), job training counseling (23%), and homemaker services (23%). Programs reported that it was often difficult for families to locate or gain access to these services.

Why do difficulties in service coordination persist? When asked to identify local barriers to interagency collaboration, respondents in the Roberts, Behl, et al. (1996) survey reported that the greatest barriers were insufficient time for service coordination activities, large caseloads, and agencies' being too protective of their turf. In fact, turf protection, or the need to maintain agency autonomy, has been cited repeatedly as a causative factor (Harbin, 1996; Harbin & McNulty, 1990; Kagan & Neville, 1993). Having few resources to contribute to causes that may not be related to their primary mission or population served, agencies are reluctant to commit money or time to interagency efforts. Permanent commitments to joint efforts with other agencies denote a release of power or authority over an agency's resources and may, thus, be perceived as threatening.

STRATEGIES FOR IMPROVING SERVICE COORDINATION

Given the fragmented nature of services in communities, what can agencies and individual practitioners do to improve services for undernourished children and their families? Unfortunately, there are no definitive answers regarding the most effective models of service coordination, and the most effective strategies for facilitating improved communication and coordination among agencies have not been identified. Even so, some general guidelines for achieving improved service coordination have been offered and are presented in the remaining sections of this chapter. Based on the earlier work of Black and Kase (1963), Swan and Morgan (1993) proposed three levels of interagency relationships that may describe services within communities: 1) *interagency cooperation,* 2) *interagency coordination,* and 3) *interagency collaboration.* These terms represent a hierarchy of sophistication in interagency relationships from least to most. A brief description of each of these three levels is provided next, along with suggestions for improving service coordination for children and families.

Interagency Cooperation

At the level of *interagency cooperation,* agencies are aware of each other's existence, share general information, and refer children and families from one agency to another; however, agencies are completely autonomous with respect to their policies and practices (Swan & Morgan, 1993). This level of interagency interactions most closely resembles what Roberts, Behl, et al. (1996) referred to as a linked services model—the primary model used for service coordination by 63% of the nominated home-visiting programs that were polled in their national study.

What can be done to improve access, use, and coordination of services to undernourished children and their families in communities that function at this level? Individual service coordinators or case managers may help to make families aware of existing services, facilitate access to needed services, and promote at least rudimentary levels of service coordination for children and their families. Service coordination activities may be performed by nurses, social workers, early interventionists, or other qualified professionals or paraprofessionals. Several factors should be kept in mind, however, when deciding who will conduct service coordination activities. First, are frequent contacts with families possible? Frequent contacts (e.g., weekly) are conducive to establishing trusting family–professional relationships and identifying the unique needs of each family served. Second, service coordinators must be knowledgeable about a broad spectrum of services that are available both within the community and outside the community. This includes both child and family services and services to improve service utilization (e.g., transportation, financial assistance). Third, service coordinators need sufficient time to conduct activities that are related to service coordination (e.g., ongoing communication with families, planning meetings, contacting other agencies, locating services).

In addition to these features, ongoing research on effective qualities of service coordinators (e.g., Dinnebeil, Hale, & Rule, 1996; Dinnebeil & Rule, 1994; Dunst, Johanson, Rounds, Trivette, & Hamby, 1992) has indicated that the attitudes and interpersonal skills of service coordinators are important. For example, a nationwide qualitative study of families and service coordinators (Dinnebeil et al., 1996) revealed that, although the knowledge and professional skills of service coordinators were perceived as being important to the development of collaborative relationships, attitudes that were reflective of family-centered beliefs and interpersonal skills were far more often identified by study participants as important to effective family–professional collaboration. Specific attributes of service coordinators that are related to these factors included a nonjudgmental attitude, trust, mutual respect, honesty, genuine caring, enthusiasm, a willingness to listen, establishing a positive atmosphere, and being dependable.

Service coordination is no small undertaking. Effective service coordination—especially for families who have extensive needs—can be extremely time-consuming. If service coordination is added to the agendas of staff members who already have a full schedule of direct service responsibilities, then one or the other is likely to be compromised. Caution should also be taken to ensure that those who are given responsibility for service coordination have the necessary skills. Few professionals receive adequate preservice preparation in the areas of service coordination and working with families, so additional training may be necessary.

Another option that programs have is to refer families to other agencies that do provide effective service coordination. Home-based intervention programs are particularly promising in this regard. For example, in a study of 539 families who were receiving early intervention services in North Carolina (McWilliam et al., 1995), only 19% of families who were receiving home-based services believed that they were not getting all of the help that they wanted for their child, whereas 36% of families of children in special classroom programs reported that their children were not getting all of the help that they needed. Families in home-based programs also were more satisfied with the amount of family-level help that they were getting (79% reported that they were getting enough) than families whose children were receiving special classroom services.

Professionals who are not functioning as service coordinators or case managers also can play an important role in coordinating services for children and families. Their efforts are especially important when service coordination across agencies relies solely on voluntary cooperation. Opening the lines of communication is the key, and getting to know people from other agencies is a good way to start. This can be accomplished by attending special-interest groups in the community or by actively participating in local or state professional associations—any activity that provides opportunities to meet and talk with professionals from other community agencies. It also can be done more directly, such as by arranging to have lunch with a clinician who works in another agency. Establishing a relationship with at least one clinician in another agency *before* problems arise can do much to prevent defensiveness when difficulties do need to be worked out at a later time. Such relationships can also serve as a means for gaining a clearer understanding about how other agencies operate.

Another strategy that is important for any clinician to use is to share with direct services providers in other agencies information about the children and families with whom they are working. This may be done by periodic telephone calls, e-mail, or letters. The information shared should provide an update about which services you have been providing, the purpose or goals of your contacts with the child and the family, progress that has been achieved, and any difficulties or additional concerns that have emerged since your last communication. Copies of reports or intervention plans may also be sent if this is appropriate. Such updates need not be formal or detailed; a note consisting of a few short paragraphs may be all that is needed and is more likely to be read than a longer document. When sharing information with other agencies, several things should be kept in mind. First, be certain that families authorize information sharing with other agencies and are aware of the content of these communications. Second, make certain that the information that is shared is going to the right person. Rather than send it to the agency, where it may end up in a file that no one reads, send it directly to the clinician in the agency who provides direct services to the child and the family. In the case of doctors' offices or clinics, it may be best to ask to whom the information should be sent so that it is seen and used by those who have direct contact with the child and the family. Third, provide periodic updates. Brief monthly or quarterly communications may be better than semiannual or yearly updates because, with longer intervals, the information may be quickly outdated. Fourth, do not expect reciprocity on behalf of other agencies. Just because other clinicians do not send you updates about their services does not mean that they are not reading yours.

In summary, good service coordination may do much to alleviate the confusion that many families face in trying to secure services in a fragmented system. Even the best service coordination, however, will not solve some issues, such as the unavailability of services, restrictive eligibility criteria, long waiting lists, or the manner in which services are provided by other agencies. Solving these issues requires the active participation of agency leaders and movement toward the next level of interagency relationships.

Interagency Coordination

At the level of *interagency coordination,* two or more agencies recognize commonalities in their missions and the population that they serve. Agencies discuss difficulties and gaps

in service delivery and, more important, respond by adapting their policies, procedures, and allocation of resources to improve services for children and families. Through joint problem solving, agencies can eliminate unnecessary duplication of services, streamline the referral process from one agency to another, improve access to client records, or make available services that previously had been in short supply or that had not existed at all (Swan & Morgan, 1993).

Given the broad spectrum of agencies that serve undernourished children and their families, joint problem solving may involve a large number of representatives within a community. Although not exhaustive, the list may include public health agencies, hospitals and medical clinics, feeding and nutrition services, child care agencies, social services, Special Supplemental Nutrition Program for Women, Infants and Children (WIC), child protective services, employment or vocational rehabilitation services, mental health centers, Part C (PL 105-17) early intervention services, and so forth. Whereas front-line staff work to coordinate the services of such agencies on behalf of individual children and families when agency interactions are less sophisticated (i.e., interagency cooperation), interagency coordination requires the initiative and leadership of higher-level administrative staff. Staff who have the authority to make decisions on behalf of their own agencies must be actively involved in efforts to coordinate services at this level.

In communities where little interagency communication exists, starting small by initiating conversations with one or two other agencies may be best. Other agencies may then be asked to join the group as work proceeds. Another strategy is to initiate a special task force, comprising representatives from various community agencies, to address a few specific issues that are related to services for children and families. Following completion of the group's original objectives, members could discuss the possibility of continuing to meet and identifying new tasks. In other communities, existing interagency work groups may provide a place for initiating conversations specifically about services for undernourished children and their families. For example, under the Individuals with Disabilities Education Act (IDEA) of 1990 (PL 101-476) and its amendments, all states that receive federal funds for birth-to-3 early intervention services are mandated to have a state-level interagency coordinating council (ICC). In addition, many communities have established local interagency coordinating councils (LICCs) that comprise representatives from a variety of community agencies that serve young children who have disabilities or who are at risk for developmental disabilities and their families. Joining such a group may be preferable to starting a new one, provided, of course, that group membership includes representatives from at least some agencies that are involved in services to undernourished children and their families.

In addition to improving the structure and efficiency of service delivery, agencies that work together can open new options for conducting service coordination. For example, two of the eight structural models for conducting service coordination described by Friesen and Briggs (1995) rely on community services' being at least at the level of sophistication of interagency coordination. Both of these models involve the use of interagency teams. One model involves the establishment of a standing committee that comprises representatives from a variety of community agencies. The primary function of this committee is to plan and authorize services for children who have very complex needs. The second model uses an ad hoc team rather than a standing committee. Team members represent the various agencies with whom the child and the family are involved and usually, but not always, are those professionals who provide direct services to the child and the family. Together, team members discuss service needs and develop a joint service plan. In some instances, the group may also meet periodically to review progress and the continued appropriateness of the service plan.

The advantage of both of these models is that resources to meet child and family needs are identified and authorized by multiple agencies at one time rather than individually at separate times through the family's or the service coordinator's seeking out services from one agency to another. Among the disadvantages, however, are that these models are very time-consuming and that, without formal written agreements, their success relies heavily on the goodwill of agencies to follow through on their commitments (Friesen & Briggs, 1995). It should also be mentioned that these models do not eliminate the need for individual service coordinators or case managers.

In summary, at the level of interagency coordination, the community service system is viewed as a whole rather than as merely a conglomeration of independent parts, and improvements in the system can be made through joint efforts among agencies. Even so, at this level, agencies still are relatively autonomous, establishing their own independent policies and procedures and deciding for themselves how their resources will be allocated. Furthermore, with each agency providing its own services, families with multiple service requirements may have numerous professionals working with them and may have to go to a variety of locations within the community to receive services.

Interagency Collaboration

Interagency collaboration is the most sophisticated level of agency relationship. At this level, agencies no longer operate independently but rather pool their resources and engage in shared decision-making to accomplish common goals. According to Swan and Morgan, interagency collaboration

> Is characterized by teamwork, mutual planning, shared ownership of problems, shared vision of goals, adjustments of policies and procedures, integration of ideas, synchronization of activities and timelines, contribution of resources, joint evaluation, and mutual satisfaction and pride of accomplishment in providing quality and a comprehensive service delivery system. (1993, p. 22)

The needs of children and families rather than the needs of individual agencies or programs guide decision-making at this level, resulting in services that are easier for families to gain access to and perhaps also resulting in the creation of new services.

Interagency collaboration has been advocated by many, and numerous federal and state policies have been rewritten to facilitate its occurrence (e.g., Strickland & McPherson, 1994), but this level of interagency relationship is difficult to achieve. Mandates alone are not sufficient to make it happen, and, even though written contracts and agreements among participating agencies are necessary for effective collaboration, they, too, offer no guarantees. This is not to say that interagency collaboration cannot happen, but it requires intensive effort and commitment by agency leaders and their boards of directors (Melaville et al., 1993; Swan & Morgan, 1993).

Family support programs offer some of the best examples of successful interagency collaboration at the community level. Many of these programs are specifically targeted at families in poverty whose children are at high risk for developmental delays and behavior problems and, thus, are applicable to a large proportion of children who have been diagnosed as undernourished. Although there is considerable variation among family support programs, several basic tenets drive their existence and the manner in which services are organized (Melaville et al., 1993). First, family support programs are based on the principle of *prevention*—helping families before problems occur. This might include well-baby health care, child care, job training, education, prenatal care, after-school programs, and programs to prevent teen pregnancies. Second, services are *comprehensive,* attending to the needs of all family members. Third, services are *integrated* by such methods as shared intake and determination of eligibility and having a single service coordinator develop a plan that addresses the needs of all family members. Fourth, services are *easily accessible* by families by having hours of operation that are convenient to families, by providing services at locations that are close to where families live and work (e.g., in schools), or by providing transportation. Finally, there is sufficient *flexibility* that services may change with the changing needs of families, and, in some cases, there may even be discretionary funds to help families who are in crisis.

Examples of such community-based prevention approaches to services are increasingly becoming available (e.g., Chamberlin, 1994; Melaville et al., 1993), and reports of their effectiveness are impressive. For example, after 7 years of operation, a program in Addison County, Vermont, showed significant reductions in the incidence of child abuse, teenage pregnancy, low birth weights, school dropout, and welfare dependency (Chamberlin, 1992). Teenage pregnancy rates fell from 70 per 1,000 teenage girls to 45 per 1,000, and only 13% of the teenagers who were served by the program had subsequent pregnancies within 5 years. Furthermore, fewer than 1% of these teenage mothers delivered low birth weight babies, as compared with 8.9% across the rest of the state. Also impressive was the finding that the percentage of teenage parents who received a high school diploma or its equivalent (general equivalency diploma) increased from 30% to 71%. But perhaps most impressive was that this program's success led to the establishment of similar programs in all Vermont counties, and state legislation was passed that appropriated funds to cover a portion of the operating budgets of these programs (Chamberlin, 1994).

Although there are no cookbooks that provide step-by-step procedures for developing a collaborative family support system of service delivery, some helpful guidelines are available (e.g., Chamberlin, 1994; Epstein, Larner, & Halpern, 1995; Melaville et al., 1993). A particularly useful guide is *Together We Can: A Guide for Crafting a Profamily System of Education and Human Services* (Melaville et al., 1993). This publication presents a five-stage process for moving from a traditional service delivery system toward genuine interagency collaboration (see Table 1). The process begins with identifying key players in the community and getting them together, then moves through the building of trust among group members, to developing and implementing a small-scale plan (a service prototype), and, finally, to strengthening the prototype and expanding it to include other sites. The authors pointed out that the process is not linear but, rather, cyclical, and groups that attempt to change the service delivery system frequently must move back and forth through the process as they proceed.

CONCLUSION

The fragmented service delivery systems found in most U.S. communities make it difficult for many families of young children to find and secure the services that they need. The assistance of a knowledgeable and skilled service coordinator may help to alleviate some of the difficulties, but even this may not be enough to prevent the long-term consequences of undernutrition for some children. There is increasing realization that service delivery systems are in need of radical change. Chamberlin (1994) aptly explained the problem using a river analogy that was developed by people who were working in international health programs:

> Downstream state agencies and human service providers are trying to rescue "drowning" children by providing neonatal intensive care for low birth weight and sick newborns; family counseling and foster care for children who have been abused or neglected; medical care for those

Table 1.   Moving toward interagency collaboration: A five-stage process

Stage One: Getting Together. In this stage, a small group comes together to explore how to improve services for children and families. They identify other community representatives with a stake in the same issue, make a joint commitment to collaborate, and agree on a unifying theme. They also establish shared leadership, set basic ground rules for working together, secure initial support, and determine how to finance collaborative planning.

Stage Two: Building Trust and Ownership. Next, partners establish common ground. They share information about each other and the needs of families and children in their community. Using this information, they create a shared vision of what a better service delivery system would look like, and they develop a mission statement and a set of goals to guide their future actions.

Stage Three: Developing a Strategic Plan. Here, partners begin to explore options that flow from their common concerns and shared vision. They agree to focus on a specific geographic area, and they design a prototype delivery system that incorporates the elements of their shared vision. Partners also develop the technical tools and interagency agreements needed to put their plan into action. During this stage, the group may go back to preceding stages to bring in new partners and to continue building ownership.

Stage Four: Taking Action. Partners begin to implement the prototype. They use the information it provides to adjust the policies and practices of the organizations that comprise the prototype service delivery system. Partners design an ongoing evaluation strategy that helps them to identify specific systems-change requirements, make mid-course corrections, and measure the results.

Stage Five: Going to Scale. Finally, partners take steps to ensure that systems-change strategies and capacities developed in the prototype are adapted, expanded, and re-created in locations throughout the community where pro-family systems are needed. To do this, partners continue to develop local leadership, strengthen staff capacity by changing preservice and inservice training, and build a strong constituency for change.

From Melaville, A.I., Blank, M.J., & Asayesh, G. (1993). *Together we can: A guide for crafting a profamily system of education and human services* (p. 20). Washington, DC: U.S. Government Printing Office; reprinted by permission.

exposed to lead, injured in an accident, or pregnant out of wedlock; special education services for those having trouble learning in school; mental health programs for those with behavioral or emotional problems; and "reform" school for those who have come into contact with the law because of delinquency or crime.

Upstream there is less activity, but people are trying to ascertain whether children swimming in the river are "at risk" for "drowning" and should be rescued. . . . Still further upstream, children are jumping or falling into the river because of some combination of family and community dysfunction. . . . Very little is being done either to teach these children to swim or, more importantly, to keep them from falling into the river. (Chamberlin, 1994, pp. 36–37)

Extending the river analogy, improved coordination among agencies is needed to prevent children who are undernourished from going too far downstream before rescue efforts are initiated. Moreover, the better that agencies work together, the more organized and effective that rescue efforts of these children are likely to be. Ideally, however, agencies would combine their resources to remove as many risk conditions as possible upstream and, thus, significantly reduce the number of children who fall into the river at all. This reduction or elimination of risk conditions is the ultimate goal of collaborative family support initiatives.

REFERENCES

Black, J., & Kase, M. (1963). Interagency cooperation in rehabilitation and mental health. *Social Service Review, 37*(1), 26–32.

Black, M.M., Dubowitz, H., Hutcheson, J., Berenson-Howard, J., & Starr, R.H. (1995). A random-ized, clinical trial of home intervention for children with failure to thrive. *Pediatrics, 95*(6), 807–814.

Chamberlin, R.W. (1992). Preventing low birth weight, child abuse, and school failure: The need for comprehensive, community-wide approaches. *Pediatrics in Review, 13,* 64–71.

Chamberlin, R.W. (1994). Primary prevention: The missing piece in child development legislation. In R.J. Simeonsson (Ed.), *Risk, resilience, and prevention: Promoting the well-being of all chil-dren* (pp. 33–52). Baltimore: Paul H. Brookes Publishing Co.

Dinnebeil, L.A., Hale, L.M., & Rule, S. (1996). A qualitative analysis of parents' and service coordi-nators' descriptions of variables that influence collaborative relationships. *Topics in Early Child-hood Special Education, 16*(3), 322–347.

Dinnebeil, L.A., & Rule, S. (1994). Variables that influence collaboration between parents and ser-vice coordinators. *Journal of Early Intervention, 18*(3), 349–361.

Dunst, C.J., Johanson, C., Rounds, T., Trivette, C.M., & Hamby, D. (1992). Characteristics of parent–professional partnerships. In S.L. Christenson & J.C. Conoley (Eds.), *Home–school col-laboration: Enhancing children's academic and social competence* (pp. 157–174). Silver Spring, MD: National Association of School Psychologists.

Epstein, A.S., Larner, M., & Halpern, R. (1995). *A guide to developing community-based family sup-port programs.* Ypsilanti, MI: High/Scope Press.

Friesen, B.J., & Briggs, H.E. (1995). The organization and structure of service coordination mecha-nisms. In B.J. Friesen & J. Poertner (Eds.), *From case management to service coordination for children with emotional, behavioral, or mental disorders* (pp. 63–94). Baltimore: Paul H. Brookes Publishing Co.

Harbin, G.L. (1996). The challenge of coordination. *Infants and Young Children, 8*(3), 68–76.

Harbin, G.L., & McNulty, B.A. (1990). Policy implementation: Perspectives on service coordination and interagency cooperation. In S.J. Meisels & J.P. Shonkoff (Eds.), *Handbook of early interven-tion* (pp. 700–722). New York: Cambridge University Press.

Individuals with Disabilities Education Act (IDEA) of 1990, PL 101-476, 20 U.S.C. §§ 1400 *et seq.*

Individuals with Disabilities Education Act Amendments of 1997, PL 105-17, 20 U.S.C. §§ 1400 *et seq.*

Kagan, S.L., & Neville, P.R. (1993). *Integrating services for children and families: Understanding the past to shape the future.* New Haven, CT: Yale University Press.

McWilliam, R.A., Lang, L., Vandivere, P., Angell, R., Collins, L., & Underdown, G. (1995). Satis-faction and struggles: Family perceptions of early intervention services. *Journal of Early Inter-vention, 19*(1), 43–60.

Meisels, S.J., Harbin, G., Modigliana, K., & Olson, K. (1988). Formulating optimal state early child-hood intervention policies. *Exceptional Children, 55,* 159–165.

Melaville, A.I., Blank, M.J., & Asayesh, G. (1993). *Together we can: A guide for crafting a profam-ily system of education and human services.* Washington, DC: U.S. Government Printing Office.

Parker, S., Greer, S., & Zuckerman, B. (1988). Double jeopardy: The impact of poverty on early child development. *Pediatric Clinics of North America, 35*(6), 1227–1240.

Roberts, R.N., Akers, A.L., & Behl, D.D. (1996). Family-level service coordination within home vis-iting programs. *Topics in Early Childhood Special Education, 16*(3), 279–301.

Roberts, R.N., Behl, D.D., & Akers, A.L. (1996). Community-level service integration within home visiting programs. *Topics in Early Childhood Special Education, 16*(3), 302–321.

Strickland, B., & McPherson, M. (1994). Maternal and child health: A collaborative agenda for pre-vention. In R.J. Simeonsson (Ed.), *Risk, resilience, and prevention: Promoting the well-being of all children* (pp. 53–73). Baltimore: Paul H. Brookes Publishing Co.

Swan, W.W., & Morgan, J.L. (1993). *Collaborating for comprehensive services for young children and their families: The local interagency coordinating council.* Baltimore: Paul H. Brookes Pub-lishing Co.

Section VII

Policy and Advocacy

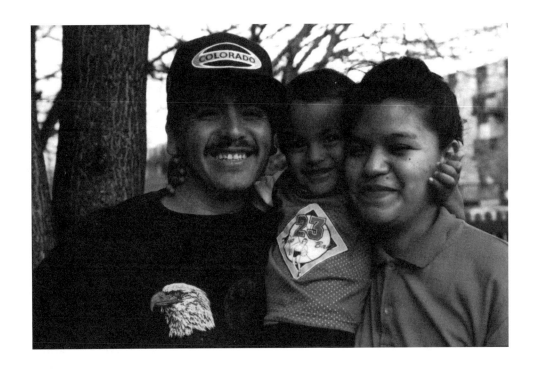

Chapter 36

Advocacy for Children and Families

Joshua Greenberg

Advocacy has become an increasingly important component of providers' work with undernourished children; however, many providers are not trained in effective advocacy techniques as part of their education. As an attorney who has worked in a pediatric setting, including extensive involvement with a hospital-based growth clinic, the author of this chapter offers concrete suggestions for improving advocacy on behalf of these children.

LEVELS OF ADVOCACY

Advocacy occurs at two levels: the individual and the systemic. Individual advocacy is perhaps more familiar. It happens whenever a social worker evaluates a child's eligibility for the Special Supplemental Nutrition Program for Women, Infants and Children (WIC) and makes an appropriate referral. Medical providers engage in individual advocacy when they write letters in support of a child's application for Supplemental Security Income (SSI) benefits. Individual advocacy probably feels like something that you already do on behalf of undernourished children.

Advocacy at the systemic level involves attempts to influence policy through several mechanisms. In addition to providing public information through a variety of media, systemic advocacy efforts may include legislative reform, defensive efforts to protect funding for important support programs, or undertaking research that has broad policy implications. Historically, providers have frequently engaged in these efforts through participation with the local chapters of their professional organizations, such as the National Association of Social Workers, the American Academy of Pediatrics, or the American Nurses Association.

Individual and systemic advocacy are interrelated. Experience with individual cases helps one to recognize public policy trends and to persuade a legislator or a reporter with a real-life story. Likewise, an understanding of policy helps one understand troublesome individual cases.

Individual Level

Individual advocacy usually involves helping clients or patients get through a bureaucratic maze. This process is complicated by the many support programs that are available to families, which have differing eligibility criteria, administering agencies, and rules. The provider's role in individual advocacy is attenuated: Although the provider can play a critical role in facilitating a patient's or client's access to benefits, ultimate decisions about whether and how to proceed must be made by the family.

Diagnosis, Assessment, Referral, and Tracking: The DART Model

Steps in individual advocacy follow a very typical problem-solving model that is familiar to a wide range of clinicians. When working with an undernourished child, most clinicians naturally proceed through four steps: diagnosis, assessment, referral, and tracking (DART). For example, the physician looks for the causes of undernutrition, devises a treatment plan, makes appropriate referrals for services that she or he cannot provide, and schedules a follow-up appointment to ensure that the child's condition is improving. The advocacy model differs little from this general approach. It is worth mentioning that in the medical treatment of undernutrition, advocacy is often an important component of clinical care.

In the *diagnosis* stage, the advocate, like the physician, tries to determine the causes of the child's undernutrition. In advocacy, diagnosis involves identifying unmet social support needs—for example, inadequate food resources, inadequate preventive medical care, and overcrowded or chaotic housing situations. Once the diagnosis has been made, *assessment* of the condition and development of a treatment plan can occur. The advocate seeks to identify unused social supports, including nutrition programs such as food stamps, school breakfast and lunch programs, and WIC. Educational deficits may need to be addressed through the early intervention and special education systems. If the child needs substantial medical intervention, then his or her insurance status becomes especially significant. Assessment, therefore, involves matching the family's unmet needs with available community and government resources.

The third step in the process is *referral*. For supports or interventions that are not provided directly in the clinical setting, providers must rely on subspecialists, outside agencies, and public systems. In linking families with social and governmental supports, one must usually make referrals. Making consistent, well-targeted referrals is an art in itself. Finally, *tracking* involves following up with clients or patients to ensure that the assessment and referral process is working. In the medical setting, tracking may involve simply scheduling the next appointment. When referring to outside agencies, tracking frequently involves timely telephone or written follow-up at critical junctures. For example, a family who is referred by the social worker to a local welfare office for food stamp benefits has a right to receive those benefits within 30 days of the completion of the application; therefore, following up approximately 45 days after making the referral will be most effective in identifying violations of mandated time lines.

Individual advocacy requires four special kinds of effort. First, identifying problems necessitates asking about them. This is most effectively done through use of a structured screening instrument. Screening tools can be as simple as a structured set of interview questions about family resources or as complicated as a menu-driven computer program, but they should attempt to gather basic information about family participation in social support programs, financial means, and needs. It is remarkable the number of families who receive some but not all of the benefits for which they are eligible.

Second, one must learn the available community resources and the basic eligibility criteria for various programs. Inappropriate referrals are not only ineffective but also frustrating for families, and they divert parental attention from more constructive efforts. Of course, the amount of time that is devoted to learning more about programs' rules and requirements is necessarily a question of time management and the allocation of staff resources. In large clinics, division of labor is an effective method for ensuring competence across a number of important programs; each person can be assigned the task of learning the basic rules and requirements for an individual program. Most agencies produce explanatory materials about the programs that they administer. Many states have advocacy organizations that conduct in-depth training about key programs. At a minimum, clinicians who work with undernourished children should have a basic understanding of the major nutrition programs, including food stamps, WIC, and the school breakfast and lunch programs. They also should know the criteria for obtaining SSI and early intervention benefits, as well as the locations of the nearest food pantries. They should know who can gain access to the benefits, what the benefits are, where to apply, and whom to call for help.

Third, effective follow-up is impossible without a tickler system, which is designed to prevent families from falling through the cracks by providing a scheduled reminder to check in with the family. In addition to making sure that the family has not encountered unforeseen barriers, follow-up helps move public systems by showing that someone is watching.

Fourth, you must keep the child's parent(s) involved. As with clinical care generally, an uninvolved parent poses nearly insurmountable barriers to successful outcomes. Explaining the process and the options in gaining access to social supports is critical because it enables parents to recognize when the process is getting derailed. Assigning specific tasks to the parent and making a list of them helps involve the parent in the process. It is one method of alleviating the fatigue and frustration that many clinicians experience when they do everything for a family, and it will empower the parent at the same time.

Improving Individual Advocacy Outcomes

The next steps will enable you to make individual advocacy more effective.

Play by the Rules

Is an undernourished child entitled to food stamp benefits? If you ask a lawyer, then the correct answer to any question that is phrased in this manner is almost always "maybe." The answer depends on a variety of factors, including the size and the composition of the household, the household's income and assets, and some of the household's expenses. The failure to appreciate how application of program rules can affect eligibility is one of the biggest gaps in provider advocacy efforts. A surgeon who wants to get paid probably would not appeal an insurer's denial of authorization for a procedure without some understanding of the utilization rule that was applied. Yet providers often implore public agencies to provide benefits without comprehending the eligibility requirements or type of verification that would be helpful in winning the case.

Rules are generally found in agency regulations and program handbooks. Agency workers should be able to provide copies of the rules that are being applied in a given situation. If the worker refuses, then call his or her supervisor or ask to speak with the agency's legal department. Local legal aid or legal services organizations should also be able to assist you with this basic research; it is worth developing a contact in one of these offices for backup purposes.

Some general rules about social support programs are worth mentioning. Almost all social support programs require one to apply before any substantive or procedural rights accrue. For example, there is no basic "right" to food stamps, to a timely determination of eligibility for food stamps, or to challenge a denial of food stamp benefits until an application has been submitted. The one right that everyone has is the right to *apply*; thus, administrative factors in local offices, such as staffing, waiting times, and the availability of translators, can make a critical difference in whether people who are in need receive benefits because they can affect whether an application is completed. If a parent leaves before filing an application, then he or she has no really effective means of later advocating that he or she should have received the benefit. Providers should be suspicious any time a client or a patient reports that he or she was turned away at an office because he or she "wouldn't be eligible."

Almost every program mandates a time line for decisions. It is usually a violation of the program's rules not to meet the deadlines. In addition, many programs, including food stamps and Medicaid, make provisions for the emergency issuance of benefits. If the application is an emergency, then it is important for the agency to know it; otherwise, the standard time line will apply.

Finally, almost all programs give an applicant the right to challenge adverse outcomes, including the denial, termination, or reduction of benefits. This critical opportunity may be an applicant's first chance to give his or her side of the story before a relatively impartial hearing officer. The right can be lost if the applicant does not file a request for a hearing within a prescribed time, which varies from program to program; thus, if a client or a patient indicates that his or her family was cut off from food stamp benefits, then it is essential to determine the date of the termination notice and to file an appeal as soon as possible.

Winning the Paper Chase

The second way to improve individual advocacy outcomes is to develop an appreciation of how important *proper* verification of eligibility can be. Most families who are denied public benefits are denied because they did not submit sufficient verification of their eligibility, not because they were technically ineligible. For example, a Massachusetts resident who fails to submit proof that he or she lives in Massachusetts (e.g., a letter from a landlord, a utility bill) can be denied food stamp benefits, even though he or she really does live in Massachusetts. Most programs have elaborate verification requirements that are designed, theoretically, to reduce fraud. The result is a morass of paper pushing for clients who do not understand what is being asked of them.

A good example is "the letter," which providers frequently are asked to write for clients or patients. It rarely is helpful to write a two-line letter that asks or implores an agency to provide a benefit to the family; however, it often is immensely helpful to write a letter that addresses a specific verification issue. For example, children who lived with relatives other than the parents historically could not receive Aid to Families with Dependent Children (AFDC) (now Temporary Assistance for Needy Families [TANF]) unless they could prove that they were related. The verification requirement in Massachusetts states that records from social services agencies are acceptable proof of relationship as long as they are dated at least 6 months prior to application; thus, a letter that complies with this rule would meet the verification requirement.

In structuring such letters (or telephone calls or hearing arguments), a good practice derived from first-year legal writing courses is to use the IRAC (Issue, Rule, Analysis, Conclusion) method. Based on the preceding example, it may be helpful to review a sample letter (see Figure 1). Contrast the letter in Figure 1 with the letter in Figure 2. The structure of the first letter follows a logical pattern. It tells the worker that the provider knows the applicable rule and informs the worker of the rule if she or he does not know it. It provides precisely the evidence that is necessary to comply with the rule. Finally, it informs the worker of the result that is expected. It leaves little room for deviation on this issue by the worker. In contrast, the second letter really does not comply with the standards in the welfare department's regulations. An unsympathetic welfare worker is unlikely to find that it provides acceptable proof of relationship and likely will deny the application.

Systemic Level

Much of the preceding section has been devoted to an appreciation of how program rules can dramatically affect client or patient eligibility for social support programs. Left unstated is a significant problem: What do you do when the "rules" are not advantageous to your clients or patients? Systemic change involves modifying programs, rules, or procedures to better serve vulnerable children.

Systemic change has become an increasingly important advocacy arena, given the political atmosphere of budget cuts and block grants and the devolution of federal authority to the states. Systemic advocacy can be either proactive (making positive changes to the system) or defensive (protecting important social programs from destructive changes). One thing is clear: Professionals can make a critical difference when they add their understanding and expertise about undernourished children to the policy debates that affect those children.

Successful systemic initiatives require careful consideration of both policy and politics (broadly defined). As a general rule, professionals who work with undernourished children, such as children's advocates, are quite comfortable with formulating effective policy but are less experienced with engaging in political activities. There are several good reasons for engaging in systemic advocacy. First, it can be fun! Professionals who feel beaten down by the bureaucratic run-around often find it empowering to work on systemic concerns. Second, systemic work presents an excellent opportunity to involve children and families in advocacy campaigns. Like professionals, parents often feel quite energized when given the opportunity to tell their stories to government officials or the media.

A Framework for Systemic Advocacy: Assessing Opportunities, Time Commitment, and Effectiveness

With any systemic work, it is useful to examine your goals and commitment carefully. First, determine whether there is a preexisting opportunity to accomplish your objectives. If legislation that addresses your concerns has already been proposed, then it can be both ineffective and disruptive to pursue an alternative path. Second, evaluate the time commitment that is required to accomplish goals. Effective systemic work requires someone with the time, energy, and inclination to follow it through. Third, determine why the input of a person who works with undernourished children is especially important to the policy maker. Finally, determine which of the methods of advocacy are the most effective for traveling your particular path—legislative, administrative, or media. Each has different institutional agendas, styles, and pressure points to which the effective advocate pays attention.

Legislative Advocacy

Legislative advocacy can occur at the federal, state, or local level. As authority over many of the critical programs that support undernourished children is being devolved to the states, there may be a strong rationale for state and local—as opposed to federal—legislative advocacy.

October 28,1998

Department of Public Welfare

9999 Any Street

Anytown, USA 99999

RE: Sandra JONES; SSN 999-99-9999

Dear Department of Public Welfare:

Sandra Jones is my client at the Anytown Multiservice Center. Her aunt, Felicia Smith, has been told that she cannot receive TANF benefits for Sandra unless she can verify that they are related [Issue]. Your regulations state that acceptable verification includes any of the following, provided that they are dated at least 6 months prior to the date of application: voluntary social service records, etc. [Rule].

Our records reflect that Ms. Smith has brought her niece here for counseling since 1994 (see attached case intake notes). As these records from more than 2 years ago note, "Sandra resides with her aunt, Felicia Smith. Her mother's whereabouts are currently unknown." Ms. Smith has been the only adult to bring Sandra to her counseling appointments over the past 2 years and has actively participated in Sandra's care [Analysis].

Based on your rules, our records from over 2 years ago, which discuss Sandra's living situation, should be sufficient to verify their familial relationship and render Sandra eligible for TANF benefits [Conclusion]. I will assume that this information is sufficient for your purposes unless I hear otherwise. If you have any questions, then please feel free to call.

Sincerely,

Maria Faulkner, Counselor

(999) 999-9999

Figure 1.   Applying the IRAC method in a letter for public services.

October 28,1998

Department of Public Welfare

9999 Any Street

Anytown, USA 99999

RE: Sandra JONES; SSN 999-99-9999

Dear Department of Public Welfare:

Sandra Jones is my client at the Anytown Multiservice Center. Her aunt, Felicia Smith, really needs to receive TANF benefits for Sandra as the family does not have enough money to buy food. Please help her receive TANF benefits, as this money will be critical to Sandra's care.

If you have any questions, then please feel free to call.

Sincerely,

Maria Faulkner, Counselor

(999) 999-9999

Figure 2.   An ineffective letter for public services.

The primary opportunity to influence the legislature is through garnering support for or opposition to pending legislation. While stand-alone bills can be important, most social programs require funding through the yearly process of budget appropriations; therefore, the single most important piece of legislation to follow is the yearly state budget. Budgets frequently contain "outside sections," which make changes in eligibility criteria, scope of benefits offered, and operational procedures for specific programs. Because the budget is a lengthy and confusing document, it is difficult initially to get a handle on how your program is funded. Committee staff, professional associations, and local advocacy organizations can usually help with this process. Substantively, you should pay attention to the same programs that you care about on the individual level: food stamps, WIC, and school nutrition programs. The critical thing to recognize in this process is how many opportunities there are to kill legislation and how many barriers must be overcome to get it passed.

The time commitment for getting involved in the legislative process can vary. The range of opportunities for legislative advocacy includes testifying at hearings, making legislative visits, and calling and writing legislators. Any successful legislative campaign requires the coordination of multiple grass-roots actions. The more contentious the proposed legislation, the greater the need for sustained organizing and advocacy; thus, the time commitment for doing legislative work may be as brief as writing a letter or as long as making numerous legislative visits to key members of a legislative committee. Whether you choose to participate as a foot soldier or as a general, the point is to take direct actions.

From the perspective of the professional working with undernourished children, several legislative pointers should make your efforts more effective. First, no one likes to hear about hungry children in his or her district. While supporting data are useful, most legislators learn from anecdote, not from detailed data analysis. It is especially important to tie these issues to things that are happening in the legislator's own district. The first thing that many staff members do when they receive a call regarding legislation is to determine whether the caller is a registered voter in the district; thus, insofar as is possible, it is important to match constituents with their own representatives.

In effectiveness, legislative visits carry the most weight. When possible, visits should be arranged in advance and carefully planned. It is usually more enjoyable to make visits in small groups. This allows people to have assigned, prepared roles, without carrying the burden of the whole visit. It can be especially powerful to bring a parent along or to have the legislator visit your clinic, agency, or workplace. If you have a lobbyist at your disposal, for example through your professional organization, then ask that person to attend the meeting with you to facilitate introductions. Letters are somewhat less compelling but still effective. Legislators and their staff pay attention to detailed, original letters but do not count form letters as very significant. Professional organizations can play an important role in organizing letter-writing campaigns and providing guidance on the key points to make in the letter. Many legislators are now going on-line, so electronic mail may be an option in your state. Telephone calls are useful as an immediate method of contacting an elected official, but they often fail to convey the detail of a letter or the face-to-face value of a meeting.

However you choose to contact your legislator, make sure that you have a fairly specific agenda (e.g., passage of a specific bill or line item in the budget). Recognize that the legislative process is largely about compromise and making deals, with legislators trading votes to get bills passed. If you have an all-or-nothing attitude, then you will not get very far with your elected official; it is better to know the areas on which you are willing to compromise.

Few issues are so clear-cut that there is no counter argument. It is far better to give and refute the counter arguments to your proposal than to pretend that they do not exist. Try to cast yourself as reasonable and as a reliable expert. You should also be cognizant of the cost of your proposal and possible funding streams. We live in an era of perpetual budget crunches, with the clear bias toward program cuts rather than expansions. You should provide supporting written information to the legislator and offer to send him or her anything else that would be helpful. Last, remember to follow up. If the legislator votes the way you wanted, then thank him or her. No one likes to receive constant criticism, but this is all too frequently the legislator's lot in life. He or she remembers letters of thanks.

Administrative Advocacy

The executive branch is responsible for implementing legislation and running programs on a day-to-day basis. Consequently, there are a number of ongoing opportunities to work with administrative agencies. Many states have advocacy coalitions or groups that monitor administrative issues; for example, there are WIC oversight groups in many jurisdictions. In addition, legislation frequently calls for the establishment of agency advisory groups. Frequently, agencies are quite happy to add your name to their membership list if you have an interest in attending. Agency staff often are required to make site visits or gather information about implementation issues; usually, you can get a staff person to make a site visit to your workplace for a meeting. Finally, it is worth paying some attention to new regulations. Many states have administrative procedures acts, which require the solicitation of public comment before implementation of new regulations. There is nothing more infuriating than working to get new legislation passed only to have its intent eviscerated through poor regulatory implementation.

As a general rule, you need to show that it is in the bureaucrats' interest to make the changes that you are recommending—because of either administrative simplification or cost savings. If you are advocating things that are administratively more complicated, such as a program that requires substantial interagency collaboration or a redesign of the agency's computer system, then you are unlikely to get very far without a legislative or judicial helping hand. Never underestimate the effects of bureaucratic inertia when dealing with the executive branch. While top-echelon administrators turn over with some frequency as a result of elections, mid-level managers and line staff generally do not. Consequently, all change, whether positive or negative, is viewed with some suspicion.

Because administrative agencies are responsible for the day-to-day operation of specific programs, they will be more susceptible to two kinds of information. First, concrete examples of how the program works (or does not work), barriers encountered, and ways to simplify the administration of the program all can grab the attention of bureaucrats.

Second, statistics and scientific data may take on increased meaning with some agency staff. An increasing number of administrators involved with these social support programs have public policy or public health backgrounds and are taught to think in terms of data, not people. Of course, much social policy is being driven by ideology that ignores both the human side of the issue and the scientific data. It may be possible to press some of the ideological buttons (e.g., cost savings, government downsizing, state and local flexibility) to your own advantage, however.

Media Advocacy

The media provide a useful alternative route for systemic change that is frequently overlooked. A media strategy should be part of any long-term systemic campaign. All elected and appointed public officials read the newspaper, and none of them like to be embarrassed or have shortcomings subjected to intense scrutiny.

It is important to consider the type of medium that is appropriate for a given story. Print media reach most policy makers and present the clearest opportunities to develop ongoing relationships with individual journalists and to speak "directly" to the public without going through a journalist's interpretation (through the use of op-ed pieces or letters to the editor). Television is best suited to stories in which the visual content is critical. Radio provides the best opportunity for spontaneous discourse and for clients to speak for themselves.

The time frame for media work can be very quick. It is typical for a reporter to call about a story (e.g., impending food stamp cuts) and want to speak that day with a recipient family. This poses particular problems unless agencies keep files of good stories that they can pull. It also helps to discuss with clients in advance the possibility of speaking with the media.

Sometimes, the media will call you. Reporters like to have a set of reliable, somewhat opinionated experts whom they can call for quotes and context as they go about their work. Sending in advance a press kit that details your expertise and outlines some relevant stories is one way to foster this relationship. When speaking with reporters, try to craft your message ahead of time; the plea that you have been misquoted or had your comments taken out of context rarely is persuasive after the fact. In crafting your message, try to be brief and use accessible language. If you do not know the answer to a question, then it is better to say so and offer to call back after you have done some research.

When seeking media coverage, recognize that the primary interest of any journalist is a good story. "Will it sell papers?" is a common cliché but a good rule of thumb. There are a number of elements that make a good story from a reporter's perspective. Stories about real people are always more readable because they put a human face on a systemic issue. The issue itself should be timely. The story should be demonstrative of a larger problem and should be something that people do not generally know. Last, journalists are self-interested and want to know that you will call them personally the next time a good story comes up. If possible, try not to shop your stories; rather, develop an ongoing relationship with a sympathetic journalist.

Organizing Your Workplace

The workplace provides the best institutional setting for dealing with systemic concerns that involve undernourished children because it brings together a critical mass of informed, experienced, and like-minded people. Workplaces do not always provide the opportunity to discuss systemic or policy concerns, however, and have disadvantages in terms of working with the legislature: The group members are likely to live in different districts and may be viewed as self-serving if they only speak in favor of their own programs.

The first step in organizing the workplace is to establish a regular time to discuss policy issues that is sacrosanct. Meetings will draw in people only when they are scheduled consistently and accomplish things. When possible, working in interdisciplinary or multidisciplinary groups is most effective because it brings a broad set of perspectives and external connections to your initiatives. If at the end of the meeting someone can speak with the nurses' association, someone else with the medical society, a third person with the teachers' union, and a fourth with the social workers' organization, then you will know that you have arrived! The personal touch in getting people involved always works best. It is amazing how many more people come to meetings or write letters to legislators when you explain face-to-face what you are trying to accomplish rather than put a flier in their mailbox. You should always check the rules about doing systemic advocacy work on company time. Although discussing policy issues and changes within the workplace does not violate federal or state rules, there are restrictions on the amount and type of lobbying that non-profit organizations can undertake. A nonprofit organization should never support an individual candidate during an election campaign.

As mentioned previously, the most effective grass-roots approach to involvement in the legislative process is mobilizing an elected official's *constituents*. This means that in organizing the workplace, it is important to categorize people by legislative district (state representatives, state senators, federal representatives, federal senators). This breakdown enables you to target individual legislators who may be ambivalent on a critical issue. Playing the inside game through the use of a paid lobbyist can be an effective counterpart to the grass-roots efforts. Your lobbyist will be able to get information about which representatives are undecided, enabling you to more strategically target individual legislators. Of course, there is nothing like holding a sign or distributing fliers for your representative during the election season to build a relationship with the candidate and her or his staff; just make sure that you are not on company time.

Establishing ongoing connections with the national and state professional associations, unions, and advocacy groups within your community will keep the information about critical systemic advocacy issues flowing into your organization. (See the Resources section at the end of this chapter for some useful national resources. For readers with the capacity and inclination, some useful World Wide Web sites are contained in that section.)

CONCLUSION

Advocacy on the individual and systemic levels is becoming increasingly critical as a result of the substantial changes in public social support programs. There are a number of reasons that advocacy must become part of the treatment plan for undernourished children. First, undernourished children need all the help that they can get. Children cannot vote, so it is more difficult to organize for them a political response to things such as budget cuts than it is for adults. Parents of undernourished children are usually dealing with a great deal of stress as a result of the child's condition and of the social, environmental, and financial factors that may have led to it. Second, professionals have a great deal to offer. Clinical information can be critical to securing positive individual outcomes for families; likewise, bringing a professional, real-life perspective to some of the ongoing ideologically driven debates can help to shift the rhetoric toward a more reasoned approach to systemic issues. Third, advocacy is energizing, personally and professionally. Engaging in advocacy can empower both parents and professionals when it is successful. All of these reasons speak to the powerful role of advocacy and the professional's obligation to engage in it.

RESOURCES

General Materials on Advocacy

Bagwell, M., & Clements, S. (1985). *A political handbook for health professionals.* Boston: Little, Brown.
Berkelhamer, J. (Ed.). (1995). Child political advocacy. *Pediatric Annals, 24,* 396–433.
Meredith, J. (1990). *Lobbying on a shoestring* (2nd ed.). Newton, MA: Auburn House Publishing Co.

Advocacy Organizations

Center on Budget and Policy Priorities
820 First Street, NE
Suite 510
Washington, DC 20002
(202) 408-1080
www.cbpp.org
Useful and timely information on federal budget issues in general and the food stamps and Medicaid programs in particular.

The Children's Defense Fund
25 E Street, NW
Washington, DC 20001
(202) 628-8787
www.childrensdefense.org
The publication *CDF Reports* is an especially good source of information on national policies that affect children. CDF also has written several excellent Advocates Guides to using the media, using data, and so forth. CDF can send you regular action alerts and legislative updates by e-mail.

Food Research and Action Center
1875 Connecticut Avenue, NW, #540
Washington, DC 20009
(202) 986-2200
www.frac.org
Publishes useful information and analyses of policies and changes that affect all of the important child nutrition programs.

Professional Organizations

American Academy of Pediatrics
National Office
141 Northwest Point Boulevard
Post Office Box 927
Elk Grove Village, IL 60009-0927
(847) 228-5005
www.aap.org

Washington, DC, Office:
The American Academy of Pediatrics
Department of Government Liaison
601 13th Street, NW
Suite 400 North
Washington, DC 20005
(202) 347-8600

American Dietetic Association
216 West Jackson Boulevard
Chicago, IL 60606
(800) 877-1600
www.eatright.org

American Nurses Association
600 Maryland Avenue, SW
Suite 100 West
Washington, DC 20024-2571
(800) 274-4ANA
www.ana.org

Association of Maternal and Child Health Programs
1220 19th Street, NW
Suite 801
Washington, DC 20036
(202) 775-0436
www.amchp1.org

National Association of Social Workers
750 First Street, NE, #700
Washington, DC 20002
(202) 408-8600
www.socialworkers.org

National Association of WIC Directors
1627 Connecticut Avenue, NW
Suite 5
Post Office Box 53355
Washington, DC 20002
(202) 232-5492
www.wicdirectors.org

Chapter 37

Pediatric Undernutrition and Public Policy

J. Larry Brown

Since at least the mid-1960s, the American public has expressed concern about domestic hunger, and the Congress and various presidents have debated its significance and cure. In 1968, in response to the report of the Citizens' Board of Inquiry into Hunger and Malnutrition, *Hunger USA,* President Richard Nixon joined a Democratic Congress to fashion a policy response for the millions of citizens who reportedly were experiencing hunger in the world's wealthiest nation.

These bipartisan efforts produced several monumental policy initiatives that still stand: the food stamp program, which had been expanded from a pilot status by President Kennedy, was extended further to cover more than 20 million citizens by 1969; the school breakfast program was created to add one additional meal during the school day for high-risk children; the summer food program was instituted to provide some modicum of nutritional protection for poor children during the summer months when they otherwise would lose the benefits of the breakfast and lunch programs; and the Special Supplemental Food Program for Women, Infants and Children (WIC) was created to reach at-risk mothers and children during the critical prenatal and preschool years.

OUTCOMES OF FEDERAL NUTRITION POLICY

Since the creation of this nutritional policy framework, evidence has amassed to indicate that, in general, these programs are highly effective. In 1976, many of the same physicians who only a decade before had discovered and reported on widespread hunger, defined as endemic undernutrition that resulted from insufficient income to purchase an adequate diet, found that these new programs were working (Citizens' Board of Inquiry into Hunger and Malnutrition, 1977). They reported to Congress that in the same communities where they had found hunger on a widespread basis in 1967 and 1968, people had food to eat. To be sure, poverty still was widespread and families still lived in dilapidated housing on the margins of society, but most of them had food in their pantries.

Successes of Federal Food and Nutrition Programs

Since the doctors reported to Congress, the scholarly community has amassed a substantial body of data on the successes of these same programs. It is now established that children who are covered by the food stamp program have significantly better dietary intakes, as measured for a number of specific nutrients, than do their nonparticipating, low-income peers (Cook, Sherman, & Brown, 1995). Children who participate in the school breakfast program have fewer absences, less tardiness, and higher scores on standardized achievement tests than do eligible children who are not covered by the program (Meyers, Sampson, Weitzman, Rogers, & Kayne, 1989). Mothers who participate in the WIC program, which is perhaps the most widely studied nutrition program of all, have infants who are less likely to have low birth weights, the single highest correlate of infant mortality, and more likely to have larger head circumferences (Rush, Kurzon, Seaver, & Shanklin, 1988).

By most objective standards, the policy initiatives that are represented by these programs are a national success story. The problem of undernutrition, particularly among children, was identified, plans were formulated to address it, and the plans made a significant difference. But many observers know that this story represents truth with a small "t." In other words, it is not the full story.

Failures of Political Resolve

During the early part of the 1980s, another Republican president, again joined by a Democratic Congress, instituted serious cutbacks in the very programs that had decreased hunger in America. From 1982 through 1985, $12.2 billion was cut from the food stamp and child nutrition programs, including school lunch and breakfast (Physician Task Force on Hunger in America, 1985). Although Congress subsequently added back a small amount of funding to the food stamp program, it still was cut by $7.0 billion, and school meal programs were cut by $5.0 billion (Physician Task Force on Hunger in America, 1985). The impact was immediate. Three million children were dropped from the school lunch program, and 2,700 schools across the country had to discontinue serving noon meals. More than 400,000 children were pushed out of the school breakfast program, and 800 schools stopped the program in response to federal policy changes. More than 22 million food stamp recipients saw their already meager benefits cut (Physician Task Force on Hunger in America, 1985).

These policy changes, in conjunction with a troubled economy that had begun under President Carter and extended well into the Reagan Administration, had dramatic results. Bread lines and soup kitchens sprung up around the nation. Where typically there had been only a handful of emergency food programs, usually located in inner-city neighborhoods, hundreds were established in response to local need. Boston saw the number of facilities rise from fewer than 40 to more than 450 within 5 years; Pittsburgh saw an increase from about 25 to more than 320; Houston reportedly had 420 facilities serving food to the hungry; and Los Angeles saw a similar increase, along with the largest food bank in the world to distribute food to the feeding facilities. By 1985, some 20 million Americans were experiencing hunger, meaning the chronic underconsumption of food and nutrients associated with insufficient income (Physician Task Force on Hunger in America, 1985). In its report to the nation, the Harvard-based Physician Task Force on Hunger in America termed hunger "a growing epidemic," one that was manmade due to policy changes and policy failures that were bipartisan in nature. In only 20 years, the nation had been treated to the best and the worst forms of bipartisanship—the former producing singularly positive improvements and the latter returning the country to widespread hunger, the dimensions of which had not been seen since the Great Depression.

This, too, however, is only the second part of the policy mosaic that constitutes the picture of undernutrition in the United States. There is a third component: Even the successful programs that were fashioned during the 1960s were not entirely sufficient to eliminate hunger. The programs succeeded in terms of making a significant difference, but they neither reached all of the people who needed them during the 1970s and 1980s nor adequately ensured nutrient sufficiency. Food stamps, the largest program and the one that packed the most wallop insofar as nutrient intake, reached only 70% of estimated eligible households at its pinnacle. Research shows that the program's coverage was limited by bureaucratic barriers, client harassment by program administrators (excessive documentation) and political leaders (campaigns against fraud and abuse), and the resulting stigma that chilled the application levels of otherwise needy and eligible clients (Physician Task Force on Hunger in America, 1986). Moreover, even when they did reach the needy, food stamp benefits were quite inadequate, ranging from 49 cents per person per meal in 1985 to 82 cents per person per meal in 1996. Under the welfare law that was adopted in 1996, however, average food stamp benefits are expected to drop to 68 cents per person per meal in coming years. The school breakfast program had not been instituted in more than half of the schools of the nation, so less than 50% of the needy children for whom it was intended were protected by its benefits. Summer food programs still reach less than 20% of needy children, and the highly touted WIC program served only two thirds of those who were eligible during the 1980s and approximately 80% of those who were eligible in 1998 (U.S. Department of Agriculture, 1998). In some instances, these program deficiencies result from inadequate federal funding and, in others, from bureaucratic resistance at the local level, including a stigma associated with program administration that frightens away otherwise eligible families and their children.

TREATMENT VERSUS PREVENTION: THE POLICY FRAMEWORK

The history of the diminution and return of hunger to America is an instructive story insofar as guiding policy for the future. Perhaps most poignant, it counters the argument that policy never works and that government is not an answer to major social ills. This experience with hunger shows that this argument is not true. The nation's experience also speaks to the need to maintain national resolve and to do so on a bipartisan basis. As a people, American citizens are capable of rising above partisan bickering, just as they are susceptible to bipartisan short-sightedness. But perhaps what the experience with hunger reveals more than anything is how deeply intertwined it is with the problem of poverty and economic insecurity and that to eliminate hunger, as most Western nations have done, requires income security among the poor. In other words, the problem of hunger can be *treated* fairly effectively with nutrition programs, but to *prevent* hunger requires that its root cause be addressed: poverty.

More than 34 million Americans live in poverty—nearly 14% of the population. Children have the highest rate of poverty of any population group, at more than 21%. Although the rate fluctuates from year to year, the rate of child poverty has been on an upward trend since 1970 (Cook & Brown, 1993). Moreover, child poverty is growing fastest among white children and in the suburbs of the nation, but the dimensions of child poverty mask a problem of even larger dimensions. The poverty level means that a household lives below the federal standard ($12,516 for a family of three [Lamison-White, 1997]) throughout the year. Yet, when one considers how many Americans live in impoverished households for at least 2 months or more during the year—a measure of the general economic vulnerability that fuels poverty—the answer is more than 50 million people: over one fifth of the U.S. population (Shea, 1995).

That such a large proportion of citizens experience economic deprivation is the result of the downscaling of the economy; average weekly earnings were lower in 1995 ($254, in constant dollars) than they were in 1979 ($315). It also is the result of tax and other policy changes that leave the richest quintile of the population with a greater share of the distribution of household income, at the expense of the poor, blue-collar households and even the middle class. From 1974 to 1994, the share of aggregate household income for the richest quintile increased from 43.5% to 49.1% (Cook & Brown, 1995). At the same time, the aggregate income of the lowest two quintiles (40% of the population) fell from 14.9% to 12.5% (Cook & Brown, 1995). In fact, during this 20-year period, aggregate income shares declined for every quintile, including the middle class, except for the wealthiest one. Although the shift of income up the economic scale works to the detriment of 80% of the population, its impact on the poor is greatest because they start with so little and government policy does so much less to assist them.

Research comparing Western and other industrial nations, known as the Luxembourg Income Study (LIS), reveals that the United States has the worst rate of child poverty (Rainwater & Smeedling, 1995). Compared with eight other industrial nations—Australia, Belgium, Canada, Finland, Netherlands, Norway, Sweden, and the United Kingdom—the United States' rate of child poverty is double or triple the rate elsewhere. Some 21.5% of American children lived in poverty in 1990, more than one in every five. This compares with 14.1% in Australia, the nation with the next highest rate, and 2.7% in Sweden, a nation whose rate is among the lowest. By comparison, the rates in most other countries range from 2.5% to 10%. The U.S. child poverty rate is the outcome of poor distribution of income. LIS analyses reveal that of 25 industrial countries, including Russia, Poland, Hungary, Spain, Ireland, Italy, and virtually all other countries of Western Europe, U.S. income disparity is greater than that in every other nation except Russia. Income inequality, the ratio of incomes of people at or above the 90th percentile to those at or below the 10th percentile, ranged from 2.25:1 in the Slovak Republic to 6.84:1 in Russia. The second highest ratio in the United States stood at 5.67:1 (Smeedling & Gottschalk, 1996), meaning that although Americans enjoy one of the world's highest standards of living, rich people in the United States typically are far better off than elsewhere, and poor people comparatively are worse off than in other industrial countries. No major Western democracy presses such hard conditions upon its poor, seemingly batters them with such contempt, or demonstrates so little resolve to assist rather than ridicule them as does the United States. LIS researchers were able to obtain comparative data from 17 industrial nations to analyze their relative successes in reducing child poverty. The analysis compares the percentage of children who are in poverty in each country both before and after taxes and government benefits. Several other countries have higher child poverty rates than the United States before taxes and benefits come into play, but the United States has the worst child poverty rate of any nation *after* government programs and tax policies come into play. France, for example, reduces its child poverty rate from 25% to 7%, the United Kingdom from 30% to 10%, Ireland from 30% to 12%, and Israel from 24% to 11%. By contrast, the U.S. rate, which began at 26%, was reduced to only 22%—the highest of the industrial world (Rainwater & Smeedling, 1995). Even when researchers held constant for race and family structure, the U.S. rate remained singularly high.

What the United States lacks and what many other countries have is an effective policy infrastructure to promote greater income security among the poor, including the development of assets. Assets are tangibles that help to improve economic security for households—a home, a college education, a car, health care, a retirement plan. Middle-class and wealthy Americans have such assets, and they were built largely through direct policies of the federal government. The G.I. Bill made it possible for millions of veterans to attend college with government subsidies; tax-deductible, government-secured home mortgages made the United States a nation of homeowners; and pretax retirement accounts, such as 403(b)s and 401(k)s, are government-subsidized benefits to promote a secure future for families (Sherraden, 1991).

Yet what is a benefit for the nonpoor can be a crime for the poor:

Grace Capitello, a mother on welfare with one child, collected bottles and cans for the eventual college education of her daughter; yet this model of virtue was arrested because the $2,200 that she had saved over 7 years had placed her over the asset limit for public assistance.

Sergeant Doggett returned from the Gulf War to face unemployment. He packed his wife and children in a van to do odd jobs and search for work in several states. Living in their van and hungry, Mrs. Doggett prevailed upon her husband to apply for food stamps. This penniless family was denied benefits because the value of their van was above government-approved asset standards for the poor; yet if they sold the vehicle, then they would have no home and no way to get to work if a job turned up.

Mary Johnson cared for her son and her elderly mother in her home. Longing to get off welfare, Ms. Johnson arranged for a loan to purchase a computer to operate a medical billing service from her living room. Her plans were dashed when she was informed that computer equipment would place her over the eligibility limit for federal welfare assistance, and she would lose benefits and health care before she would be able to get on her feet through her attempts to achieve self-employment.

NUTRITION AND WELFARE POLICY: REFORM OR DEFORM?

For the United States to address in any meaningful way undernutrition and other outcomes that are associated with poverty, it will have to contend with the double standard that was illustrated in the vignettes in the previous section. Many policy analysts believe that what the poor need is exactly what the middle class needed and received in past decades—a little help and a real opportunity for the Grace Capitellos, Sergeant Doggetts, and Mary Johnsons of the nation. The U.S. government subsidizes the middle class and the wealthy to the tune of about $599 billion annually in federal benefits such as home mortgage deductions and pretax retirement accounts (Center on Hunger, Poverty and Nutrition Policy, 1996). By contrast, the much-maligned and recently abolished AFDC program cost the federal government under $14 billion annually—less that 1% of the federal budget and less than 3% of the subsidies that are given to the nonpoor. It is patently unfair for a nation to invest so much of its government largesse to the benefit of the wealthy and the middle class but to do so little to help "even the deck" for the poor. To provide greater assistance to those whose needs are less while actually denying such assistance to those whose needs are more is a policy that is based neither on fairness nor, arguably, on the long-term interest of the nation.

President Clinton and the Congress purportedly took a major step toward rectifying this imbalance through passage of the Personal Responsibility and Work Opportunity Reconciliation Act of 1996 (PL 104-193). The most sweeping change in federal policy in the 60 years since Franklin Roosevelt's New Deal, this law for the first time in modern history removed the protection of welfare benefits for poor children. States rather than the federal government decide whether an impoverished child will receive assistance for food, shelter, and clothing, making assistance the "luck of the draw" based on the vagaries of state politics and state boundaries rather than the hallmark of a federal policy that is designed to protect all children. With great bipartisan fanfare, supporters of the new law say that it will provide an opportunity for the poor, a chance to be productive rather than idle. But a substantial body of empirical evidence, based on research into poverty and welfare since the mid-1970s, indicates that this "reform" is not likely to work and that the political invective about motivating the poor to be self-sufficient rather than lazy will neither reduce poverty nor improve the lives of its victims.

Research suggests that the twin pillars of welfare reform are fatuous (Center on Hunger, Poverty and Nutrition Policy, 1995a). The first pillar is that welfare leads to illegitimacy, and the second is that increasing illegitimacy is the chief factor behind rising poverty in the United States. Evidence indicates that there is no truth to either argument. Numerous studies, for example, demonstrate *no* relationship between welfare and fertility decisions (Center on Hunger, Poverty and Nutrition Policy, 1995c). Welfare benefits have no impact on child-bearing decisions. This was the outcome of a monumental 1994 study by The Urban Institute (Acs, 1994), which closely mirrored the findings of the Panel Study of Income Dynamics (Duncan & Hoffman, 1990), which was conducted 4 years earlier. These outcomes are consistent with research findings that were released in 1993 by the Institute on Poverty at the University of Wisconsin and in 1994 by the School of Public Policy at the University of California, Berkeley (Mauldon & Miller, 1994), which also found that welfare has no significant effect on fertility decisions. Moreover, these outcomes are consistent with analyses that show that although out-of-wedlock births have increased in the United States, welfare benefits actually have declined significantly (over 40%), and that the growth of single-parent families is among primarily the nonpoor a result of changes in social mores and increased options for women through improved wages and greater employment opportunities.

Because the first pillar of the new welfare reform law is fatuous, so is the second on which it is based: that the 2-decade rise in U.S. child poverty is due to out-of-wedlock births. Here, too, the empirical evidence points to the fallacy of the argument (Center on Hunger, Poverty and Nutrition Policy, 1995c). A 1993 Bureau of the Census study (Hernandez & Myers, 1993) found that the post-1959 rise in single-parent families accounted for 2–4 percentage points of the child poverty rate in 1988. Similarly, The Urban Institute reported in 1993 that research shows that changes in family structure account for only 1–4 percentage points of the increase in child poverty. Data do show that the chief factors behind increasing child poverty are economic in nature. The Bureau of the Census found that economic factors such as low-wage jobs accounted for more than 85% of child poverty in 1988, and other research points to recessions and wage inequality as significant factors (Bane, 1986; Bianchi, 1993). In summary, the new welfare reform policy is built on a house of cards, supported neither by empirical evidence amassed by nearly 2 decades of research nor by the experience of other industrial nations.

For these reasons, the new welfare law is unlikely to help reduce child poverty, and the policy framework that it represents is likely to be a failure in terms of both reducing child poverty and enhancing healthy child development. Many policy observers recognize that a nation cannot remedy perceived social problems without investing additional resources to do so. This principle is reflected in the LIS: Nations that invest most heavily in the reduction of child poverty show the most success, whereas the United States and other nations that invest far less show the least success. During the debate over welfare reform, most experts in the scholarly community advanced this same principle: Reducing child poverty requires investments over current expenditures (Center on Budget and Policy Priorities, 1995). Political leaders did not heed this principle; instead, they reduced the nation's investment dramatically. Between 1997 and 2002, some $55 billion less will be spent on assistance for the poor. From the critical food stamp program, 80% of the benefits of which go to low-income families with children, Congress and the President agreed to cut $27 billion (Greenstein, 1996). Research reported by the Center on Hunger, Poverty and Nutrition Policy at Tufts University (Cook & Martin, 1995) shows that poor children who are covered by the food stamp program have significantly higher dietary intakes of 10 of 16 specific nutrients than do their nonparticipating peers. For overall dietary energy, for example, children who are covered by the program have 31.7% fewer deficiencies. For folate and magnesium, the reduction of deficiencies is over 50% (Cook & Martin, 1995).

Under the new welfare law, the typical food stamp benefit of 80 cents per person per meal will drop to 66 cents. Reimbursements for the important summer food program for children also will decrease, as will investments that enable schools to begin a school breakfast program. It is such disinvestments in the poor that lead to the conclusion that welfare reform is not really about reform but about welfare reduction, a politically motivated gambit to ingratiate elected officials with their perceived political base. Any genuine effort to reduce child poverty in the nation almost certainly would bring American policy closer to the standard that is evinced by other industrial countries, which have achieved much greater success than the United States.

CHILDHOOD HUNGER: COSTS AND SOLUTIONS

The United States may be prompted to better protect and invest in its children by a relatively recent body of evidence referenced by several authors in this book. Since the early 1980s, understanding of the link between nutrition and cognitive development in children has expanded dramatically (Brown & Pollitt, 1996). Research outcomes have required modification of the long-held concept of a critical period in brain development. Although the period from conception to the age of about 3 years is still critical, particularly with respect to formation and growth, **morphological plasticity** is greater than previously appreciated, making intervention and rehabilitation even more crucial in the lives of deprived children. This relatively good news is offset by the knowledge that even moderate to mild undernutrition—the kind that is evinced among the low-income pediatric population in the United States—produces long-term cognitive impairments. Insufficient dietary energy interferes with environmental or social interactions to impede cognitive function, and it is this process that appears to mediate impairments more powerfully than morphological insult per se. Moreover, the period of risk for developmental impairments that are associated with undernutrition has been extended over a longer period of time, requiring surveillance and intervention beyond the preschool years. Finally, cognitive impairments occur through a less linear and more multifactorial interaction than previously appreciated. Empirical outcomes have found that children who experience undernutrition alone often catch up once the period of risk has remitted, whereas children who experience both undernutrition *and* environmental insults more often succumb to impairments in cognitive function (Center on Hunger, Poverty and Nutrition Policy, 1995b).

This body of evidence is rich in terms of policy significance (Brown & Sherman, 1995). It means that nutrition is a far more significant factor in child development than was previously considered, and it means that poverty and undernutrition, combined, are a deadly combination in terms of limiting development and function. Income is such a powerful correlate of both behavior and cognitive function in children that the correlation remains even when family structure is controlled.

Although undernutrition that occurs in isolation (e.g., illness, war) frequently is remediated, dietary deficiency in the United States typically covaries with conditions of poverty. Poor housing, limited health care, and substandard schools are interactive factors that are mediated by inadequate income and that combine with undernutrition to limit cognitive function. In many instances, this rich and powerful interaction is dominated by specific conditions that are endemic in the low-income pediatric population and that have concrete applications. Iron deficiency anemia, for example, is sufficiently high in the United States, affecting nearly one quarter of poor children (Pollitt, 1994), as to constitute a serious public health problem. This deficiency lends itself to relatively simple and effective remediation through screening and supplementation, yet the problem remains endemic in the at-risk population and covaries with still other disorders—lead poisoning, for example. Iron deficiency anemia places children at greater risk of neurological impairment as a result of lead poisoning because poor children are more likely to have diets that are deficient in iron and more likely to live in leaded environments.

Aside from pediatric iron deficiency and its relationship to lead poisoning, other policy implications flow from empirical outcomes that link nutritional status with behavior, growth, and cognitive function. In terms of health status and educational readiness, the research suggests that undernutrition exacts a stiff toll. Pollitt (1994), for example, has reported that nutritional deficiencies are among the chief causes of absenteeism, poor classroom performance, and early dropout rates. Poor nutrition and infection have a synergistic interaction, which makes their respective impact difficult to decipher, but it is known that illness-related school absences correlate with cognitive outcomes on standardized measures and that frequency of illnesses in the early years of school is a strong predictor of standardized test outcomes during adolescence. In terms of school readiness, the evidence suggests that policies to ensure the nutritional well-being of children are critical. This evidence suggests the efficacious utilization of child nutrition programs, such as school breakfast, school lunch, and summer food. Meyers and his colleagues (Meyers et al., 1989) demonstrated this point with their pioneering study of the breakfast program, which found fewer absences, less tardiness, and higher standardized test scores among school breakfast participants. Such outcomes suggest that, from the perspective of public policy, when billions of dollars are invested in the education of children each year, school nutrition program investments may be offset many times over because they protect a substantially larger investment in the nation's schools. In terms of other nutrition policies, the most significant nutrition program, bar none, is food stamps. In terms of the volume of people that it protects (23 million per month in FY 1997), federal expenditures ($25 billion appropriated for FY 1998) (United States Department of Agriculture, Food and Nutrition Program, 1997), and the nutritional protections that it provides (cited previously), the food stamp program is the nation's chief weapon in its arsenal of nutrition programs. That it has been cut so dramatically to pay for federal budget cuts that are associated with the new welfare reform act is counterintuitive—in keeping neither with scientific evidence nor with any policy framework based on the premise that a government should reduce rather than exacerbate dietary deficiencies among its people.

Ultimately, however, even the maximum utilization of these programs still would mean that they work only "at the margins" and will produce only marginal gains in terms of child well-being, unless the paramount factor of poverty is tackled. Poverty has such a powerful influence on child development, one so directly and strongly linked to dietary deficiencies and adverse health outcomes, that any efforts to improve the nutritional status of children will require direct efforts to improve the economic well-being of the families in which they live. Science has clarified the mechanisms through which undernutrition interferes with human capital formation, the cornerstone of the nation's social development and economic growth. The challenge now is to apply this knowledge in the federal policy arena. New policy applications typically take place within a policy era, and many observers believe that the United States is making a major transition. The most significant policy era for the United States in terms of social programs, including nutritional interventions, began with the New Deal in the 1930s. Out of this era, the nation fashioned a policy framework, amended over the decades, based on the premise that in a wealthy democracy vulnerable people should neither die prematurely nor suffer unnecessarily as a result of want. The chosen vehicle for ensuring implementation of this collective consensus had been the federal government. Although this framework has been altered significantly by the new welfare law, whether the nation will abide an even greater shift remains an open question and, if so, to what is the nation shifting. The opposing extremes of policy transition that Americans are experiencing could hardly be greater. On the one hand, it is possible that an "era of limits" may become the hallmark of public policy, ushering in a new framework that is akin to the new welfare legislation. Under this scenario, the predominating forces in the policy arena will hold that America cannot do much about social inequality, that it is caused largely by individual deviance and personal choices. The extension of this position is that government should do little to remedy the worst excesses, in part because people choose to be poor and in part because tax dollars are limited and should not be wasted on social experimentation. That this position was manifest during an earlier period in U.S. history and exacerbated human suffering in the years prior to and during the Great Depression is not a paramount consideration by its proponents. Arguing that America is a land of opportunity—and virtually equal opportunity at that—adherents to this viewpoint propose both a diminished federal policy role and a diminished use of the purse strings of government. On the other hand, the period of policy transition in which the nation now finds itself, certainly its more regressive manifestations, may be but the short-term costs and pain of repositioning itself more in keeping with other industrial democracies. Under this scenario, the New Deal framework provided a sound hallmark for decreasing the worst extremes of pain and suffering, but it proved to be insufficient to remedy poverty itself. The poor were kept alive, but too few were helped to get out of poverty. Whether this is because programs were not permitted to work to their full extent or because they had built-in flaws, the poor, unlike the middle class, were not able to acquire assets and other means to improve their economic security. Perhaps without discarding central elements of the New Deal, a new framework—one that both encourages and supports efforts of the poor to become self-sufficient—will be created.

It is this latter policy alternative that seems most in keeping with empirical findings in the fields of child development, nutrition, education, and poverty. The conditions of hunger and poverty interfere dramatically in the development of human capital, exacting serious and direct tolls on the victims and extracting great costs from the nation itself. Chief among these costs are poor returns on investments such as education and health care and the limited productivity of the work force resulting from the burden of a large number of workers who are undereducated, underprepared, and, therefore, underperforming. That this situation has enormous significance for the competitiveness of the United States in an increasingly competitive globalized market may shift the discussion of public policies to address undernutrition, poverty, and educational readiness from the realm of moral diatribe to that of the economic future of the nation and its leadership in the world.

REFERENCES

Acs, G. (1994, May). *The impact of AFDC on young women's childbearing decisions.* Washington, DC: The Urban Institute.

Bane, M.J. (1986). Household composition and poverty. In S.H. Danziger & D.H. Weinberg (Eds.), *Fighting poverty: What works and what doesn't.* Cambridge, MA: Harvard University Press.

Bianchi, S.M. (1993). Children in poverty: Why are they poor? In J.A. Chafel (Ed.), *Child poverty and public policy.* Washington, DC: The Urban Institute Press.

Brown, J.L. (1970). Hunger USA: The public pushes Congress. *Journal of Health and Social Behavior, 11*(2), 115–126.

Brown, J.L., & Pollitt, E. (1996, February). Malnutrition, poverty and intellectual development, *Scientific American,* 38–43.

Brown, J.L., & Sherman, L.P. (1995). Policy implications of new scientific knowledge, *Journal of Nutrition, 125,* 2281S–2284S.

Center on Budget and Policy Priorities. (1995). *Welfare and out of wedlock births: A research summary.* Washington, DC: Author.

Center on Hunger, Poverty and Nutrition Policy. (1995a). *Statement on key welfare reform issues: A review of the empirical evidence.* Boston: Tufts University.

Center on Hunger, Poverty and Nutrition Policy. (1995b). *Statement on the link between nutrition and cognitive development in children.* Boston: Tufts University.

Center on Hunger, Poverty and Nutrition Policy. (1995c). *Statement on welfare reform: The empirical evidence.* Boston: Tufts University.

Center on Hunger, Poverty and Nutrition Policy. (1996). *Four levels of welfare.* Boston: Tufts University.

Citizens' Board of Inquiry into Hunger and Malnutrition in the U.S. (1968). *Hunger USA.* Boston: Beacon Press.

Citizens' Board of Inquiry into Hunger and Malnutrition in the U.S. (1977). *Hunger USA revisited.* Boston: Beacon Press.

Cook, J.T., & Brown, J.L. (1993). *Alternative futures for child poverty in the U.S.: National and state projections to the year 2010.* Boston: Tufts University, Center on Hunger, Poverty and Nutrition Policy.

Cook, J.T., & Brown, J.L. (1995). *Asset development among America's poor: Trends in the distribution of income and wealth.* Boston: Tufts University, Center on Hunger, Poverty and Nutrition Policy.

Cook, J.T., & Martin, K.S. (1995). *Differences in nutritional adequacy among poor and non-poor children.* Boston: Tufts University, Center on Hunger, Poverty and Nutrition Policy.

Cook, J.T., Sherman, L.P., & Brown, J.L. (1995). *Impact of food stamps on the dietary adequacy of poor children.* Boston: Tufts University, Center on Hunger, Poverty and Nutrition Policy.

Duncan, G.J., & Hoffman, D.S. (1990). Welfare benefits, economic opportunities, and out-of-wedlock births among black teenage girls. *Demography, 27*(4), 519–535.

Greenstein, R. (1996). *Food assistance provisions of the final welfare bill.* Washington, DC: Center on Budget and Policy Priorities.

Hernandez, D.J., & Myers, D.E. (1993). *America's children: Resources from family, government and economy.* New York: Russell Sage Foundation.

Lamison-White, L. (1997). *U.S. Bureau of the Census current population reports: Poverty in the United States, 1996.* Washington, DC: U.S. Government Printing Office.

Mauldon, J., & Miller, S. (1994, August). *Child-bearing desires and sterilization among United States women: Patterns by income and AFDC recipiency* (Working Paper No. 209). Berkeley: University of California–Berkeley, Graduate School of Public Policy.

Meyers, A.F., Sampson, A., Weitzman, M., Rogers, B., & Kayne, H. (1989). School Breakfast Program and school performance. *American Journal of Diseases of Children, 143,* 1234–1239.

Personal Responsibility and Work Opportunity Reconciliation Act of 1996, PL 104-193, 8 U.S.C. §§ 1621 *et seq.*

Physician Task Force on Hunger in America. (1985). *Hunger in America: The growing epidemic.* Middletown, CT: Wesleyan University Press.

Physician Task Force on Hunger in America. (1986). *Increasing hunger and declining help: Barriers to participation in the food stamp program.* Boston: Harvard School of Public Health.

Pollitt, E. (1994). Poverty and child development: Relevance of research in developing countries to the United States. *Child Development, 65,* 283–295.

Rainwater, L., & Smeedling, T.M. (1995, August). *Doing poorly: The real income of American children in a comparative perspective* (Working Paper No. 127). Syracuse, NY: Syracuse University, Maxwell School of Citizenship and Public Affairs.

Rush, D., Kurzon, M.R., Seaver, W.B., & Shanklin, D.S. (1988). The national WIC evaluation: Evaluation of the Special Supplemental Food Program for Women, Infants and Children. *American Journal of Clinical Nutrition, 47,* 412–511.

Shea, M. (1995). *U.S. Bureau of the Census current population reports: Dynamics of economic well-being. Poverty, 1991–1993.* Washington, DC: U.S. Government Printing Office.

Sherraden, M. (1991). *Assets and the poor: A new American welfare policy.* Armonk, NY: M.E. Sharp.

Smeedling, T.M., & Gottschalk, P. (1996, March). *International evidence on income distribution in modern economies: Where do we stand?* (Working Paper No. 137). Syracuse, NY: Syracuse University, Maxwell School of Citizenship and Public Affairs.

U.S. Department of Agriculture. (1998). *Special Supplemental Nutrition Program for Women, Infants and Children (WIC): Eligibility and coverage estimates 1998 update—U.S. and outlying areas.* Washington, DC: Author.

U.S. Department of Agriculture, Food and Nutrition Program. (1997, December). *Nutrition program facts: Food Stamp Program* [On-line]. Available: http://www.usda.gov/fcs/stamps/fspfor~1.htm

Appendix A

Glossary

achalasia: failure to relax; specifically refers to obstruction that develops in the terminal esophagus just above the junction with the stomach; abnormal contractions of the esophagus also are associated

achondroplasia: abnormal bone formation resulting in a congenital dwarf, with disproportionately short extremities and relatively large head and body

acidosis: state characterized by actual or relative increase of acid content in body fluids; the pH may be normal or decreased, depending on compensation; tissue function often is disturbed; opposite of alkalosis

adenoidectomy: surgical removal of the adenoids

alkali treatment: treatment with a base to raise the pH and reduce acidosis

aminoaciduria: the urinary excretion of amino acids

anaphylaxis: a rapid, generalized, and often unanticipated immune-mediated (e.g., **IgE** antibody) event that occurs after exposure to certain foreign substances in previously sensitized persons; life-threatening and affects most commonly the lungs, blood vessels, and skin

anemia: low supply of red blood cells in the blood, measured as **hemoglobin** or **hematocrit**; can be due to **iron deficiency** or other causes

anomaly: a structural defect, especially congenital, of blood or body parts

anorexia: loss of appetite

anteroposterior: looking at a body from the front to the back

antral: in the antrum of the stomach, which is an area at the far end of the stomach leading to the duodenum

apnea: cessation of breathing

arterovenous malformation: an abnormal collection of blood vessels with characteristics of both arteries and veins

aspiration: sucking (during inspiration) into the airways of fluid or foreign body, as of vomitus or milk

515

ataxia: incoordination of muscular action, often with unsteady gait

atresia: absence of a normal opening or normally hollow organ

atrial septal defect: an opening (hole) in the wall between the two upper chambers of the heart called the atria

autosomal recessive inherited disorder: a condition that is inherited; requires that both parents carry the abnormal gene

bilious: relating to or containing bile

bolus: a soft mass of chewed food

cachexia: weakness and emaciation

candida: a type of fungus that can cause infection

cariogenic: favorable to the development of dental caries

catch-up growth: an increase in growth velocity following a period of impaired growth due to undernutrition or illness

cerebral: pertaining to the cerebrum (brain)

cerebral palsy: a neurodevelopmental condition that is associated with impairment of motor skills; usually the result of brain injury

cheilosis: crusted or fissured lesions grouped at corners of mouth; associated with vitamin deficiency

cholecystitis: inflammation of the gall bladder

ciliary motility: the movement of the microscopic hairs in the nose and the airway

circadian rhythm: biological rhythm that has an approximate 24-hour period

cirrhosis: a condition whereby the normal liver cells are replaced by fibrous tissue and the liver loses its ability to help in digestion and body chemistry

cleft lip and palate: a deformity characterized by a cleft or fissure in the formation of the lip or palate; may be unilateral or bilateral and involve the lip or the palate or both

clubbing: a change in the contour of the fingernails that occurs when there is not enough oxygen present in the body over a long period of time

congestive heart failure: the inability of the heart to keep up with the demands of the body; characterized by rapid heart rate, rapid breathing, and accumulation of fluid in the body

contingent interactions: reciprocal interactions in which the actions of one person respond to those of the other

contrast studies: imaging studies in which agents are introduced into the body to better show an area (e.g., barium is swallowed to outline the stomach)

cubitus valgus: a deformity of the elbow; with the elbow extended, the arm down, and the palm facing forward, the elbow deviates away from the body

Cushing syndrome: a condition resulting from hyperfunction of the adrenal cortex resulting in excessive production of glucocorticoids or from the administration of excessive amounts of exogenous glucocorticoid; clinical manifestations are related to the effects of excessive glucocorticoid production (weight gain, central obesity, rounded facies), excessive androgen production (excessive hair, acne, and masculinization), and excessive mineralocorticoid production (edema, hypertension)

cyanosis: a blue color that develops when there is not enough oxygen in the blood

cystic fibrosis: a chronic disease of the lungs and the pancreas

DEXA scan: a type of X-ray scan used to assess bone density and lean body mass

diaphragmatic hernia: a condition in which the diaphragm, the muscle that helps in respiration and separates the lungs from the abdominal cavity, has an abnormal opening in it and the stomach and the intestines move into the chest

diastole: the portion of the heart cycle when the heart is filling with blood that is returning from circulating through the body

diencephalon: the part of the brain that includes the thalami and third ventricle

DiGeorge syndrome: a genetic disorder involving malformations of the thymus, parathyroids, and major blood vessels arising from the heart

digitalis: a medication to help the heart contract efficiently

diplegia: paralysis of the lower extremities

diplopia: double vision

diuretics: a group of medications to help the body get rid of excess water

dolichocephaly: long, narrow head

dysentery: severe diarrhea

dysmorphic: poorly or abnormally formed

dysmotility: abnormal motor activity and propulsion of the gastrointestinal tract, which may result from disorders of the neural, motor (muscle), or hormonal systems

dysplasia: abnormal growth of cells, tissues, or organs

ECG: electrocardiogram; a diagnostic study done to assess the electric functioning of the heart

echocardiogram: a diagnostic study that makes an image of the heart using ultrasonic technique

edema: swelling that occurs when fluid leaks out of the blood vessels and into the surrounding tissue; may be associated with congestive heart failure or renal failure

elemental formula: refers to formula that has been treated by processes that mimic protein digestion; the resulting product has proteins broken down into their smallest or simplest elements: amino acids; such formulas usually have also had the carbohydrate and fat components specially treated to make them easy to digest and absorb

empacho: an illness in many Latino ethnic groups that features gastrointestinal symptoms and lack of appetite; onset is attributed to change in a child's formula or milk, saliva swallowing during teething, or dietary indiscretion

endogenous: originating or produced within the organism or one of its parts

endotracheal intubation: the placement of a tube into the trachea (windpipe) to assist a patient who is having difficulty breathing

energy expenditure: amount of energy utilized in maintaining body functioning and to support level of activity

enteral: of feedings, provided by mouth or gastrostomy tube so that the intestines will digest them

enteric: relating to the small intestine

enterocolitis: inflammation of the small and large intestines

eosinophil: a specialized form of a white blood cell, or leukocyte, that can be found in the peripheral circulating blood or in tissue, often associated with allergy

epicanthal fold: redundant fold of skin over the inner corner of the eye

epigastric: in the upper-middle region of the abdomen

epinephrine: (adrenaline) a hormone that is used in the medical treatment of acute allergic disorders

epiphyses: centers of new bone formation at the ends of long bones

erythema: redness

esophageal varices: dilated veins in the esophagus that bleed easily; this condition usually develops in patients who have cirrhosis

Eustachian tube dysfunction: the Eustachian tube connects the nasal passages to the middle ear and helps keep pressure in the ear normal; if the Eustachian tube is malfunctioning, then the pressure in the middle ear becomes abnormal and fluid accumulates

exogenous: originating or produced from outside the body

ferritin: the chief form of storage iron in the body; its measurement in the blood is used as an indicator of the level of body iron stores

fetal alcohol syndrome: a disorder that develops when a mother drinks during pregnancy; characterized by growth impairment, characteristic facies, and brain damage

flaccid: characterized by a decrease in muscle tone; flabby or lacking firmness

follicle stimulating hormone (FSH): a hormone produced by the anterior portions of the pituitary gland, which stimulates the Graffian follicles of the ovary and assists in their maturation and the secretion of estrogen hormones

free erythrocyte protoporphyrin: a precursor of hemoglobin; becomes elevated in the blood when there is an inadequate supply of iron for hemoglobin production or when lead is present to interfere with the process

frontal bossing: prominence and thickening of the frontal bones of the skull

fundoplication: surgical suture of the fundus of the stomach around the esophagus to prevent reflux

gastrostomy tube: a tube that is surgically inserted through the abdominal wall into the stomach; food and liquids are delivered directly into the stomach by this tube

glucocorticoid: any steroid-like compound that is capable of significantly influencing intermediary metabolism

glucose polymers: a compound made up of glucose molecules; easy to digest

glycogen: starch that is stored in the body for energy

glycosuria: the urinary excretion of glucose

Hashimoto's thyroiditis: an autoimmune disease that is characterized by infiltration of the thyroid gland with lymphocytes, resulting in progressive destruction of the glandular tissue and hypothyroidism

hematocrit: the percentage of the blood that is made up of red blood cells

hemiparesis: paralysis of one side of the body

hemoglobin: the compound in red blood cells that carries oxygen

hepatic glycogen: starch that is stored in the liver

hepatosplenomegaly: enlarged liver and spleen

herpetic stomatitis: a viral infection involving the mouth

hiatal hernia: protrusion of the stomach through the opening (hiatus) in the diaphragm through which the esophagus normally passes

hives: (urticaria) localized swollen, itchy skin patches typically caused by IgE-mediated allergic reactions

homeostasis: the development of steady cycles of sleeping, waking, feeding, and alertness during the first few months of life

human milk fortifier: a powdered product used for nutrient fortification of human milk; contains protein, vitamins, and minerals and is low in osmolarity

hyperchloremic: an abnormally large amount of chloride ions in the circulating blood

hyperglycemia: elevated blood sugar

hypermetabolic state: a state related to some abnormal condition such as fever in which caloric needs are increased

hypersensitivity: heightened or exaggerated sensitivity to stimuli

hypochloremic alkalosis: a disturbance in the normal balance of electrolytes and acid in the body; there are insufficient levels of chloride and acid

hypochondroplasia: a bone disorder with radiographic changes similar to but less pronounced than achondroplasia

hypoglycemia: low blood sugar

hypogonadism: small ovaries or testes

hypokalemic alkalosis: a disturbance in the balance of electrolytes and acid in the body characterized by low potassium and low acid levels

hyposensitivity: low or diminished sensitivity to stimuli

hypoxemic: inadequate levels of oxygen in the blood

IgE: an antibody involved in immediate hypersensitivity (allergic) reactions

immune function: functioning of the immune system, which protects the body from infection

immunodeficiency: defect in the immune system

intercostal retractions: the sinking in of the tissue between the ribs; it is a sign of the use of these rib muscles to help in breathing and is associated with respiratory difficulty

intraventricular hemorrhage: bleeding into a chamber in the brain

intussusception: the infolding of one segment of the intestine within another

iron deficiency: insufficient quantity of iron in the body

iron deficiency anemia: anemia due to an insufficient quantity of iron in the body

ketone: an organic acid that is produced under certain metabolic conditions; associated especially with a high rate of burning fat for fuel (instead of carbohydrates)

ketosis: condition characterized by increased production of **ketones**

lactose: sugar found in milk

linear growth: a normal process of increase in length or height of an infant, child, or adolescent

lumen: the interior space of a tubular structure, such as the intestine

luteinizing hormone (LH): a hormone that stimulates the final ripening of the ovarian follicles and their secretion of progesterone

macroorchidism: enlarged testes

malabsorption: inadequate absorption of the ingredients in food; leads to insufficient calories and large, bulky or diarrheal stools

marasmus: severe wasting most commonly due to prolonged dietary deficiency of energy (i.e., simple starvation)

MCT oil: a specially formulated oil that contains medium chain triglycerides, which are digested more easily

mechanical ventilation: breathing that is produced artificially using a machine (ventilator)

meconium ileus: blockage of the small intestine that occurs because of thick, sticky meconium, which is the first type of stool that is present in the intestine of newborns; associated with cystic fibrosis

metabolic acidosis: an abnormal condition in which blood and body fluids are acid because of metabolic causes (e.g., diabetes mellitus, renal failure)

metabolic pathways: chemical and physical processes by which food is built up into protoplasm (essential living material in cells) and broken down into simpler substances with release of energy

microcephaly: small head

micronutrient: nutrients required in very small quantities; this term primarily is used to describe a category that includes all vitamins, minerals, and trace elements

monosaccharide: a carbohydrate that cannot form any simpler sugar by simple hydrolysis (digestion)

morphological plasticity: the capacity of the brain to alter its normal developmental trajectory, typically as a result of external insult

mucosa: the lining of the gastrointestinal or respiratory tract

murmur: a noise that the heart makes when the blood flow going through it is affected by areas of widening or narrowing within the heart

mycobacterium avium intracellulare: a bacterium that can infect the lungs or the gastrointestinal tract of people with AIDS

narcissistic resolution: maturing from the infant's position of being gratified and the center of attention to that of the older child with limits and social participation

nasal polyps: growths that appear in the nose, are attached by a stalk, and are a reaction to chronic inflammation

nasogastric: from the nose to the stomach

nasogastric tube: a tube that is placed through the nose into the stomach; may empty the stomach or assist in feeding

necrotizing enterocolitis: a condition of the prematurely born infant in which the tissue of the colon and small intestine becomes inflamed and destroyed

NICU: neonatal intensive care unit

nocturnal: pertaining to the hours of darkness

Noonan syndrome: a genetic condition characterized by webbing of the neck, congenital heart disease, and short stature

numeracy, test of: assesses one's numerical ability

nutrient: substance offering nourishment, which is necessary for growth, body functioning, and maintaining life

nystagmus: jerking of the eyes

obstructive sleep apnea: abnormal pauses in breathing during sleep caused by an obstruction to air flow

open oral rest posture: the mouth is held in an open position at rest rather than closed with the lips together

optic atrophy: loss of tissue in the optic nerve

optic nerve hypoplasia: defective formation of the optic nerve

osmolarity: concentration of active particles in a liter of solution

osmotic diarrhea: diarrhea caused by excessive water being drawn into the small intestine because of the presence of unabsorbed small particles or compounds, such as nutrients (e.g., simple sugars, amino acids) or electrolytes (salts)

ossification centers: areas of the bony skeleton where new bone is formed

osteosclerosis: abnormal increased density of bone occurring in a variety of disease states

otitis media: ear infection; refers to inflammation, usually due to viral or bacterial infection, of the middle ear

pancreatic insufficiency: inadequate secretion of the enzymes that are necessary for the normal digestion of proteins and fats; present in cystic fibrosis

pandemic: worldwide epidemic

parenteral: given by intravenous tube or another route other than the gastrointestinal tract

pathogen: a bacterial, viral, or parasitic agent that causes disease

pathology: the essential nature, causes, and development of abnormal conditions, as well as the structural and functional changes that result from disease processes

peripheral pulmonic stenosis: a narrowing of the caliber of the blood vessels that supply the lungs; such narrowing results in the presence of a sound called a murmur when the lungs are evaluated using a stethoscope

peristalsis: movement of the gastrointestinal tract; the waves of alternate circular contraction and relaxation by which contents are propelled forward

periumbilical: area on abdomen around navel

pertussis: whooping cough

phosphaturia: the urinary excretion of phosphates

polycose: a powder or liquid product made of hydrolyzed cornstarch to increase caloric density of liquid or solid food; contains no lactose and no residue but has a relatively low renal solute load

polyphagia: excessive food intake

polyunsaturated: of a fatty acid, having more than one bond between carbon atoms that is not saturated with hydrogen atoms; polyunsaturated fatty acids usually come from vegetable sources and are liquid at room temperature

protein hydrolysate formula: a formula in which the major protein source (e.g., casein in cow milk) has been enzymatically digested into smaller protein fragments; the intent is to provide a formula with fewer allergenic properties (i.e., hypoallergenic)

protein-energy malnutrition (PEM): malnutrition of young children resulting from deficits in protein or energy or both; same as protein-calorie malnutrition; includes marasmus, which tends to occur in the first year of life as a result of energy deficiency, and kwashiorkor, which tends to affect toddlers as a result of protein deficiency, but the two conditions overlap

proximal: close to the midline of the body

ptosis: droopy eyelid

pulmonary hypertension: elevated pressure of blood as it flows through the blood vessels that supply the lungs; places a strain on the heart

quadriplegia: paralysis of all extremities

rachitic rosary: the costochondral junctions (where the ribs meet the chest plate) become prominent, and the beading of the ribs becomes palpable and visible

radioallergosorbent test (RAST): a blood test capable of detecting IgE antibody directed at specific allergens

radionuclide: a particular atomic species with defined characteristics and properties (nuclide) of artificial or natural origin that exhibits radioactivity

rales: abnormal sounds heard when a physician examines the chest; due to the presence of fluid in the air sacs of the lung; occurs with congestive heart failure and pneumonia

rectal prolapse: a condition in which the rectum (lower end of the large intestine) protrudes through the anal opening; associated with cystic fibrosis

renal solute load: the electrolyte and metabolic end product of protein metabolism, which must be excreted in urine; requires water for urinary excretion

resting energy expenditure: calories consumed at rest

reticuloendothelial system: a group of cells in the liver, spleen, bone marrow, and lymph nodes that take up and rid the body of undesirable particles

review of systems: a careful review of a patient's history by inquiring for symptoms that are associated with each system or anatomic region of the body

rhonchi: a noise that is made as air moves through the airways of the lungs when mucus is present; heard when the patient is examined with a stethoscope

rickets: a disease due to an inborn biochemical error or a concurrent lack of vitamin D and insufficient exposure to ultraviolet radiation (sunlight), resulting in abnormal bone growth and, in more severe cases, skeletal deformities

ring: a circular band surrounding a wide central opening

rubella syndrome: a disorder that develops when a woman contracts rubella (German measles) during pregnancy; associated with growth impairment, cataracts, congenital heart disease, and mental retardation in the child

rumination: repeatedly regurgitating food, then chewing it again

satiety: state of being satisfied, of having enough; having had enough to eat

scoliosis: curvature of the spine

semi-elemental formula: refers to a formula that has been treated by processes that *partially* digest its protein, which results in smaller peptides or protein building blocks of two or more amino acids; this is in contrast to more completely digested formulas that contain individual amino acids; such formulas also *may* have had the carbohydrate and fat components specially treated to make them easy to digest and absorb

sensory integration: the ability to take in sensory information from the environment, to process and integrate these sensory inputs within the central nervous system, and to use this sensory information to plan and organize behavior

sepsis: presence of pathogenic organisms or their toxins in the blood or tissues

serous otitis media: the presence of fluid in the middle ear, usually associated with Eustachian tube dysfunction

shunts: blood vessels that change the usual path of circulation; these may occur naturally or be created surgically to treat a defect such as would occur with congenital heart disease

sino-pulmonary: referring to the sinus and lung

sinusitis: an inflammation or infection of the sinuses, the air-filled cavities in the bones of the face

skin tests: a procedure, usually by prick or puncture, to detect specific IgE antibodies to a given allergenic extract (e.g., cow milk, dust mite, ragweed)

somatopsychological differentiation: distinguishing among feelings, thoughts, and sensations

sphincter: a ring of muscle that constricts a passage or a tube

stenosis: narrowing of a normally open tube

strabismus: crossed eyes

stricture: a circumscribed narrowing or stenosis of a hollow structure, such as esophagus or intestine

stunted: linear growth retardation resulting in a height- or length-for-age that is substantially lower than the age- and gender-specific reference data (below the 5th percentile for age on the growth charts commonly is used as an indicator of stunting)

submucous cleft: a separation of the muscle layers of the palate with the overlying mucous membrane tissue being normal

supplement: a food-based or pharmaceutical item that serves as an additional source of nourishment

systole: the portion of the heart cycle when the muscular portion of the heart is contracting and pushing out blood to the body

tachypnea: abnormally rapid breathing

tetralogy of Fallot: a combination of congenital structural defects involving the heart, which include narrowing of the pulmonary artery and a ventricular septal defect

thrill: a vibration that an examiner feels over the heart or blood vessels due to turbulent blood flow; a murmur that can be felt

tonsillectomy: surgical removal of the tonsils

transferrin saturation: used as an indicator of iron transport in the blood, which is calculated by dividing serum iron by the transferrin (the primary iron transport protein) value (expressed as a percentage)

transposition of the great vessels: a congenital reversal of the major blood vessels that arise from the heart; the blood vessel that goes to the lungs (pulmonary artery) comes off from the left side of the heart, and the aorta (the blood vessel that supplies the body) comes off from the right side of the heart

tremor: involuntary trembling

trisomy: the presence of a third chromosome where there should be a pair; for example, trisomy 21 causes Down syndrome

Turner syndrome: a genetic disorder in females in which there is only one X (female) chromosome; associated with short stature as well as other structural abnormalities including undeveloped ovaries

tympanocentesis: a procedure in which fluid is removed from behind the eardrum

tympanogram: a test of the mobility of the eardrum (tympanic membrane); poor mobility may imply fluid in the middle ear (serous otitis media)

tympanostomy tube: a surgically implanted tube, placed through the eardrum (tympanic membrane), that allows middle-ear fluid to drain into the ear canal and out of the ear

ventricular septal defect: an opening (hole) in the wall between the two muscular chambers of the heart, called ventricles

vesicoureteral reflux: abnormal reverse flow of urine from bladder to ureter

volvulus: a twisting of the intestine, causing obstruction

web: a tissue or membrane bridging a space

wheeze: a noise that is heard in the lungs when there is narrowing of the airways; it is characteristically present in asthma

Williams syndrome: a genetic disorder characterized by prominent lips, hoarse voice, and cardiac anomalies

Appendix B

PROCESS
Pediatric Review and Observation of Children's Environmental Support and Stimulation

Patrick H. Casey

Clinicians and researchers have documented that the general well-being of children, including their health, growth, and development, is affected to a significant degree by the environment in which they live (Sameroff, 1986). The quality of the early home environment generally predicts long-term child status better than do early child biological characteristics (Casey & Bradley, 1982; Cohen & Parmalee, 1983). Most of the influences of the environment on infant well-being are mediated through the social and nonsocial experiences that are incurred directly by the child in the home, most directly by the parenting process (Bradley & Casey, 1992). Aspects of the home environment that are known to affect children's long-term status include the physical environment, such as the availability of age-appropriate toys and learning materials, stable adults with whom the child can interact, and organization of the home; and the socioemotional environment, such as parental nurturing, responsiveness, encouragement, and stimulation.

An understanding of these aspects of the child's home environment is clinically relevant because child health clinicians most often influence the well-being of children by

The PROCESS may be obtained from the author at the following address: Patrick H. Casey, M.D., Department of Pediatrics/CARE Slot 900, Arkansas Children's Hospital, 800 Marshall Street, Little Rock, AR 72202-3591; (501) 320-3300.

their impact on the parenting process. Although researchers have generally used prolonged home visits or extensive parent interviews to assess the home environment, such approaches are of little utility in a pediatric clinical setting for practical reasons. In addition, medical office encounters provide an excellent opportunity to observe parent–child behaviors. For example, child health clinicians often note whether the parent talks to the child during the examination, responds to the child's vocalizations, comforts the child if upset, or expresses annoyance or strikes the child.

PROCESS: ITS PURPOSE AND USEFULNESS

The Pediatric Review and Observation of Children's Environmental Support and Stimulation (PROCESS) (Casey, Bradley, Nelson, & Whaley, 1988) was developed to be used by child health clinicians during clinic visits to assess social and inanimate aspects of the home environment of infants who are younger than 18 months (Casey & Bradley, 1988). The PROCESS provides child health clinicians a brief, easy-to-score, clinically useful, reliable, and valid method to measure children's home environments in a clinical setting. The instrument consists of a written questionnaire to assess the organization and developmental stimulation quality of the physical environment and an observation rating instrument of the socioemotional support that is available in the parent–child interaction, as noted during the clinical encounter (see Figure 1).

The PROCESS was not developed as a screening test to predict long-term outcomes; rather, it was developed to function as part of an informal, ongoing data-gathering process for use at the time of data collection for case-finding and clinical intervention by the interested clinician.

DEVELOPMENT AND PSYCHOMETRIC PROPERTIES OF THE PROCESS

The original items for the PROCESS were derived from an initial instrument by Casey from Bradley's work on the Home Observation for the Measurement of the Environment (HOME) (Caldwell & Bradley, 1984), a widely used inventory of the home environment that requires a home visit (Bradley, 1993); from reviewing other published inventories; and from conducting several item-generation sessions. The instrument was revised twice after experience with two separate varied samples of approximately 50 mother–child pairs seen in various clinical settings. Items were eliminated and revised based on clinical acceptability and standard item analyses. The third and final version of the PROCESS was based on technical properties of individual items and subscales. The PROCESS now consists of a 24-item questionnaire that is completed by the parent and 20 items that are rated by the clinician based on observation of the parent and the child.

Final reliability and validity analyses were based on a sample of 76 mother–infant pairs, seen in both a private pediatric setting and a subspecialty clinic in a teaching hospital. Interobserver reliability for the total scale was 0.92 based on the Kappa coefficient. Internal consistency of the socioemotional support observation scale was 0.76 as determined by the Alpha coefficient. The internal consistency for the entire PROCESS was 0.76. Concurrent validity was assessed by administering the HOME within 3 weeks after completion of the PROCESS, as well as a laboratory observation of mother–child interaction in a subsample of the validation sample. Pearson product-moment correlations were performed with the total PROCESS and subscales against the HOME and the parent–child interaction scores. The total PROCESS score, for example, correlated 0.86 with the parent–child interaction and 0.84 with the HOME. Controlling for income and education, Pearson correla-

CLINICAL OBSERVATION

Child's name _____

Child's age _____ Gender _____ Race _____ Observation date _____

Observer _____

____ 1. Mother asks questions that are relevant to and appropriate about the child.
- ____ irrelevant or no questions asked
- ____ few questions are relevant
- ____ most questions are relevant
- ____ all questions are relevant

____ 2. Mother shows interest in child's behavior.
- ____ little or no interest
- ____ only somewhat interested
- ____ moderately interested
- ____ very interested

____ 3. Mother reports how smart or how good child is.
- ____ never
- ____ once
- ____ 2 or 3 times
- ____ many times

____ 4. Mother talks, sings, or otherwise vocalizes to child.
- ____ never
- ____ once
- ____ 2 or 3 times
- ____ many times

____ 5. Mother is comfortable in caring for child.
- ____ very uncomfortable/awkward
- ____ somewhat uncomfortable
- ____ comfortable
- ____ very comfortable

____ 6. Mother responds to child's social initiations with social response (e.g., smile, eye contact, laugh).
- ____ never
- ____ once
- ____ 2 or 3 times
- ____ many times

____ 7. Mother initiates verbal interchanges with observer (e.g., asks questions, makes spontaneous comments).
- ____ never
- ____ once
- ____ 2 or 3 times
- ____ many times

____ 8. Mother expresses ideas freely and easily, uses statements of appropriate length for conversation (more than brief answers).
- ____ very poor expressive skills— one- or two-word answers
- ____ poor expressive skills
- ____ appropriate expressive skills
- ____ very expressive skills

____ 9. Mother is eager to pat or pick up crying child to quiet or comfort.
- ____ ignores child, needs prompting
- ____ slow response
- ____ adequate response
- ____ monitors child during distress and is eager to respond

____10. Mother attends to child's responses during the examination.
- ____ never
- ____ once
- ____ usually
- ____ almost always

Figure 1. Sample items from the PROCESS clinical observation form. (Copyright © 1988 by Patrick Casey; reprinted by permission.)

tion of the PROCESS with the HOME was 0.63 and with the total score for parent–child interaction was 0.77. Low scores on the PROCESS identified 77% of low HOME scores, whereas high scores on the PROCESS identified 90% of the high HOME scores (Casey, Bradley, Nelson, & Whaley, 1988).

In a separate sample of low birth weight, preterm children, the clinical observation scale of the PROCESS was correlated with concurrent and follow-up HOME and child developmental status scores (Casey, Barrett, Bradley, & Spiker, 1993). The clinical observation data that were collected at 8 months of age in this low birth weight, preterm sample correlated with 12-month HOME at 0.62 and 36-month HOME at 0.67. The 8-month clinical observation correlated with the 36-month Stanford-Binet Intelligence Scale (Terman & Merrill, 1973) at 0.53, whereas the HOME collected at 12 months correlated with the 36-month Stanford-Binet at 0.51. In summary, the PROCESS has adequate reliability and validity.

USING AND SCORING THE PROCESS

The written questionnaire is completed by the parent typically in the waiting room or in the examination room prior to the clinician visit. The clinical observation, a typical 15- to 20-minute semistructured health maintenance clinic visit, assesses the socioemotional support that is available in the parent–child relationship. Any child health clinician who has experience in such health maintenance visits, whether nurse clinician, family physician, or pediatrician, can learn to use this observation instrument. It was not designed for use by other clinicians, such as dietitians or social workers, who do not use a physical examination as part of their data-gathering process. The parent's behavior is initially observed by the clinician while taking a medical history. The child should be placed on the parent's lap during the history and should remain on the lap during the less obtrusive parts of the physical examination, such as examination of the extremities and the abdomen. The child then is separated from the parent and placed on the examination table for the more invasive aspects of the physical examination, such as examination of the eyes, ears, and throat. This semistructured format, which is typical of health maintenance visits, allows observation of the parent–child relationship in increasingly stressful situations. The 15–20 minutes used for such a visit provide an opportunity for a wide array of parent behaviors to occur and for parents to exhibit the kinds of behaviors that are typical of their behavior at home. Some of the items in the observation may occur spontaneously during the interview (e.g., "mother reports how smart or how good baby is"; "mother asks questions that are relevant to and appropriate about the child"). Some of the items monitor the parent's response to events in the exam (e.g., "mother responds to child's social initiations with social response [smile, eye contact, laugh]"; "mother eager to pat or pick up crying baby to quiet or comfort"). Other items require subjective interpretation of events by the clinician (e.g., "mother is comfortable in caring for baby"; "mother is detached and/or inwardly absorbed"). With practice, the clinician develops comfort in soliciting responses and observing directly for items that require scoring. The clinician scores the items in the observation scale immediately after the completion of the clinic visit.

Twenty items are scored in the clinical observation of the socioemotional support. Each item is scored on a 4-point Likert scale from the least positive response (score 1) to the most positive response (score 4). A clinical observation guide is provided to assist the clinician with scoring the observation items. The parent questionnaire consists of 24 items, each with a 1–4 Likert scale scored in the same fashion as the observation scale. In addition, a toy checklist consisting of 40 options is completed by the parent (see Figure 2). These are checked, and the total is summed.

TOY CHECKLIST

We are interested in finding out which kinds of toys children have in their home. The items below are for children of different ages. Please check any of the following that you have in your home and that your child is allowed to play with. Do not check the ones that you do not have or that are broken.

____ doll	____ stuffed animal	____ toy animals
____ stroller	____ push or pull toy	____ walker
____ toy telephone	____ mobile	____ ball
____ children's books	____ plastic snap-together beads	____ building toys
____ crib gym	____ shape-sorting ball or box	____ blocks
____ squeeze toys	____ musical toy or music box	____ swing
____ car, truck, or train	____ shovel or other digging toy	____ pounding toy
____ teething ring	____ homemade toys (e.g., doll)	____ mirror
____ stacking rings	____ boxes or plastic containers	____ bathtub toys
____ surprise box	____ pots and pans	____ bucket or pail
____ plastic keys on a ring	____ jump seat or door swing	____ rattles
____ children's records	____ record player	____ busy box
____ measuring cups	____ toy dishes	____ pacifier
	____ busy bath	

THANK YOU FOR YOUR RESPONSES AND TIME

Figure 2. Toy checklist. (Copyright © 1988 by Patrick Casey; reprinted by permission.)

A scoring procedure guideline is provided, and scores are recorded on the PROCESS recording form. This provides for a summation of the scores in both the developmental stimulation and the organization subscales of the parent questionnaire along with a total score. The total score of the clinical observation and number of toys based on a weighted scale is calculated. Finally, a total PROCESS score is calculated by summing the parent questionnaire total, the weighted toys total, and the clinical observation total.

CLINICAL USEFULNESS

The PROCESS was not intended to be a screening instrument like the Denver Developmental Screening Test (Denver II) (Frankenburg, Dodds, Archer, Shapiro, & Bresnick, 1992), whereby a score below a certain level is interpreted as suspect and is used to suggest further developmental evaluation. The PROCESS is conceived as a standardized part of a dynamic assessment that is useful for normal and abnormal children. The use of the PROCESS may sensitize and attune the clinician to specific facets of the parenting process so that clinical counseling may be directed to specific parent actions. Because the PROCESS is a clinical instrument for use at the time of data collection for case finding by the interested clinician, along with other data such as medical history and physical, the authors do not recommend the use of a cutoff score at any level for interpretation as normal or abnormal.

Parents often appreciate and enjoy input from expert child health clinicians regarding how they may positively affect their child's well-being. Information gathered by the PROCESS provides a natural entree to dialogue with parents during which information can be provided that will foster favorable development of the child. The clinician may affect parent–child interaction by pointing out infant social skills as efforts to communicate, such as eye contact or smiling, and by encouraging the parent to be sensitive to these skills and to provide nurturing, timely responses when possible. Modeling sensitive and responsive interactions may be helpful for some parents. For example, undernourished infants with failure to thrive are more likely to have asynchronous interactions with their parents, as either cause or effect (see Chapter 8). Such a parent–child dyad may score low on the clinical observation scale. The child health clinician may choose to intervene with parent–child interaction beginning with these items. In addition, information collected by the PROCESS regarding the child's home environment may help the child health clinician adopt appropriate management and treatment plans. For example, an infant who grows up in a deficient environment, despite functioning normally in the first year of life, may be expected eventually to display less than normal skills. The child health clinician monitoring this child may adopt an aggressive follow-up plan that may include nurse home visits and referrals to early intervention programs before the child develops such delays.

The National Center for Education in Maternal and Child Health has published guidelines for health supervision for infants and children (Green, 1994). Those guidelines place significant emphasis on observation of parent–child relationships during health supervision visits and on providing information to promote mutually satisfying parent interactions. Childhood clinicians often observe positive and negative parent behaviors in child health visits, which may be indicative of parent behaviors that occur at home.

Information collected by the PROCESS provides data that can be used in counseling and management planning. The PROCESS provides data that help the clinician focus clinical observations on specific positive or negative interactions during the clinical visit and objectify and quantify observations. These observations may then help the clinician determine how best to intervene.

REFERENCES

Bradley, R.H. (1993). Children's home environments, health, behavior, and intervention efforts: A review using the HOME Inventory as a marker measure. *Genetic Social and General Psychology Monographs, 119,* 437–490.

Bradley, R.H., & Casey, R.H. (1992). Family environment and behavioral development of low birth weight children. *Developmental Medicine and Child Neurology, 34,* 822–826.

Caldwell, B.M., & Bradley, R.H. (1984). *Home Observation for the Measurement of the Environment.* Little Rock: University of Arkansas, Center for Child Development and Education.

Casey, P.H., Barrett, K., Bradley, R.H., & Spiker, D. (1993). Pediatric clinical assessment of mother–child interaction: Concurrent and predictive validity. *Journal of Developmental and Behavioral Pediatrics, 17,* 313–317.

Casey, P.H., & Bradley, R.H. (1982). The impact of the home environment on children's development: Clinical relevance for the pediatrician. *Journal of Developmental and Behavioral Pediatrics, 3,* 146–152.

Casey, P.H., Bradley, R.H., Nelson, J.Y., & Whaley, S.A. (1988). The clinical assessment of a child's social and physical environment during health visits. *Journal of Developmental and Behavioral Pediatrics, 9,* 333–339.

Cohen, S.E., & Parmalee, A.H. (1983). Prediction of five year Stanford-Binet scores in pre-term infants. *Child Development, 54,* 1242–1253.

Green, M. (Ed.). (1994). *Bright futures: Guidelines for health supervision of infants, children, and adolescents.* Arlington, VA: National Center for Education in Maternal and Child Health.

Frankenburg, W.K., Dodds, J., Archer, P., Shapiro, H., & Bresnick, B. (1992). The Denver II: A major revision and standardization of the Denver Developmental Screening Test. *Pediatrics, 89,* 91–97.

Sameroff, A.J. (1986). Environmental context of child development. *Journal of Pediatrics, 109,* 192–200.

Terman, L.M., & Merrill, M.A. (1973). *Stanford-Binet Intelligence Scale: Manual for the third revision, Form L-M.* Boston: Houghton Mifflin.

Appendix C

The NCAST Feeding Scale

Madeleine U. Shalowitz and Ida S. Mabry

The Nursing Child Assessment Satellite Training (NCAST) feeding and teaching scales were first developed in the early 1970s by Barnard and colleagues (Sumner & Spietz, 1994) to help identify children who are at risk for adverse developmental outcomes. At the time, a formal review of the available instruments did not reveal an instrument that could conveniently and reliably assess the interaction of caregiver, infant, and environment. Although the instrument initially was developed for the purposes of research, its applicability now extends into the clinical setting to identify areas of strength and need, to tailor intervention to the caregiver–infant dyad, and to monitor progress. Whether the observer plans to use the instrument for research or clinical work, an extensive training program must be completed to ensure reliability on the scales.

The original (1972) scales, NCAF (feeding) and NCAT (teaching), represented assessments of caregiver (usually mother) and infant interaction focused on a routine, frequently occurring task (feeding) and on a novel task (teaching). The NCAST scales represented separately the contributions of the mother and the infant to the quality of the interaction, recognizing that the mother bears the added responsibility for identifying the infant's cues and responding in a contingent manner.

In 1979, Barnard and her colleagues modified the format of the scales to increase the ease of use so that the instrument better suited community health nurses. The latest version (Sumner & Spietz, 1994) contains changes that are intended to clarify meaning and to simplify wording. The item content remains unchanged.

To learn more about the NCAST scales and to arrange training in their administration, contact NCAST Publications, University of Washington, Box 357920, Seattle, WA 98195-7920; (206) 543-8528, Fax: (206) 685-3284.

STRUCTURE

The feeding scale consists of 76 binary (yes-no) items that cluster into six conceptually derived subscales. Four of these subscales represent the maternal contribution to the interaction: 1) Sensitivity to Cues, 2) Response to Distress, 3) Social-Emotional Growth Fostering, and 4) Cognitive Growth Fostering. Two subscales represent the infant's contribution to the interaction: 1) Clarity of Cues and 2) Responsiveness to Caregiver (see Figure 1). A yes or no response refers to whether the evaluator observed the specific item content during the course of the feeding. Instrument scoring includes the sum of items observed (the number scored "yes") as follows: 1) total score, 2) caregiver total, 3) infant total, and 4) six subscale scores. Observers may score the interaction in real time or retrospectively from videotape.

SETTINGS AND SUBJECTS

The NCAST scales have been used in home observations and in a variety of settings, including hospitals and clinical laboratories. The scales apply to the assessment of any caregiver–infant interactions, although most of the accumulated data consist of observations with the mother. The Feeding Scale assesses infants who are between the ages of 2 weeks and 12 months and can be used for older children if their cognitive level is less than 12 months (Padgett, 1994). The Teaching Scale may be more useful for assessing older

I. Sensitivity to Cues

5. Caregiver allows child to explore the task material for at least five seconds before giving the first task related instruction.

10. Caregiver changes position of child and/or materials after unsuccessful attempt by the child to do the task.

II. Response to Distress

14. Caregiver changes voice volume to softer or higher pitch.

18. Caregiver avoids making negative comments to child.

III. Social-Emotional Growth Fostering

25. Caregiver laughs or smiles at child during the teaching interaction.

30. Caregiver avoids vocalizing to child at the same time child is vocalizing.

IV. Cognitive Growth Fostering

38. Caregiver describes perceptual qualities of the task materials to the child.

48. Caregiver uses the teaching loop at least once.

V. Clarity of Cues

53. Child changes intensity or amount of motor activity when task material is presented.

58. Child grimaces or frowns during the teaching episode.

VI. Responsiveness to Caregiver

66. Child smiles at caregiver within five seconds after caregiver's verbalization.

72. Child physically resists or responds aggressively when caregiver attempts to intrude physically in child's use of the task materials.

Figure 1. Sample subscale observation criteria. (From Sumner, G., & Spietz, A. [Eds.]. [1994]. *NCAST caregiver/parent–child interaction feeding manual.* Seattle: University of Washington, School of Nursing, NCAST Publications; reprinted by permission.)

children with their caregivers. Because the observer assesses strengths and areas of need for the caregiver and the infant separately, the NCAST feeding scale can identify variations that modify interactions of children or caregivers who have physical limitations or medical or emotional impairments. When the observer presents the results of the assessment in an informative, supportive (nonevaluative) fashion, caregivers can accept the observation without feeling intimidated.

PSYCHOMETRIC PROPERTIES

According to the revised feeding manual (Sumner & Spietz, 1994), the current database contains 1,914 feeding cases derived from videotapes scored to 85% agreement by partners during reliability training. Although this database contains the collected observations of many trained evaluators in a variety of clinical situations, it does not strictly represent a normative sample. The ethnic breakdown of 1,523 cases is 791 Caucasian, 431 black, and 301 Hispanic. The mothers averaged 28 years of age and had 12–14 years of schooling. The majority were married.

Concurrent Validity

The NCAST feeding scale and the Home Observation for the Measurement of the Environment (HOME) (a well-established measure of the developmentally nurturing qualities of the home environment) (Bradley & Caldwell, 1978) were scored on 286 videotapes, which were used to establish rater reliability (Sumner & Spietz, 1994). The HOME total score showed the highest correlation with the following caregiver scores on the NCAST feeding scales: Social-Emotional Growth Fostering, .47, $p < .01$; Cognitive Growth Fostering, .50, $p < .01$; and Caregiver Total Score, .48, $p < .01$. These subscales of the NCAST and the HOME tap similar qualities of the parent–child interaction and the home environment (Sumner & Spietz, 1994).

Predictive Validity

Three-month feeding scales did not predict 24-month Bayley Mental Development Index (MDI) (Bayley, 1993); however, the total scores from the 10-month feeding scales ($N = 45$) correlated significantly with the MDI at 24 months (.46, $p < .01$) (Sumner & Spietz, 1994). The subscale that showed the greatest correlation with the MDI at 24 months was Cognitive Growth Fostering (.50, $p < .01$); thus, the parent's demonstration of qualities that promote cognitive growth on the NCAST at 10 months are associated with cognitive testing results at age 2.

Test-Retest Reliability

Repeated measures reveal changes over time (weeks to months), suggesting the dynamic nature of dyadic relationships. Overall, the Caregiver or Parent Total Score (which represents the mother's contribution to the interaction) shows greater stability than the Infant Total Score (which represents the infant's contribution to the interaction) (Sumner & Spietz, 1994). Test-retest reliability over a shorter time period to assess stability of the measure has not been published.

EXPERIENCE

Studies using the NCAST scales support the need to assess 1) both the parent's and the infant's contributions to the interaction, 2) the mutuality or the contingency of the interaction, and 3) the adaptations and changes in interactions over time (Barnard & Kelly, 1990).

In comparisons of parent–child interactions, level of education explained more of the variation in group differences than did ethnicity. The NCAST scales have been used to describe a variety of mother–infant pairs: no identified risk, medically at risk, socially at risk, or a combination of risk factors (Sumner & Spietz, 1994). Examples of medically at-risk samples include premature infants with and without complications, infants with cleft lips and palates, and infants with congenital heart disease. Examples of social risk include low socioeconomic status, adolescent parents, and caregiver substance abuse. Studies that examine diverse ethnic groups are limited (e.g., MacDonald-Clark & Harney-Boffman, 1992; Seideman, Haase, Primeaux, & Burns, 1992). Sample sizes in these studies generally were small. Further work should extend the current experience in larger samples with greater cultural diversity.

USE FOR UNDERNOURISHED CHILDREN

As part of a multidisciplinary program, the NCAST feeding scales can be a useful adjunct to the assessment and management of children with undernutrition and their caregivers (Lobo, Barnard, & Coombs, 1992; Mabry, 1994). The infant subscale directs the observer to note many of the interactional characteristics that are associated with malnutrition: poor eye contact, gaze aversion, withdrawal behavior, irritability especially with handling, feeding difficulties, preference for objects instead of people, and aversion to cuddling. In addition, the caregiver subscale may identify such areas of concern as poor parenting skills, poor recognition of the infant's cues, inability to handle the infant's stress, and poor feeding skills. Assessment in the home often reveals more information than in an isolated clinic session. For clinical purposes, the NCAST scales will suggest an intervention tailored to the family's needs and can serve as a tool to monitor the family's progress over time. To use the tool for research purposes, however, the interactions should be videotaped and scored by an independent observer.

SUMMARY

The NCAST feeding and teaching scales offer a structured view of parent–child interaction. Observations using the scales can be valuable for understanding the process of development, mechanisms of risk, and protective factors (Barnard, Morisset, & Spieker, 1993). As part of a multidisciplinary program, the NCAST feeding scales can be a useful adjunct to the management of children with undernutrition.

REFERENCES

Barnard, K.E., & Kelly, J.F. (1990). Assessment of parent–child interaction. In S.J. Meisels & J.P. Shonkoff (Eds.), *Handbook of early childhood intervention* (pp. 278–302). New York: Cambridge University Press.

Barnard, K.E., Morisset, C.E., & Spieker, S. (1993). Preventive interventions: Enhancing parent–infant relationships. In C.H. Zeanah, Jr. (Ed.), *Handbook of infant mental health* (pp. 386–401). New York: Guilford Press.

Bayley, N. (1993). *Bayley Scales of Infant Development* (2nd ed.). San Antonio, TX: The Psychological Corporation.

Bradley, R.H., & Caldwell, B.M. (1978). Screening the environment. *American Journal of Orthopsychiatry, 48,* 114–130.

Lobo, M.L., Barnard, K.E., & Coombs, J.B. (1992). Failure to thrive: A parent–child interaction perspective. *Journal of Pediatric Nursing, 7,* 251–261.

Mabry, I.S. (1994). Incorporating the NCAST feeding scale in team management of children with failure to thrive. In G. Sumner & A. Spietz (Eds.), *NCAST caregiver/parent–child interaction feeding manual* (pp. 159–161). Seattle: University of Washington, School of Nursing, NCAST Publications.

MacDonald-Clark, N.J., & Harney-Boffman, J.L. (1992). Using the NCAST and the HOME with a minority population: The Alaskan Eskimos. *Pediatric Nursing, 20,* 481–489.

Padgett, D. (1994). Using the feeding scale with a handicapped child. In G. Sumner & A. Spietz (Eds.), *NCAST caregiver/parent–child interaction feeding manual* (pp. 154–155). Seattle: University of Washington, School of Nursing, NCAST Publications.

Seideman, R.V., Haase, J., Primeaux, M., & Burns, P. (1992). Using NCAST instruments with urban American Indians. *Western Journal of Nursing Research, 14,* 308–321.

Sumner, G., & Spietz, A. (Eds.). (1994). *NCAST caregiver/parent–child interaction feeding manual.* Seattle: University of Washington, School of Nursing, NCAST Publications.

Appendix D

The Feeding Scale

Irene Chatoor

During infancy, feeding is an activity that often reflects the nature of the relationship between mother and child. The observation of feeding provides a window through which patterns of the mother–child relationship can be assessed. Although a variety of different methods to assess infant and parent behaviors during feeding have been developed, most of the instruments can be used only for research purposes (Drotar, Eckerle, Satola, Pallotta, & Wyatt, 1990; Haynes, Cutler, Gray, & Kempe, 1984; Sanders & Le Grice, 1989) or they cover certain age periods only (Sumner & Spietz, 1994).

The purpose of the Feeding Scale is threefold: 1) to identify maladaptive patterns of interaction that characterize mother–infant dyads with specific feeding disorders and that differentiate them from healthy mother–infant dyads and from each other (Chatoor, 1993), 2) to assess the effect of treatment on mother–infant interactions (Chatoor, Hirsch, & Persinger, 1997), and 3) to assist in training professionals in the observation of mother–infant interactions and in the assessment of feeding disorders.

DESIGN OF THE FEEDING SCALE

The Feeding Scale was designed to be used for research and clinical practice to assess mother–child interactions in infants and toddlers ages 1 month to 3 years (Chatoor, Getson, et al., 1997). All observations for the development of the Feeding Scale were made in the

The development of the Feeding Scale was supported by grants to Dr. Chatoor from the National Institute of Mental Health (1KO7 MH00791-01A1), the Children's Hospital Research Foundation, and the Board of Lady Visitors.

Information on how to order the Feeding Scale can be obtained from Irene Chatoor, M.D., Children's National Medical Center, 111 Michigan Avenue, NW, Washington, DC 20010.

laboratory at a children's hospital and coincided with the time when the child normally would feed at home, most commonly during lunchtime. The mother was instructed to bring food that she normally would feed her child at home. The room for the feeding at the laboratory was furnished in a standard way. It provided the mother with a comfortable chair for herself, a highchair for infants, and a small chair and a low table for toddlers. The mother was asked to choose the furniture that she was accustomed to using at home. The room was then set up accordingly. Mother and child were left alone in the room for feeding, and the first 20 minutes of the feeding were videotaped from behind a one-way mirror. Two trained observers, who were blind to the child's diagnosis, independently rated the mother–infant/toddler interactions from the videotape of each child.

PSYCHOMETRIC PROPERTIES OF THE FEEDING SCALE

The development and the psychometric properties of the Feeding Scale are described in Chatoor, Getson, et al. (1997).

A series of studies have been conducted to first create and then assess the psychometric properties of the Feeding Scale. Through factor analysis, a scale with 46 items (26 maternal items and 20 infant items), which are grouped into five subscales, was developed. The five subscales are 1) Dyadic Reciprocity, 2) Dyadic Conflict, 3) Talk and Distraction, 4) Struggle for Control, and 5) Maternal Non-Contingency.

Discriminant function analysis was used for each of the five subscales to assess the ability of the Feeding Scale to predict group membership of normal infants/toddlers versus infants/toddlers with feeding disorders. Correct group classification by the five subscales ranged from 69% for Maternal Non-Contingency to 82% for Dyadic Reciprocity.

Further analyses were used to determine the ability of the Feeding Scale to discriminate three clinically defined groups of infants and toddlers with feeding disorders from three control groups and from each other. The classification of feeding disorders according to a developmental framework was first described by Chatoor and colleagues (Chatoor, Dickson, Schaefer, & Egan, 1985; Chatoor, Schaefer, Dickson, & Egan, 1984) and has been further developed by Chatoor (1997a, 1997b).

The Feeding Scale identified distinct patterns of interaction of the three groups of mothers and infants/toddlers with developmental feeding disorders, which, in agreement with the clinical assessment, differentiated them from the control groups and from each other. Mothers and infants with feeding disorders of homeostasis showed low Dyadic Reciprocity. The somewhat older infants with feeding disorders of attachment showed the same difficulty in Dyadic Reciprocity, and there was significant Maternal Non-Contingency during feeding. The toddlers with feeding disorders of separation (later described as infantile anorexia [Chatoor, 1989]) also lacked pleasurable Dyadic Reciprocity compared with their control group. The most striking characteristic of the infantile anorexia group, however, was intense Dyadic Conflict, which differentiated them from their control group (Chatoor, Egan, Getson, Menvielle, & O'Donnell, 1988) and the other two groups of infants with feeding disorders (Chatoor, Getson, et al., 1997).

Both interrater and test-retest reliability were examined. Two observers, who were blind to the diagnosis of the individual children, were trained to independently rate videotapes with the Feeding Scale. Interrater reliability for the various subscales of the Feeding Scale ranged from .82 for the subscale Talk and Distraction to .92 for the subscale Dyadic Conflict. If there is disagreement of more than one point on an item, then the raters should repeat the observation of relevant sections of the videotape and discuss their observations until they reach consensus.

DYADIC RECIPROCITY

MOTHER	None	A Little	Pretty Much	Very Much	Item Score
1. Positions infant for reciprocal exchange	0	1	2	3	
2. Talks to infant	0	1	2	3	
3. Makes positive remarks to infant	0	1	2	3	
4. Makes positive statements about infant's food intake	0	1	2	3	
5. Waits for infant to initiate interactions	0	1	2	3	
6. Shows pleasure towards infant in gaze, voice or smile	0	1	2	3	
7. Appears cheerful	0	1	2	3	
8. Appears sad	3	2	1	0	
9. Appears detached	3	2	1	0	
10. Positions infant without needed support	3	2	1	0	
11. Holds infant stiffly	3	2	1	0	

INFANT	None	A Little	Pretty Much	Very Much	
12. Looks at mother	0	1	2	3	
13. Smiles at mother	0	1	2	3	
14. Appears cheerful	0	1	2	3	
15. Avoids gaze	3	2	1	0	
16. Falls asleep and stops feeding	3	2	1	0	

Dyadic Reciprocity Subscale Score

Figure 1.   Sample page from the Feeding Scale. (From Chatoor, I. [1998]. *The Feeding Scale.* Washington, DC: Children's National Medical Center; reprinted by permission.)

Forty infants and toddlers, ranging in age from 7 months to 3 years, were videotaped during two visits to the laboratory at the hospital within a 2-week period. Two observers coded independently all of the items of the Feeding Scale for each infant during the first and second visits. Pearson correlations were determined to assess test-retest reliability, which was found to be somewhat variable. It ranged from .46 for Dyadic Conflict to .72 for Dyadic Reciprocity. The subscale scores for some mother–infant pairs were quite variable when the first and the second visits were compared; however, no trend was noted. Some mother–infant pairs seemed to experience more conflict during the first visit, whereas the opposite was true for others. The means for the total group of 40 children for each of the five subscales for Time 1 and Time 2 were remarkably consistent.

DEVELOPMENTAL CONSIDERATIONS

Considering the developmental changes that occur between the ages of 1 month and 3 years, it was expected that these changes would be reflected in the scores of the five subscales of the Feeding Scale. To address this issue, 146 healthy infants and toddlers without feeding problems, ranging in age from 1 month to 3 years, were assessed. The children were broken down into seven age groups of approximately 20 infants or toddlers each, and the means and the standard deviations of each subscale for each age group were determined.

Infants younger than 3 months showed significantly less Dyadic Reciprocity than older infants, and mothers showed the highest Non-Contingency during these early months. The subscale Talk and Distraction increased in a linear fashion with age. The oldest children showed the highest scores on this subscale. The other four subscales showed considerable stability between 3 months and 3 years of age with one exception during the period between 12 and 18 months, when most toddlers in this culture make the transition to self-feeding. During this age period, an increase in Dyadic Conflict and in Struggle for Control was noted.

To be able to consider these developmental changes in mother–infant/toddler interactions, the means and standard deviations of the five subscales for the seven age groups were transformed to T-scores and represented in graphic display for each age group. This allows clinicians to compare the scores of a particular child with the T-scores of children of the same age group. In research, it is advisable to match control groups by age to deal with the developmental changes in mother–child interactions in the first years of life.

SUMMARY AND CONCLUSIONS

The Feeding Scale is a global rating scale with a total of 26 mother items and 20 infant items. It was standardized for the observation of mother–infant/toddler interactions during 20 minutes of feeding in a laboratory setting. At the end of the observation, the items are rated along four points and yield five subscales.

The Feeding Scale has good predictive validity. It identifies four of five infants or toddlers with and without feeding disorders, and it differentiates three types of infants/toddlers with developmental feeding disorders from healthy control subjects without feeding disorders and from each other.

Learning how to use the Feeding Scale is easy. In general, raters can be trained to excellent interrater agreement by rating an average of 10 training videotapes. To prevent observer drift, two observers should rate the feeding independently and compare their ratings of each of the 46 items.

The videotaping of feeding on two separate occasions revealed that there can be considerable variation for some mother–infant/toddler pairs. In order to establish a more stable profile of their interactions, multiple assessments are recommended. In clinical situations that may not allow for more than one diagnostic assessment, it is important to ask the parent how representative the feeding in the laboratory was of most feedings at home. In previous studies, less than 15% of the mothers believed that the feeding in the laboratory was substantively different from feedings in the home (Chatoor, Getson, et al., 1997).

In summary, the Feeding Scale is a practical, easy-to-learn assessment tool for mother–infant/toddler interactions spanning the age period from 1 month to 3 years. It can be used in research and in clinical practice for the diagnostic assessment and treatment of feeding disorders.

REFERENCES

Chatoor, I. (1989). Infantile anorexia nervosa: A developmental disorder of separation and individuation. *Journal of the American Academy of Psychoanalysis, 17,* 43–64.

Chatoor, I. (1993). Mother–infant interactions in three developmental feeding disorders associated with failure-to-thrive. *Abstracts for the 60th Anniversary Meeting of the Society for Research in Child Development, 28.*

Chatoor, I. (1997a). Feeding and eating disorders of infancy and early childhood. In J. Wiener (Ed.), *Textbook of child and adolescent psychiatry* (2nd ed., pp. 527–542). Washington, DC: American Psychiatric Press, Inc.

Chatoor, I. (1997b). Feeding and other disorders of infancy or early childhood. In A. Tasman, J. Kay, & J. Lieberman (Eds.), *Psychiatry* (pp. 683–701). Philadelphia: W.B. Saunders.

Chatoor, I. (1998). *The Feeding Scale.* Washington, DC: Children's National Medical Center.

Chatoor, I., Dickson, L., Schaefer, S., & Egan, J. (1985). A developmental classification of feeding disorders associated with failure-to-thrive: Diagnosis and treatment. In D. Drotar (Ed.), *New directions in failure-to-thrive: Research and clinical practice* (pp. 235–258). New York: Plenum.

Chatoor, I., Egan, J., Getson, P., Menvielle, E., & O'Donnell, R. (1988). Mother–infant interactions in infantile anorexia nervosa. *Journal of the American Academy of Child and Adolescent Psychiatry, 27,* 535–540.

Chatoor, I., Getson, P., Menvielle, E., O'Donnell, R., Rivera, Y., Brasseaux, C., & Mrazek, D. (1997). A feeding scale for research and clinical practice to assess mother–infant interactions in the first three years of life. *Infant Mental Health Journal, 18,* 76–91.

Chatoor, I., Hirsch, R., & Persinger, M. (1997). Facilitating internal regulation of eating: A treatment model for infantile anorexia. *Infants and Young Children, 9,* 12–22.

Chatoor, I., Schaefer, S., Dickson, L., & Egan, J. (1984). Nonorganic failure-to-thrive: A developmental perspective. *Pediatric Annals, 13,* 829–843.

Drotar, D., Eckerle, D., Satola, J., Pallotta, J., & Wyatt, B. (1990). Maternal interactional behavior with non-organic failure-to-thrive infants: A case comparison study. *Child Abuse and Neglect, 14,* 41–51.

Haynes, C.F., Cutler, C., Gray, J., & Kempe, R. (1984). Hospitalized cases of non-organic failure-to-thrive: The scope of the problem and short-term lay health visitor intervention. *Child Abuse and Neglect, 8,* 229–242.

Sanders, M.R., & Le Grice, B. (1989). *Mealtime Observational Schedule: An observational manual.* Unpublished technical manual, University of Queensland, Herston, Queensland, Australia.

Sumner, G., & Spietz, A. (Eds.). (1994). *NCAST caregiver/parent–child interaction feeding manual.* Seattle: University of Washington, School of Nursing, NCAST Publications.

Appendix E

AIMS
Developmental Indicators of Emotional Health

Jayne D.B. Marsh

One of the major challenges for professionals in all disciplines who work with young children is assessing and evaluating emotional health and making appropriate interventions within the contexts of their existing service delivery activities. Professionals who work with young children and their families need to be trained and supported in emotional health assessment and intervention skills, and they need to be knowledgeable in data collection for assessment and intervention purposes. Green (1985) identified the need to develop and implement new models of care that include a focus on the emotional, psychosocial aspects of health care. The ability to address psychosocial-emotional development is critical to overall successful child health supervision (Sharp, Pantel, O'Murphy, & Lewis, 1992). Training programs and assessment methodologies need to explicate a philosophical foundation that can guide assessment and early intervention (Brown & Thorp, 1992).

PURPOSE

The AIMS (Attachment-Interaction-Mastery-Support) System of Practice is a set of parent questionnaires that was developed to assist child health care providers, early interventionists, nurses, mental health practitioners, child care providers, and physicians in supporting the emotional development and well-being of young children (ages birth–5) and their families. This emotional development and well-being is characterized by the central child, parent, and family concepts, or domains, on which this system is based:

1. Attachment: Family feelings
    - Special and unique ties among parents and children
    - Learning to express trust and feel secure
    - Being emotionally tuned in to each other
2. Interaction: Family behaviors
    - Parent–child communication
    - Parent teaching and guidance
    - Limit setting
    - Establishing routines
    - Quality of caregiving
3. Mastery: Family capabilities
    - Accomplishment of basic skills
    - Sense of competence
    - Ability to learn
    - Problem solving
4. Support: Family resources
    - Seeking help when needed
    - Using help when needed
    - Making and keeping friends
    - Maintaining contact with family, friends, and the community

BACKGROUND

A 14-member, multidisciplinary instrumentation team worked for more than 4 years to develop the AIMS System of Practice. On the team were professionals from the fields of nursing, social work, psychology, pediatrics, adult education, early childhood, speech therapy, and human services administration, as well as parents.

To construct parent questionnaires that would address child, parent, and family emotional health, the team identified hundreds of phrases that exemplify attachment, interaction, mastery, and support, such as "mother picks up crying baby." These phrases became roots of questions, or items, in the parent questionnaires. All of the roots were then rated on a seven-point scale and ranked as to how central they were to the team's definition of emotional health and to each of the AIMS domains. The roots that were ranked the highest were then analyzed by computer. Approximately 40 themes, or groupings of similarly ranked items, resulted from factor analysis. The team then wrote drafts of questionnaire items from these.

AIMS project staff reviewed and revised the drafts and constructed 12 parent questionnaires, or indicators, tailored for families of children from 2 weeks through 5 years of age. Staff also consulted the literature on parenting, family theory, child development, and other topics and sources to determine any themes or developmentally appropriate behaviors that were overlooked in the team's drafts. After this process, the team reviewed, edited, and finally approved all of the parent questionnaires as developmental indicators of emotional health. The team then distributed the indicators to professionals and parents in Maine and across the United States for review and incorporated feedback from these various sources and improved readability to a fifth-grade level. To accompany and support the parent questionnaires, or indicators, the team additionally developed the following:

1. Intake Forms
   - Family Information (demographics and history)
   - Family Concerns Indicator (stress inventory)
2. Parent Questionnaires
   - Developmental Indicators corresponding to the specific child wellness assessment ages of 2 weeks; 2, 4, 6, 9, 12, 15, and 18 months; and 2, 3, 4, and 5 years (to promote parent–professional dialogue and data collection for assessment and intervention)
3. General Interview Questions and Points of Observation: Guidelines
   - Suggestions for general parent–child interviews and observations (for additional assessment information toward intervention)
4. Focused Interview Questions and Brief Psychosocial Interventions
   - Suggestions for focused parent–child interviews toward clinical profile development around psychosocial issues
   - Suggestions for brief parent–child interventions to strengthen or to pursue concerns around attachment, interaction, mastery, and support

INTENDED USE

The AIMS System of Practice was designed for use in many types of settings: well-child care (e.g., pediatrics, family practice, well-child clinics), early intervention programs, community and mental health agencies, home visiting, child care centers, and other broader-based child services. The AIMS Indicators are intended to aid professional assessment and intervention of young children in the following ways:

1. To facilitate a dialogue between parents and the professional to promote healthy emotional development
2. To provide multiple points of entry for discussion and discovery of information
3. To identify and facilitate strengths in four areas of emotional health: attachment, interaction, mastery, and social support
4. To identify and intervene in possible areas of concern around the development and emotional health of young children

The developers of the AIMS System of Practice recommended that professionals use a variety of methods to collect information in conducting brief psychosocial assessments. Professionals are encouraged to use the complete AIMS System of Practice. Limited, less than full use of the system is acceptable; however, the more regularly the parent questionnaires and supportive materials are used, the more complete the professional's understanding of the child in the context of the family will be.

It is recommended that the parent questionnaires be used at regular intervals, ideally at each specific age interval. The Family Information form can be used annually and updated periodically as needed. It is recommended that the Family Concerns Indicator also be implemented at least annually; if stressors are unusual or great, then the professional should implement the appropriate parent questionnaire and conduct a more extended interview using the focused interview questions and brief psychosocial interventions. Questionnaires, observations, and interviews are not sufficient by themselves; each method of collecting data adds depth and detail to the overall assessment process.

The AIMS materials do not constitute a comprehensive identification of psychopathology, and no attempt is made to cover *all* relevant areas of emotional development.

The AIMS Indicators *do not* produce a score or a label. They are *not* intended to provide a measure of emotional health; they are intended as aids to intervention. The items on the parent questionnaires are a sample of the entire range of emotional health factors and, thus, are limited in the depth of information that they can provide. The materials do attempt to pinpoint selected potential areas of concern that are common in children of certain ages. This is done through the use of probes, which are always given as numbers 5 and 9 in each domain on all of the parent questionnaires. The probes look at behaviors, feelings, attitudes, and/or beliefs that are thought to be problematic or likely to indicate problems or concerns. If the parent indicates through the probes some possible concerns or issues, then the professional can readily address them.

Concerns that emerge from use of the AIMS System of Practice should be followed up and validated before any diagnosis or label is given. This may involve more in-depth assessment using psychological tests, further parent interviews, child observation and interview, and so forth over time.

Training in use of the AIMS System of Practice is recommended for the most effective implementation. Training generally consists of an AIMS history, the AIMS conceptual framework and a definition of the AIMS domains, interactive slides to put AIMS into practice, a presentation of the component parts of the AIMS System of Practice, and a composite case exercise with development of a clinical profile and various supportive topical areas (self-care, early childhood emotional development, character or moral development, resiliency in children, early childhood clinical assessment, therapeutic communication, temperament issues, parent awareness, and child abuse). An AIMS User's Manual also is available to assist and support use of the AIMS System of Practice.

PARENT RESPONSE

Parents have reported gaining valuable information about development and parenting from completing the parent questionnaires of the AIMS System of Practice; feeling validated and affirmed as a parent; becoming more reflective about their parenting skills and abilities; being more prepared to have a discussion with their child's provider; and being more in partnership with their professional provider. Parents have also reported that a professional's use of the AIMS System of Practice represented a commitment to them, their child, and their family. Overall, parents seemed to enjoy completing the questionnaires and did not believe that they were time-consuming. They believed that the questionnaires were helpful, even when the provider did not discuss them, but even more helpful when the provider did so.

PROFESSIONAL RESPONSE

A variety of professionals have used the AIMS System of Practice, including physicians, public and community health nurses, early interventionists, social workers, and clinicians, and have responded on different levels based on their individual settings and fields of practice. Those interviewed have found the AIMS System of Practice very useful in collecting information in a more intentional way, providing multiple points of entry with the family, especially in establishing a relationship and a dialogue. They reported an increased awareness and understanding of emotional health in early childhood as well as an increase in their ability to respond to psychosocial issues in the families they see. They believed that the AIMS System of Practice gave them words and methods with which to incorporate emotional health assessment and brief intervention into their practice.

Professionals indicated how the AIMS System of Practice helped them to organize information, identify strengths and possible areas of concern, clarify options, and highlight parental priorities. The AIMS materials provided them a method for recognizing the dynamics of family situations, especially in identifying child, parent, and family strengths, and a means to establish a connection with families. Use of the AIMS System of Practice among colleagues also assisted in encouraging case discussions, clinical profile development, peer reflection, and collaboration.

PSYCHOMETRIC PROPERTIES

Psychometric research was initiated in the original AIMS project through field testing at six sites in Maine. As each of the 12 age-specific parent questionnaire forms is made up of distinct items, they essentially are 12 separate instruments. Analyses were done on the 6-month and 24-month parent questionnaires, as the numbers for completed questionnaires were greatest at those ages (68 and 72 respectively). Confirmatory factor analysis showed that the four-factor model hypothesized for the AIMS indicators (Attachment-Interaction-Mastery-Support) was represented in the 6- and 24-month data. This provides initial evidence of construct validity.

Although these studies establish the significant potential of the AIMS Indicators, further psychometric analysis is needed on the additional age-specific forms to further confirm the validity and reliability of all of the AIMS Indicators. There also has been very limited use of the AIMS Indicators in diverse ethnic cultures. The AIMS System of Practice has been used mainly with typical families, as well as with single parents and families with low income, social-behavioral issues, and children who have special needs.

QUALITATIVE ANALYSIS

Analysis involving matched pre- and posttest data of professionals who received training and used the AIMS Indicators showed that training and use of the system have the desired effect of improving psychosocial practice in early childhood. With training and use of the AIMS System of Practice, these professionals were better able to describe emotional health, using more detail and identifying child, parent, and family strengths as well as areas of possible concern. Findings indicated a more open-ended, exploratory style with parents and a greater sense of partnership with them.

Analysis of satisfaction surveys from professionals who were trained to use the AIMS System of Practice also is positive. These professionals indicated that content areas of the AIMS methodology were extremely useful. Narrative comments supported that the AIMS framework increased professionals' understanding of the parents and children in the context of the family and the community; increased their awareness of infant mental health and the emotional health of families; provided strategies for increasing communication, partnership, intervention, and support to families; and provided a means for better planning around child, parent, and family needs and objectives and for better use of time by dovetailing emotional health with developmental issues to give a more complete picture of the family.

SUMMARY

The AIMS System of Practice is a developmentally specific, family-oriented, wellness-focused, preventive intervention assessment methodology. It can be used by a variety of professionals in diverse settings to increase their awareness and understanding of the emotional development and health of the child–parent–family system. It provides a means for enhancing dialogue and establishing a partnership with families using multiple points of entry. It serves to strengthen the foundations of emotional health in early childhood.

REFERENCES

Brown, C.W., & Thorp, E.K. (1992). Individual training for early intervention practitioners. In E. Fenichel (Ed.), *Mentorship to support development of infants, toddlers and their families: A sourcebook* (pp. 42–48). Washington, DC: ZERO TO THREE: National Center for Infants, Toddlers and Families.

Green, M. (1985). The adaptation of children and families: The new pediatric agenda. In M. Green (Ed.), *The psychosocial aspects of the family* (pp. 1–12). Lexington, MA: Lexington Books.

Sharp, L., Pantel, R.H., O'Murphy, L.O., & Lewis, C.C. (1992). Psychosocial problems during child health supervision visits: Eliciting, then what? *Pediatrics, 89*(4), 610–623.

FURTHER INFORMATION

The AIMS System of Practice and other supportive materials are available from the University of Southern Maine, Edmund S. Muskie School of Public Service, Child and Family Institute, National Clearinghouse, One Post Office Square, Post Office Box 15010, Portland, Maine 04112; (800) HELP-KIDS/(207) 780-5813. Call for a catalog, to place an order, or for more information. Training is available by contacting Jayne D.B. Marsh at the Child and Family Institute or at (207) 780-5822; jaynem@usm.maine.edu, for a brochure or for further information.

ORDERING

AIMS Developmental Indicators of Emotional Health/System of Practice (complete set of forms) F010091 $50.00

AIMS User's Manual (implementation/use of the materials) B050071 $30.00

AIMS Handbook for Practitioner's (review of the literature supporting the framework and philosophical concepts of AIMS) B050103 $20.00

AIMS Training Manual for Professionals in Well-Child Care Settings (presenting topical areas supporting use of the AIMS System) B050104 $20.00

Full complement of AIMS materials (as listed above) F050105 $110.00

Appendix F

Food Diary (English and Spanish)

Questionnaire About Growth and Nutrition
(English and Spanish)

Growth Plotting Aid

Reference Data on Weight Gain During the
First 2 Years of Life

Conversion of Pounds and Ounces to Grams and of
Inches to Centimeters

Growth Charts for Low Birth Weight Infants

Parent-Specific Adjustments for Evaluation of
Length

Food Diary
(English and Spanish)

FOOD DIARY

Please write down everything that your child has to eat or drink for three normal days (two week days and one weekend day). Include snacks as well as meals. Measure liquids in ounces and solids in teaspoons or quarter cups. Write down things that you add to food, such as butter on bread; describe how it was prepared (e.g., raw, boiled, fried).

Child's name _____

Date/time	Food	Amount	Do not write here						
			grain	fruit	veg	pro	dairy	fat	cal

Failure to Thrive and Pediatric Undernutrition: A Transdisciplinary Approach
edited by Daniel B. Kessler and Peter Dawson
© 1999 by Paul H. Brookes Publishing Co.

DIARIO ALIMENTICIO

Por favor escriba todo lo que su niño normalmente come durante tres días (dos días de la semana y un día del fin de semana). Incluya bocadillos así como las comidas. Mida los líquidos en onzas y los sólidos en cucharaditas o cuartos de taza. Escriba también las cosas que le pone a la comida, como mantequilla en el pan, etc. Mencione como preparó la comida (por ejemplo; frita, cocida, cruda).

Nombre del niño _____

Fecha/ hora	Comida	Cantidad	No escriba en este espacio						
			gran	frut	verd	pro	láct	gras	cal

Failure to Thrive and Pediatric Undernutrition: A Transdisciplinary Approach
edited by Daniel B. Kessler and Peter Dawson
© 1999 by Paul H. Brookes Publishing Co.

Questionnaire About Growth and Nutrition (English and Spanish)

QUESTIONNAIRE ABOUT GROWTH AND NUTRITION

Child's name _____ Your name _____ Date _____

What do you think about your child's growth? _____

_____

_____

Are you concerned about it? (circle)   yes, a lot   yes   not much   no

Why or why not? _____

_____

_____

FOOD CHOICES

Are you using: breast   bottle   both

If not breast, then which type of milk or formula do you use? _____

    How many ounces does your child take at a time? _____

    Please estimate the ounces per day that your child takes: _____

Do you give your child (circle):

    water   juice   soda pop   Kool-Aid   fruit drink

    How many times per day do you give each of them to your child? _____

    How many ounces does he or she take at a time? _____

    Estimate ounces per day: water _____   juice _____   other _____

Do you give your child vitamins? _____

What solid foods does your child like? _____

What solid foods does your child not like? _____

Do you prefer to give your child or your family special kinds of food? _____

HOW YOUR CHILD EATS

Does your child like to eat? _____

Is your child using (circle):

    tippy cup   regular cup   fingers   spoon   fork

Which one is the best description? (circle)

    mostly I feed   both   mostly my child
    my child   does the eating

How long does a normal meal for your child last? _____

Do you have any trouble getting him or her to eat? _____ If yes, then what do you do

when your child doesn't eat? _____

Where is your child when eating? _____

Does someone usually sit with him or her? _____ Who? _____

Failure to Thrive and Pediatric Undernutrition: A Transdisciplinary Approach
edited by Daniel B. Kessler and Peter Dawson
© 1999 by Paul H. Brookes Publishing Co.

Do you add food to your child's bottle? _____

Does your child take a bottle to bed at nap or bedtime? _____

Would you like something to read about feeding children? _____

How would you describe this child's personality? _____

What is your favorite time together with your child? _____

Do you have any concerns about your child's development or behavior? _____

CHEWING AND SWALLOWING

Does he or she make noises when sucking? _____

Does he or she lose milk from the mouth while sucking? _____

Does your child often gag, cough, or choke on foods? _____ Which ones? _____

Does he or she spit out food or vomit certain foods or textures? _____

Does he or she have trouble with chewing? _____

Does he or she cry or seem uncomfortable during or after eating? _____

DAILY ROUTINES

Who feeds your child most of his or her meals? _____

Who else feeds your child? _____

How does your family handle meals?

_____ unplanned, everyone gets his or her own

_____ unplanned, food is fixed whenever someone is hungry

_____ planned, with foods cooked but not always served at regular times

_____ planned, with foods cooked and served at regular times every day

When does your child usually eat?

_____ whenever he or she is hungry

_____ at the same general times each day

_____ on a regular schedule

Including snacks and nursing, at what time does your child usually eat? _____

FAMILY HISTORY

Who lives in your home?

Name	Age	Relation to you

Failure to Thrive and Pediatric Undernutrition: A Transdisciplinary Approach
edited by Daniel B. Kessler and Peter Dawson
© 1999 by Paul H. Brookes Publishing Co.

_____

_____

_____

About the child's parents:

	Name	Last grade of school completed	Type of work	Height	Weight
Birth mother					
Birth father					

Are your child's parents (circle):   married   living together   single   separated   divorced

Are the child's mother and father related to each other in ways other than by being married (for example, are they cousins)? _____

Were either of the child's parents small when they were growing up? _____

What were meals like for you when you were growing up? _____

If you have other children, how have they grown? _____

Has anyone in your family had an eating disorder? _____

In the past few years, have any of these things happened in your family?

(Circle if yes)   Family moved   Injury or illness   Loss of work
                  Financial stress   Drug or drinking problems   Feeling depressed
                  Arguments   Violence   Trouble with the law

Other: _____

With whom do you talk about feeding and taking care of children? _____

What do they think about your child's growth? _____

Would you like to know about places where you can meet other parents of young children like yours? _____

Is your child on WIC? _____

Do you get food stamps? _____

How often do you run out of food or formula or add water because you do not have enough money to buy a new supply? (circle)   never   occasionally   most months

How often do you cut the size of your children's meals or skip meals because there is not enough money for food?   (circle)   never   occasionally   most months

How often do you run out of money to buy food for a meal?   (circle)

    never   occasionally   most months

Failure to Thrive and Pediatric Undernutrition: A Transdisciplinary Approach
edited by Daniel B. Kessler and Peter Dawson
© 1999 by Paul H. Brookes Publishing Co.

How often do your children say that they are hungry because there is not enough food in the house? (circle)   never   occasionally   most months   does not apply

PREGNANCY (Questions for the child's mother)

How did you feel when you found out that you were pregnant? _____

Was the pregnancy planned? _____

How far along were you when you started prenatal care? _____

Did you try to change your eating habits? _____ What did you do? _____

Did you take any medicines? _____

Did you drink alcohol? _____ How many drinks per week? _____

Did you use street drugs? _____ Which ones? _____

Were there stressful events during the pregnancy? _____

Do you need information about birth control? _____

BIRTH

Where was your child born? _____

Was he or she born early, on time, or late? _____

What did he or she weigh at birth? _____ Birth length? _____

Were there any problems during labor or delivery? _____

How many days did your child stay in the hospital? _____

Did he or she have any medical problems as a newborn? _____

CHILD'S MEDICAL HISTORY

What medical problems has your child had? _____

How many ear infections has he or she had? _____

Are you giving him or her any medications? _____

Has your child stayed in the hospital overnight?   yes   no

Has your child had any operations?   yes   no

Does your child live in or regularly visit a house or child
care facility built before 1950?   yes   no

Does your child live in or regularly visit a house or child
care facility built before 1978 that is being or has been
renovated or remodeled (within the past 6 months)?   yes   no

What places do you take him or her when he or she is sick? _____

What places do you take him or her for shots or checkups when he or she is well? _____

Failure to Thrive and Pediatric Undernutrition: A Transdisciplinary Approach
edited by Daniel B. Kessler and Peter Dawson
© 1999 by Paul H. Brookes Publishing Co.

CHILD'S SYMPTOMS

Has your child had any of these symptoms? (circle)

Sick a lot	yes	no
Vomiting	yes	no
Diarrhea	yes	no
Stomachache	yes	no
Stomach looks too big	yes	no
Food allergies or bad reactions to foods	yes	no
Cannot breathe through nose	yes	no
Snoring or noisy breathing	yes	no
Problems with teeth	yes	no
Trouble sleeping	yes	no

Failure to Thrive and Pediatric Undernutrition: A Transdisciplinary Approach
edited by Daniel B. Kessler and Peter Dawson
© 1999 by Paul H. Brookes Publishing Co.

CUESTIONARIO SOBRE LA NUTRICIÓN Y EL CRECIMIENTO

Nombre del niño _____ Su nombre _____ Fecha _____

¿Qué piensa sobre el crecimiento de su niño? _____

_____

_____

¿Esto le preocupa? (circule)   si, mucho   si   no tanto   no

Explique por que: _____

_____

_____

COMIDA

Usted lo alimenta con: pecho   biberón   los dos

Si no da pecho, ¿Qué tipo de leche o fórmula usa? _____

   ¿Cuántas onzas toma cada vez que come el niño? _____

   ¿Cuántas onzas cree que toma el niño durante todo el día? _____

¿Qué le da de tomar a su niño? (circule)

   agua   jugo   refresco   Kool-Aid   bebida de fruta

   ¿Cuántas veces al día le da estos líquidos? _____

   ¿Cuántas onzas toma cada vez? _____

   ¿Cuántas onzas cree que toma durante todo el día? agua _____ jugo _____ otro: _____

¿Le da vitaminas al niño? _____

¿Qué tipo de comidas sólidas le gustan al niño? _____

¿Qué tipo de comidas sólidas no le gustan al niño? _____

¿Qué comidas prefiere su familia o le gusta darle al niño? _____

COMO COME SU NIÑO

¿Le gusta comer a su niño? _____

¿Qué usa el niño para comer? (circule)

   vaso con tapadera   taza   con los dedos   cuchara   tenedor

¿Cuál de las siguientes es la mejor descripción? (circule)

   regularmente yo le doy de comer   los dos   regularmente el niño come sin ayuda

¿Normalmente cuanto tiempo dura el niño comiendo? _____

¿Usted ha tenido problemas para que el niño coma? _____ Si la respuesta es sí, ¿Qué

hace usted cuando el niño no quiere comer? _____

Failure to Thrive and Pediatric Undernutrition: A Transdisciplinary Approach
edited by Daniel B. Kessler and Peter Dawson
© 1999 by Paul H. Brookes Publishing Co.

¿Dónde está el niño cuando come? _____

¿Alguien se sienta a comer con el? _____ ¿Quién? _____

¿Le pone otros alimentos o adhiere otra comida en el biberón? _____

¿Se duerme el niño con el biberón o cuando duerme la siesta? _____

¿Le gustaría obtener más información sobre la alimentación del niño? _____

¿Cómo describe la personalidad de su niño? _____

¿Cuál es la hora que usted disfruta más con su niño? _____

¿Tiene alguna preocupación sobre la conducta o desarrollo de su niño? _____

MASTICAR Y TRAGAR

¿El niño hace ruido cuando mama? _____

¿Mientras mama, al niño se le derrama la leche de la boca? _____

¿Regularmente el niño se atraganta, tose o parece ahogarse con la comida? _____

¿Con cuáles comidas? _____

¿El niño escupe o vomita con ciertos tipos de comida o texturas? _____

¿El niño tiene problemas para masticar? _____

¿El niño llora o parece estar incómodo durante o después de comer? _____

RUTINA DIARIA

¿Quién le da de comer al niño la mayor parte del tiempo? _____

¿Quién más le da de comer al niño? _____

¿Cómo planean las comidas en su familia?

_____ nadie prepara, cada quien come lo que prepara

_____ nadie prepara, la comida se prepara cuando alguien tiene hambre

_____ se planea, la comida se prepara pero no se sirve a una hora específica

_____ se planea, la comida se prepara y se sirve a una hora específica

¿Regularmente cuándo come el niño?

_____ a la hora que tiene hambre

_____ generalmente a la misma hora todos los días

_____ en un horario regular

¿A qué hora del día su niño come regularmente? Incluya bocadillos y cuando le da pecho. _____

_____

Failure to Thrive and Pediatric Undernutrition: A Transdisciplinary Approach
edited by Daniel B. Kessler and Peter Dawson
© 1999 by Paul H. Brookes Publishing Co.

HISTORIA FAMILIA

¿Quién vive en su casa?

Nombre	Edad	Parentesco

Información de los padres del niño:

	Nombre	¿Hasta que año fue a la escuela?	¿A qué se dedica?	Estatura	Peso
Madre					
Padre					

¿Los padres del niño están?   casados   viven juntos   solteros   separados   divorciados

¿El padre y la madre del niño tienen algún parentesco aparte de estar casados? (Por ejemplo; primos, etc.) _____

¿Alguno de los padres del niño eran bajos de estatura durante su niñez? _____

¿Durante su niñez, como recuerda las comidas en la casa, a la hora de comer? _____

Si usted tiene otros niños, ¿Cómo es su desarrollo y crescimiento? _____

¿Alguien en su familia tiene problemas para comer? (Desorden Alimenticio) _____

¿Hay otros niños en su familia que han tenido una enfermedad grave o han muerto? _____

¿En los últimos años que eventos han pasado en su familia? (circule)

Se cambiaron de casa   Lesiones o enfermedades   Pérdida de empleo   Problemas
                        Problemas con alcohol   Depresión   económicos
                           o drogas   Discusiones   Tristeza
                        Violencia   Problemas legales   Pleitos

Otro: _____

¿A quién le pide consejos sobre la alimentación o como cuidar a su niño? _____

¿Qué piensan ellos del desarrollo y crecimiento de su niño? _____

¿Quisiera información de otros lugares donde usted puede conocer otros padres de familia que tengan hijos de la misma edad que el suyo? _____

¿Su niño esta en el programa del WIC? _____

Failure to Thrive and Pediatric Undernutrition: A Transdisciplinary Approach
edited by Daniel B. Kessler and Peter Dawson
© 1999 by Paul H. Brookes Publishing Co.

¿Usted recibe estampillas para la comida? _____

¿Qué tan seguido se le acaba la comida o le pone más agua a la fórmula, porque se la acabó el dinero para comprar más comida para el niño? (circule)   nunca   a veces   casi siempre

¿Qué tan seguido tiene que reducir las porcións de comida o no le da comida al niño cuanda es hora de comer, porque se le acabo el dinero para comprar comida? (circule)

    nunca   a veces   casi siempre

¿Qué tan seguido se le acaba el dinero para comprar comida? (circule)

    nunca   a veces   casi siempre   no se aplica

¿Qué tan seguido sus niños le dicen que tienen hambre porque no tiene suficiente comida en la casa? (circule)

    nunca   a veces   casi siempre

EMBARAZO (Preguntas para la madre del niño)

¿Cómo se sintió cuando supo que estaba embarazada? _____

¿El embarazo fue planeado? _____

¿Cuánto tiempo tenía de embarazo cuando empezó con los cuidados prenatales? _____

¿Trató de cambiar sus hábitos alimenticios? _____ ¿Qué fue lo que hizo? _____

¿Tomó medicinas? _____

¿Consumió alcohol? _____ ¿Cuántas bebidas por semana? _____

¿Usó drogas ilegales? _____ ¿Cuáles y cuántas veces? _____

¿Durante el embarazo, tuvo problemas o presiones emocionales? _____

_____

¿Necesita información para el control de la natalidad? _____

NACIMIENTO

¿Dónde nació su bebé? _____

¿Nació el bebé antes de tiempo, a tiempo, o después de la fecha estimada? _____

¿Cuánto pesó el bebé al nacer? _____ ¿Estatura? _____

¿Tuvo problemas durante el trabajo de parto o durante el nacimiento? _____

_____

¿Cuántos días estuvo el bebé en el hospital? _____

¿El bebé tuvo problemas médicos de recién nacido? _____

HISTORIA MÉDICA DEL NIÑO

¿Qué tipo de problemas médicos ha tenido el niño? _____

¿Cuántas infecciones del oído ha tenido? _____

¿Esta tomando alguna medicina? _____

¿Su niño ha pasado la noche en el hospital?	si	no
¿Su niño ha tenido operaciones?	si	no
¿Su niño vive, visita con regularidad, o asiste a un lugar donde lo cuidan que haya sido construído antes de 1950?	si	no
¿Su niño vive, visita con regularidad, o asiste a un lugar donde lo cuidan que haya sido construído antes de 1978 y que lo estén renovando o haya sido remodelado durante los últimos 6 meses?	si	no

¿A qué lugares ha llevado al niño cuando se enferma? _____

¿A qué lugares ha llevado al niño para las vacunas y revisiones de rutina? _____

SÍNTOMAS DEL NIÑO

¿Su niño ha tenido alguno de los siguientes síntomas? (circule)

Se enferma mucho	si	no
Vomito	si	no
Diarrea	si	no
Dolor de estómago	si	no
Estómago inflamado	si	no
Reacciones severas o alergias a la comida	si	no
No puede respirar por la nariz	si	no
Ronca o hace ruido cuando respira	si	no
Problemas dentales	si	no
Problemas para dormir	si	no

Failure to Thrive and Pediatric Undernutrition: A Transdisciplinary Approach
edited by Daniel B. Kessler and Peter Dawson
© 1999 by Paul H. Brookes Publishing Co.

Growth Plotting Aid

This graphing aid makes it much easier to plot growth data accurately. Photocopy it onto a transparency, as thick as possible. Drill a tiny hole in the center circle.

To use the graphing aid, line up the vertical line with the child's age. Line up the horizontal line with the child's length, weight, or head circumference. Put a pencil into the center circle, and mark a dot. Use the aid in a similar manner to plot weight for height.

If you use a pencil, then you can erase errors.

Based on the Accuplot Growth Plotting Aid © 1983 Ross Laboratories. Included with permission of Ross Products Division, Abbott Laboratories, Inc.

Failure to Thrive and Pediatric Undernutrition: A Transdisciplinary Approach
edited by Daniel B. Kessler and Peter Dawson
© 1999 by Paul H. Brookes Publishing Co.

Reference Data on Weight Gain During the First 2 Years of Life

These tables show percentile distributions of weight gain for normal infants. They were published to aid the early detection of inadequate or excessive weight gain. They may also be used to follow children after treatment has begun.

The authors of these tables used fairly long age intervals to reduce the likelihood that variations from day to day, which could be due to feedings, urination, or bowel movements, would be misleading. The authors chose intervals so that "the difference between the 5th and 50th percentiles . . . would be less than 180 grams—about a single feeding" (Fomon, 1991, p. 415).

The data are based on infants from the 1977 NCHS growth charts and from the University of Iowa. Infants were white, and the sample included both breast-fed and formula-fed infants. The original study included length as well as weight.

REFERENCES

Fomon, S.J. (1991). Reference data for assessing growth of infants. *Journal of Pediatrics, 199,* 415–416.

Guo, S., Roche, A.F., Fomon, S.J., Nelson, S.E., Chumlea, W.C., Rogers, R.R., Baumgartner, R.N., Ziegler, E.E., & Siervogel, R.M. (1991). Reference data on gains in weight and length during the first two years of life. *Journal of Pediatrics, 119,* 355–362.

One-month increments in weight (gm/day) from birth to 6 months

Age (months)	n	Weight (g/day)[a]	Percentile						
			5th	10th	25th	50th	75th	90th	95th
Boys									
Up to 1	580	30 ± 9.4	15	18	24	30	36	42	45
1–2	580	35 ± 8.5	22	25	29	35	40	46	50
2–3	580	27 ± 7.9	15	18	22	26	31	36	41
3–4	298	20 ± 3.6	15	16	18	20	22	24	26
4–5	298	17 ± 3.4	12	14	15	17	19	21	23
5–6	298	16 ± 3.5	11	12	14	15	17	19	21
Girls									
Up to 1	562	26 ± 8.4	11	16	20	26	32	36	39
1–2	562	29 ± 7.7	18	20	24	29	34	39	42
2–3	562	23 ± 7.2	12	14	19	23	28	32	35
3–4	298	19 ± 5.3	13	15	17	19	21	23	26
4–5	298	16 ± 5.0	11	13	14	16	18	20	22
5–6	298	15 ± 4.7	10	11	13	14	16	18	18

Two-month increments in weight from birth to 12 months

Age (months)	n	Weight (g/day)[a]	Percentile						
			5th	10th	25th	50th	75th	90th	95th
Boys									
Up to 2	580	33 ± 7.0	21	24	28	32	38	42	44
1–3	580	31 ± 6.9	20	22	27	31	35	39	43
2–4	65	23 ± 4.7	—	17	19	23	26	29	—
3–5	298	19 ± 3.2	14	15	17	18	20	22	24
4–6	298	16 ± 2.9	12	13	14	16	18	20	21
5–7	233	15 ± 2.4	11	12	13	15	16	18	18
6–8	233	13 ± 2.4	10	11	12	13	15	16	17
7–9	233	12 ± 2.4	9	10	11	12	14	15	16
8–10	233	12 ± 2.4	9	9	10	11	13	15	15
9–11	233	11 ± 2.3	8	8	9	11	12	14	14
10–12	233	10 ± 2.3	7	8	9	10	12	13	14
Girls									
Up to 2	562	28 ± 6.5	17	20	23	28	32	36	38
1–3	562	26 ± 6.3	16	19	22	26	30	34	37
2–4	74	22 ± 5.4	—	16	19	21	24	27	—
3–5	298	18 ± 4.7	13	14	16	17	19	21	22
4–6	298	15 ± 4.6	11	12	14	15	17	18	19
5–7	224	14 ± 4.7	11	11	13	14	15	17	17
6–8	224	13 ± 4.6	10	10	12	13	14	16	16
7–9	224	12 ± 4.5	9	10	11	12	13	15	15
8–10	224	12 ± 4.5	8	9	10	11	13	14	14
9–11	224	11 ± 4.4	8	8	9	10	12	13	14
10–12	224	10 ± 4.3	7	8	9	10	11	13	13

From Guo, S., Roche, A.F., Fomon, S.J., Nelson, S.E., Chumlea, W.C., Rogers, R.R., Baumgartner, R.N., Ziegler, E.E., & Siervogel, R.M. (1991). Reference data on gains in weight and length during the first two years of life. *Journal of Pediatrics, 119,* 355–362; reprinted by permission.

Note: From birth through 3 months, Iowa data; from 3 through 6 months, combined data; from 6 through 12 months, Fels data.

[a] Values expressed as mean ± SD.

Three-month increments in weight from birth to 24 months

Age (months)	n	Weight (g/day)[a]	Percentile						
			5th	10th	25th	50th	75th	90th	95th
Boys									
Up to 3	580	31 ± 5.9	21	23	27	31	34	38	41
1–4	65	27 ± 5.1	—	21	23	27	30	34	—
2–5	65	21 ± 4.3	—	15	17	21	23	27	—
3–6	298	18 ± 2.9	13	14	16	18	19	21	23
4–7	233	16 ± 2.4	12	13	14	15	17	18	19
5–8	233	14 ± 2.4	11	11	13	14	15	17	18
6–9	233	13 ± 2.4	10	10	11	13	14	16	17
7–10	233	12 ± 2.4	9	9	10	12	13	15	16
8–11	233	11 ± 2.4	8	9	10	11	12	14	15
9–12	233	11 ± 2.3	8	8	9	10	12	14	14
10–13	233	10 ± 2.3	7	8	9	10	11	13	14
11–14	233	10 ± 2.3	7	7	8	9	11	12	13
12–15	233	9 ± 2.3	6	7	8	9	10	12	13
13–16	233	9 ± 2.3	6	6	7	9	10	12	13
14–17	233	8 ± 2.2	6	6	7	8	10	11	12
15–18	233	8 ± 2.2	5	6	7	8	9	11	12
16–19	233	8 ± 2.2	5	6	7	8	9	10	12
17–20	233	8 ± 2.2	5	5	6	7	9	10	12
18–21	233	7 ± 2.2	5	5	6	7	8	10	11
19–22	233	7 ± 2.1	4	5	6	7	8	10	11
20–23	233	7 ± 2.1	4	5	6	7	8	9	11
21–24	233	7 ± 2.1	4	5	6	7	8	9	11
Girls									
Up to 3	562	26 ± 5.5	17	20	23	26	30	33	36
1–4	74	24 ± 5.1	—	19	21	24	27	30	—
2–5	74	20 ± 3.9	—	16	17	19	21	25	—
3–6	298	17 ± 4.6	12	13	15	17	18	20	21
4–7	224	15 ± 4.8	11	12	13	15	16	17	18
5–8	224	14 ± 4.7	10	11	12	13	15	16	17
6–9	224	13 ± 4.6	10	10	11	12	14	15	16
7–10	224	12 ± 4.5	9	9	10	12	13	14	15
8–11	224	11 ± 4.4	8	9	10	11	12	14	14
9–12	224	11 ± 4.3	8	8	9	10	12	13	14
10–13	224	10 ± 4.2	7	8	9	10	11	12	13
11–14	224	10 ± 4.2	7	7	8	9	11	12	13
12–15	224	9 ± 4.1	7	7	8	9	10	12	12
13–16	224	9 ± 4.0	6	7	8	8	10	11	12
14–17	224	9 ± 3.9	6	6	7	8	9	11	12
15–18	224	8 ± 3.9	6	6	7	8	9	10	11
16–19	224	8 ± 3.8	6	6	7	8	9	10	11
17–20	224	8 ± 3.8	5	6	7	7	9	10	11
18–21	224	8 ± 3.7	5	5	6	7	8	10	11
19–22	224	7 ± 3.6	5	5	6	7	8	9	10
20–23	224	7 ± 3.6	5	5	6	7	8	9	10
21–24	224	7 ± 3.5	5	5	6	7	8	9	10

From Guo, S., Roche, A.F., Fomon, S.J., Nelson, S.E., Chumlea, W.C., Rogers, R.R., Baumgartner, R.N., Zielgler, E.E., & Siervogel, R.M. (1991). Reference data on gains in weight and length during the first two years of life. *Journal of Pediatrics, 119,* 355–362; reprinted by permission.

Note: From birth through 3 months, Iowa data; from 3 through 6 months, combined data; from 6 through 12 months, Fels data.

[a] Values expressed as mean ± SD.

Conversion of
Pounds and Ounces to Grams
and of Inches to Centimeters

Conversion of pounds and ounces to grams

Pounds		Ounces														
	0	1	2	3	4	5	6	7	8	9	10	11	12	13	14	15
0		28	57	85	113	142	170	198	227	255	283	312	340	369	397	425
1	454	482	510	539	567	595	624	652	680	709	737	765	794	822	850	879
2	907	936	964	992	1021	1049	1077	1106	1134	1162	1191	1219	1247	1276	1304	1332
3	1361	1389	1417	1446	1474	1503	1531	1559	1588	1616	1644	1673	1701	1729	1758	1786
4	1814	1843	1871	1899	1928	1956	1984	2013	2041	2070	2098	2126	2155	2183	2211	2240
5	2268	2296	2325	2353	2381	2410	2438	2466	2495	2523	2551	2580	2608	2637	2665	2693
6	2722	2750	2778	2807	2835	2863	2892	2920	2948	2977	3005	3033	3062	3090	3118	3147
7	3175	3203	3232	3260	3289	3317	3345	3374	3402	3430	3459	3487	3515	3544	3572	3600
8	3629	3657	3685	3714	3742	3770	3799	3827	3856	3884	3912	3941	3969	3997	4026	4054
9	4082	4111	4139	4167	4196	4224	4252	4281	4309	4337	4366	4394	4423	4451	4479	4508
10	4536	4564	4593	4621	4649	4678	4706	4734	4763	4791	4819	4848	4876	4904	4933	4961
11	4990	5018	5046	5075	5103	5131	5160	5188	5216	5245	5273	5301	5330	5358	5386	5415
12	5443	5471	5500	5528	5557	5585	5613	5642	5670	5698	5727	5755	5783	5812	5840	5868
13	5897	5925	5953	5982	6010	6038	6067	6095	6123	6152	6180	6209	6237	6265	6294	6322
14	6350	6379	6407	6435	6464	6492	6520	6549	6577	6605	6634	6662	6690	6719	6747	6776
15	6804	6832	6860	6889	6917	6945	6973	7002	7030	7059	7087	7115	7144	7172	7201	7228
16	7257	7286	7313	7342	7371	7399	7427	7456	7484	7512	7541	7569	7597	7626	7654	7682
17	7711	7739	7768	7796	7824	7853	7881	7909	7938	7966	7994	8023	8051	8079	8108	8136
18	8165	8192	8221	8249	8278	8306	8335	8363	8391	8420	8448	8476	8504	8533	8561	8590
19	8618	8646	8675	8703	8731	8760	8788	8816	8845	8873	8902	8930	8958	8987	9015	9043
20	9072	9100	9128	9157	9185	9213	9242	9270	9298	9327	9355	9383	9412	9440	9469	9497
21	9525	9554	9582	9610	9639	9667	9695	9724	9752	9780	9809	9837	9865	9894	9922	9950
22	9979	10007	10036	10064	10092	10120	10149	10177	10206	10234	10262	10291	10319	10347	10376	10404
23	10433	10461	10489	10518	10546	10574	10603	10631	10659	10688	10716	10744	10773	10801	10830	10858
24	10886	10915	10943	10971	11000	11028	11057	11085	11113	11141	11170	11198	11226	11255	11283	11311
25	11340	11368	11397	11425	11453	11482	11510	11538	11567	11595	11623	11652	11680	11708	11737	11765
26	11793	11822	11850	11878	11907	11935	11963	11992	12020	12049	12077	12105	12134	12162	12190	12219

27	12247	12275	12304	12332	12360	12389	12417	12445	12474	12502	12530	12559	12587	12616	12644	12672
28	12701	12729	12757	12786	12814	12842	12871	12899	12927	12956	12984	13012	13041	13069	13097	13126
29	13154	13183	13211	13239	13268	13296	13324	13353	13381	13409	13438	13466	13494	13523	13551	13579
30	13608	13636	13664	13693	13721	13750	13778	13806	13835	13863	13891	13920	13948	13976	14005	14033
31	14061	14090	14118	14146	14175	14203	14231	14260	14288	14317	14345	14373	14402	14430	14458	14487
32	14515	14543	14572	14600	14628	14657	14685	14713	14742	14770	14798	14827	14855	14884	14912	14940
33	14969	14997	15025	15054	15082	15110	15139	15167	15195	15224	15252	15280	15309	15337	15365	15394
34	15422	15450	15479	15507	15536	15564	15592	15621	15649	15677	15706	15734	15762	15791	15819	15847
35	15876	15904	15932	15961	15989	16017	16046	16074	16103	16131	16159	16188	16216	16244	16273	16301
36	16329	16358	16386	16414	16443	16471	16499	16528	16556	16584	16613	16641	16670	16698	16726	16755
37	16783	16811	16840	16868	16896	16925	16953	16981	17010	17038	17066	17095	17123	17151	17180	17208
38	17237	17265	17293	17322	17350	17378	17407	17435	17463	17492	17520	17548	17577	17605	17633	17662
39	17690	17718	17747	17775	17804	17832	17860	17889	17917	17945	17974	18002	18030	18059	18087	18115

From 0 to 22 pounds from Avery, G.B., Fletcher, M.A., & MacDonald, M.G. (1994). *Neonatology: Pathophysiology and management of the newborn* (4th ed., p. 1422). Philadelphia: Lippincott-Raven Publishers; reprinted by permission. From 23 to 39 pounds from Chisholm, L.J. (1967). *Units of weight and measure (metric) and U.S. customary* (National Bureau of Standards Miscellaneous Publication 286). Washington, DC: U.S. Department of Commerce, National Bureau of Standards, Superintendent of Documents, U.S. Government Printing Office.

Conversion of inches to centimeters

Inches	0	$^1/_4$	$^1/_2$	$^3/_4$	Inches	0	$^1/_4$	$^1/_2$	$^3/_4$
12	30.5	31.1	31.7	32.4	48	121.9	122.6	123.2	123.8
13	33.0	33.7	34.3	34.9	49	124.5	125.1	125.7	126.4
14	35.6	36.2	36.8	37.5	50	127.0	127.6	128.3	128.9
15	38.1	38.7	39.4	40.0	51	129.5	130.2	130.8	131.4
16	40.6	41.3	41.9	42.5	52	132.1	132.7	133.3	134.0
17	43.2	43.8	44.4	45.1	53	134.6	135.3	135.9	136.5
18	45.7	46.4	47.0	47.6	54	137.2	137.8	138.4	139.1
19	48.3	48.9	49.5	50.2	55	139.7	140.3	141.0	141.6
20	50.8	51.4	52.1	52.6	56	142.2	142.9	143.5	144.1
21	53.3	54.0	54.6	55.2	57	144.8	145.4	146.0	146.7
22	55.9	56.5	57.1	57.8	58	147.3	148.0	148.6	149.2
23	58.4	59.1	59.7	60.3	59	149.9	150.5	151.1	151.8
24	61.0	61.6	62.2	62.9	60	152.4	153.0	153.7	154.3
25	63.5	64.1	64.8	65.4	61	154.9	155.6	156.2	156.8
26	66.0	66.7	67.3	67.9	62	157.5	158.1	158.7	159.4
27	68.6	69.2	69.8	70.5	63	160.0	160.7	161.3	161.9
28	71.1	71.8	72.4	73.0	64	162.6	163.2	163.8	164.5
29	73.7	74.3	74.9	75.6	65	165.1	165.7	166.4	167.0
30	76.2	76.8	77.5	78.1	66	167.6	168.3	168.9	169.5
31	78.7	79.4	80.0	80.6	67	170.2	170.8	171.4	172.1
32	81.3	81.9	82.5	83.2	68	172.7	173.4	174.0	174.6
33	83.8	84.5	85.1	85.7	69	175.3	175.9	176.5	177.2
34	86.4	87.0	87.6	88.3	70	177.8	178.4	179.1	179.7
35	88.9	89.5	90.2	90.8	71	180.3	181.0	181.6	182.2
36	91.4	92.1	92.7	93.3	72	182.9	183.5	184.1	184.8
37	94.0	94.6	95.2	95.9	73	185.4	186.1	186.7	187.3
38	96.5	97.2	97.8	98.4	74	188.0	188.6	189.2	189.9
39	99.1	99.7	100.3	101.0	75	190.5	191.1	191.8	192.4
40	101.6	102.2	102.9	103.5	76	193.0	193.7	194.3	194.9
41	104.1	104.8	105.4	106.0	77	195.6	196.2	196.8	197.5
42	106.7	107.3	107.9	108.6	78	198.1	198.9	199.4	200.0
43	109.2	109.9	110.5	111.1	79	200.7	201.3	201.9	202.6
44	111.8	112.4	113.0	113.7	80	203.2	203.8	204.5	205.1
45	114.3	114.9	115.6	116.2	81	205.7	206.4	207.0	207.6
46	116.8	117.5	118.1	118.7	82	208.3	208.9	209.5	210.2
47	119.4	120.0	120.6	121.3	83	210.8	211.5	212.1	212.7

Growth Charts for Low Birth Weight Infants

Growth of low birth weight (LBW, 1,501–2,500 g) premature ($\leq$ 37 weeks' GA) infants differs from that of normal birth weight term infants during infancy and early childhood. Because these infants may not catch up to term infants in growth during the early years, their growth should be compared with that of premature infants of similar birth weight.

The growth percentiles presented here are based on a large sample of infants enrolled in the Infant Health and Development Program (IHDP). Some infants most likely to experience growth problems from biologic or environmental causes were excluded. Also excluded were premature infants with birth weights greater than 2,500 g and small-for-gestational-age term infants, but these infants can be plotted on these graphs. Study infants are representative of premature infants who receive modern neonatal intensive care.

INSTRUCTIONS FOR USE

1. Measure and record weight, length, and head circumference.
2. Calculate gestation-adjusted age by subtracting Adjustment for Prematurity in weeks from postnatal age in weeks. Adjustment for Prematurity equals 40 weeks minus GA. For example, at 12 weeks' postnatal age, an infant born at 30 weeks' GA would be 2 weeks' (0.5 months) gestation-adjusted age.
3. Plot data at the gestation-adjusted age on the appropriate graph.
4. When possible, plot serial data on the same graph to permit detection of change in growth percentiles with age.

INTERPRETATION

These graphs permit comparison of an LBW premature infant's growth relative to current reference data. Further investigation may be indicated when the plotted measurements are markedly different from the 50th percentile, or growth percentile changes rapidly.

Reprinted by permission of Ross Products Division, Abbott Laboratories.

These charts can be used with infants whose birth weight is 1,500–2,500 grams. Charts for very low birth weight infants (less than 1,500 grams) are available from Ross Products Division, Abbott Laboratories.

Name_____

Record #_____

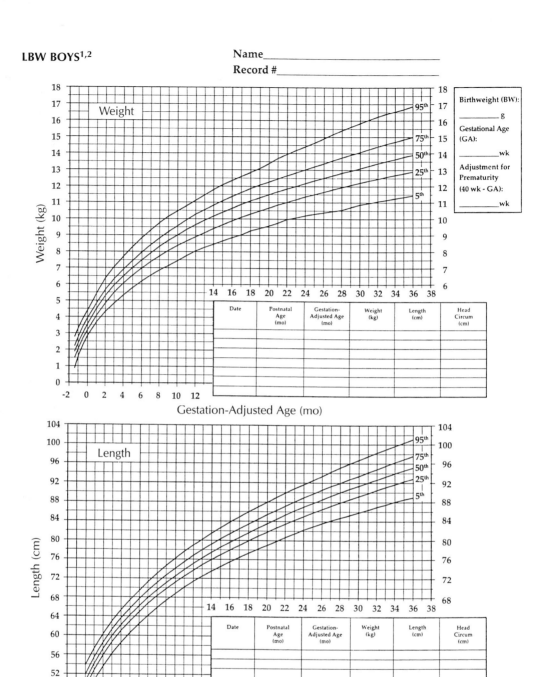

[1] The Infant Health and Development Program. (1990). Enhancing the outcomes of low-birth-weight, premature infants. *JAMA, 263*(22), 3035–3042.

[2] Casey, P.H., Kraemer, H.C., Bernbaum, J., et al. (1991). Growth status and growth rates of a varied sample of low birth weight, preterm infants: A longitudinal cohort from birth to three years of age. *Journal of Pediatrics, 119,* 599–605.

Reprinted by permission of Ross Products Division, Abbott Laboratories.

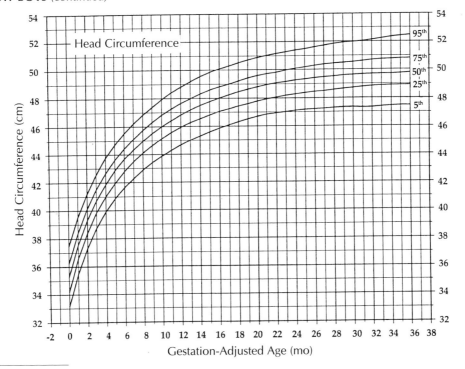

Reprinted by permission of Ross Products Division, Abbott Laboratories.

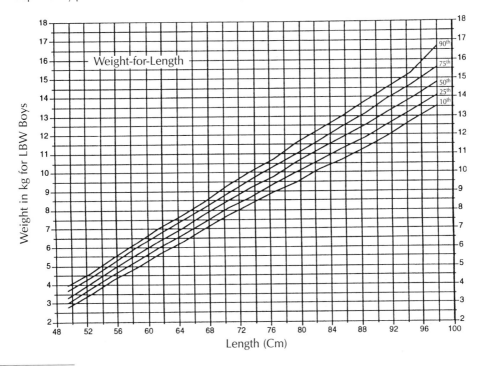

From Guo, S.S., Wholihan, K., Roche, A.F., Chumlea, W.C., & Casey, P.H. (1996). Weight-for-length reference data for preterm low-birthweight infants. *Archives of Pediatrics and Adolescent Medicine, 150,* 964–970; reprinted by permission. Copyright 1996, American Medical Association.

Failure to Thrive and Pediatric Undernutrition: A Transdisciplinary Approach
edited by Daniel B. Kessler and Peter Dawson
© 1999 by Paul H. Brookes Publishing Co.

LBW GIRLS[1,2]

Name_____

Record #_____

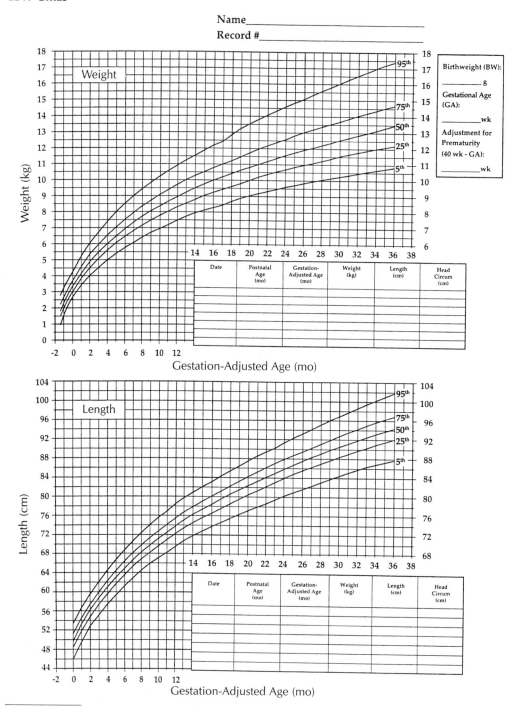

[1] The Infant Health and Development Program. (1990). Enhancing the outcomes of low-birth-weight, premature infants. *JAMA, 263*(22), 3035–3042.

[2] Casey, P.H., Kraemer, H.C., Bernbaum, J., et al. (1991). Growth status and growth rates of a varied sample of low birth weight, preterm infants: A longitudinal cohort from birth to three years of age. *Journal of Pediatrics, 119,* 599–605.

Reprinted by permission of Ross Products Division, Abbott Laboratories.

Failure to Thrive and Pediatric Undernutrition: A Transdisciplinary Approach
edited by Daniel B. Kessler and Peter Dawson
© 1999 by Paul H. Brookes Publishing Co.

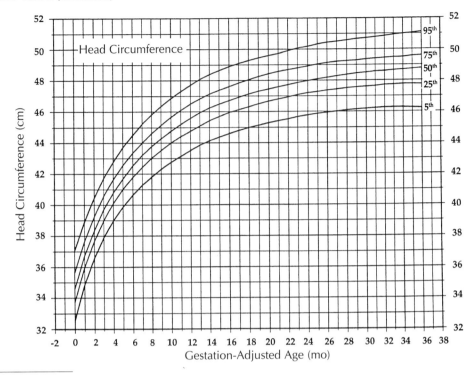

Reprinted by permission of Ross Products Division, Abbott Laboratories.

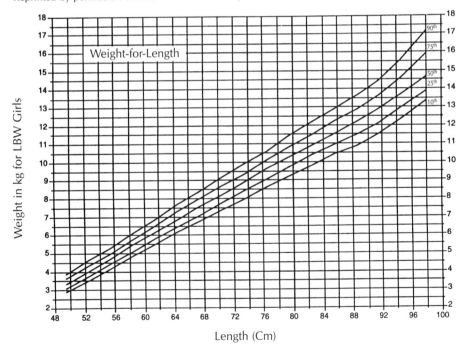

From Guo, S.S., Wholihan, K., Roche, A.F., Chumlea, W.C., & Casey, P.H. (1996). Weight-for-length reference data for preterm low-birthweight infants. *Archives of Pediatrics and Adolescent Medicine, 150,* 964–970; reprinted by permission. Copyright 1996, American Medical Association.

Failure to Thrive and Pediatric Undernutrition: A Transdisciplinary Approach
edited by Daniel B. Kessler and Peter Dawson
© 1999 by Paul H. Brookes Publishing Co.

Parent-Specific Adjustments for Evaluation of Length

Recumbent length and stature (standing height) are affected by both genetic and non-genetic factors. The genetic component should be considered when concern arises that diet or disease may have retarded or accelerated growth. Adjustment of length or stature to take parental stature into account may help identify or explain the nature of a growth problem. Such adjustment may prompt diagnostic studies or suggest a genetic basis for the growth problem.

Parent-specific adjustment procedures have been developed for U.S. children by Himes, Roche, and Thissen.[1,2] The accompanying tables of adjustments are adapted from their research. Parent-specific adjustments need not be done routinely but should be considered when a child has unusual length or stature. As a guideline for applying parent-specific adjustments, "unusual" may be defined as below the 5th percentile or above the 95th percentile in length or stature for age.

Occasionally, a child's length or stature may appear normal, but the parents (one or both) are very tall or very short. Under such circumstances, parent-specific adjustment also is appropriate. Rapid decrease or increase in a child's percentile for length or stature generally is not an indication for applying parent-specific adjustments because the cause is more likely to be nongenetic than genetic.

The following tables for children younger than 3 years are based on recumbent length, not height.

---

[1] Himes, J.H., Roche, A.F., & Thissen, D. (1981). Parent-specific adjustments for assessment of recumbent length and stature. *Monographs in Paediatrics, 13.*

[2] Himes, J.H., Roche, A.F., Thissen, D., & Moore, W.M. (1985). Parent-specific adjustments for evaluation of recumbent length and stature of children. *Pediatrics, 75,* 304–313.

Reprinted by permission of Ross Products Division, Abbott Laboratories.

These tables are based on the 1977 NCHS growth charts. The original study goes up to 18 years.

INSTRUCTIONS

1. Measure and record mother's stature.
2. Measure and record father's stature.
3. When one parent's stature cannot be measured, the measured parent's estimate of the other parent's stature (in cm) can be substituted for measured stature, and midparent stature can be calculated as in instruction 4. Alternatively, the measured parent's perception of the other parent's stature (short, medium, or tall) can be used to determine midparent stature directly from Table 1.
4. Calculate midparent stature by adding the mother's stature and the father's stature in cm and dividing by two. Metric equivalents for stature are shown on p. 578.
5. Measure, record, and plot the child's length (birth to 36 months) in cm on the appropriate growth chart that displays the National Center for Health Statistics (NCHS) percentiles. Metric equivalents for length are shown on p. 578.
6. Calculate the child's adjusted length by using the parent-specific adjustments from Table 2 (for boys) or Table 3 (for girls).
    a. Locate the age closest to that achieved by the child.
    b. For that age, locate the horizontal row that includes the child's length.
    c. Locate the vertical column closest to the midparent stature for the child's mother and father.
    d. The parent-specific adjustment (in cm) appears at the row-column intersection.
    e. Add the parent-specific adjustment to the child's length if the factor has no sign; subtract the adjustment if it has a minus sign.
7. Determine the child's parent-specific adjusted percentile by plotting adjusted length on the appropriate NCHS growth chart. Clearly label plotted measurements as being actual or adjusted values.

INTERPRETATION

A child at a low percentile for actual length whose parents are short probably is genetically short. However, his or her shortness, particularly if it is extreme, may have additional contributing factors that should be considered.

If the child's adjusted percentile is low, his or her growth probably has been slowed by nongenetic factors, and diagnostic studies should be considered. If the parents are tall, the child's adjusted percentile will be lower than his or her actual percentile, and his or her shortness is more likely due to malnutrition or disease.

A child at a high adjusted percentile for length most often will be found to have accelerated maturation. Rarely, a specific disorder such as Marfan's syndrome or pituitary gigantism may be responsible for the child's unusual length.

FOLLOW-UP

Counseling may be advisable when a child is judged to be genetically short or tall. Additional contributing factors should be considered and growth monitored to confirm the relative stability of the child's length or stature percentile.

Further investigation and modification of diet or specific therapy are indicated for a child with unusual length due to malnutrition or disease. Growth should be monitored to evaluate the effectiveness of dietary management or drug therapy.

Table 1. Midparent stature (cm) when measured parent reports other parent's stature as short, medium, or tall

Measured parent's stature (cm)	Midparent stature (cm)[a]					
	When mother reports father's stature as			When father reports mother's stature as		
	Short[b]	Medium[b]	Tall[b]	Short[c]	Medium[c]	Tall[c]
146	156	162	166	150	154	158
148	158	162	166	152	156	160
150	158	164	168	152	156	160
152	160	164	168	154	158	162
154	160	166	170	154	158	162
156	162	166	170	156	160	164
158	162	168	172	156	160	164
160	164	168	172	158	162	166
162	164	170	174	158	162	166
164	166	170	174	160	164	168
166	166	172	176	160	164	168
168	168	172	176	162	166	170
170	168	174	178	162	166	170
172	170	174	178	164	168	172
174	170	176	180	164	168	172
176	172	176	180	166	170	174
178	172	178	182	166	170	174
180	174	178	182	168	172	176
182	174	180	184	168	172	176
184	176	180	184	170	174	178
186	176	182	—	170	174	178
188	178	182	—	172	176	180
190	178	184	—	172	176	180
192	180	184	—	174	178	182
194	180	—	—	174	178	182
196	182	—	—	176	180	184
198	182	—	—	176	180	184

[a]All midparent statures are rounded to the nearest 2 cm to facilitate use of Tables 2 and 3.

[b]Values for father's stature used in calculations of midparent stature: short, 167.6 cm (5 ft 6 in.); medium, 176.3 cm (5 ft 9½ in.); tall, 185.4 cm (6 ft 1 in.).

[c]Values for mother's stature used in calculations of midparent stature: short, 154.9 cm (5 ft 1 in.); medium, 162.8 cm (5 ft 4 in.); tall, 170.7 cm (5 ft 7¼ in.).

Example #1.   Girl aged 12 months, length 27¼ inches, mother's stature 60½ inches, and father's stature 65¼ inches.

Daughter's actual length in cm is 69.2 (from p. 578).
Daughter's actual percentile is below the 5th (from NCHS growth chart).
Mother's stature in cm is 153.7 (from p. 578).
Father's stature in cm is 165.7 (from p. 578).

Midparent stature is $\dfrac{153.7 + 165.7}{2} = 159.7$ cm.

Adjustment is 2 cm (from Table 3).
Daughter's adjusted length is 69.2 cm + 2 cm = 71.2 cm.
Daughter's adjusted percentile is between the 10th and 25th (from NCHS growth chart).

Interpretation: Probably genetically short. Consider additional contributing factors.

Example #2.   Boy aged 31 months, length 35 inches, mother's stature 68½ inches, and father's stature reported as "tall."

Son's actual length in cm is 88.9 (from p. 578).
Son's actual percentile is 10th (from NCHS growth chart).
Mother's stature in cm is 174.0 (from p. 578).
Midparent stature is 180.0 cm (from Table 1).
Adjustment is −4 cm (from Table 2).
Son's adjusted length is 84.9 cm.
Son's adjusted percentile is below the 5th (from NCHS growth chart).

Interpretation: Probably nongenetically short. Further investigation may be indicated, especially if growth is dropping across percentiles.

Table 2. Parent-specific adjustments (cm) for length of boys from birth to 36 months

Age (months)	Length (cm)	150	152	154	156	158	160	162	164	166	168	170	172	174	176	178	180	182	184
Birth	40.0– 43.9	2	1	1	1	1	1	1	0	0	0	0	0	0	-1	-1	-1	-1	-1
	44.0– 52.9	2	2	1	1	1	1	1	0	0	0	0	0	0	-1	-1	-1	-1	-1
	53.0– 56.9	2	2	1	1	1	1	1	1	0	0	0	0	0	-1	-1	-1	-1	-1
1	40.0– 44.9	2	2	1	1	1	1	1	0	0	0	0	-1	-1	-1	-1	-1	-2	-2
	45.0– 48.9	2	2	2	1	1	1	1	0	0	0	0	0	-1	-1	-1	-1	-2	-2
	49.0– 52.9	2	2	2	1	1	1	1	1	0	0	0	0	-1	-1	-1	-1	-2	-2
	53.0– 56.9	2	2	2	2	1	1	1	1	0	0	0	0	-1	-1	-1	-1	-1	-2
	57.0– 62.9	2	2	2	2	1	1	1	1	1	0	0	0	0	-1	-1	-1	-1	-2
3	52.0– 56.9	3	2	2	2	1	1	1	1	0	0	0	-1	-1	-1	-1	-2	-2	-2
	57.0– 60.9	3	2	2	2	2	1	1	1	0	0	0	0	-1	-1	-1	-2	-2	-2
	61.0– 66.9	3	3	2	2	2	1	1	1	1	0	0	0	-1	-1	-1	-1	-2	-2
	67.0– 68.9	3	3	2	2	2	2	1	1	1	0	0	0	0	-1	-1	-1	-2	-2
6	62.0– 64.9	3	3	2	2	2	1	1	1	0	0	0	-1	-1	-1	-2	-2	-2	-3
	65.0– 66.9	3	3	3	2	2	2	1	1	1	0	0	-1	-1	-1	-2	-2	-2	-3
	67.0– 73.9	3	3	3	2	2	2	1	1	1	0	0	0	-1	-1	-1	-2	-2	-2
	74.0– 76.9	4	3	3	3	2	2	2	1	1	1	0	0	0	-1	-1	-1	-2	-2
9	66.0– 68.9	3	3	3	2	2	1	1	1	0	0	0	-1	-1	-2	-2	-2	-3	-3
	69.0– 72.9	4	3	3	3	2	2	1	1	1	0	0	-1	-1	-1	-2	-2	-2	-3
	73.0– 76.9	4	3	3	3	2	2	2	1	1	0	0	0	-1	-1	-2	-2	-2	-3
	77.0– 80.9	4	4	3	3	3	2	2	1	1	1	0	0	0	-1	-1	-2	-2	-2
12	67.0– 71.9	4	3	3	2	2	2	1	1	0	0	-1	-1	-1	-2	-2	-3	-3	-3
	72.0– 74.9	4	4	3	3	2	2	1	1	1	0	0	-1	-1	-1	-2	-2	-3	-3
	75.0– 78.9	4	4	3	3	2	2	2	1	1	0	0	0	-1	-1	-2	-2	-3	-3
	79.0– 82.9	4	4	3	3	3	2	2	1	1	1	0	0	-1	-1	-1	-2	-2	-3
	83.0– 84.9	4	4	4	3	3	2	2	2	1	1	0	0	0	-1	-1	-2	-2	-3

Midparent stature (cm)

(continued)

Table 2. *(continued)*

Age (months)	Length (cm)	Midparent stature (cm)																	
		150	152	154	156	158	160	162	164	166	168	170	172	174	176	178	180	182	184
18	73.0– 75.9	4	4	3	3	2	2	1	1	0	0	−1	−1	−2	−2	−2	−3	−3	−4
	76.0– 80.9	4	4	3	3	2	2	2	1	1	0	0	−1	−1	−2	−2	−3	−3	−4
	81.0– 84.9	5	4	4	3	3	2	2	1	1	0	0	0	−1	−2	−2	−3	−3	−3
	85.0– 88.9	5	4	4	3	3	2	2	1	1	1	0	0	−1	−1	−2	−2	−3	−3
	89.0– 92.9	5	5	4	4	3	3	2	2	1	1	0	0	−1	−1	−2	−2	−2	−3
24	78.0– 82.9	5	4	4	3	3	2	2	1	0	0	−1	−1	−2	−2	−3	−3	−4	−5
	83.0– 86.9	5	5	4	4	3	2	2	1	1	0	0	−1	−2	−2	−3	−3	−4	−4
	87.0– 92.9	6	5	5	4	3	3	2	2	1	1	0	−1	−1	−2	−2	−3	−3	−4
	93.0– 96.9	6	5	5	4	4	3	3	2	1	1	0	0	−1	−1	−2	−3	−3	−4
30	85.0– 88.9	6	5	5	4	3	3	2	1	1	0	−1	−1	−2	−3	−3	−4	−4	−5
	89.0– 92.9	6	5	5	4	4	3	2	2	1	0	0	−1	−2	−2	−3	−3	−4	−5
	93.0– 96.9	6	6	5	4	4	3	3	2	1	1	0	−1	−1	−2	−3	−3	−4	−5
	97.0–100.9	7	6	5	5	4	3	3	2	2	1	0	0	−1	−2	−2	−3	−4	−4
36	88.0– 90.9	6	6	5	4	3	3	2	1	1	0	−1	−1	−2	−3	−4	−4	−6	−6
	91.0– 94.9	6	6	5	4	4	3	2	2	1	0	−1	−1	−2	−3	−3	−4	−5	−5
	95.0– 98.9	7	6	5	5	4	3	3	2	1	1	0	−1	−1	−2	−3	−4	−4	−5
	99.0–102.9	7	6	6	5	4	4	3	2	1	1	0	−1	−1	−2	−3	−3	−4	−5
	103.0–106.9	7	7	6	5	5	4	3	2	2	1	0	0	−1	−2	−2	−3	−4	−4

Reprinted by permission of Ross Products Division, Abbott Laboratories. Originally adapted from Himes, Roche, & Thissen (1981).

Table 3. Parent-specific adjustments (cm) for length of girls from birth to 36 months

Age (months)	Length (cm)	Midparent stature (cm)																	
		150	152	154	156	158	160	162	164	166	168	170	172	174	176	178	180	182	184
Birth	40.0– 42.9	1	1	0	0	0	0	0	0	0	0	0	0	0	0	0	0	0	–1
	43.0– 50.9	1	1	1	0	0	0	0	0	0	0	0	0	0	0	0	0	0	–1
	51.0– 54.9	1	1	1	0	0	0	0	0	0	0	0	0	0	0	0	0	0	0
1	46.0– 56.9	1	1	1	1	1	1	0	0	0	0	0	0	0	0	–1	–1	–1	–1
	57.0– 58.9	1	1	1	1	1	1	1	0	0	0	0	0	0	0	–1	–1	–1	–1
3	52.0– 54.9	2	2	1	1	1	1	1	0	0	0	0	0	–1	–1	–1	–1	–2	–2
	55.0– 60.9	2	2	2	1	1	1	1	1	0	0	0	0	–1	–1	–1	–1	–1	–2
	61.0– 66.9	2	2	2	2	1	1	1	1	0	0	0	0	0	–1	–1	–1	–1	–1
6	58.0– 60.9	3	2	2	2	1	1	1	1	0	0	0	–1	–1	–1	–2	–2	–2	–3
	61.0– 63.9	3	3	2	2	2	1	1	1	0	0	0	–1	–1	–1	–1	–2	–2	–2
	64.0– 68.9	3	3	3	2	2	1	1	1	1	0	0	0	–1	–1	–1	–2	–2	–2
	69.0– 72.9	3	3	3	2	2	2	1	1	1	0	0	0	–1	–1	–1	–1	–2	–2
9	64.0– 66.9	4	3	3	2	2	2	1	1	0	0	0	–1	–1	–2	–2	–3	–3	–3
	67.0– 70.9	4	3	3	3	2	2	1	1	1	0	0	–1	–1	–1	–2	–2	–3	–3
	71.0– 73.9	4	4	3	3	2	2	2	1	1	0	0	0	–1	–1	–2	–2	–2	–3
	74.0– 76.9	4	4	3	3	3	2	2	1	1	1	0	0	–1	–1	–1	–2	–2	–3
12	66.0– 68.9	4	4	3	3	2	2	1	1	0	0	–1	–1	–2	–2	–3	–3	–4	–4
	69.0– 72.9	4	4	3	3	2	2	1	1	0	0	0	–1	–1	–2	–2	–3	–3	–4
	73.0– 77.9	5	4	4	3	3	2	2	1	1	0	0	–1	–1	–2	–3	–3	–3	–4
	78.0– 82.9	5	5	4	4	3	3	2	2	1	1	0	0	–1	–1	–2	–2	–3	–3
18	74.0– 76.9	5	4	4	3	2	2	1	1	0	0	–1	–1	–2	–2	–3	–4	–4	–5
	77.0– 80.9	5	4	4	3	3	2	2	1	1	0	0	–1	–2	–2	–3	–3	–4	–4
	81.0– 84.9	5	5	4	4	3	3	2	2	1	0	0	–1	–1	–2	–2	–3	–3	–4
	85.0– 88.9	6	5	5	4	4	3	2	2	1	1	0	0	–1	–1	–2	–2	–3	–4

(continued)

591

Table 3. (*continued*)

Age (months)	Length (cm)	Midparent stature (cm)																	
		150	152	154	156	158	160	162	164	166	168	170	172	174	176	178	180	182	184
24	77.0– 80.9	5	4	4	3	3	2	1	1	0	0	−1	−2	−2	−3	−3	−4	−5	−5
	81.0– 84.9	5	5	4	4	3	2	2	1	1	0	−1	−1	−2	−2	−3	−4	−4	−5
	85.0– 88.9	6	5	5	4	3	3	2	2	1	0	0	−1	−1	−2	−3	−3	−4	−4
	89.0– 92.9	6	6	5	4	4	3	3	2	1	1	0	0	−1	−2	−2	−3	−3	−4
	93.0– 94.9	7	6	5	5	4	4	3	2	2	1	1	0	−1	−1	−2	−2	−3	−4
30	83.0– 84.9	6	5	4	4	3	2	2	1	0	0	−1	−2	−2	−3	−4	−4	−5	−6
	85.0– 89.9	6	5	5	4	3	3	2	1	1	0	−1	−1	−2	−3	−3	−4	−5	−5
	90.0– 94.9	7	6	5	5	4	3	3	2	1	1	0	−1	−1	−2	−3	−3	−4	−5
	95.0– 97.9	7	6	6	5	4	4	3	2	2	1	0	0	−1	−2	−2	−3	−4	−4
36	87.0– 88.9	6	5	5	4	3	3	2	1	0	0	−1	−2	−2	−3	−4	−5	−5	−6
	89.0– 92.9	6	6	5	4	4	3	2	1	1	0	−1	−2	−2	−3	−4	−4	−5	−6
	93.0– 96.9	7	6	5	5	4	3	2	2	1	0	0	−1	−2	−3	−3	−4	−5	−5
	97.0–100.9	7	7	6	5	4	4	3	2	1	1	0	−1	−1	−2	−3	−4	−4	−5
	101.0–104.9	8	7	6	6	5	4	4	3	2	1	0	0	−1	−1	−2	−3	−4	−4

Reprinted by permission of Ross Products Division, Abbott Laboratories. Originally adapted from Himes, Roche, & Thissen (1981).

592

Index